# THE UNIQUE HERBAL

## NEW INSIGHTS INTO ANCIENT MEDICINES

VOLUME THREE (I-L)

ROBERT DALE ROGERS (RH) AHG

# CONTENTS

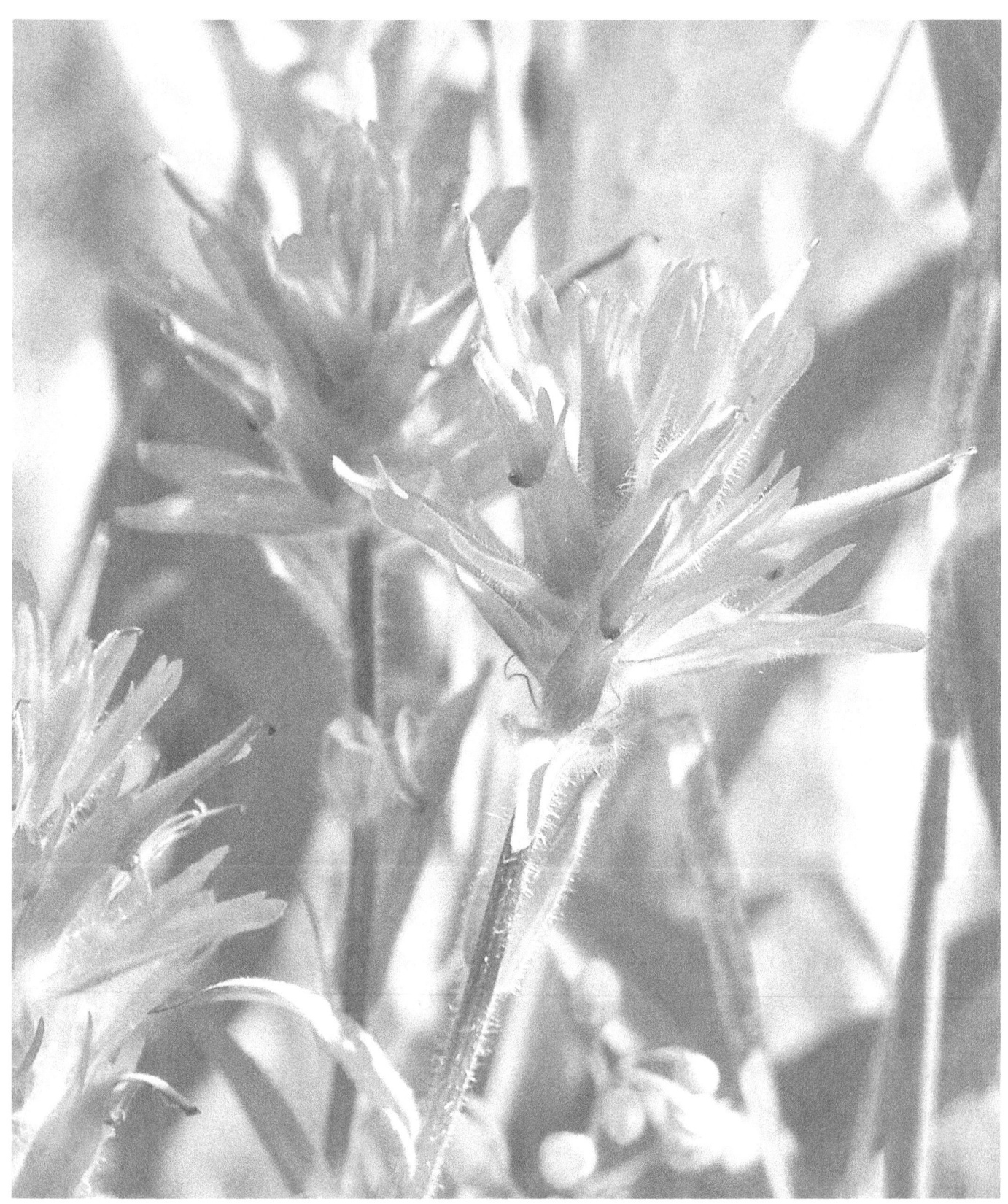

INDIAN PAINTBRUSH

# INTRODUCTION

Over the years,I have accumulated some information, a bit of knowledge and even a little wisdom about medicinal plants.

Many of the healing herbs in this volume set are relatively unknown; and some are little used in day-to-day clinical practice. Some are well known, but not utilized to their full extent of possibilities.

It is my hope that these pages may lead to a new and expanded materia medica, and a wider appreciation of many, often neglected, overlooked, and useful medicinal plants.

North American herbals tend to repeat, with increasingly useful additions, the same hundred or so plant medicines. The purpose of this book is to expand that awareness and hope that other herbalists will begin to look at the plants in their backyard and explore, observe and experience for themselves.

In turn, we could reconnect and continue the work begun in past centuries by the Eclectics and other plant people.

Like some of my previous publications, this book records indigenous use of medicinal herbs, garnered respectfully from the oral tradition, as well as work by various cultures around the world, the Eclectic physicians, modern herbalists, and recent scientific findings on various plant constituents.

It also includes homeopathic usage, essential oils, hydrosols, gemmotherapy, flower essences, personality traits, spiritual properties and astrological correspondences.

Please contact me if you wish to contribute;I am always learning.

Some Other Books by Robert Dale Rogers - www.amazon.com/author/robertdalerogers

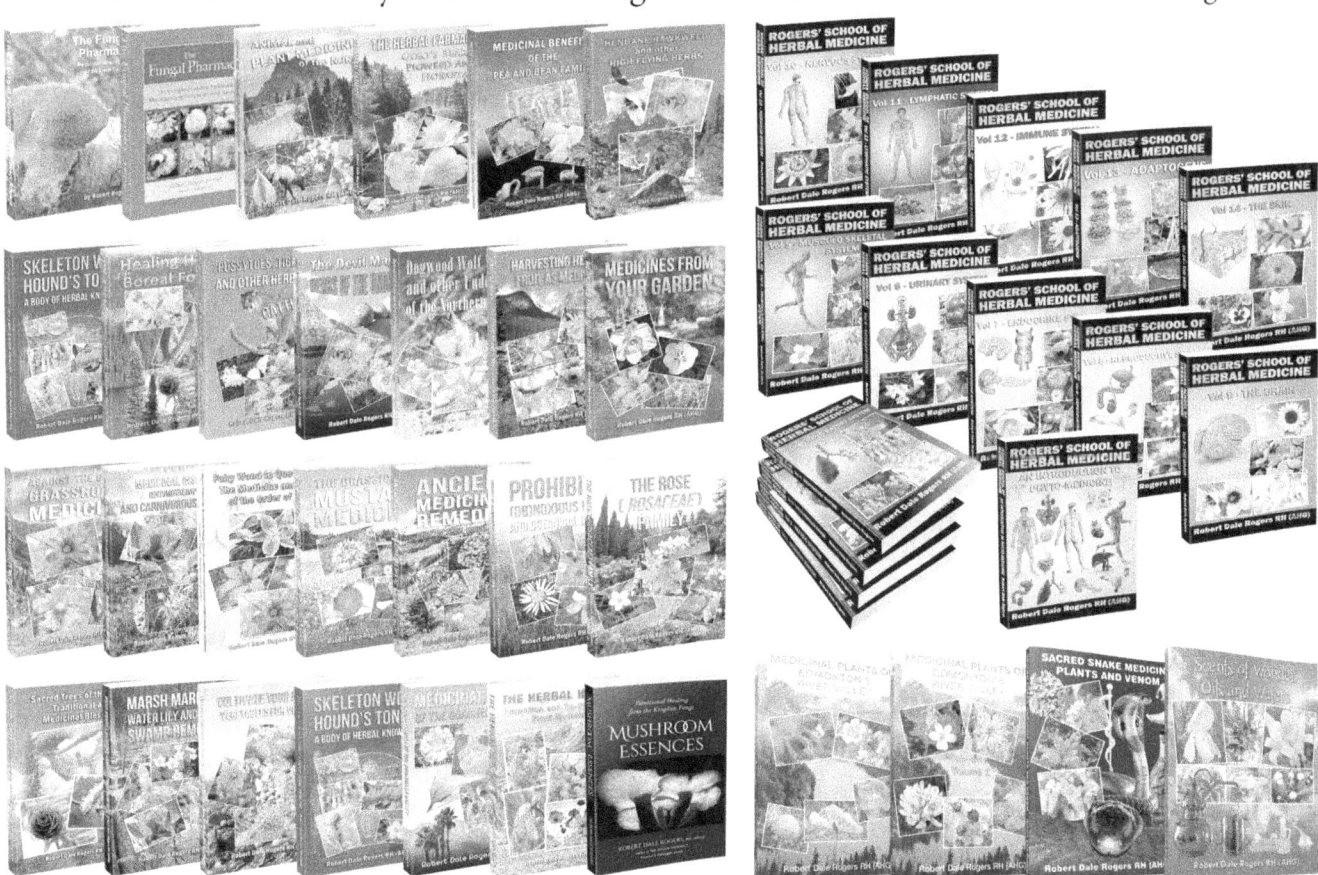

www.selfhealdistributing.com or www.scentsofwonder.ca - email: scents@telusplanet.net - Fax: 1 780-439-9540

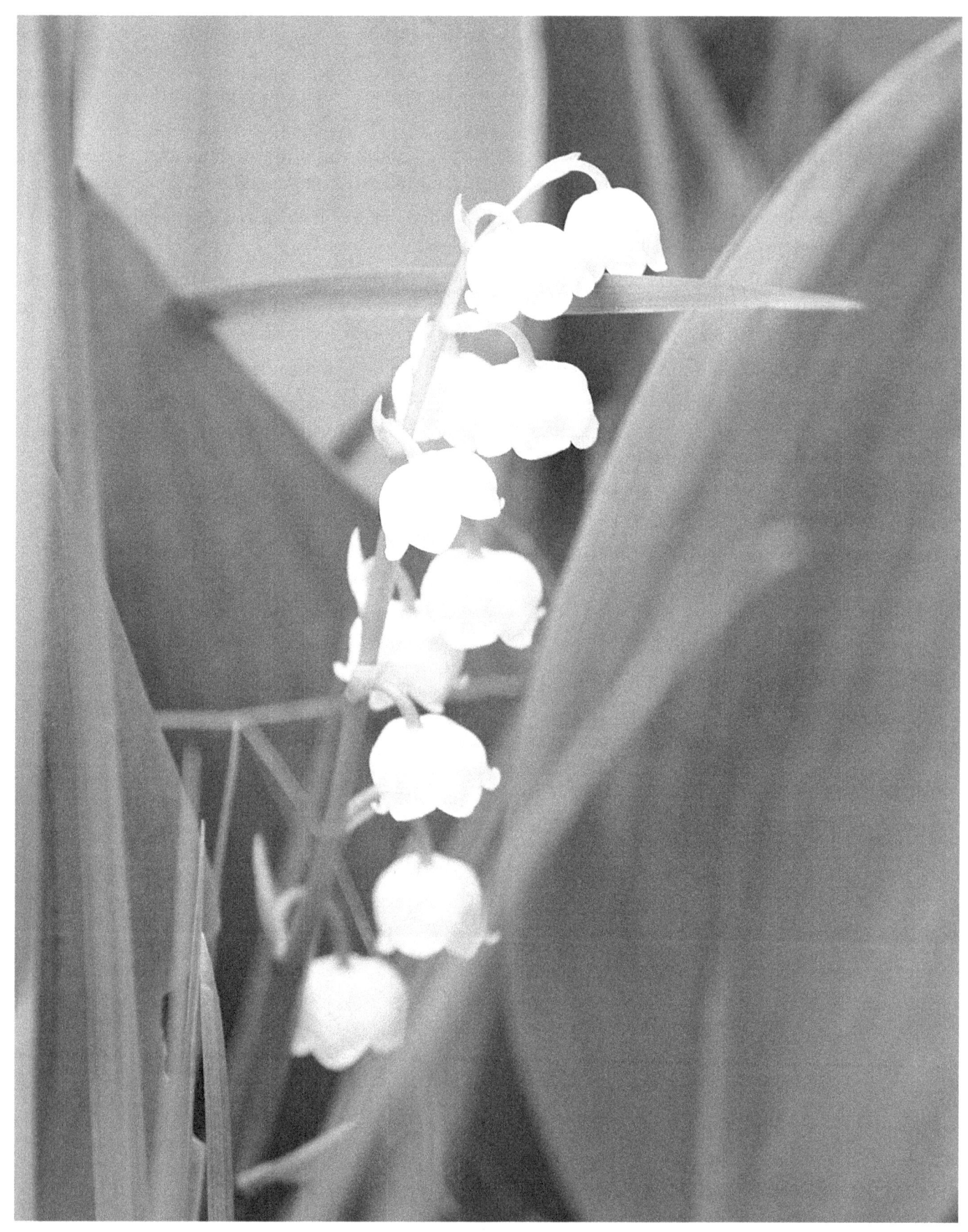

LILY OF THE VALLEY

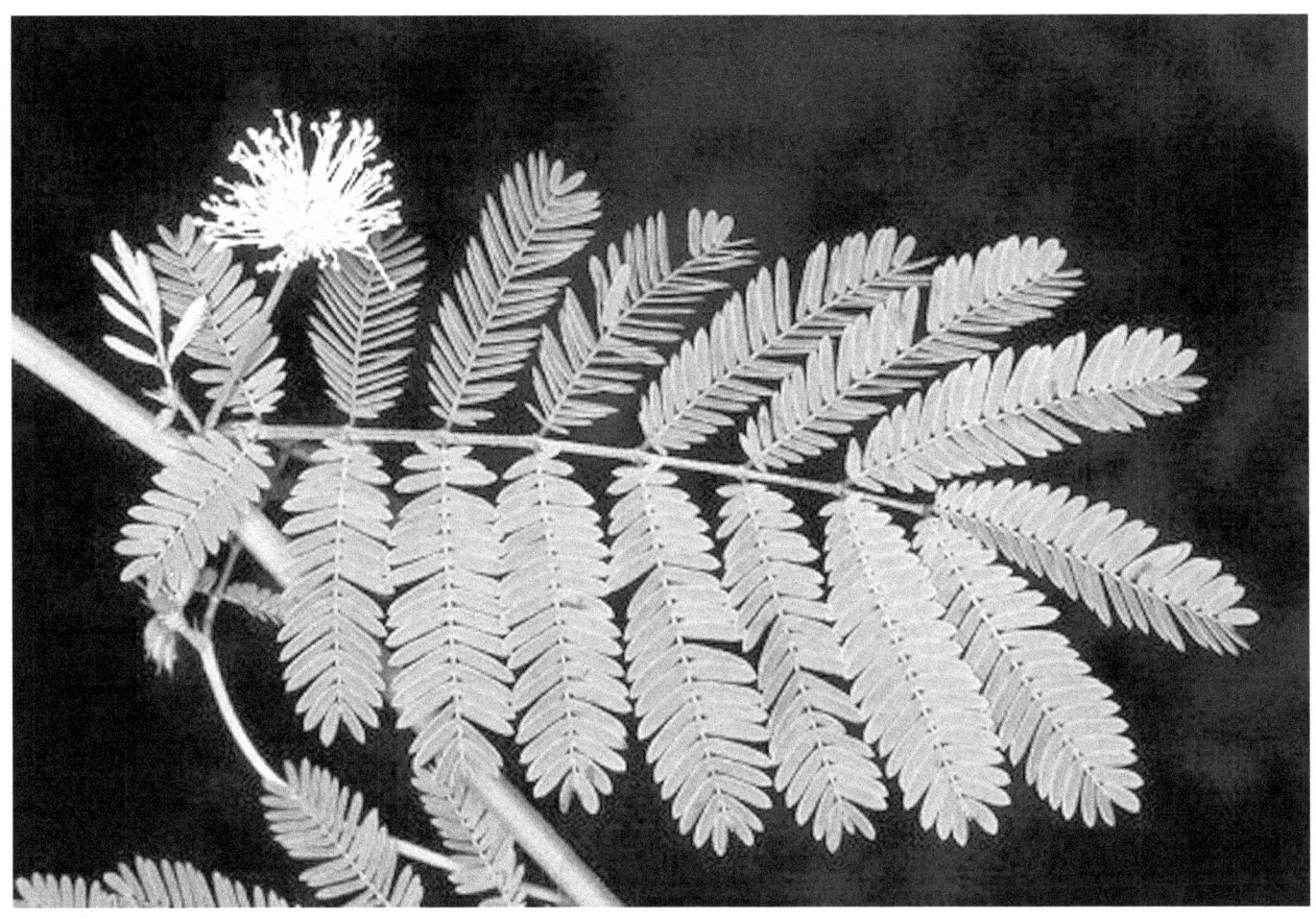

ILLINOIS BUNDLE FLOWER (Courtesy of southeasternflora.com)

**ILLINOIS BUNDLE FLOWER**
**SPIDER BEAN**
(***Desmanthus illinoensis*** [Michx.] MacMill ex B. L. Rob. & Fernald)
**PARTS USED**- root

Laws are spider webs through which the big flies pass and the little ones get caught.  **HONORE DE BALZAC**

We're all just a bundle of habits shaped by our memories.                    **JOSHUA FOER**

Illinois Bundle Flower grows from three to five feet tall in the western tallgrass of Manitoba. It is not common, but is sometimes used in prairie restoration and is an important food plant for livestock and wildlife.

The bundled white flowers create an attractive starburst effect, that later develop into curved, brown wafer-like seedpods.

The Paiute placed five seeds in the eye at night to cure trachoma, washing them out in the morning.

The Pawnee decocted the leaves as a wash for skin itch.

Bundle Flower is being investigated as a prairie perennial that produces around 800 pounds of seed per acre. Wes Jackson, director of the Land Institute, and author of New Roots for Agriculture, believes "we have to farm the way nature farms".

Breeding programs with Bundle Flower may increase yields by five, ten or twenty fold in the hands of talented agronomists and breeders.

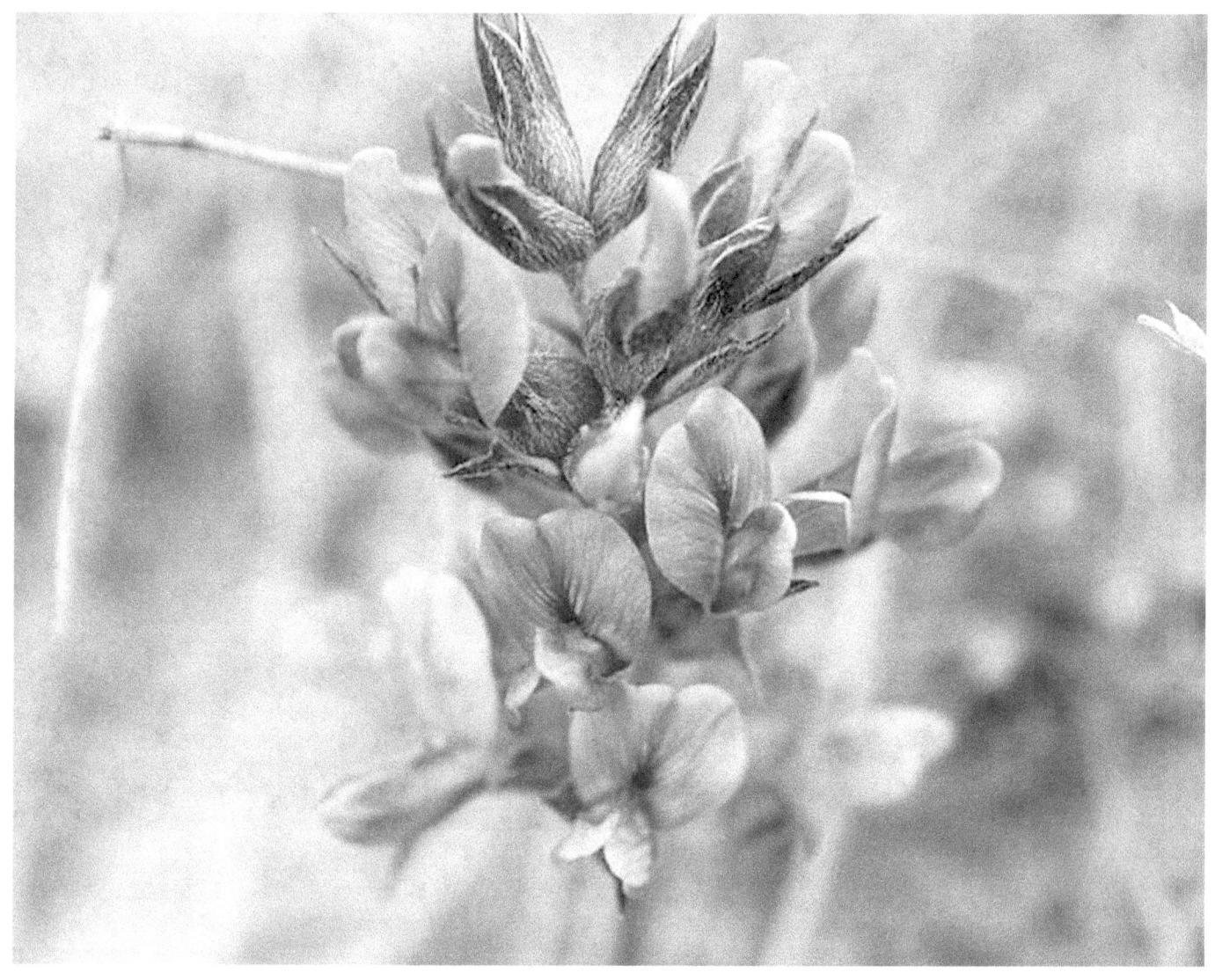

PRAIRIE TURNIP

Soil nitrogen levels in four year old stands in poor soil were nearly identical to that of better soil sites despite initial differences, suggesting plants that yield a good harvest and simultaneously fertilize the soil, is the way to go. *Rhizobium giardinii* is microsymbiont.

The root is a treasure trove of tryptamines, and as a source of DMT contains 200 mg/100 grams dry weight, with the root bark a whopping 340 mg/100g DMT. The constituent NMT is also present in the root at 0.5% and root bark at 8%.

The root also contains both N-hydroxy-NMT and 2-hydroxy-MNT.

Both are pharmacologically unknowns, but it is of interest that N-hydroxy-NMT has the same relationship to NMT that N-hydroxy-MDMA does to MDMA.

And because N-HO-MDMA has a potency equal to MDMA, it is possible that N-HO-NMT, may have potency equal to NMT. More research would of course, help sort out the human activity of NMT.

The Shulgins, in their book TIKHAL: The Continuation, write. "To my knowledge there have been no reports of oral activity of NMT, although its wide availability from botanic sources has encouraged some explorers to assay it. I have had one report that the smoking of 50-100 mg gave visuals that lasted for maybe 15 seconds."

**INDIAN BREADROOT**
**PRAIRIE TURNIP**
**CREE POTATO/TURNIP**
(*Psoralea esculenta* Pursh.) not accepted
(*Pediomelum esculentum* [Pursh] Rydb.)
**SILVER LEAF PSORALEA**
(*P. argophylla* Pursh.) not accepted
(*P. collina*)
(*Psoralidium argophyllum*)
(*Pediomelum argophyllum* [Pursh] J. W. Grimes)
**LANCE LEAVED PSORALEA**

**LEMON SCURF PEA**
(*P. lanceolata*) not accepted
(*P. stenostachys* Rydb.) not accepted
(*P. scabra* Nutt.) not accepted
(*Psoralidium lanceolatum* [Pursh] Rydb.)
**FEW-FLOWERED PSORALEA**
**SLENDER FLOWERED SCURF PEA**
(*Psoralidium tenuiflorum* [Pursh] Rydb.)
**SCURF PEA**
(*P. corylifolia* L.) not accepted
(*Cullen corylifolia* [L.] Medik.)
**PARTS USED-** root

*Psoralea* is from the Greek **PSORA**, meaning itch, scab or mange, or **PSORALEOS**, warted; and refers to the rough texture, or glandular dots that cover the plant. The original genus name *Pediomelum* means Plains Apple.

Esculenta means edible. Lanceolata means lance-leaved, and argophylla means silver leaf. Tenuiflora means thin, slight or few flowers.

Indian Breadroot, at one time, was plentiful all along the Battle River of central Alberta. It was a staple, prized for its sweet, crisp flavour, but becoming increasingly rare due to modern agriculture methods.

It was said to be a favorite of the now extinct Prairie Grizzly Bear.

Breadroot was dug by the women with fire-hardened chokecherry sticks, and considered tastiest when harvested as blooms fade. It is worth noting that the tops detach as seedpods ripen and blow across the prairies in June, making identification difficult.

It was then peeled and eaten raw, or dried and coated with fat for winter supplies. They taste sort of like yams. They were ground dry into meal and made into cakes baked over fire coals.

The taste is sweet when freshly dug from ground and later like corn. Some authors suggest the flavour is of raw green beans or unroasted peanuts.

The tough outer skin must be peeled while fresh or it becomes like leather. Peel from the long tail of the root back to the fat part. The young, thin roots are best tasting, sweet and crisp.

The Plains Cree liked a pudding made of flour, breadroot and saskatoon berries. They call the tuber **MISTASKUCIMINA**, meaning Grass Berry.

Northern Cree know it as **MISH TAS KO SHE MIN** meaning "large fruit plant". I have also seen **MIX TAS COOS SE NENA**. All are similar, linguistically.

Root Woman, from Saskatchewan, says it is also known as **SOWKAAS**, or **MIX TAS COOS SE NENA**.

The Blackfoot dried pieces of the root, and attached it to clothing and robes or ornamentation and medicine. Sometimes the root was scraped and used to replace pieces of diamond willow fungi that were attached to "weasel robes". To the Blackfoot it is known as Elk Food or **MAHS** or **MAS'**, a general term for root.

The thick brown-barked roots are dug up shortly before the flowers drop. They often boiled the two together to treat coughs, or breadroot was simply chewed to relieve sore throats.

The spittle was inserted for ear or eye problems, and then covered with a heated cloth or soft hide.

The root decoction relieves gastroenteritis, and is mildly diuretic. The chewed roots were applied to sprains and fractures.

When necessary, the root was chewed and juice blown into a baby's rectum, using an eagle bone, to treat colic. Pieces of dried root were given to teething infants.

The Cheyenne used it as a diarrhea medicine, internally, and a burn medicine as a wash made from the root and June Grass (*Koeleria macrantha* or *K. cristata*).

**MO?OHTA?ENO** was one of the most important Cheyenne foods, either fresh, or cut thin and dried for winter use as soup thickeners. The Sioux and Dakota also used the tuber of **TIP SI NA**, for food, as did the Osage tribe, who called it **TAAHGU**.

The Crow call the plant **ESHARUSHA**.

Indian Breadroot, woven into four arm's length braids, once traded for a good quality buffalo robe. A high price indeed! Wild Turnip Hill, on the Blood Reserve, was called **MAS'-ETOMO** or Turnip Butte because it grows so well on the well- drained, sandy soil.

Another site near Cowley, Alberta was known as **AKAI SOWKAAS** meaning "many prairie turnips".

Early Canadian voyageurs called it pomme de prairie, or pomme blanche.

In France, under the name of **PICQUOTIANE** it was cultivated as a potato substitute.

Breadroot is a cold-tolerant plant that possesses the ability to grow in crude oil-contaminated soil. Robson DB et al, *Int J Phytoremediation* 2003 5(2):105-23.

Silver Leaf Psoralea was used by the Cheyenne as a febrifuge, decoctions of the plant used for fever; and salves of the plant also applied in high fever states. They call it Devil's turnip **HESTAMOA?KANO** or To Make Cold Medicine, **TO'WAN I YUHKTS**.

For fevers, the leaf and stem are ground into a powder, combined with animal fat and rubbed into the skin.

Just to the south of the Blackfoot, the Montana tribe decocted the plant as a wash for wounds. The dark blue purple flowers have a sweet scent that lingers.

The Chippewa used the root as a wash that they applied to the chest and legs of their horses as a stimulant.

The Fox, or Mesquakie, considered root infusions to cure chronic constipation, while the Dakota used it as horse medicine.

The Lakota name is **TI'CANICAHU** (long billed curlew stem), which somehow refers to "one that doesn't have a home".

In times of famine and scarcity, the less desirable Silver Leaf was eaten by the Montana and other Plains tribes. The tuber is smaller, more difficult to collect, more fibrous and less suitable for making flour, and lower in carbohydrates and source of energy.

Scurf Pea was traditionally used by the Cheyenne in ceremonial medicine. The Navaho applied plant lotions and poultices to itch and sore skin. They used cold infusions for stomachache and menstrual pain, as well as a ceremonial chant lotion for protection from witches.

The Arapaho dried the leaves and powdered them for snuff, chewed the fresh leaves for sore throat and made a leaf infusion as a wash for headache.

They rubbed the aromatic leaves on their skin as a moisturizer.

The Zuni ate fresh flowers for stomach pain.

The root was used for more serious conditions such as venereal disease.

The native plant is usually found on sand dunes or sandy soil.

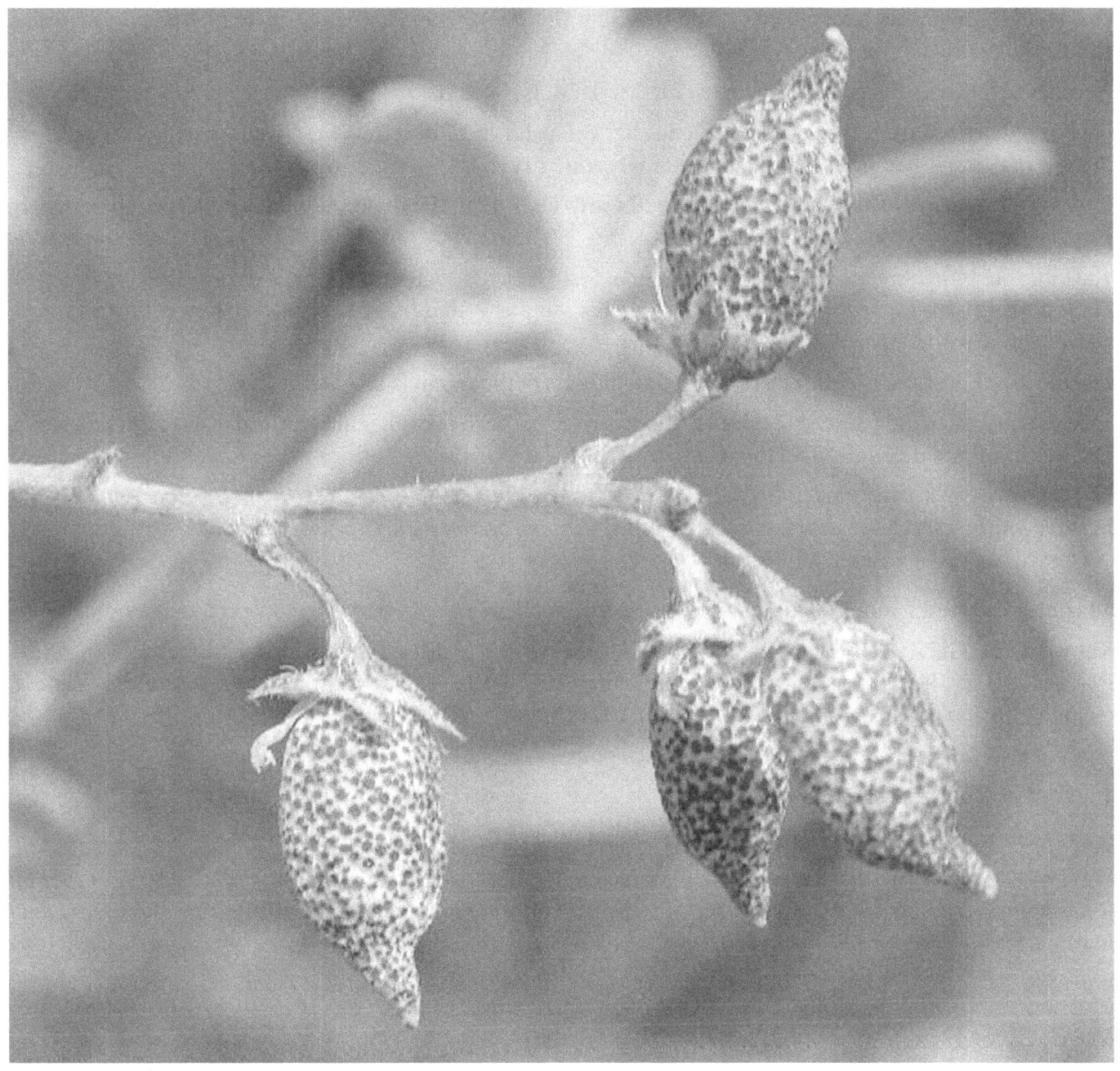

FEW-FLOWERED PSORALEA- MATURE FRUIT

The related California Tea (*P. physodes*) has leaves, that when dry, make an acceptable tasting beverage; also possessing antispasmodic action for menstrual cramps. If you hold the leaf up to light, numerous semi-transparent dots will be noted. These carry the aromatic oils that carry the pleasant, characteristic scent.

Rooibos tea, made from the dried, fermented leaves of *P. linearis* is a popular beverage in Africa. It is caffeine free, with a higher fluoride content than oriental green tea. Japanese research in the 1980s showed Rooibos contains compounds similar to SOD, an anti-oxidant compound that retards aging.

Medically, the leaf tea is given for allergies, especially eczema, as well as hay fever and asthma in children.

A liqueur called Buchenbosch contains the herb; as well as fruit drinks, soup bases, sauces and baked goods.

Our own prairie plants have not even been tested for this constituent. Synonyms include *Aspalathus linearis*, and *A. contaminatus*.

Another member of the genus, distributed further south is *P. juncea*.

Plicatin B, isolated from the leaves and stems, has been shown to have anti-mutagenic activity, in studies by Menon et al, published in the *Journal of Natural Products* 1999.

*Psolalea melitotoides* is found in Ohio and southward. Dr. King mentioned the roots and leaves possess mild stimulating and bitter tonic properties.

The infusion or tincture has been used in languor or feebleness associated with mental or physical over-exertion, in certain forms of chronic dyspepsia, to relieve anorexia and as a stimulating tonic in affections of the mesentery, accompanied with diarrhea and painful abdomen.

Few-flowered Psoralea is quite scarce, but found in parts of the foothills in Alberta.

Various tribes, including the Dakota, used the root decoctions, with two other unidentified plants for tuberculosis. The Navaho, far to the south, used the root to treat sheep's cough. Plant infusions were drunk, the leaves smoked for influenza; and even used as a wet poultice for purification.

Further south, it is one of several species classified as *Contrayerba Blanco*, or Drake's Foot. The root powders are mixed with cool water to induce vomiting.

Of course the most famous of this genus is the Scurf Pea (*C. corylifolia*) from China.

Known as **BU GU ZHI**, this annual can be grown easily on the prairies, for its seed. It is sometimes known as **PU KU CHIH**. The name is derived from the Indian **HAKUCK**, which was transliterated into the Chinese, meaning "torn old paper". I have also seen **COT CHU**, and **PO KU CHI**.

The blackish yellow seeds are found in oval black pods, surrounded by a persistent calyx.

The seeds are pungent and bittersweet.

It has a multitude of uses in Traditional Chinese and Ayurvedic medicine.

Work by Zobel et al, at Trent University in Ontario, found linear furanocoumarins on the surface of seeds from *P. bituminosa* totaling about 1%. Psoralen and xanthotoxin were present, with very little bergapten. *Canadian Journal of Botany* 1991 69:8.

The related *P. glandulosa* from Chile contains compounds with anti-inflammatory and anti-pyretic activity.

## MEDICINAL

**CONSTITUENTS**- *C. corylifolia* seed- flavonoids including coryfolin, coryfolinin, and havachromene, phenol bakuchiol, angelicin, bavachin, bavachinin, isobavachin, isobava-chalcone, raffinose, and furano-coumarins such as psoralen, isopsoralen, and psoralidin, fatty and essential oils, phytosterols, resins.
Leaf- genistein.
*P. esculenta* root- various amino acids including 1.2% glutamic acid, 7-42% protein, 3.6% fat, and 57% water.
*P. argophylla*- (-)glyceollin

In the Traditional Chinese approach to medicine, Scurf Pea seed is a tonic and astringent of the uro-genital system in cold and deficient conditions. That is, it tones the Kidneys and promotes Yang. It is widely used in Ayurvedic medicine as well.

It is not dissimilar to Dodder (*Cuscuta*) Seed in its action on the reproductive system of both men and women. Low sex drive or interest, impotence, premature ejaculation all fit the picture pattern.

It has been used to prevent miscarriage and correct menorrhagia, and heavy bleeding.

It probably has some form of hormonal activity not fully understood, but with apparent androgenic and estrogenic influence.

Dribbling urination, with frequent nighttime visits, or daytime incontinence may be relieved.

It is a coronary and bronchial relaxant, useful in treating acute asthma, angina pectoris and overall cardiovascular tonic. In animal hearts, both in vivo and in vitro, it dilates coronary arteries, but has no effect on oxygen consumption of heart muscles. It also stimulates the heart and increases heart rate and function. The main activity is due to corylifolinin, which opens coronary arteries and stimulates heart contractions.

The seeds act as a norepinephrine-dopamine reuptake inhibitor, *in vitro*. Zhao G et al, J Ethnopharm 2007 112(3):498-506.

Corylifolinin, bavachinin and psoralen all inhibit osteosarcoma and secondary lung cancer.

Bavachinin is both a potent PPARgamma agonist, associated with blood sugar regulation, and hMAO inhibitor that may be useful in Parkinson's disease. Zarmouh NO et al, *Evid Based Complement Alternat Med* 2015:852194.

The seed, known as Bauchee seed, is used for infections, or cases of low white blood counts in leukopenia. Ethanol extracts inhibit the tuberculosis mycobacterium.

It exhibits anti-oxidant properties as well as anti-allergenic activity.

The seeds has been shown to artificially inhibit tumours; probably due to the furanocoumarins, likely psoralidin. The dried, ripe fruit inhibits proliferation of colon cancer cell lines. Park GH et al, *BMC Complement Altern Med* 2016 16(1):373.

It is often called "Restore Bone Resin" in Chinese, for its fracture healing properties similar to garden cress and comfrey. Osteoporosis after menopause may be due, in part, to hormonal influence, and the seed has been found to be one of the world's richest sources of daidzein and genistein, two well-studied phytoestrogen compounds.

The seed possesses slow hemostatic action, but is still effective.

For various skin problems both internal use and external decoctions are utilized. Psoriasis, vitiligo, alopecia, solar urticaria, and skin cancers all respond to the double-seated action. External use promotes the production of melanin, as well as calloused skin and warts. Work by Hussain I et al, *Drug Des Devel Ther* 2016 found ointment containing crushed seed powder effective for small, circular white lesions of vitiligo.

Psoralen has been found to possess therapeutic activity against *Tinea versicolor* and psoriasis. Psoralen from seeds show potential benefit in Alzheimer's disease. Choi YH et al, *Planta Medica* 2008 74(11):1405-8.

Glycyrhetinic acid from licorice root may increase the kidney toxicity of bakuchiol. Li A et al, *PeerJ* 2016 Nov 22;4:e2723. They should not be used together.

A mini review of this genus, but mainly *P. corylifolia*, was recently published by Li CC et al, *Evid Based Complement Altern Medicine* 2016 November 17.

Our native species on the prairies have been vastly understudied.

Recent work by Borchardt et al, *J Med Plants Res* 2008 2:4 shed some light on the seeds of Indian Breadroot. Extracts were found to possess activity against *Pseudomonas aeruginosa*, and to have high anti-oxidant level of 43,182 TE/100 grams. Blueberries, by comparison are rated at only 3,300.

Indian Breadroot is diuretic, but usually used as an emergency food.

Silver Leaf Psoralea contains glyceollin, a compound that shows novel mechanisms of estrogen receptor positive breast cancer. Bratton MR et al, *J Steroid Biochem Mol Biol* 2015 150:17-23. Not surprisingly, this phytoalexin is found in stressed soybeans.

The compound glyceollin I inhibits ZEB1, suggesting use in letrozole resistant breast cancer. Carriere PP et al, *Int J Environ Res Public Health* 2015 13(1).

The compounds exert anti-tumor activity on triple negative breast carcinoma cells. Rhodes LV et al, *Oncol Lett* 2012 3(1): 163-71. Animal studies suggest inhibition of prostate cancer cells. Kim HJ et al, *Proc Nutr Soc* 2012 71(1): 166-74.

Glyceollins regulate cancer cell growth by inhibiting vascular endothelial growth factor. Lee SH et al, *J Cell Physiol* 2015 230(4): 853-62.

Recent work suggests glyceollins show potential to improve clinical outcomes in patients with osteoporosis. Bateman ME et al, *Phytomedicine* 2017 27: 39-51.

Glyceollins up-regulate glucose transporters, and may be useful in pre-diabetic conditions by increasing glucose uptake by adipocytes. Boue SM et al, *J Agric Food Chem* 2012 60(25): 6376-82.

The closely-related Samson Snakeroot, or Congo Root, (*P. melilotoides*) from Kentucky and Ohio, was used by the Eclectics. Dr. King wrote, "the root and leaves of these plants (*P. esculenta* and *P. melilotoides*) appear to possess the properties of a mild, stimulating, bitter tonic, and have been advantageously employed in cases of languor or feebleness from mental or physical exertion, in certain forms of chronic dyspepsia, to relieve anorexia and as a stimulating tonic in strumous affections of the mesentery, accompanied with diarrhea, tumid abdomen, etc."

The related *P. glandulosa* from Chile contains bakuchiol, which has shown activity against gram-positive bacteria. It was at one time erroneously called Paraguay Tea or Yerba Mate.

## INDIAN BREADROOT

### CONSTITUENTS

| | |
|---|---|
| Dry matter (% of fresh wt) | 43.02 |
| Total protein (% of dry wt) | 4 ?? |
| Starch (% of dry wt) | 69.84 |
| Calcium (% of dry wt) | 0.51 |
| Magnesium (% of dry wt) | 0.14 |
| Lysine (grams/100 g) | 6.5 |

Indian Bread root is higher than Yampa (see volume 5) in calcium, magnesium and iron, with slightly less starch.

However, it does have high levels of lysine, a limited amino acid in cereal grains.

## SPIRITUAL PROPERTIES

The Cheyenne call it Devil's Turnip. A long time ago, some maidens went looking for wild turnips (*P. esculenta*). Whenever they thought they had found one, it turned out to be a false one. Finally, when they were far away from camp, a medicine man from the village, realizing that the girls were being led away by the devil in the form of this plant, warned some of the people who then went to rescue the girls.               **WILLARD**

Indian Turnip has powerful medicinal properties, especially when one is working with the flowers. The herb has the interesting property of helping an individual awaken to their spiritual purpose. This can even be beyond life purpose, as if understanding more of what God has intended for them or what they elected for their lives before coming here. When an individual works on a spiritual project, it will be greatly enhanced by this plant.

The signature relates to the flowers, their unique shape and way it seems to hold back energy, as if waiting to be welcomed.               **GURUDAS**

# RECIPES

**TINCTURE** (*P. corylifolia*)- 2-4 ml

**DECOCTION**- 3-6 grams.

**CAUTION**- Scurf Pea- Do not use in cases of yin deficient conditions with heat, during pregnancy or breastfeeding. Very large doses have been shown to possess tetrogenic effects. Do not combine with licorice root.

The seeds may create a carboxylesterase 1 (CES1) deficiency that may activate or deactivate various drugs. CES1 is responsible for activitation of ACE inhibitors. It also has the ability to metabolize heroin and cocaine, suggesting therapeutic roles for this enzyme. A deficiency is associated with non-Hodgkin lymphoma and B-cell lymphocytic leukemia, suggesting caution using this herb in certain situations.

**INDIAN PAINTBRUSH, RED**
(***Castilleja miniata*** Dougl. ex Hook.)
**ALPINE RED PAINTBRUSH**
(***C. rhexifolia*** Rydb.)
**CUSICK'S PAINTBRUSH**
(***C. cusickii*** Greenm.)
**STIFF YELLOW PAINTBRUSH**
**LABRADOR PAINTBRUSH**
(***C. lutescens*** [Green.] Rydb.)
(***C. septentrionalis*** Lindl.)
**SCARLET PAINTBRUSH**
**PAINTED CUP**
(***C. coccinea*** [L.] Spreng.)
**SESSILE PAINTBRUSH**
(***C. sessiliflora*** Pursh.)
**PURPLE PAINTBRUSH**
(***C. raupii*** Pennell)

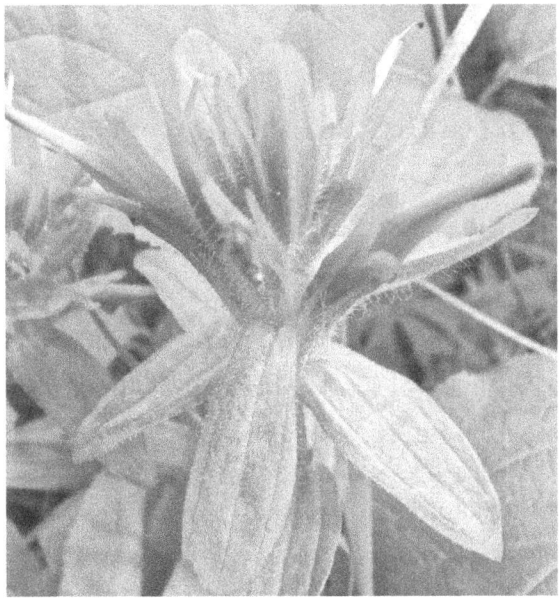

COMMON RED INDIAN PAINTBRUSH

Scarlet tufts are glowing in the green like flakes of fire; the wanderers of the prairie know them well, and call that brilliant flower the Painted Cup.                    **BRYANT**

It is startling to see a leaf thus brilliantly painted, as if its tips were dipped in some scarlet tincture, surpassing most flowers in intensity of colour.                    **THOREAU**

Castillcja was named in honour of the Spanish botanist, from Cadiz, Domingo Castillejo by Jose Celestino Mutis. He was physician to the Viceroy of New Granada (Columbia), where two indigenous varieties grow. Miniata is named for the lead oxide colour minium, which is scarlet red, and was used to illustrate medieval manuscripts. Lutescens means yellowish. Raupii is named in honor of the 20th century botanist Hugh Raup.

The Paintbrushes are all semi-parasitic, which stands them in good stead in times of stress, and drought.

The showy, leaf bracts look like a paintbrush, hence the common name. This particular red species has an affinity for south facing slopes with good drainage.

The flowers can be eaten, and in particular, the long white corolla tubes are rich in nectar.

The Blackfoot mixed the plant with warm water to be taken as a diuretic. Children rubbed the flowers on their arrows for color and shine.

Arrow feathers were dyed a light yellow by pressing them together with the bright yellow flowers.

The Blackfoot believed that the colors were the effect of age; the youngest white, then red and finally yellow.

9

The flowers were used to waterproof and shine hides. The Zuni, for example, used the root of *C. integra* with minerals to dye buckskin black.

A Metis elder from the Elizabeth Colony in Alberta said he added the dried flower heads to wild chamomile to make a tea for headaches and to relax nerves.

Some paintbrushes were mixed with Beard Tongue, infused in warm water, and applied to centipede stings.

Women bleeding from their vagina, but not during menstruation, drank large quantities of the plant infusion and rubbed it into their abdomen.

A tea was given to those spitting blood, the brew rubbed as well into the chest with a rag.

The Gitksan of British Columbia used *C. miniata* for a wide variety of ailments. Decoctions of the entire plant, including root, were taken for lame back, stiff lungs, coughs, nosebleeds, and sore eyes. It is both purgative and diuretic.

They used the seeds as a specific decoction for coughs.

This plant is called **IHLLEE'EM TS'AK**, or bleeding nose, the same as Red Columbine, with the former distinguished short, and the latter, tall.

Indian Paintbrush (*C. linariaefolia*) is the state flower of Wyoming.

The Nevada tribe decocted small amounts of *C. linariafolia* as a venereal disease remedy. They called the plant Snake's Friend, because they found it near rocks where rattlesnakes lived, and believed the rattler distilled its venom from the flowers. The Hopi, Navaho, Shoshoni and Tewa all used this plant as a contraceptive. The Navaho, or Navajo used *C. integra* root decoctions to purify the blood after accidents.

The Quileute used infusions of *C. angustifolia* to normalize menstrual periods, while the Costanoan washed infected sores with strong decoctions of *C. affinis*. Various tribes macerated paintbrush in bear grease as a hair oil to invigorate and make it glossy.

Sessile Paintbrush was especially prized for this, with both flowers and leaves used in the maceration.

The Chippewa made flower decoctions of Scarlet Paintbrush (*C. coccinea*) to treat colds, rheumatism and paralysis. The Chippewa name translates roughly as "Winabojo's Grandmothers Hair". This plant is found as far west as Manitoba.

The Menomini used it as a love charm, the object being to place the flower upon the person of affection.

The Cherokee used Scarlet Paintbrush as part of ceremonies to "do combat with the enemy". The Cree used various species for protection and allaying spells.

# MEDICINAL

**CONSTITUENTS-senecionines,** quinolizidines and other alkaloids due mainly to their semi-parasitism on roots of *Senecio, Lupinus, and Thermopsis* species.
*C. rhexifolia*- stems and leaves- senecionine, its N-oxide
blossoms and seeds- rhexifoline (a newridine monoterpene alkaloid)
*C. tenuiflora*- aerial- tenuifloroside, apigenin, lutein 5-methyl ether, verbascoside, isoverbascoside, geniposide, caryoptoside, 8-epi-loganin, mussaenoside, bartioside and aucubin.

Studies conducted at Arizona State University in Tempe have discovered two cytotoxic compounds in the closely related *C. linariaefolia*. Acetoside and isoacetoside show *in vivo* activity against murine P-388 lymphocytic leukemia. Mannitol was found in this species. Obviously, more research is required. Pettit GR et al, *J Nat Prod* 1990 53(2).

Michael Moore says that two or three cups of moderately strong Indian paintbrush tea a day is a remedy for water retention associated with weather and temperature changes.

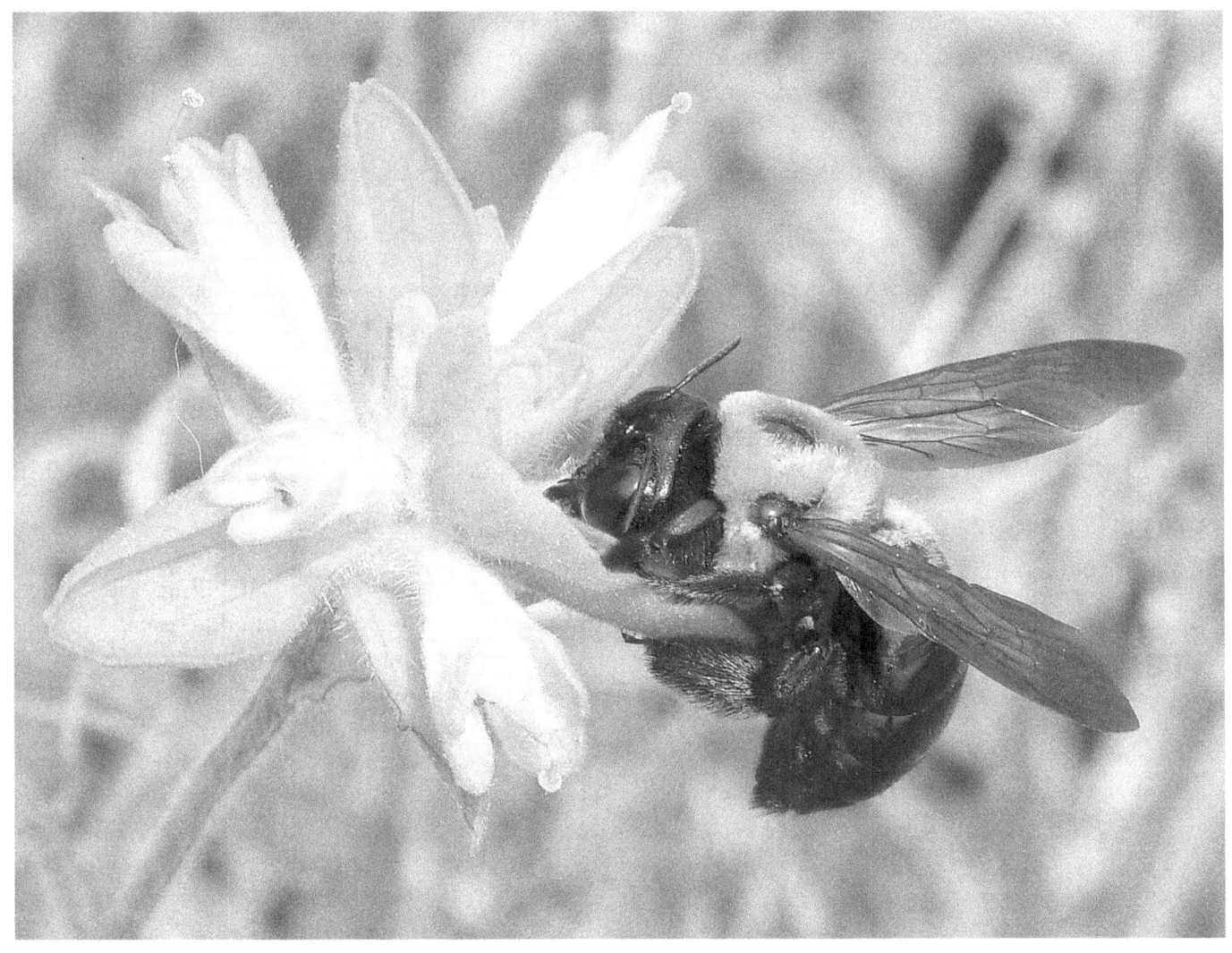

INDIAN PAINTBRUSH AND BEE

A reported hybrid between *C. rhexifolia* and *C. miniata* was found to contain sarracine and three new alkaloids, 7-angelylplaynecine, 9-angelylplaty-necine, and its N-oxide in the leaves and stems; with a trace of senecionine. The hybrid seed contains rhexifoline and deoxy-rhexifoline.

The related *C. tenuiflora* has been studied in Mexico. Water extracts were found to increase the rate of heart activity at doses as low as 0.1 mg/ml. The plant shows anti-inflammatory and anti-ulcerogenic activity. Sanchez et al, *J Ethnopharm* 2013 150(3) 1032-7. Water extracts showed moderate anti-inflammatory activity similar to dexamethasone. Also studied was the related *C. canescens*.

Work by Professor Lazo de la Vega and Dr. Galindo have found the plant therapeutic for liver and gastrointestinal complaints. The plant has been used traditionally in Mexico for cough, dysentery, anxiety, nausea and vomiting.

Geniposidic acid was found more potent than indomethacin. Carrillo-Ocampo D et al, *Molecules* 2013 18(10):2109-18. It is known by several common names including Bella Inés, "Cola de Borrego", or Mirto Cimarrón, meaning roughly, Wild Myrtle.

Geniposidic acid is the main constituent in *Gardenia jasminoides*, traditionally used for inflammation, jaundice and hepatic disorders.

Recent work found *C. tenuiflora* may have benefit in depression. Work by Herrera-Ruiz M et al, *Molecules* 2015 20(7):13127-43 identified and isolated compounds via methanol extraction.

The bitter principles have an affect on the glands, stimulating their secretion. This is especially useful in dyspepsia due to hypoacidity, and there is need for more gastric juices and pepsins. It stimulates the secretion of saliva, helping ensure better digestion of starches and sugars. The action is one of stimulation and toning that helps regulate the function of the stomach, and correct anemia of various origins.

It is also a diuretic, not only one that increases water flow, but helps discharge excessive toxins from the body.

## FLOWER ESSENCES

Indian Paintbrush (*C. miniata*) flower essence helps the soul to learn how to use creative potential in a manner which is richly resonant with the physical world. **FLOWER ESSENCE SOCIETY**

Indian Paintbrush flower essence encourages us to take the time to be still and to relax into the silence to regain our energy. It connects our creative aspect with the grounding of our earth roots. It helps us find abundant energy to meet our daily survival needs so that we can live a fuller and more creative life. It lets us love our Mother Earth and all of her creatures. It connects heaven and earth. **WILD ROSE**

## SPIRITUAL PROPERTIES

Once upon a time, a Blackfoot maiden fell in love with a wounded prisoner she was attending. The maiden realized that the tribe was only nursing him in order to torture him later. She planned an escape for the

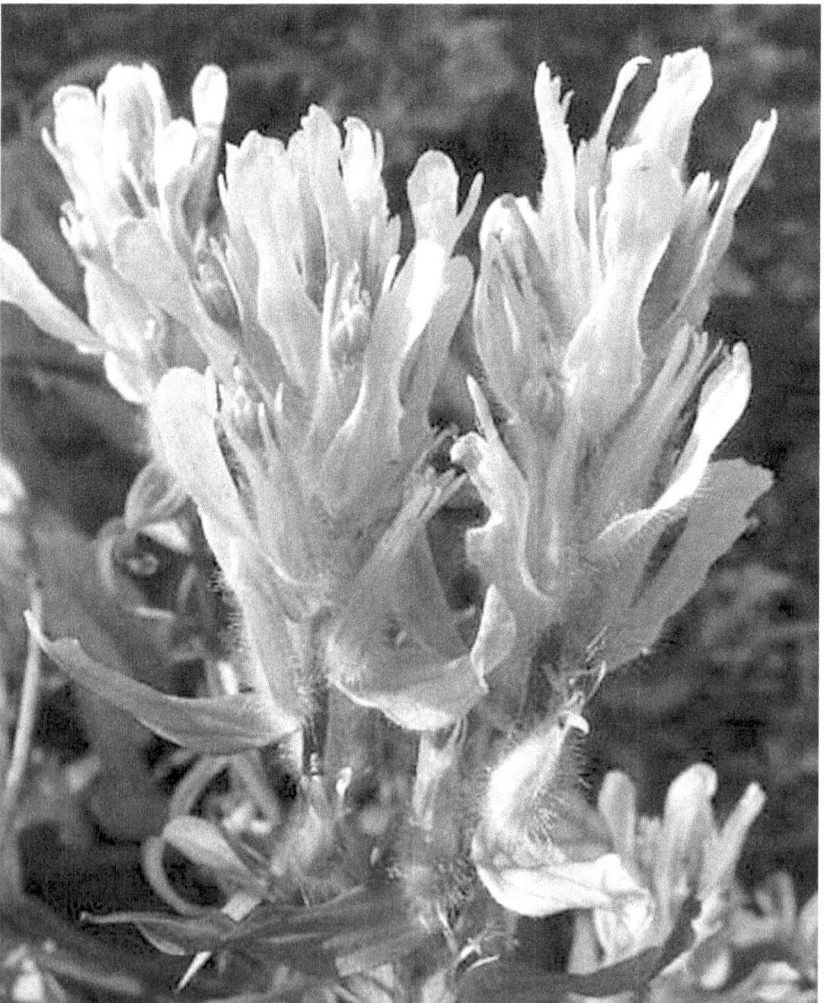

PURPLE PAINTBRUSH

prisoner, accompanying him for fear of the punishment for such a deed. After some time in her lover's camp she grew homesick for a glimpse of her old home. She went to the site and hid in the bushes and overheard two young braves discussing what would happen to the maiden that betrayed them.

Knowing she could never return, she took a piece of bark and drew a picture of the camp upon it with her own blood with a stick. She then threw the stick away and returned to her lover's camp. Where the stick landed, a little plant grew with a brush-like red flower, dyed with the blood of this girl. This became the first Indian paintbrush. **ANNORA BROWN**

Bluejay was an important tribal god. He was sent on a journey equipped with five buckets of water to extinguish five burning fields through which he would have to pass. Mistaking a brilliant field of red paintbrush for a fire, he wasted much of the water on it.

Later when he got to the real fires, he didn't have enough left to put them out, and he died in the blaze. **CHINOOK LEGEND**

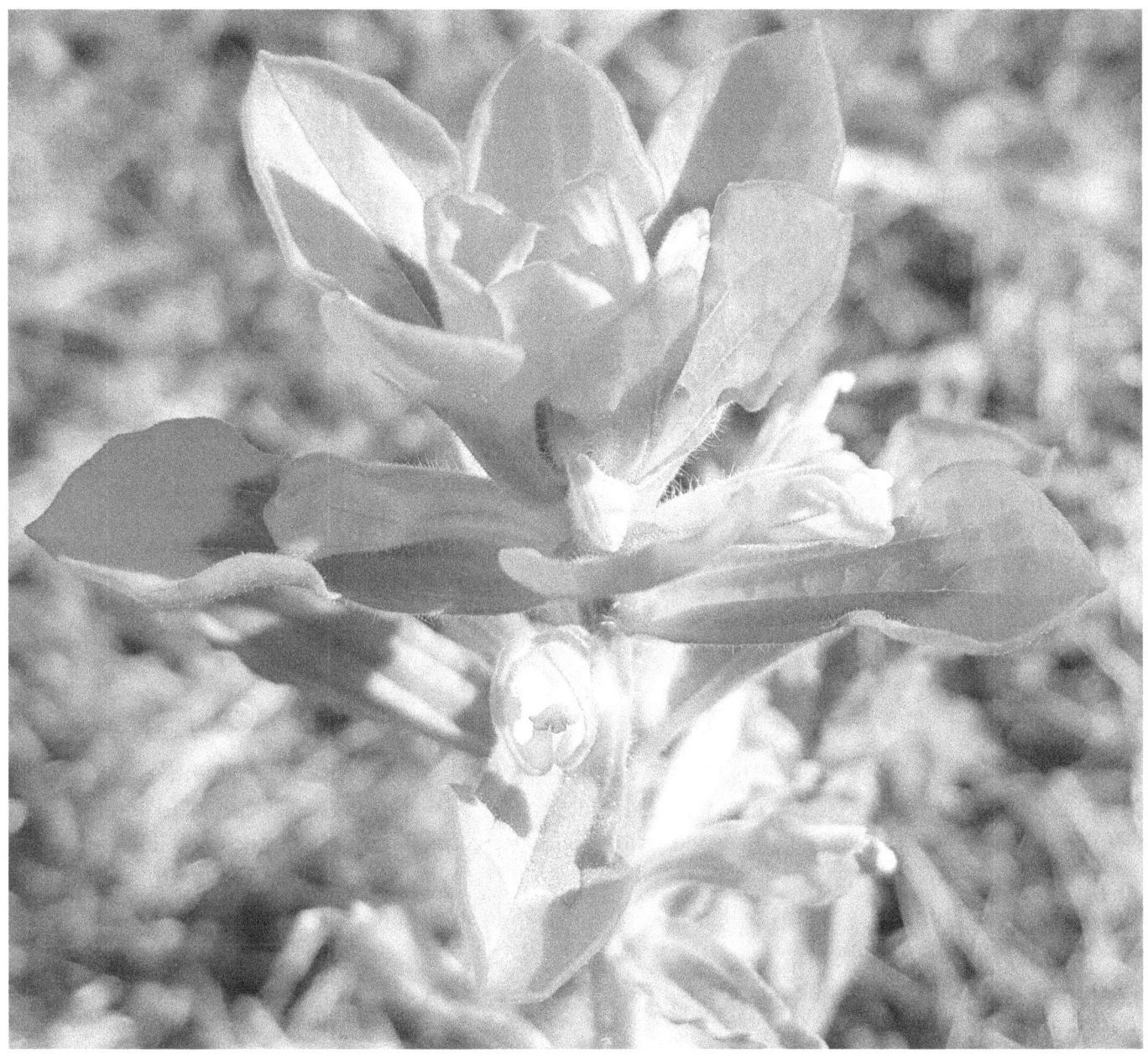

SCARLET PAINTBRUSH (*C. coccinea*)

## DOCTRINE OF SIGNATURES

Indian Paintbrush's dependency on other plants demonstrates its low vitality, physical weakness, and energy depletion. Even though the plant steals nutrients form host plants, it has the ability to integrate with and give something to the plant that it has taken from.

As people, we often need compassion from others to assist us with survival needs. Once these basic needs are dealt with, we can then feel the relief to live more freely and creatively. The significance of root burrowing into the roots of other plants and the reddish orange colour of the bracts corresponds with the root chakra; this gives attention to understanding and identifying the roots that connect us to our spiritual heritage. From this vantage point, an awareness of dysfunctional patterns from this and past lives may surface for examination and dissolution. The sharing of the host plant's vital nutrients, with seemingly no loss or harm to themselves, is an example of the law of supply: humble receiver and unconditional, compassionate giver.

13

The hidden, pale green flowers correspond to the heart chakra and the brightly coloured reddish orange bracts show a direct connection between the heart and the first and second chakras. The soft fuzzy, delicate leaves and flowers stretch outward as if to receive and give the life force.

The corolla tube inside the flower petal has a sweet nectar, when you eat a few flower petals and sit in silence, Indian Paintbrush will provide visions, imagery, and spiritual insights if you are open to receive its gifts. This signature is indicative of the sixth chakra. **PALLASDOWNEY**

### RECIPE

**INFUSION**- Take four grams of dried aerial parts to 120 grams of hot water. Steep ten minutes. Drink a half cup before each meal.

**IRONWOOD**
**HOP HORNBEAM**
(***Ostrya virginiana*** [Mill.] K. Koch.)
**AMERICAN HORNBEAM**
**BLUE BEECH**
**IRONWOOD**
(***Carpinus caroliniana*** Walter.)

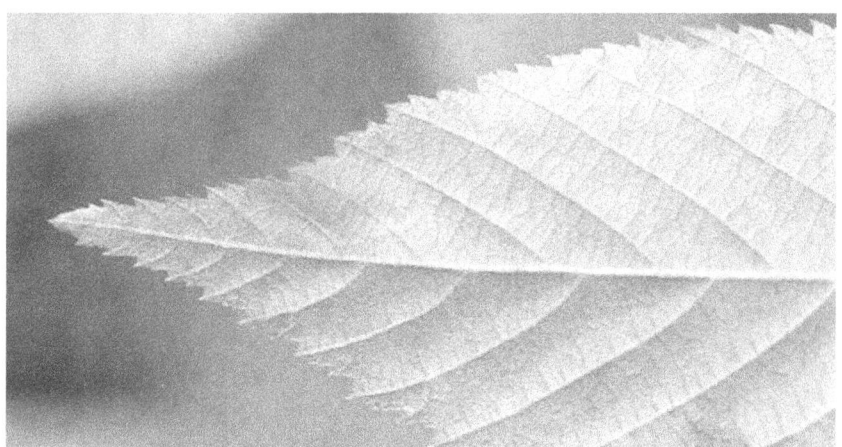

IRONWOOD LEAF (Courtesy of southeasternflora.com)

**CONSTITUENTS**- *O. virginiana* bark- (2S)dhurrin, (2R)-taxiphyllin

A sincere diplomat is like dry water or wooden iron. **JOSEPH STALIN**

Ostrya is from the Greek meaning shell, in reference to the inflated, cream colored flower bracts.

Ironwood, as the name suggests, was used for tool handles, sleigh runners, levers, cogwheels and other projects where a tough wood was required. The wood is very dense weighing nearly 49 pounds per cubic foot, and a specific gravity of 0.779.

The name Hop Hornbeam comes from the fall strobili that look, smell and taste like beer, and hops. And yet it is a member of the Birch family.

The leaves, when under attack by caterpillars, release cis-alpha-bergamotene, which attracts predator insects to feast on the invaders.

It has an outer layer of white wood, surrounding a dense centre of dark wood.

Native to eastern Canada, this deciduous hardwood is fully hardy to zone three on the prairies. In work at Morden, fifteen trees planted in 1939 showed a hardiness rating of 9.8. It has been successfully grown in the Patterson Gardens of the U of Saskatchewan, which is considered zone two.

Forestry concerns in Ontario have in the past cut the tree down to improve stands of maple. Ironically, it is an understory tree to mature maples and oaks, and protect them from strong winds.

It is only propagated by seed, which appears when tree is around twenty-five years old. The little nutlets are harvested and planted in fall with light covering of soil. They require double stratification to break dormancy, a warm and then cold treatment, and still may take up to two years to germinate, with low 25% rate.

The inner bark is boiled with potassium dichromate to produce an orange dye for wool. Adding alum will give a bright yellow color.

The eastern Chippewa combined the heartwood with hazelnut and white oak root and the inner bark of chokecherry to stop lung hemorrhages. They called the tree **MA'NANOUS'**.

It was combined with spruce and pine needles, along with the green tip heads of club moss (*Lycopodium obscurum*) as a decoction and steam for rheumatism, and with Eastern Cedar (*Thuja occidentalis*) for cough syrup. The Onondaga used a 1:3 decoction slowly decreased to one-third volume over low heat for coughs and catarrh.

The Iroquois and Mohawk decocted the bark to treat cancer of the rectum, and combined it with other herbs including white oak, American beech and blue beech (*Carpinus caroliniana*) to treat consumption. It was decocted in half and taken one cup at a time starting on the second day before the full moon and continued until finished.

The Potawatomi call this one of their cramp barks and used infusions to cure the flux. They call it **MÎANOO'S** meaning hornbeam.

Millspaugh mentioned, "a decoction of the heart-wood of this tree has long been used by the laity as an anti-periodic in intermittent fever, and as a tonic and alterative in scrofulous dycrasias and dyspepsia."

The cyanogenic glycosides in bark, create a similar effect as those from Prunus species.

Dhurrin and prunasin appear useful in external treatment of psoriasis, in the form of a wash or fomentation. Paoletti I et al, *Inflammation* 2013 36(6): 1316-26.

Dhurrin is found in sorghum, and taxiphyllin is present in *Triglochin maritima*, mentioned in chapter on Grass (volume 2). The latter is also found in Yew (*Taxus* genera) and raw bamboo shoots, which should be cooked for human consumption.

The tree is high in calcium and nitrogen and low in potassium and phosphorus.

Millspaugh wrote that either the powder or decoction caused headaches, loss of appetite, nausea, flatulence, colic, biliousness, aching extremities, exhaustion and sweating.

## HOMEOPATHY

Increased appetite, awakening at 4 am with the desire to eat. Right side is more affected, including the temple, teeth and abdomen.

Light sensation in head is worse from walking. Bowels and stomach feel congested, heavy as if bound by lead poisoning. Slimey copper taste is present in mouth.

**DOSE**- Tincture to third potency. Burt did original proving by self- experimentation with powdered heartwood at 2x and 3x in 1867.

King did a proving with three males with tincture, 1x and 3x in 1868.

A mother tincture is made of the fresh dark heartwood, by powdering and covering with five parts alcohol for at least a week. The tincture will have a brilliant orange red color, bitter taste and peculiar astringency.

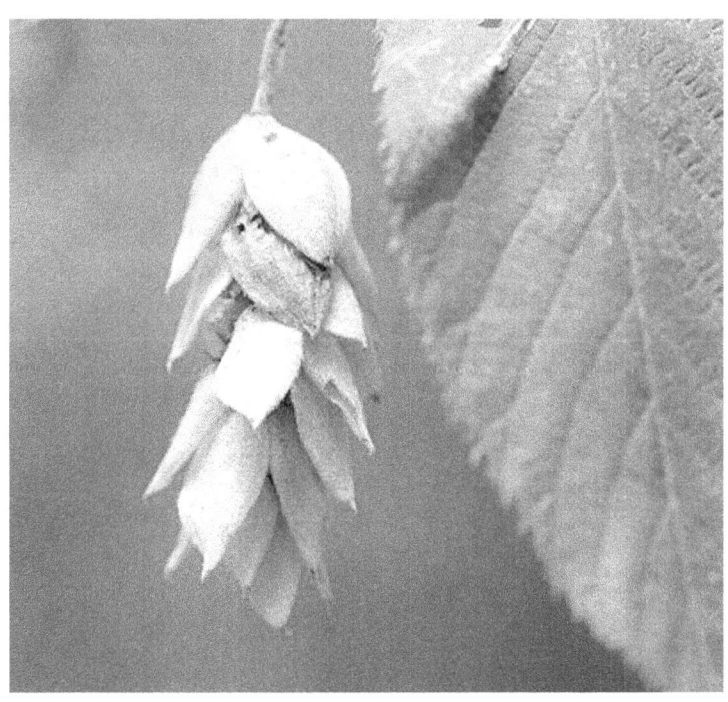

IRONWOOD (*O. virginiana*) FLOWER
(Courtesy of southeasternflora.com)

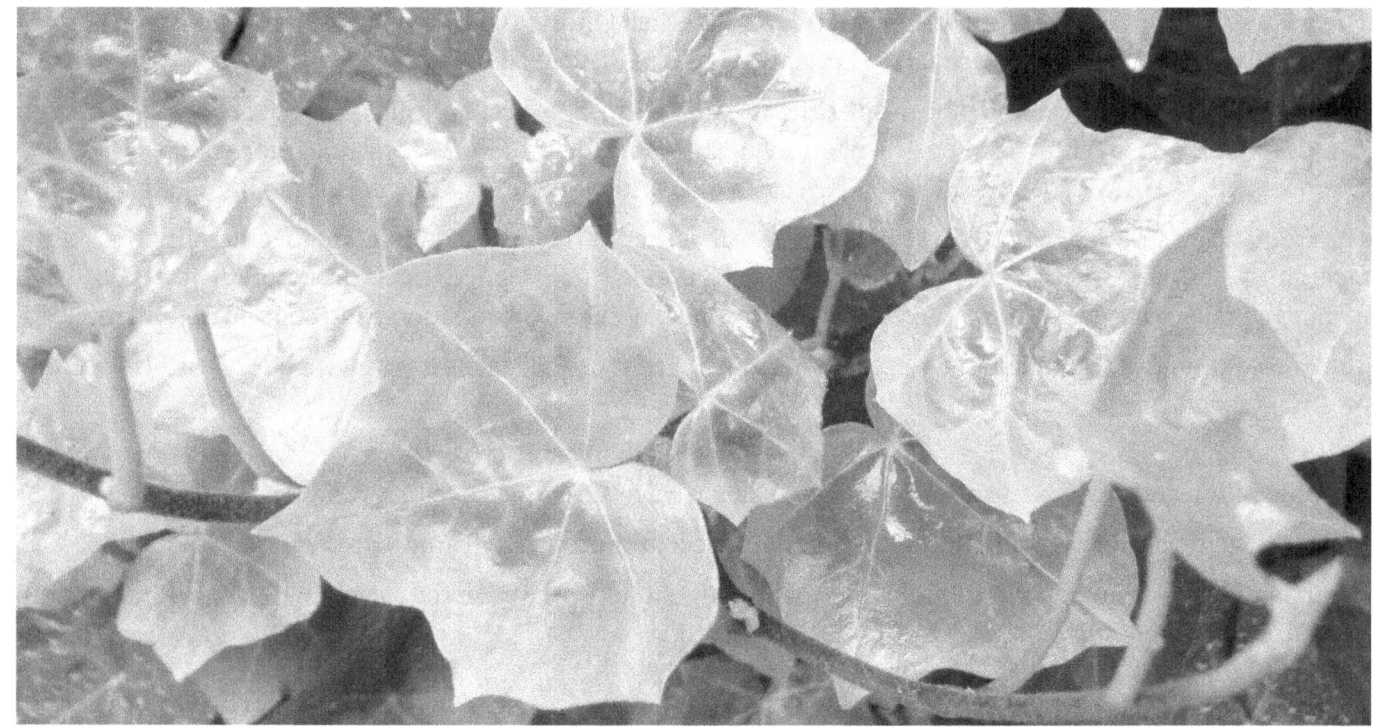

ENGLISH IVY

**ENGLISH IVY**
(*Hedera helix* L.)
**AMERICAN IVY**
**VIRGINIA CREEPER**
**WOODBINE**
(*Parthenocissus quinquefolia* [L.] Planch.)
(*Ampelopsis quinquefolia* [L.] Michx.) not accepted
(*A. hederacea*) not accepted
(*P. inserta* [Kern.] Fritsch) not accepted
**BOSTON IVY**
**JAPANESE CREEPER**
(*P. tricuspidata* [Siebold & Zucc.] Planch.)
(*A. triscupidata* Siebold & Zucc.) not accepted
**PORCELAIN VINE**
**TURQUOISE BERRY VINE**
**SEVEN LEAF CREEPER**

(*P. heterophylla* [Blume] Merr)
(*Vitis heterophylla* [Buckley] Britten) not accepted
**PORCELAIN BERRY**
**AMUR PEPPERVINE**
(*A. glandulosa* [Wall.] Momly.)
(*A. glandulosa* var. *brevipedunculata* [Maxim.] Momly.)
(*A. brevipedunculata* [Maxim] Trautv.)
(*A. heterophylla* [Thunb.] Siebold & Zucc.) not accepted
**SEVEN LEAF CREEPER**
(*P. heptaphylla* [Buckley] Britton ex Small)
**JAPANESE IVY**
**JAPANESE PEPPERVINE**
(*A. japonica* [Thunb.] Makino)
**PARTS USED**- wood, leaf, fruit

Oh roses for the flush of youth
And laurel for the prefect prime;
But pick an ivy branch for me
Grown old before my time.

**C. G. ROSSETTI**

With frantic rout and bacchanalian roar.
Their ivy-circled spears on high they bore.

**CATULLUS**

Ivy, ivy, I love you, in my bosum I put you, the first young man who speaks to me, my future husband he shall
be.
**SCOTTISH SAYING**

Hedera is from the Celtic **HOEDRA**, meaning "a cord", or from the Greek **HEDRA** meaning "a seat". In Latin it is called **ABIGA** that could be easily corrupted to **IVA**.

Some authors believe ivy is from the Anglo Saxon **IFEG**, itself of obscure origin. Helix means twisted or turned.

Parthenocissus is from the Greek **PARTHENOS,** meaning virgin; and **KISSOS** that means ivy. The generic name was derived from the old French name **VIGNE-VIERGE**, and then translated into the Greek.

Quinquefolia means five-leafed. Triscupidata means, three-pointed, referring to leaf shape, when young. Amelopsis is derived from the Greek **AMPELOS** meaning, a vine; and **OPSIS**, meaning likeness.

To the ancients, Ivy was dedicated to Dionysus, whose statues were covered with the plant, under the name of Kissos.

Kissos, or Cissus was a nymph who is said to have joyously danced herself to fatal exhaustion.

Dionysus, the Greek God of Wine, is often pictured crowned with ivy. According to myth, Dionysus as a youngster used ivy to foil some sailors who kidnapped him to sell as a slave in Egypt. But Dionysus caused the ship to be gripped by ivy so it could not sail.

Dionysus had two feasts, the Anthesterion, or Flower Uprising in spring, and Mysterion, the Toadstool Uprising in fall. (See Fly Agaric in the Fungal Pharmacy).

The worshippers decorated themselves with garlands of ivy; whereas crowns were given to Greek poets and the newly married as a sign of fidelity. The Greek name for ivy was **KISSOS**.

Dionysus had a wife Ariadne, who was an orgiastic goddess, in whose honor male human sacrifice was performed.

Ivy was a symbol of immortality and sacred to the Egyptian Osiris, the god of abundance and fertility; as well as Bacchus, the Roman God equivalent of Dionysus. According to Ovid, the young Bacchus was given to the nymphs of Nysa, who hid his cradle from Juno, by covering it with ivy. It is said that he was the son of Jupiter and Semele.

Ivy month is October, hence the numerous wine and beer festivals in Europe. A religious cult, known as Bacchae made an intoxicating brew of ivy, Fly Agaric mushroom, and pine sap. The poet Orpheus was killed by a group of ivy brew drinkers, although it is said that his head miraculously survived and continued to sing as it floated down the Hebrus river.

Ivy Ale is still brewed at Trinity College in Oxford, England.

Ivy is a broad-leaved evergreen ground cover that does well near house foundations. It has dark, green leaves, and green-yellow flowers after about ten years that turn into black berries. It is quite unusual in that it flowers in the fall, and sets seeds in the spring, the opposite of most plants.

It cannot survive the harshness of prairie winters, without some sort of micro-climate. However, in Edmonton, where I reside, I often see boston ivy sprawling away from basements, and taking over wherever it gets a chance. It thrives on full or partial shade, under trees. At the University of Alberta, there is Boston ivy some 80 years old, while in England there are English ivy plants up to 500 years of age.

In parts of the southeastern United States, it climbs hundred foot tall trees.

Ivy has an extensive history as a sacred and spiritual symbol. It was the letter G, for Gort, in the Druid alphabet. Ivy was said to represent intoxication, possibly because of the association of ivy with the Dionysian cult.

Because of it traditional connection with the Wine God, Ivy was believed to both cure and cause drunkenness. The Romans used ivy leaves boiled in wine as a "hair of the dog" remedy for hangovers.

Plutarch said the Dionysian bacchantes were intoxicated as much by the ivy as by the wine. Certain varieties of ivy do contain substances that "confuse the mind", as one 16th century writer expressed it.

The leaves and berries were decocted for severe headaches following a night of drinking. Goblets carved from the ivy wood represented this fact, and many popular tavern symbols contain the ivy bough.

Ivy's habit of entwining represents the spiraling cycles of the moon, the female menstrual cycle, fertility and such.

Yuletide celebrations in Britain often include a girl dressed in ivy representing the moon goddess, and a boy in holly representing the sun god. They would sing satirical songs and compete with one another, before strolling hand in hand down the street. The last stoke of wheat was bound with ivy as a sign of good luck, and called Ivy Girl.

*The Last Leaf* written by O. Henry features Ivy as the main character. It is worth a read.

Pliny records several uses for the plant, and in medieval times the berries were used as a cure for the plague.

The Leech Book of Bald (900 AD) has a recipe for tender ivy twigs, simmered in butter, as a sunburn salve for the face.

In the Middle Ages, it was part of the so-called Soporific Sponge, consisting of Hemlock, mandrake, poppy, lettuce, and other herbs. These were poured onto a sponge and held under a patient's nose as an anaesthetic. The poor victim could not help but pass out from the vile smell.

The berries were macerated in vinegar during the London plague. The berries were eaten for aches and pains but no longer suggested.

In Wiltshire, the leaf decoctions were traditionally used as an abortifacient.

European herbals at one time recommended ivy internally for treating upper respiratory congestion, spasmodic coughs, including whooping, delayed or absent menstruation, arthritis, phlebitis, neuraligia, cellulitis, burn wounds, rheumatism and internal parasites.

Ivy extracts are used by cosmetic companies for vasoconstriction and anti-exudative properties, reducing capillary permeability, moderating peripheral sensitivity and improving tolerance to skin massage. Ivy extracts also activate circulation, allow drainage of infiltrated tissue and reduce inflammation and edema.

Sewn together leaves in the shape of a cap were placed on the heads of children with eczema.

The roots were used as strops to sharpen knives, and the stems twisted for rope.

At one time, cups carved from ivy wood were filled with liquid and left overnight, to treat afflictions of the spleen. In Shropshire, England, the same cups were filled with milk and drank by children to prevent whooping cough.

Gilliver in 1947 tested 1915 species of plants for ability to inhibit germination of conidia of Venturia inaequalis, the organism associated with apple scab. Twenty-three percent were active but by far the most powerful was the one from ivy.

In both *in vivo* and *in vitro* testing, ivy has been shown to possess potent anthelmintic activity. Various saponin complexes showed efficacy against the *Dicrocoelium* fluke parasite in sheep after three doses; one at 500 and two at 800 mg/kg.

Alpha hederin was administered in vitro to *Fasciola hepatica* and at a rate of 0.005 mg/ml, all worms succumbed within 24 hours.

Work by Eguale et al, Exp Parasitol 116:4 found water/alcohol extracts of the fresh fruit a potent anthelmintic.

The need for safer anthelminthics for both the sheep and cattle industry is obvious; and here is another option.

The yellow mucilage that helps promote climbing vertical walls has been studied. The liquid is composed mainly of arabinogalactan proteins, that in combination with calcium driven electrosatic interactions and pectin, favor curing of an adhesive film.

Of course, nanotechnology is looking at ivy nanoparticles for application as novel scaffolds for cancer therapy and regenerative medicine.

Virginia creeper, or American Ivy is a common ornamental vine native to southern Manitoba, but introduced throughout the prairies for the shade protection it afforded early homesteads.

The plant has come to symbolize sweet neglect, and the birth date of May 4th.

The Cree call either this ivy or Porcelain Vine, **KA PISCIPOMAKAHK MISTIK-WACEKOS**.

The Chippewa used the young shoots of **MANIDO'BIMA'KWUD** for food. They cut the stalks into short lengths, which were then boiled and peeled. Between the outer bark and wood was a sweet substance that could be chewed off like corn on the cob. The water was then boiled down to syrup. When maple syrup was lacking it was sometimes used to boil wild rice.

The stems are very strong, as are the tiny adhesive disks that hold themselves to trees, and buildings. It has been estimated that a single tendril with just five disk-bearing branches can support up to ten pounds! The adhesive structure consists of debranched rhamnogalacturonan I-reactive components, callose and mucilaginous pectins.

The young shoots have been reportedly eaten cooked, and the fruit eaten raw. I cannot vouch for this, as I have also heard that the plant is considered toxic.

It has been implicated in one fatality of a child who ate the berries. In one lab study, a guinea pig fed 12 berries died within 36 hours. It also contains raphides, needle like crystals that irritate and swell tissue. Raphides are present in leaves and twigs and exude juice.

The twigs have been used as an astringent, tonic and expectorant. The leaves and twigs were sometimes made into a cough syrup.

The fruit are used to give a pink colour to wool. The sap of the closely related, Boston Ivy (*P. tricupidata*) was used in Japan as a sweetener, before the introduction of sugar.

The leaves also contain irritating raphides.

The Omaha Ponca name for the plant translates as "ghost grapes", and they of course avoided it.

The Fox tribe used the leaves, when picked green and dried, for infusion to reduce fever and cool the body. They also decocted the root to cure diarrhea.

The Cherokee used plant infusions for curing yellow jaundice.

The berries were also said to be effective; and sometimes used together for general bladder troubles

The roots were used by some Natives for various disorders of the stomach and bowel. Whether this was simply an emetic or purgative effect is not certain.

The Houma poulticed the crushed leaves and with vinegar applied them to lockjaw.

The Iroquois poulticed the vines and applied them to swellings on the wrists. A compound decoction of the bark was taken for stricture caused by a menstruating, while another formula was used for difficult urination.

The Creek used the roots to treat gonorrhea.

Woodbine, or Virginia Creeper (*P. inserta*) was at one time, considered the western form of *P. quinquefolia*, hardy to zone 2-3 and found in Manitoba as far north as Riding Mountain. Taxonomists disagree! The Navaho used infusions of the leaves and berries as a fomentation for swollen limbs. The Iroquois used it as part of a combination for difficult urination.

Boston Ivy (*P. tricuspidata*) is more vigorous than either English Ivy or *P. quinquefolia*, and despite its name, is native to China and Japan. This is the ivy referred to in the Ivy League, and is planted where true Ivy would not survive. The original name IV league, originates from the roman numeral four, as a descriptor of Harvard, Yale, Princeton and probably Columbia as universities of note. Covering the stone walls with boston ivy was a fashion of the day.

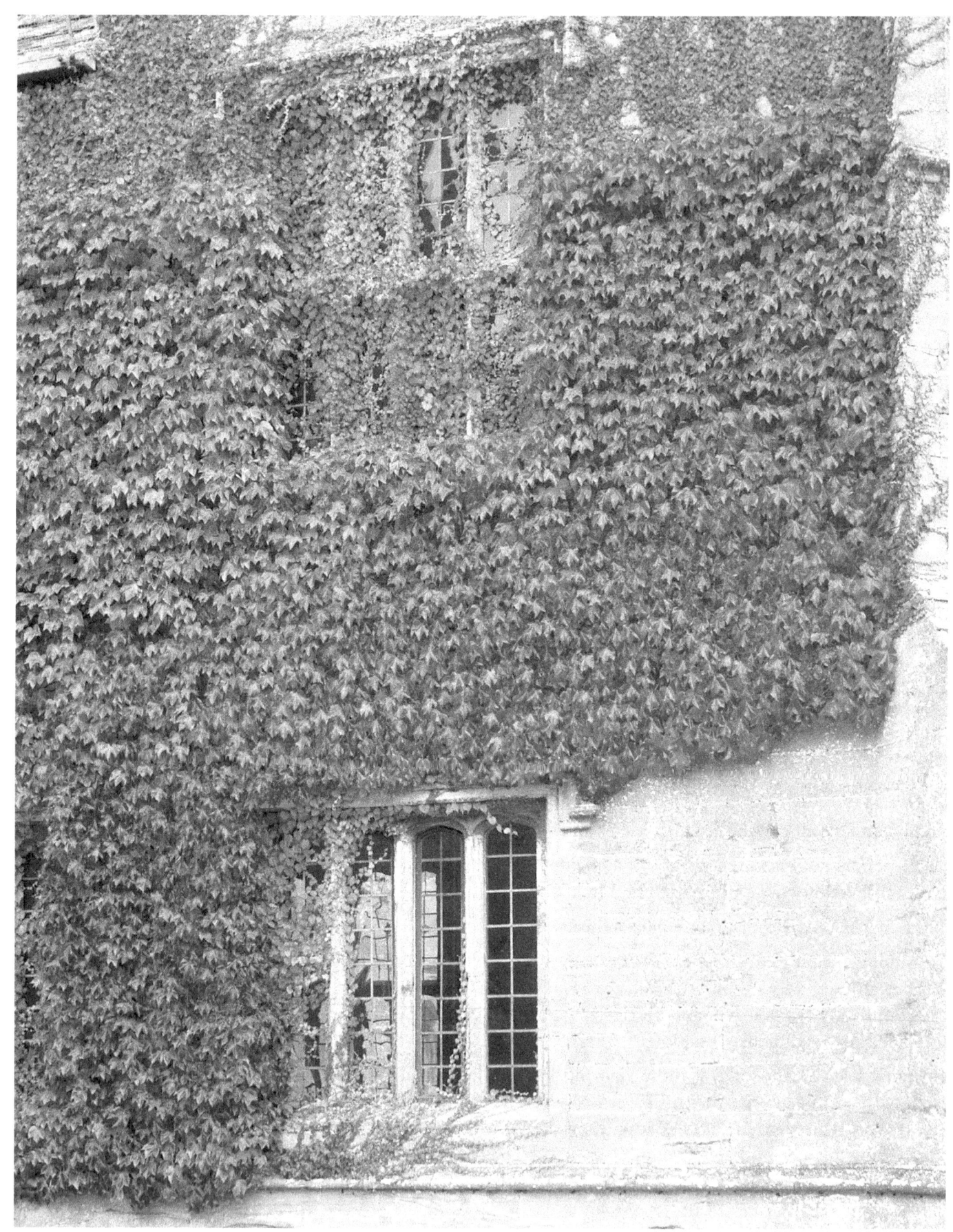

BOSTON IVY

It is known in TCM as **DI JIN**, or sometimes "wall climbing tiger. In Mandarin, the plant is known as **HAN YU PIN YIN**, or páqiáng hu. In Japan it is known as **TSUTA**.

The plant excretes calcium carbonate that acts as an adhesive pad for attachment.

Porcelain Vine, also known as Seven Leaf Creeper, is hardy to zone 3 on the prairies, and will grow 15 feet in a summer. It has grape like leaves with small greenish flowers, and berries that look like miniature grapes that ripen to turquoise and hence the other common name, Turquoise Berry Vine.

It is related to the wild Grape, which is also more common to Manitoba along riverbanks and found in the forests on occasion.

In former Indochina, the leaves were used to make medications to heal, or ease the pain of millipede stings.

Traditional Chinese Medicine has given several names to the vine, **LU P'U T'AO**, green grape, **YEH P'U T'AO**, wild grape or **SHE P'U T'AO**, snake grape, are the most common.

The related Amur Peppervine, also known as Porcelain Vine is hardy to zone 4, and also found in the eastern prairies as an introduced plant. It is widely used in traditional Asian medicine.

Seven leaf Creeper (*P. heptaphylla*) is native to Texas, but has spread to other southern United States. It is rare, and has not been well studied.

Japanese Ivy (*A. japonica*) is sometimes grown as a climbing vine on the prairies, and is hardy in sheltered areas. It is used in Traditional Chinese Medicine and called **PAI LIEN**, or **BAI LIAN,** because the root is white in color, and able to astringe furuncles and lesions; hence "white astringent".

It is also called **SSU HSIEN NAO HU-LU** meaning Gourd Hanging by a Silk Thread; **CH'I TZU MEI,** seven sisters; **YEH HUNG SHU,** wild red yam and my personal favorite **CHIU TZU PU LI NIANG,** meaning " nine sons inseparable from mother".

Other names include **QU ZI MEI**, in Mandarin, and **BAAK LIM**, in Cantonese.

# MEDICINAL

**CONSTITUENTS-** *H. helix* leaf -iodine, saponins 5% (triterpenic saponosides-Hederaoscide HOH (glucose, arabinose), hederagenine, alpha-hederin, helicin, echinocystic and oleanolic acid and 10 other triterpene glycosides, emetine, polyacetylenes, carubin, nicotiflorin, chlorogenic acid, resins, formic and oxalic acid, volatile oils; polyynes including falcarinol, and 11,12-didehydrofalcarinol, and sterols including beta sitosterol and campesterol. A natriuretic peptide has recently been found. Hederacoside C breaks down to (-)-hederin and emetine.
Leaf wax- n-alkanols 45%, monoacids 18.8%, triterpenes 9.7%, n-aldehydes 8.7%, and n-alkanes 7.7%.
Fruit- polyynes, falcarinone, falcarinol and a polyyne epoxide, calcium oxalate.
*P. quinquefolia*- leaf wax- oleanolic acid
leaf- pyrocatechin, parthenocissins A and B, resveratrol, cisso-tannic acid, tartaric acid, sodium, potassium, glycolic acid, calcium glycollate. No tartaric or potassium bitartrate in autumn leaves, but pectin and calcium glycolate detected. Also 3,4,5-trihydroxy-benzoic acid, piceatannol, resveratrol, resveratrol trans-dehydrodimer, cyphoste mmin B, pallidol, cyphostemmin A, quercitin-3-O-alpha-L-rhamnoside, myricetin-3-O-alpha-L-rhamnoside.
Stem wood- tricuspidatol A, parthenocissins M-N, miyabenol C, trans-e-viniferin.
berry- 2% oxalic acid and calcium oxalate. Same constituents as leaf except no glycolic acid, as well as beta sitosterol, methyl and ethyl 4-oxo- 1-2-dihydro quinolilne-4-carboxylate.
*A. brevipedunculata*- root and branch bark- flavonoids, phenols, beta amyrin, betulin, vanillic acid, ethyl gallate, kaempferol, 3,5 dimethoxy-4-hydroxybenzoic acid, aromadendrol, resveratrol, (+)-hopeaphenol, and (+)-vitisin.
*A. japonica*- ampelopsin, myricetin, lupeol, beta sitosterol, daucosterol, catechin, sucrose, palmitic acid.
*P. tricuspidata*- stem wood- tricuspidatol-A (a resveratrol dimer)
stem- cyanidin, lysopine, octopinic acid, fatty acids, five acetophenones, five flavonoids and nine stilbene derivatives.
Leaves- five caffeic acid derivatives, quercitin, kaempferol, beta sitosterol glucoside, 2alpha-hydroxyursolic acid and 2,24-dihydroxyursolic acid.

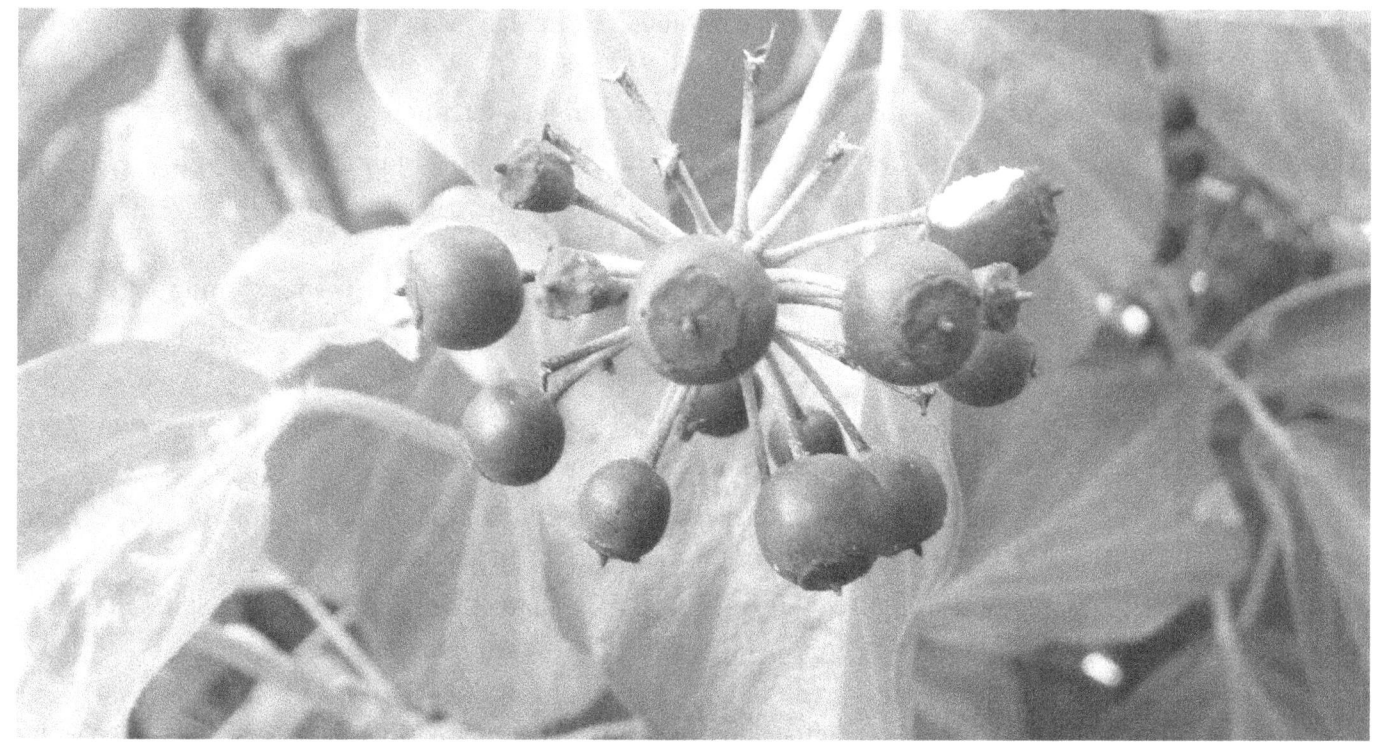

ENGLISH IVY AND BERRIES

English ivy tincture is prepared from the flowering twigs, and is often used in treating coughs, of acute or chronic catarrh. The young leaves are anti-spasmodic, expectorant and have mildly sedative properties, according to Weiss.

At least six phytochemicals are believed responsible for stopping bronchial spasms and for loosening sticky secretions so that they can be more easily coughed up. Trute et al, *Planta Medica* 1997 63:2. These are alpha hederin, and hederacosides C and D.

This makes it useful in chronic bronchitis, laryngitis, tracheitis, pertussis, and other mucus coughs.

It combines well with Sundew, in the treatment of whooping cough, and with Gum weed in chronic bronchitis.

The compounds are not water soluble, so it must be taken as an extract. Having said that, it appears that water extracts prevent or treat gastric ulcers. Mulkijanyan K et al, *Georgian Med News* 2013 224: 63-6.

Tinctures appear to reduce inflammation, and may be useful in arthritis. Rai A, *Ind J Pharm Sci* 2013 75(1): 99-102.

Ivy leaf activity is believed related to the presence of polar saponins that do not easily absorb but stimulate the bronchi via parasympathetic reflex.

Ivy leaf is a cool, bronchial relaxant and expectorant. Ivy Leaf Original Cough Syrup is now available in the United States, and marketed as a dietary supplement by NuTru, Inc.

One double-blind, placebo-controlled study of 25 children aged 10-15 with asthma demonstrated improvement in lung capacity after ten days treatment with ivy extract. Huntley & Ernst, *Thorax* 2000 55.

A larger, more well-designed study of 1350 patients by Hecker et al, *Forsch Komplement Klass Natur* 2002 9 with chronic bronchitis shows 94% of patients indicated their cough was reduced or eliminated.

A more recent, open multi-center study of 9657 patients, including 5181 children, found a syrup of the dried leaf showed 95% improvement in seven days in cases of bronchitis. With antibiotics, there was no increased efficacy, but 26% more side effects. Fazio et al, *Journal of Phytomedicine* July 2006.

In a study of 350 bronchial patients, a good outcome was found in 98.8%. Stauss-Grabo M et al, *Phytomed* 2011 18:6.

Schmidt et al, *Phytotherapy Research* 2012 26:12 1942-47 looked at 268 children aged 0-12 years of age treated with an ivy extract, syrup or cough drops for two weeks.

The global effect was good or very good in 96.5% of cases.

Prospan, a pharmaceutical marketed in Europe contains the total glycosides of ivy. In an ultrasound atomizer, twenty drops are diluted 1:5 with water three times daily for three weeks.

A double-blind, placebo-controlled, randomized cross-over study of 30 children with partial or uncontrolled mild persistant allergic asthma (despite budesonide), looked at a four week period with ivy leaf dry extract, in addition to inhaled corticosteroid therapy or placebo. This was followed by wash-out phase and switch. The study indicated children with bronchial asthma, on steroids, may benefit from this additional therapy. Zeil S et al, *Phytomedicine* 2014 21(10): 1216-20.

A dry leaf extract (EA575)® decreased IL-6, released by cytokines in response to allergens and respiratory viruses. Schulte-Michels et al, *Pharmazie* 2016 71(3): 158-61.

This preparation has been available over the counter in Europe for decades. Eighteen publications covering clinical trail of over sixty-five thousand patients are discussed in detail, in paper by Lang C et al, *Planta Medica* 2015 81(12-13): 968-74.

The extract inhibits the internalization of beta2-adrenergic receptors under stimulating conditions. Greunke C et al, *Pulm Pharmacol Ther* 2015 31:92-8.

Other work suggests alpha hederin affects IL-2 and IL-17 pathways, suggesting inflammation mediation, at least in asthma-model rats. Ebrahimi H et al, Drug Dev Res 2016 77(2): 87-93.

A 3:1 combination of ivy and goldthread root increase tracheal secretions and inhibit cough in optimal manner. Song KJ et al, *Yonsei Med J* 2015 56(3): 819-24.

Enterovirus 71 is a cause of hand foot and mouth disease. The anti-viral activity of hederasaponin B and 30% alcohol tincture of leaf showed significant anti-viral activity. Song J et al, *Biomol Ther* (Seoul) 2014 22(1): 41-6.

The leaves are useful in tracheitis, laryngitis, pharyngitis and other throat inflammations.

A natriuretic peptide is believed related to ion transportation. Maybe.

Alpha hederin acts as an indirect GRK2 (G protein-coupled receptor kinse 2) inhibitor. Schulte-Michels J et al, *Phytomedicine* 2016 23(1): 52-7.

Ivy extracts act synergistically with oseltamivir in drug-resistant influenza viral infections. Hong EH et al, *PLoS One* 2015 10(6):e131089.

Emetine is very effective against liver flukes, mollusks, intestinal parasites and fungal infections, including *Candida albicans*. J. Moulin-Traffort et al, *Mycoses* 1998 41(9-10): 411-416.

The wood, on its own, is more of an anti-spasmodic.

The leaves can be used as an emmenagogue internally; and as a topical application for relieving neuralgic pain, gout, and rheumatic conditions.

The leaves are useful in removing cellulite, mainly by external application in poultices, fomentations, and creams. They constrict veins, helping varicose veins to tighten up and disappear from the surface. The inhibition of elastase and hyaluronic acid are due to sapogenins like hederagenin and oleanolic acids.

External applications as compresses, or ointments relieve lymphadenitis, myalgia, phlebitis and edema. Skin showing seborrhoeic tendency and wherever there is need to promote drainage of dermal tissue, such as cellulite, lymphagitis and saggy eye tissue all benefit from ivy. Facino et al, *Acta Ther* 1990 16.

A poultice of the leaves, or applying the gum resin from incisions in the bark, can also be applied to sores, burns, skin eruptions, corns, calluses and parasitic conditions like scabies. The ivy leaf contains antiseptic properties, as well as saponins (hederas) that fight bacteria, fungi, worms and protozoa, according to Bisset, *Herbal Drugs and Phyto-pharmaceuticals* 1994.

Applications of the leaf decoction to children with head lice, can be helpful as part of a treatment program. The hair rinse also blackens hair.

Early German herbals suggest ivy leaf poultices for strengthening the fontanel, or soft spot, on the skull of newborns. For this, combine with pineapple weed, and apply as a warm poultice.

Nasal polyps sometimes respond to inhalations of the powdered leaf.

Various polyacetylenes have been shown analgesic as well as anti-bacterial and anti-fungal (including *Candida*) in studies conducted by Tanaka and Ikeshiro in *Arzneimittel-Forschung*, 1977. A follow up by Moulin et al, *Mycoses* 1998 41:9-10 found that alpha hederin is indeed antifungal, with a minimal inhibitory concentration of 25 ug/ml.

Alpha hederin is a potent cytotoxin, and induces apoptosis in human cancer cell lines HepG2 and AGS. Yang H et al, *Pharmacogn Mag* 2017 13(49): 118-22. Alpha hederine has protective activity against $H_2O_2$ genotoxicity in HepG2 cells by alkaline comet assay. It either scavenges free radicals or enhances catalase activity.

The same compound has been found to potentiate 5-FU, a chemotherapy drug at sub 1C50 levels by 3.3 fold. This synergistic activity may be useful in colo-rectal cancer cell therapies. Bun et al, *Phytother Res* 2008 22:10.

The gum resin can be used like spruce gum, to relieve toothache pain. Simply cut the bark, and a brown resin will exude. Roll this between your fingers until toothpick thin, and insert into the dry cavity for temporary relief. English pharmacists previously sold the remedy as Ivy Gum.

It is one of the few land-locked plants with an iodine content.

The berries are dry and bitter when ripe. Both leaf and berries alcohol extracts tested on rat prostate cancer showed inhibition of cell migration. Gumushan-Aktas H & S. Altun, *Oncol Lett* 2016 12(4): 2985-91.

Hederagenin disrupts mitochondrial membranes in human LoVo colon cancer cells. Liu BX et al, *BMC Complement Altern Med* 2014 14:412.

Ivy contains both estrogenic and gonadotropin stimulants, and excels as a pelvic decongestant. The leaf can be used alone, or added to other estrogenic formulas for treating amenorrhea, or scanty periods.

As a vaso-constrictor, it is used for phlebitis, and digestive hemorrhage. Work by deMedeiros et al, Journal of Ethnopharmacology 2000 72:1-2 found ivy extracts to exhibit anti-thrombin activity.

It relieves the menstrual pain due to analgesic and antispasmodic properties, combining well with cramp bark.

Delmas et al, *Planta Medica* 2000 66:4 suggest that three saponins, alpha hederin, beta hederin, and hederacolchiside A1, exhibit strong anti-proliferative activity on all stages of the parasite, *Leishmania infantum*. The ratio between anti-leishmanial activity on amastigotes and toxicity to human cells suggests that the saponins could be considered a possible drug for this problem. More recent work does not support the in vivo effect. Hooshyar H et al, *Jundishapur J Microbiol* 2014 7(4):e9432.

Alpha hederin and hederagenin induce autophagy and promote the degradation of neurodegenerative mutant disease proteins, *in vitro*. Wu AG et al, *Pharmacol Res* 2017 115:25-44. This may lead to therapeutic activity in Parkinson's and Huntington's disease. Earlier studies found the compounds improved motor deficits in Parkinson's disease mice.

Alpha hederin may inhibit growth and induce apoptosis in breast cancer cell lines. Cheng L et al, *Int J Oncol* 2014 45(2): 757-63.

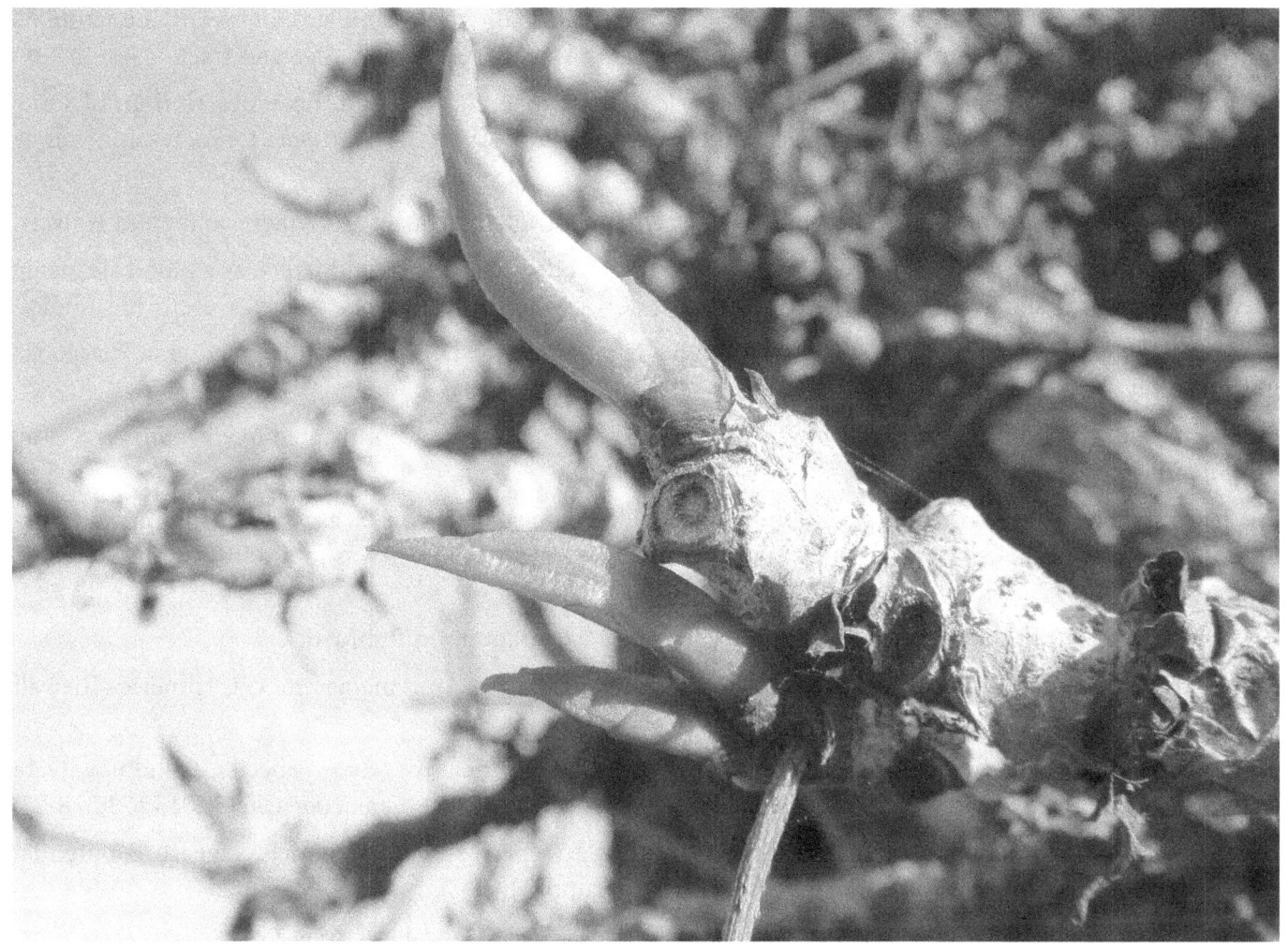

YOUNG, SPRING SHOOTS OF VIRGINIA CREEPER

Hederacoside C was long considered one of the main bioactive compounds in ivy leaf, but its bioavailability is extremely low, and poorly absorbed from gastrointestinal tract.

The yellow material used by ivy to adhere to trees and walls helps it hold two million times its weight, and consists of nanoparticles one thousand times thinner than hair. Work at the University of Tennessee, reported in Science Daily July 25, 2010 found these nanoparticles four times better than titanium or zinc for sunscreen. Patents are sure to follow.

English ivy has one final medicinal use. The live plant rapidly clears benzene contained in some car exhaust fumes. Maybe plant it around your garage. Indoors, the plant removes toluene from the environment. Dela Cruz M et al, *Environ Sci Pollut Res Int* 2014 21(13): 7838-46.

Virginia creeper, or American Ivy (*P. quinquefolia*) bark and twigs are used as an alterative, for treating colds and persistent nagging respiratory disorders.

It is a diaphoretic, astringent and tonic with some expectorating ability, combining well with spiderwort, hollyhock and wild bergamot as a fever-breaking hot infusion.

The herb improves the vigor of the lungs, with moderate expectoration.

It is used mainly in the form of syrup for scrofula, syphilitic affections, bronchitis, and other pulmonary complaints, according to Dr. King.

Sluggish lymphatic systems respond well, especially those with faulty fat assimilation. Grover Coe wrote its primary action was on the absorbents, the lymphatic tissue of the mesentery and digestive tract.

William Cook, in *A Compendium of the New Materia medica*, together with additional descriptions of some old *Remedies*, published in 1896, used the leaf infusion as an adjunct with *Aralia hispida* for increasing kidney urine production.

For scrofula he recommended four parts Rumex, two parts Celestrus, and equal parts American Ivy and Figwort.

American Ivy combines well with birch leaf, dandelion root, bittersweet twigs and violet, as a blood cleansing alterative for various skin conditions, taken cool after gentle decoction. Infusions of leaf may be useful in jaundice.

Matthew Wood mentions in *The Earthwise Herbal* that he has used the herb successfully in eczema, that looks like poison ivy rash.

Studies have found a direct correlation of glucose and insulin levels when administered *in vivo*. Kumar S et al, *J Compl Integr Med* 2011 8:1.

The plant stem and leaves contain resveratrol, found in Fleece flower and grapes, as well as pallidol and trans-e-viniferin. Activity against two human skin melanoma skin cancer cell lines was found in work by Nivelle L et al, Molecules 2017 22(3).

Resveratrol has significant anti-oxidant benefit, with over 9400 citations on PubMed.

Resveratrol is a monomeric stilbene, trans-epsilon-viniferin is dimeric, and miyabenol C is trimeric. They all down-regulate inflammation.

Parthenocissin A and pallidol are resveratrol dimers that scavenge reactive oxygen species. Pallidol activate transcription factor Nrf2, which regulates cellular anti-oxidant systems. Li C et al, *Food Chem* 2015 173:218-23.

Parthenocissin A showed neuroprotective activity in ischemic/reperfusion mice models, suggesting potential benefit in stroke therapy. He S et al, *Phytother Res* 2010 24(suppl.1): 63-70.

Pallidol and miyabenol C inhibit the growth of human colon cancer cells. Gonzalez-Sarrias A et al, *J Agric Food Chem* 2011 59(16): 8632-8.

Miyabenol C is a potent beta-secretase inhibitor, and may help prevent accumulation and deposition of amyloid-B peptide in the brain, that leads to Alzheimer's disease. Hu J et al, *PLoS One* 2015 10(1).

It also shows anti-proliferative and apoptotic effects on myeloid and lymphoid cell lines, including myeloma cell line U266. Barjot C et al, Life Sci 2007 81(23-24): 1565-74.

The compound docks to binding sites of estrogen receptors. Tian CY et al, *Sheng Wu Hua Xue Yu Sheng Wu Wu Li Xue Bao* (Shanghai) 2003 35(1): 77-81.

Some of these stilbens are found in caragana and carex species.

The cuticular wax contains oleanolic acid as the main constituents.

Both acidic and ethanol extracts of the leaf, stem and root indicate activity against yeasts and Gram positive bacteria.

Boston Ivy (*P. tricuspidata*) is used in Chinese medicine to treat arthritis, headaches, stomach problems and blood in the stool.

Recent work shows activity against the plasmodium species responsible for malaria. Park WH et al, *Antimicrob Agents Chemother* 2008 52(9): 3451-3. The novel stilbene glycoside was comparable to standard drug, choroquine.

Extracts of the leaf and flower show significant cytoxicity against both estrogen dependant and non-dependant breast cancer cell lines. *Arch Bio Sci* 2009 61:4.

Stilbene derivatives, from stems, show strong inhibition on both adipocyte differentiation and pancreatic lipase, suggesting possible benefit in treating excess fat accumulation. Lee SH et al, *Nat Prod Commun* 2013 8(10): 1439-41.

The leaves possess potent anti-oxidant activity. Saleem M et al, *Arch Pharm Res* 2004 27(3): 300-4.

Turquoise Berry Vine (*A. brevipendunculata*) root and branch bark are used in Traditional Chinese Medicine; and called **YIE PU T'AO TENG**.

Traditionally, they have been used for bathing body parts affected by abscesses, boils and skin ulcers, as well as for dispelling clots and reducing swelling from injury.

The fruit, roots and leaves have all been used for preparing baths; while the roots have generally been used for internal use.

Phenols and flavonoids, from the root and branches possess anti-cancer activity, against sarcoma 180, cancer of the alimentary tract and urinary tract, as well as malignant lymphoma.

Work cited above for Boston Ivy, found leaf and flower extracts cytotoxic against both estrogen dependant and non dependant breast cancer cell lines. Ethanol extracts of the berries show liver protection. Yabe et al, *J Ethnopharm* 1997 56:1.

The berries have been studied by Yabe et al, *Dokkyo University School of Medicine* in Japan. Several reports in both 1997 and 1998 issues (56:1 and 59:3) in the *Journal of Ethnopharmacology* suggest the berries help stimulate collagen synthesis and protect the liver from ferrous iron. This may lead to possibly helping alleviate the premature aging associated with hemachromatosis, or iron overload.

Ethanol extracts may be useful for the treatment of hepatic fibrosis, in a manner similar to silymarin, derived from milk thistle seeds. Yum MJ et al, *Pharm Biol* 2017 55(1): 1577-85. Ethanol extracts also exhibit anti-oxidant activity, which may explain, in part, the anti-inflammatory and anti-hepatoxic effects. Wu MJ et al, *Am J Chin Med* 2004 32(5): 681-93.

Two stilbenes, (+)-hopeaphenol and (+)-vitisin, derived from the bark of A. brevipedunculata var. hancei, possess remarkable ACE inhibition. The bark was tinctured with 90% alcohol. Su PS et al, *J Pharm Biomed Anal* 2015 108: 70-7.

Work by Sun X, et al reported in the March, 1986 *Journal of Traditional Chinese Medicine* shows the root effective against herpes zoster.

Research in Taiwan by Lee and Lin, found the herb containing anti-mutagenic factors with both direct and indirect activity. *Mutat Res* 1988 204:2.

Extracts may be useful for various osteoclast-associated bone diseases, based on work by Kim JY et al, *Molecules* 2014 19(11): 18465-78.

Water extracts inhibit cytokine IL-1beta and chemokine CCL-5, suggesting use in treating inflammatory conditions. Le MQ et al, *J Pharmacol Sci* 2014 126(4): 359-69.

Recent studies, by Yoshizawa et al, reported in the *Journal of Agriculture and Food Chemistry* 48 2000 looked at the effect of small fruit juices on HL leukemic cells.

The fruit of *A. brevipedunculata*, known as **NOBUDOU** in Japan, showed a NBT reducing rate of 45.3%; as compared to Black currant (*R. nigrum*) at 65%; and Raspberry fruit at 38%.

Japanese Ivy root or Pei Lien (*Bai Lian*) is used in China for its neutral properties and sour, bitter taste to clear fevers, and detoxify. The root is a bit pungent, little sweet and astringent.

It alleviates pain, and promotes greater muscle regeneration, and gaining weight.

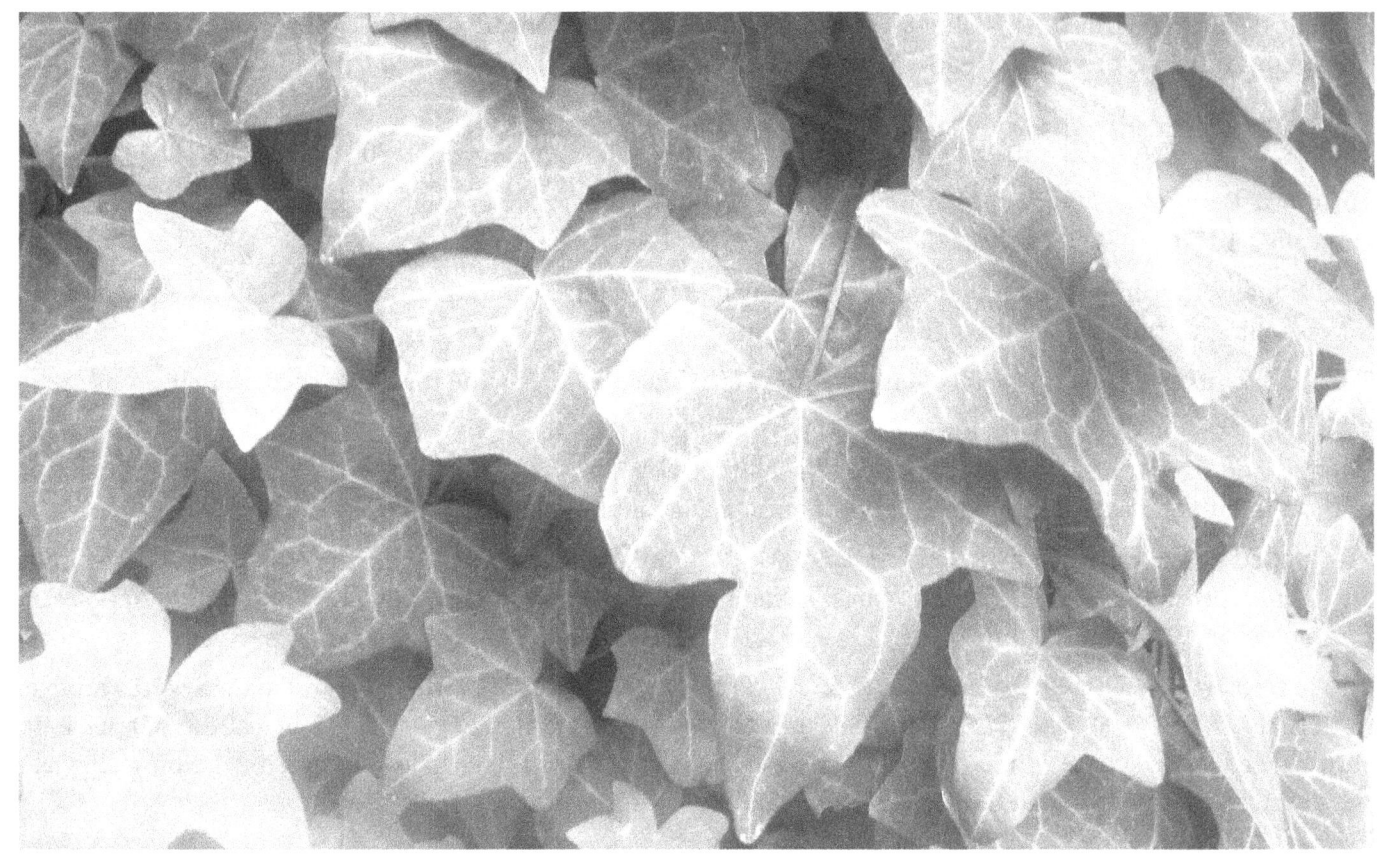

ENGLISH IVY

Due to its ability to astringe furuncles and lesions, in Mandarin it is called **PAI LIEN**, meaning "White Astringent", or **QI ZI MEI**. Its main activity is on the heart and stomach meridians, helping promote tissue regeneration and tumor dispersion. In Cantonese, the plant is known as **BAAK LIM**.

It is often used for tuberculosis of the cervical nodes, bleeding hemorrhoids, leucorrhea with blood, and injury from burns.

Momordin I induces apoptosis in promyelocytic leukemia (HL-60) cancer cell lines. Kim JH et al, *Anticancer Res* 2002 22(3): 1885-9.

Momordin I is a potent inhibitor of osteoclast differentiation and may be useful in bone disease conditions. Hwang YH et al, *Biochem Biophys Res Commun* 2005 337(3); 815-23.

Momordins from root (Momordin I, Id, and Ie) showed cytotoxicity against human cancer cell lines, and murine colon cancer. Lee DK et al, *Anticancer Res* 1998 18(1A): 119-24.

The root tincture suppresses migration and invasion in human MDA-MB-231 breast cancer cell lines. Nho KJ et al, *Mol Med Rep* 2015 11(5): 3722-8.

Topical application of the extracts reduced skin inflammation in work by Choi MR et al, *Ann Dermatol* 2016 28(3): 352-9.

Animal studies suggest the root tincture accelerate scald wound repair during the inflammation and proliferative phases of the healing process. Lee K et al, *BMC Complement Altern Med* 2015 15: 213.

A standardized extract of the root protects dopaminergic neurons in Parkinson's disease models. Park H et al, *Evid Based Complement Altern Med* 2013:346438.

Piceatannol, also found in Amur Berry Vine (above), and *Polygonum cuspidatum*, is a better anti-cancer agent than resveratrol. Lin LL et al, *J Chromatogr B Analyt Technol Biomed Life Sci* 2007 853(1-2): 175-82.

Boils, carbuncles, and a variety of weeping, suppurative sores and sloughing ulcers also benefit from both internal and external uses. It can be used as decoction for frost bite, or fungal infections such as athlete's root, tinea and ringworm.

The root is decocted, ten to fifteen grams at a time, or given as a tincture, 1-3 ml. Do not use in digestive deficiencies with chills.

## HOMEOPATHY

Ivy (*Hedera helix*) is a most interesting remedy. It has the ability to move deep seating deposition phase diseases, by a process of regressive vicariation to the acute stage.

Circulation is poor, with icy hold and moist hands and feet (frog's hands). This is accompanied with shivering and chilliness, bouts of perspiration and palpitations until 4 AM.

There may be inter-cranial pressure, as in chronic hydrocephalus, with delirium and chronic convulsions. Dr. John Clarke reports the case of Dr. Cooper.

He is said to have cured a case of hydrocephalus with a single drop of Ivy mother tincture. "Clear fluid dripped from his nostrils for three weeks".

Extreme anxiety with lives constantly in a state of unrest and worry; fresh air being the only relief.

The thyroid gland is swollen, constricted with hyperactivity and heart palpitations.

The menstrual cycle may be late, with a pre-menstrual discharge that is acrid and scorching. There may be pain in the left ovary and fallopian tubes and the patient feels somewhat better during menses.

An eruption of small white pustules can occur on the face and body.

Symptoms in the body start on the left and spread to the right. They are worse in the middle of the night, but relieved by fresh air, cool baths, movement, massage, and the afternoon and early evening.

It is the remedy of the "worn out" syndrome, according to Julian. It suits the tubercular conditions, especially of the phosphoric types.

**DOSAGE**- 3rd to 30th potency. 1x-2x for goiter. Third to sixth potency for catarrhal infections of the respiratory tract; 6-12x for biliary incoordination; 12-30x for Basedow's disease. The mother tincture is prepared from the flowering twigs and is used for coughs.

Original proving by Mezger in Germany in 1932 on 17 provers.

Ampelopsis (Virginia Creeper) is used for renal dropsy, hydrocele and chronic hoarseness in scrofulous patients. It helps alleviate choleric symptoms that are generally worse about 6 pm.

Pupils will appear dilated, with the left costal region sore and sensitive. There may be pain in the elbow joints, and the back is sore. Overall, the limbs are sore.

Vomiting, and purging with tenesmus; accompanied by abdominal rumbling may also be present.

Roof of mouth as if scalded. Measle like eruption over face, neck, arms and hands with itching, stinging and burning sensation.

Dreams of the dead, talking with dead. Flighty restless feeling.

**DOSE**- Second to 3rd potency. The mother tincture is prepared from the fresh leaf. Self experimentation by Cook and Emmerson with tincture in 1906. Intoxication of two young children who chewed leaves. Contact dermatitis in 28 year old woman reported by Haynes in 1878. Clinical observations by Boericke.

# GEMMOTHERAPY

The young shoots of Virginia Creeper (*Amelopsis weitchi* / *A. veitchi*) are a remarkable remedy for tendons and ligaments.

It effectively combats deformations and sclerosis and prevents severe C.E,P deformations.

This includes use in rheumatoid arthritis, and peri-arthritis of the shoulder.

**DOSE**- 1D glycerine macerate. 30-40 drops several times daily as needed.

# ESSENTIAL OIL

English Ivy contains essential oils including methyl ethyl ketones and methyl isobutyl ketones. It is not available commercially.

An absolute is made from the treatment of ivy leaves with alcohol. Ivy leaf absolute is a dark, green, semi solid mass with intensely herbaceous green or a bark green odour with rich, sweet, bitter foliage undertones. It will find good use in blends where a heavy, not expressly floral, green note is desired. It will modify violet leaf and hop absolutes, and is useful in forest blends, fougeres and chypres; or combined with oak moss.

*Amelopsis brevipedunculata* var. *heterophylla* has been steam distilled, with 86 compounds identified in leaves and 78 in branches. The essential oils of leaves contain palmitic acid (12.5%), phenylacetaldehyde (4.1%) and hexahydrofarnesyl acetone (3.9%). The branches contain same amount of palmitic acid, but with terpinen-4-ol (4.4%) and alpha-cadinol (3.7%). The most odorous compounds were (E,Z)-2,6-nonadienal which has a green, melon odor; (E)-2-nonenal that is grassy, phenylacetaldehyde that is honey-like, and (E)-linalool oxide that is woody in scent.

## FLOWER ESSENCE

Ivy essence represents honesty. It balances the heart chakra and its associated nadis. Take the essence to ease hidden fears and anxieties; it helps to release true feelings and identify your emotional needs.          **OLIVE**

Ivy essence helps ground us in situations where shock may otherwise make us space out and even lose the will to live.          **YORKSHIRE**

# SPIRITUAL PROPERTIES

Ivy has also long been a symbol of love and fidelity because of the way it clings to any support. This is illustrated in the tragic legend of Tristan and Iseult.

After the loss of Tristan, her bethrothed, Iseult died of a broken heart. Both were buried in the same churchyard, but by the king's command the graves were some distance apart.

However, the ivy plants soon grew on both graves and the lovers were reunited by the twining together of the vines.

The infant Bacchus was abandoned by his mother. She hid him under an ivy bush, knowing that the ivy would protect him.

When he grew to manhood, the young god Bacchus was crowned with ivy. The beautiful nymoph **KISSOS**, danced before Bacchus so delightfully that he made a feast in her honour. He summoned all the gods to the feast and bade the nymph to dance before them.

Kissos had fallen madly in love with Bacchus. She danced with such abandon and joy that all the gods marveled. Her dance became a love dance, swiftly increasing, when overcome with emotion, she fell to the ground and died. Bacchus mourned for the lovely maid and named the ivy Kissos in her honour. Ivy vines sprang up and covered her grave with verdure. An old saying is "Ivy will grow over the graves of a maid who dies for love."          **ALMA GUILLET**

Ivy's entwining habit also represents the movement and cycles of the heavenly bodies-the stars and planets-and it is symbolic of the knowledge and understanding of the way in which these movements are reflected on earth. In particular, ivy represents the spiraling cycles of the moon, of which there are just over twelve to each solar cycle...The traditional Chrismas carol the Holly and the Ivy, which is seen as a celebration of Christ's suffering, also concerns the differences between expansive male and restrictive female principles of life and the rivalries between sun god and moon goddess, as well as the pulls and influences of the perpetual cycles of the sun and the moon. The rivalry between holly and ivy can, on its simplest level, also be interpreted as symbolic of the domestic war of the sexes.                                                                                                                    **GIFFORD**

Holly is the male plant and ivy the female. The explanation seems to lie in the fact that the last sheaf in harvest was bound with ivy and was eventually called the Ivy Girl, a name that came to be synonymous with a shrewish wife, but the sentiments of this medieval song bring no emphatic confirmation with that idea.                           **WATTS**

## PERSONALITY TRAITS

Ivy is a name for a faithful, stalwart, honest, poetic, humorous person who has walked a rocky path and who has learned well from that experience.

This is the magical name of a person worthy of respect.                                                                                      **MCFARLAND**

Ivy is a terrifying force to the psyche, with its climbing tentacles that envelop buildings and trees. Ivy persistently looks for cracks to reach into. It has been known to tear buildings down, reach into the slats, pry open joints, and dig into masonry. Ivy has also been found to clean contaminants from the polluted air in its surroundings.

This is a powerful plant in many ways, and similarly for human physiology it reaches into the farthest areas of the body, reduces the inflammation of toxic buildup, binds the deposits of toxins from the tissues and helps eliminate these influences.                                                                                           **TIMOTHY LEE SCOTT**

The symbolism of the ivy rests on three facts which are that it clings, it thrives in the shade and it is an evergreen.

Its clinging has made the ivy a symbol of the traditional, albeit now unpopular, image of the helpless female clinging to her man for protections...

Like other evergreens, the ivy symbolizes eternal life and resurrection. It has been associated with the Egyptian god Osiris and the Greco-Roman god Attis; both of whom were resurrected from the dead. Medieval Christians, noticing that ivy thrived on dead trees used it to symbolize the immortal soul.

Because it thrives in the shade, ivy represents debauchery, carousing, merry making, sensuality, the flourishing of hidden desires and the enjoyment of secret or forbidden pleasures. Dionysus [Bacchus] the Greco-Roman god of wine, satyrs and Sileni are often wreathed in ivy...the Greeks crowned their poets with wreaths of this plant.                                                                                                                                **TUCKER**

## RECIPES

**INFUSION**- Pour boiling water over 0.5 grams of dried ivy leaves, steep 10 minutes, and strain. Drink up to three times daily with honey if desired.

Avoid the berries, as they may be toxic. Allergic dermatitis can occur from handling the fresh leaves or sap resin.

**TINCTURE**- *H. helix*- 15-30 drops. The fresh plant tincture is prepared at 1:2 and 60% alcohol

Gum resin- Tincture at 1:5 and 70%. Only 5-10 drops as needed.

*P. quinquefolia*- 10-30 drops 3 times daily. The bark from twigs and vine are used after berries ripen.

*A. japonica*- 1-3 ml daily

**DECOCTION**- Two tbsp every 2 hours. For American Ivy, use two ounces of bark in one litre of water, and simmer down to 500 ml. Take 2 tbsp every two hours.

*A. japonica* root decoction- 10-16 grams.

**SYRUP**- 2-4 ounces three times daily.

**CELLULITE CREAM**- Slowly simmer 2 ounces of fresh ivy leaves in 60 ml of coconut oil for two hours. A double boiler system is best. Remove from heat and as it begins to harden add 5 ml of essential oils, comprised of grapefruit, fennel, juniper berry and cypress. Rub into affected areas firmly once a day.

**POULTICE**- Take two handfuls of ivy leaves and simmer until tender. Place on corn, bind and allow to draw. Repeat until corn lifts away with root.

**CULTIVATION**- Sagogenin content of leaves is 1.5 times richer in autumn than other times of year. Hederagenin content (21.7 mg/ gram of dry weight) is highest in the fruit of flowering shoots, while oleanolic acid (14.2 mg/gram dry weight) is found in the leaves of vegetative shoots in late fall.

**SCROFULA AND GLAND ENLARGEMENT**- Take two parts each of yellow dock root, dandelion root and bittersweet (*Solanum dulcamara*) twigs; and one part each of Figwort root (*S. nodosa*) and American Ivy bark or twigs. Simmer together until reduced by one third. Sweeten with honey. Dosage is one tablespoon three times daily.

**JACK IN THE PULPIT**
**DEVIL'S EAR**
**INDIAN TURNIP**
**DRAGON ROOT**
(***Arisaema triphyllum*** [L.]Schott.)
(***Arum triphyllum*** L.) not accepted

Jack-in-the-pulpit
Preaches today
Under the green trees
Just over the way.                                                         **JOHN G. WHITTIER**

Always speak politely to an enraged Dragon.                                **STEVEN BRUST**

Arisaema is from the Greek **ARON** for arum and **HAEMA** blood, due to red spots on the leaves of some European species. Triphyllum means three leaves.

This soggy, woodland perennial is found in only Manitoba on the Canadian prairies. It is found down to Florida and westward to Kansas and Minnesota.

It is a most beautiful and striking plant and flower which can change from male to female year to year. The long spathe looks like an old-fashioned pulpit, and is really an umbrella to prevent rainwater washing away pollen, or drowning the flowers.

The plant can live for 20-100 years and will generally have male flowers early in life and then switch with age. They can be male, female, or bisexual. The latter are found in about 13% of flowers. They are attractive to deer for consumption.

Size does matter, and the probability of being female increases with size. If shocked by transplanting, they will often revert back to males.

Georgia O'Keeffe was attracted to the plant and painted six canvases starting in 1930 that explored the sensual nature of the plant. Some authors have taken to calling it Jill-in-the-pulpit when it changes sex.

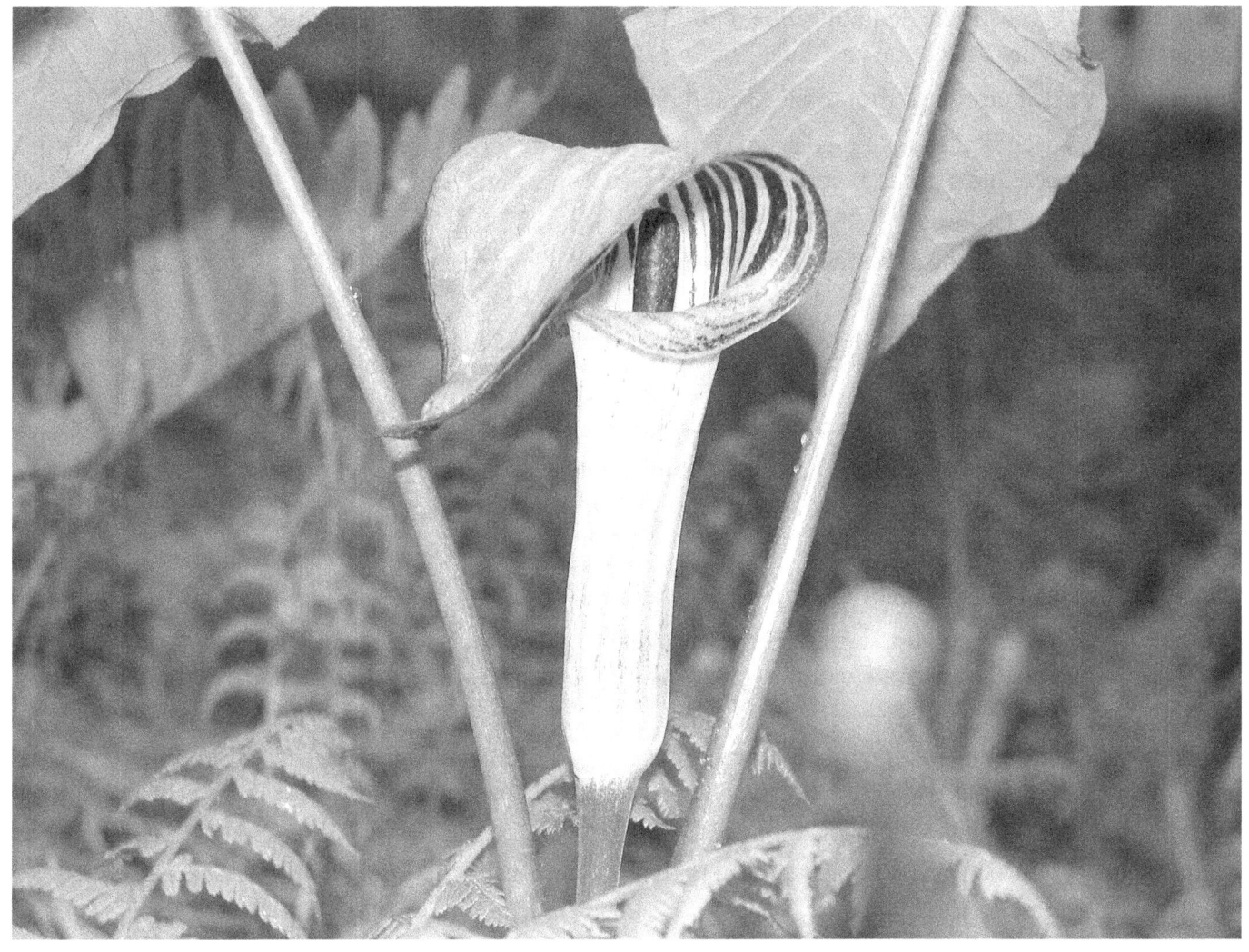

YOUNG JACK IN THE PULPIT

The female flowers turn into bright, waxy crimson berries in the fall. It is said the ripe berries were eaten, with venison by indigenous people.

The French-Canadian loggers thought the spathe looked like a log hook, or *gouet*, hence the French name gouet à trios feuilles, "hook with three leaves."

Various native tribes used the plant for healing. The Iroquois used rhizome infusions for contraception; one teaspoon of dry powdered corm in cold water to prevent conception, and two teaspoons in hot water for permanent sterility. At least, in one book. Daniel Moerman records "cold infusions of roots taken 'for nonconception caused by cold blood.'" This makes more sense, as the ground plant was put in mare's feed to induce pregnancy.

And yet for cold, deficient pelvic congestion, the corm/tuber was dried and powdered for infertility. The Iroquois name **KAHAHOOSA** means, papoose cradle.

A compound, decoction steam was used "when a person has cold sweats, not very sick."

Small amounts of dried powder were used as snuff for headaches, and congestion.

The dry, corm powder was used for colic and a cooled decoction of the rhizome was applied to sore eyes by the neighboring Chippewa.

It was used extensively for expectoration, in conditions such as asthma and bronchitis.

The fresh corm is caustic and irritating, due to oxalic acid, so only dried root should be used. After drying for six months, it can be roasted and powdered, adding a chocolate-like flavor to bread.

The Pawnee applied powdered root to the head to relieve headaches.

The Meskawaki used the seed as a medical diagnostic tool for discerning recovery or death for ailing patients. A seed was dropped into a cup of stirred water. If the seed went around clockwise four times, the patient would recover. Less time and they would not.

The Menominee placed the pulverized root into lip incisions to counteract "witchery" to face. Could this be Bell's palsy?

They would put the finely chopped, fresh root into meat for their enemies. Very small amounts were used in a combination to cure insomnia.

Snake bites were relieved by applying a poultice of root to affected area.

Numerous tribes used the corm for boils, abscesses, and liniments for swellings, rheumatism and generalized pain.

The Cherokee used it as a stimulant, expectorant, diaphoretic and carminative. Infusions were gargled for throat irritations.

Decoctions of corm were taken by Choctaw "to make blood".

Matthew Wood, noted herbalist, suggests the spirit signature is the underwater panther, a terrible, powerful but usually invisible spirit. Underwater panther medicine supports the water in the body, due to their "sumptuous, fat, water roots."

Constantine Rafinesque (1828) wrote the herb, "has been found beneficial in lingering atrophy, debilitated habit, great prostration in typhoid fevers, deep seated rheumatic pains, or pains in the breast, chronic catarrh etc,…[and] quickens circulation".

An ointment, produced from dry corm, is used for ringworm, scrofulous sores and skin abscesses.

The related *A. heterophyllum, A. amurense* and *A. consanguineum* tubers are utilized in TCM under **TIAN NAN XING**, meaning "sky's southern star". It is also known as **SHE LIU GU**. Our Jack in the Pulpit is most closely related to *A. amurense*, but not to *A. dracontium* and *A. macrophyllum*.

The bitter, warm and acrid properties help to dry dampness and dissolve phlegm. This includes coughs with white or yellow sputum or liver wind rising with phlegm stagnation resulting in vertigo, facial paralysis, seizures, epilepsy, muscle spasms and cramps.

Used topically, it reduces swelling and dissipates nodules, including sports injuries and joint pain. The herb has marked sedative and analgesic effects.

In one study of 105 patients with cervical cancer, both oral and topical application of the herb resulted in a 78% rate of effectiveness. *Chinese Herbology* 1998 1972 17:8.

An agglutinin, isolated from *A. heterophyllum*, is cytotoxic to A549 non small lung cancer cells, through apoptosis and autophagy, via inhibition of the P13K/Akt pathway and induction of ER stress. Feng LX et al, *j* 2016 14(11): 856-64.

Other work found a lectin from this plant inhibits various human cancer cell lines, especially HOP-62 (95%) and HCT-15 (92%). Kaur M et al, *Arch Biochem Biophys* 2006 445(1): 156-65.

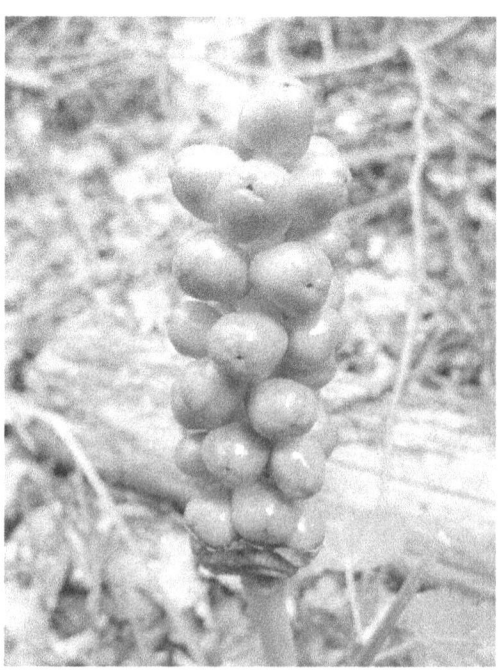

NEW BERRIES

The herb is sometimes mixed with bovine bile and called **DAN NAN XING**, or gallbladder southern star. This reduces the drying aspect and makes it more suitable for patients with underlying yin deficiency. It is used for similar purposes.

In both cases, ginger root is the antidote for over dose complications.

# HOMEOPATHY

There is an irritable disposition, and great restlessness. Absent-minded and forgetful.

Burning sensation of lips, mouth, throat, lungs and anus. Chills over body, great daytime drowsiness, and sleeplessness.

Head, throat and eyelids feel swollen, hot and irritated.

Quivering of the upper left eyelid is considered a specific indication.

Voice is hoarse or lost, worse from talking. Even one drop at highest potency has restored voice in a few hours. It is sometimes called Clergymans's Sore Throat.

**DOSE-** 3x to 30x.

# FLOWER ESSENCES

Jack in the Pulpit essence helps clear one's path to authentic spirituality and true spiritual insight. It helps one be aware of the rewards of selfless service and balanced leadership. **INJOYNOW ESSENCES**

Jack in the Pulpit essence is for developing authentic spirituality; helping one resolve conflicts between past spiritual experience and present spiritual insight. **DELTA GARDENS**

Jack in the Pulpit is one of the holiest of all flowers known for its strong visual image of someone in prayer. By taking this flower essence you will connect directly to the wisdom of the spiritual realm. For children this essence returns them to their heart and soul purpose directly and clearly. They will know they are being looked after and will feel safe and secure. **GRANDPARENTS OF THE FOREST**

# PERSONALITY TRAITS

The nose knows in Arum too. Itching for advancement and a better position, his nose becomes irritated, inflamed and aggravated. So distressing are these symptoms, that he will, in classic Arum style, bore his finger there to effect some relief.

Paradoxically, the finger-in-the-nose manoeuver is hardly the means of gaining the exalted social position he seeks. **VERMEULEN**

# SPIRITUAL PROPERTIES

This herb has the interesting property of helping an individual awaken to their spiritual purpose.

The way energy of a spiritual nature manifests in your life must follow patterns that cooperate and harmonize with the physical, mental and emotional levels. It would be wise to use a flower essence of this plant. The signature relates to the flowers, their unique shape and way it seems to hold back energy, as if waiting to be welcomed.

There is some stimulation of the root chakra and added energy in the eighth, ninth, tenth and eleventh chakras. There is a strengthening of the conception vessel meridian, and the nadis near the crown chakra are stimulated, as are the mental and causal bodies. In some individuals, the causal, soul and integrated spiritual bodies are brought into a temporary state of alignment. Press the medulla oblongata and top of head at the same time to activate the test point. **GURUDAS**

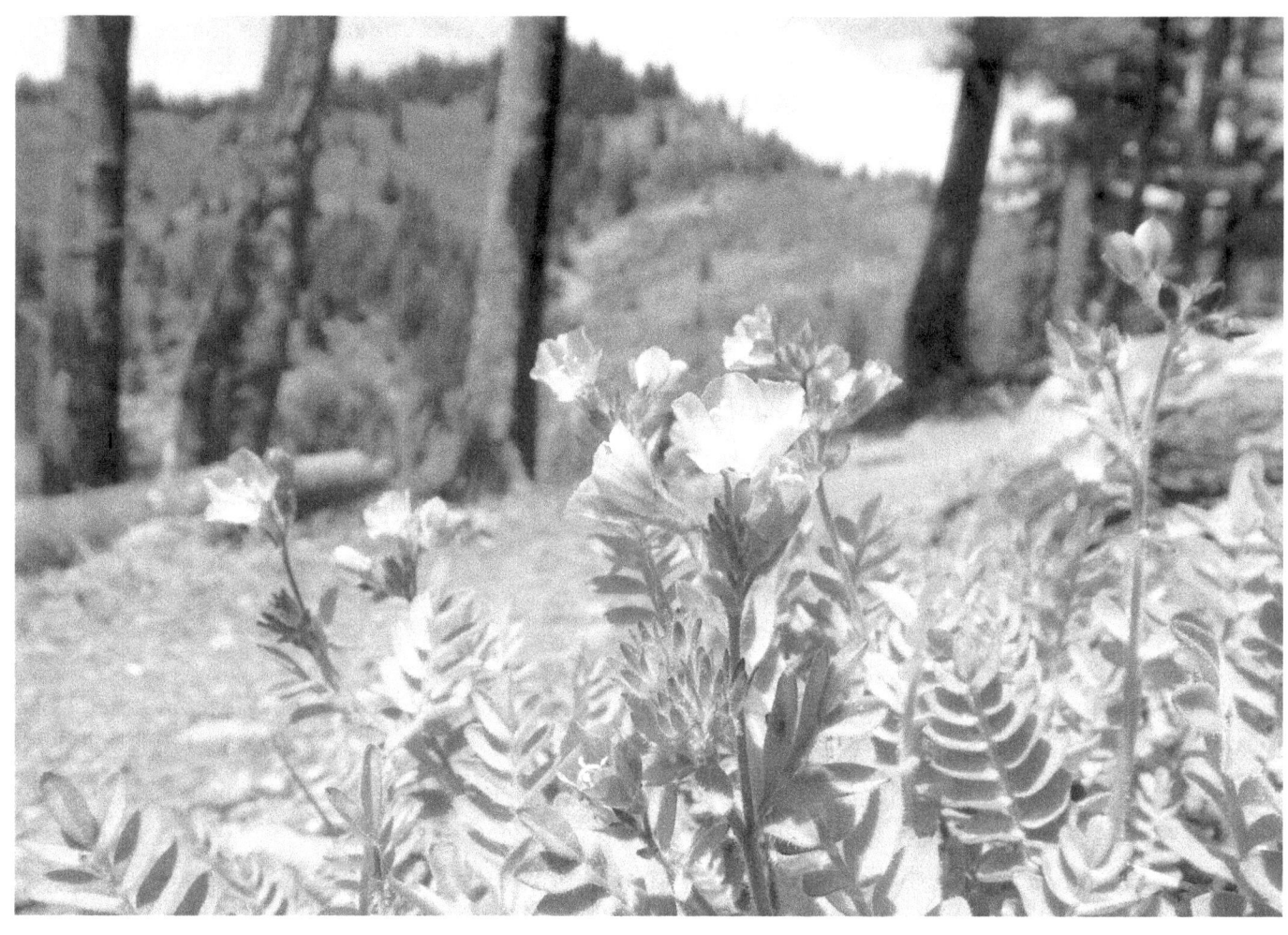

JABOB'S LADDER

**TALL JACOB'S LADDER**
(*Polemonium caeruleum* **ssp.** *villosum* [J. H. Rudolph ex Georgi] Brand)
**WESTERN JACOB'S LADDER**
(*P. caeruleum* **ssp.** *occidentale* Greene)
**SHOWY JACOB'S LADDER**
(*P. pulcherrimum* Hook.)
**SKUNKWEED**
**SKUNKY JACOB'S LADDER**
**ALPINE SKY PILOT**
(*P. viscosum* Nutt.)
**JACOB'S LADDER**
(*P. acutiflorum* Willd.)
**FALSE JACOB'S LADDER**
**GREEK VALERIAN**
**ABSCESS ROOT**
(*P. reptans* L.)
**PARTS USED** - leaves, flowers, roots

Jacob slept with a stone for a pillow, and he dreamed and behold a ladder set upon the earth and the top of it reached to Heaven and behold the Angels of God ascending and descending on it.        **GENESIS 28:12**

36

The plant not strange to Scottish skies,

Whose leaflets, ladder-like arise,

Pointing to azure vaults above—-

The Patriarch's Dream—in southern grove infrequent.

The common name alludes to Jacob's dream of angels climbing the ladder to heaven, and the plant's ladder-like placement of leaves. Jacob's ladder is also a ship's rope or chain ladder to let people come and go from smaller boats. It is also used for a steep flight of steps up a cliff.

Polemonium is from the Greek **POLEMOS**, meaning war and supposedly the result of two kings (one Polemon of Cappadocia) who went to battle over who first discovered the medicinal properties of the plant. Or, it was named in honor of Polemon, an early Athenian philosopher.

**CAERULEUM** is from the deep blue colour of the flowers, while **PULCHERRIMUM** means "very handsome, or beautiful". This may be due to the bright orange ring inside the blue flowers. Sky Pilot refers to the plants ability to thrive in high altitudes.

Tall Jacob's Ladder is most common to the aspen parkland and boreal forest of northwestern Alberta, while Skunkweed and Showy Jacob's Ladder are restricted to the western foothills.

As the name suggests, Skunkweed is particularly mephitic, especially when in flower.

Tall Jacob's Ladder has been used traditionally as a remedy for nervous complaints, headaches and heart palpitations.

Jacob's Ladder is a beautiful flowering plant, tainted in reputation by the disagreeable leaf scent. The other common name of Greek Valerian (*P. caeruleum*) gives some indication of medicinal usage, and the smelly sock odour. Cats love the plant smell, like they do honeysuckle wood and valerian root.

Researchers suggest that the foul, skunky smell may serve to repel nectar feeding ants, who can rob the sweet without pollinating the flowers.

Dioscorides suggested the root in wine for cases of dysentery, toothache and, of course, the bites of poisonous animals.

Turner, a famous 16th century English herbalist, called it "Valeriana greca, and this is oure commune Valerian that we use against cuttes". As late as 1830, it was retained in some European Pharmacopoeias, mainly for treating syphilis and rabies.

Previously known to the Greeks as **CHILODYNAMIA**, due to its valuable astringent properties. Like valerian, it had a reputation for curing epilepsy.

The plant is ruled by Mercury, and in the language of flowers symbolizes "coming down"- the ladder, I suppose.

An old English name was Make-bate, as it was said to set a married couple quarreling if put in their bed.

When the plant is slowly boiled in canola oil for an hour or more, it colours the oil black. This can be used to dye grey hair jet black, and is considered a valuable hair-dressing.

The Thompson tribe of B.C. used decoctions of the related *P. elegans* as a head and hair wash.

Tall and Western Jacob's Ladder may have numerous variations of the same species, but there is no consensus on this.

Skunkweed has different scent forms, based on the altitude at which it grows. Two out of three plants growing on lower, wooded slopes have a nasty "skunky" scent; and ironically are pollinated mainly by flies.

Up in alpine meadows, two out of three flowers have a honey-like candy scent, and are mainly visited by Bumblebees.

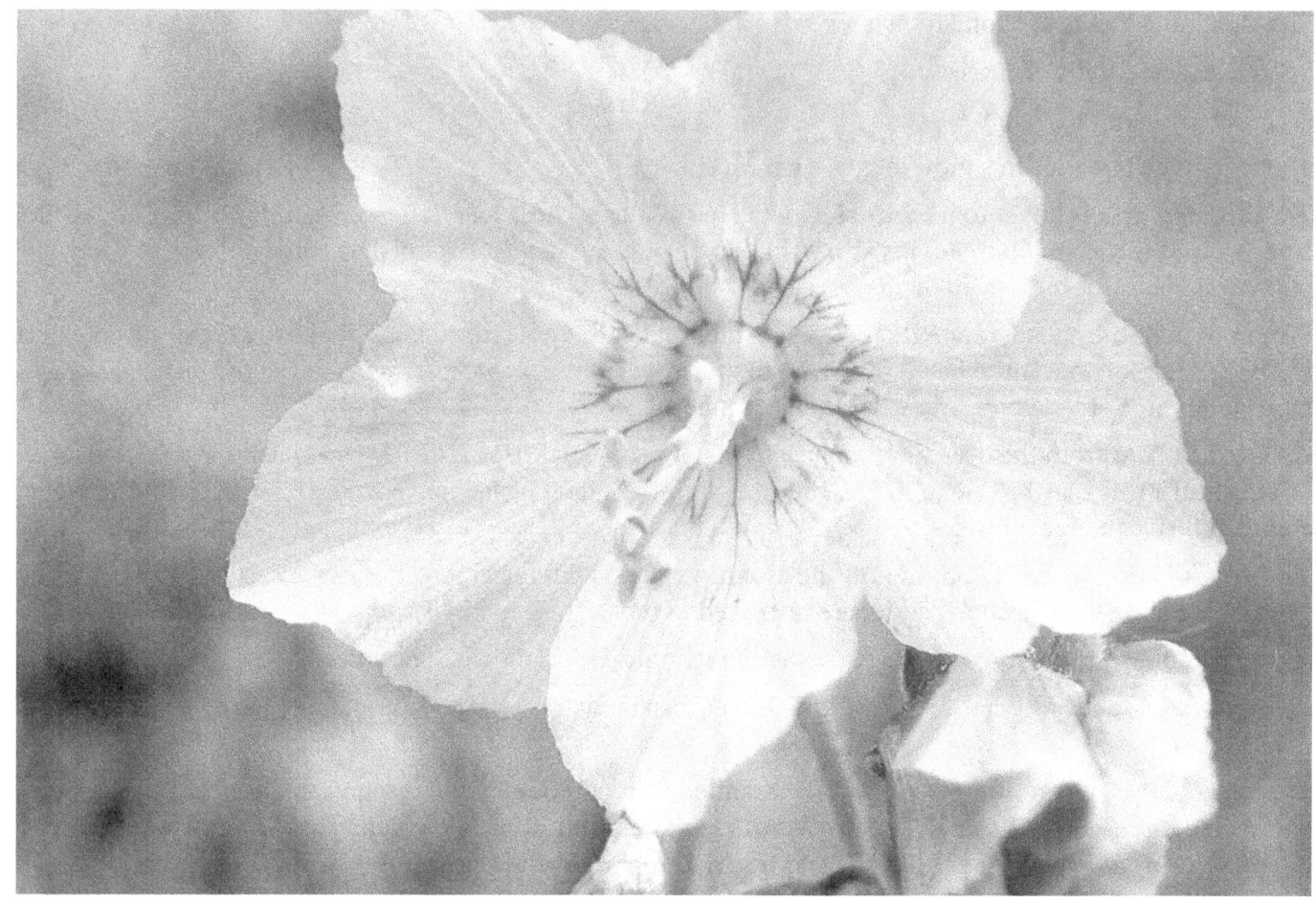

POLEMONIUM ACUTIFLORUM FLOWER

Native tribes to the south used the related Abscess root for hemorrhoids, to induce vomiting, and treat eczema. The root tea was also used to induce sweating, in fevers, pleurisy, and other bronchial afflictions.

Usually purple blue, an occasional white or yellow flowered variety is found.

Abscess root (*P. reptans*) is native to northeastern North America, and often found in prairie gardens .

It is also known as Greek Valerian, Creeping Polemonium, or Sweat root, and used with mandrake root, to increase its emetic effect. I bet!

The root is slightly bitter and astringent, increasing perspiration and expectoration.

This makes it useful for coughs, colds, bronchitis, laryngitis, tuberculosis and other feverish, inflamed conditions. It is rarely used today in herbal medicine.

If used, it is important to take extra fluids due to its extreme diaphoretic action.

## MEDICINAL

### CONSTITUENTS-

*P. caeruleum* roots- triterpene saponins including camelliagenin E and derivatives including polemoniumgenin A, a di-ester of camelliagenin E; poleomonium saponin 1, acetic/angelic/tiglic/ alpha-methyl-butyric acid as well as traces of propionic and isobutyric acid.
*P. viscosum*- baicalein, and mosloflavone (beta, 6, 7-dimethyl ether); polygalitol (1, 5-anhydro-D-sorbitol/glucitol)

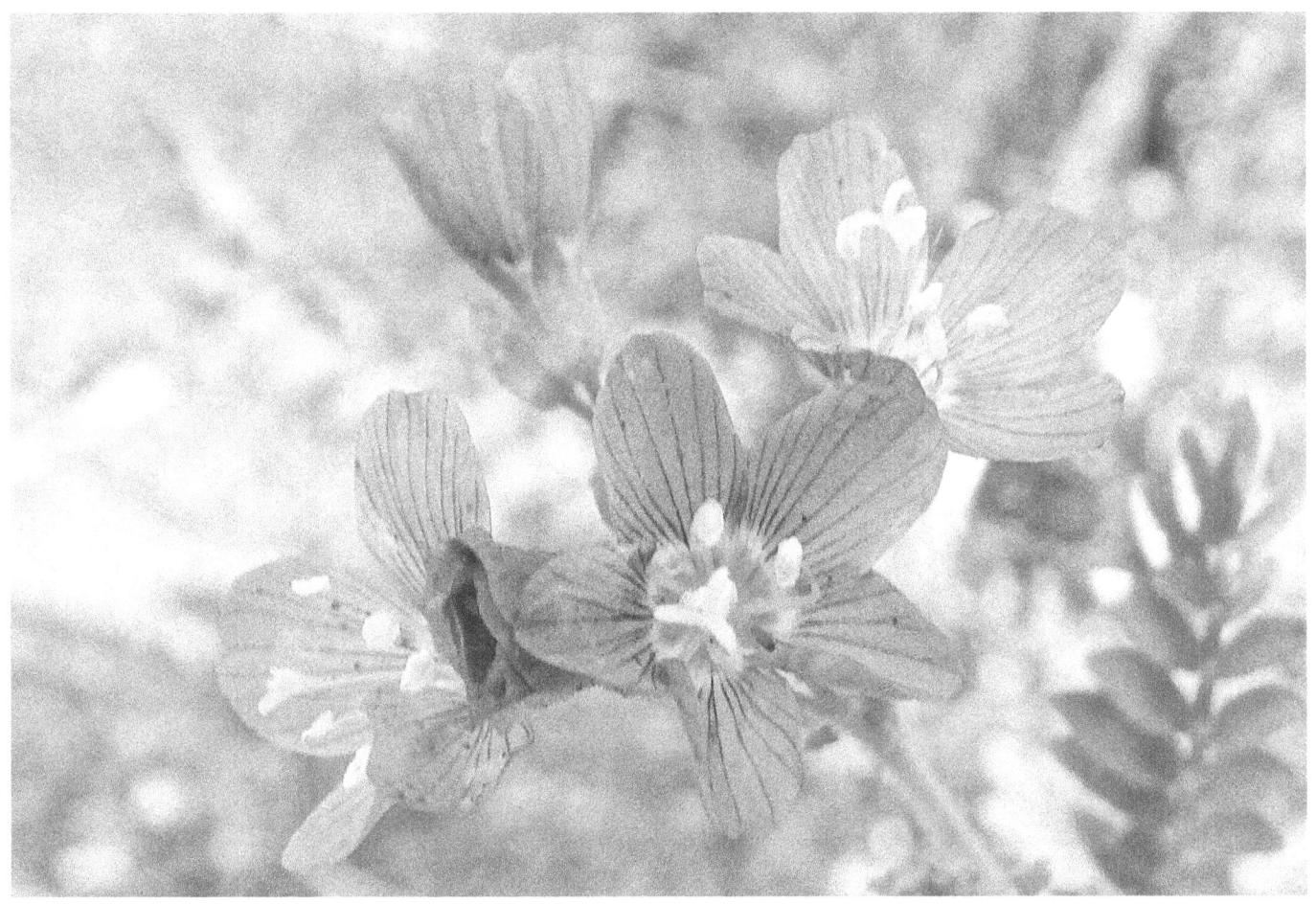

SHOWY JABOB'S LADDER

Warm infusions of Tall Jacob's Ladder root will produce copious perspiration, making it a fast-acting diaphoretic; and invaluable in pleurisy and other inflammatory conditions of the bronchials and lungs. The root saponins are a good expectorant.

Root tinctures can be used in lymphatic conditions, or other chronic congestions in the body where an alterative is indicated. The plants astringent properties also make is useful in bowel complaints like diarrhea; but not when inflamed.

Work by Loukova et al, in 1996, showed that Greek Valerian is a chromium accumulator, and therefore potentially useful in chromium deficient conditions like diabetes.

The roots exhibit anti-fungal activity against *Candida albicans, C. tropicalis, Torulopsis glabrata, Cryptococcus neoformans* and other dermatophytes; again due to their saponin content. Hiller K et al, *Pharmazie* 1981 36(2): 133-4.

Work by Grebneva et al in St. Petersburg, Russia, was reported in *Rastitel'nye-Resursy* 2000 36:3 on the anti-microbial activity of a mixture called Polestell. It consists of Tall Jacob's Ladder, Elecampane, Bergenia (*B. crassifolia*), and Chickweed (*Stellaria dichotoma*), and as an infusion was found active against gram positive bacteria such as *Bacillus subtilis, Staphylococcus aureus,* gram negative bacteria such as *E. coli* and *Pseudomonas aeruginosa*, as well as fungi, *Candida albicans*.

Camelliagenin shows significant inhibition of biofilm in amoxicillin-resistant *E. coli* and erythromycin-resistant *S. aureus*, related to the decrease of mannitol dehydrogenase activity and extracellular DNA content. It may be a useful antibiotic substitute to treat infections in chickens [and humans]. Ye Y et al, *BMC Vet Res* 2015 11:214.

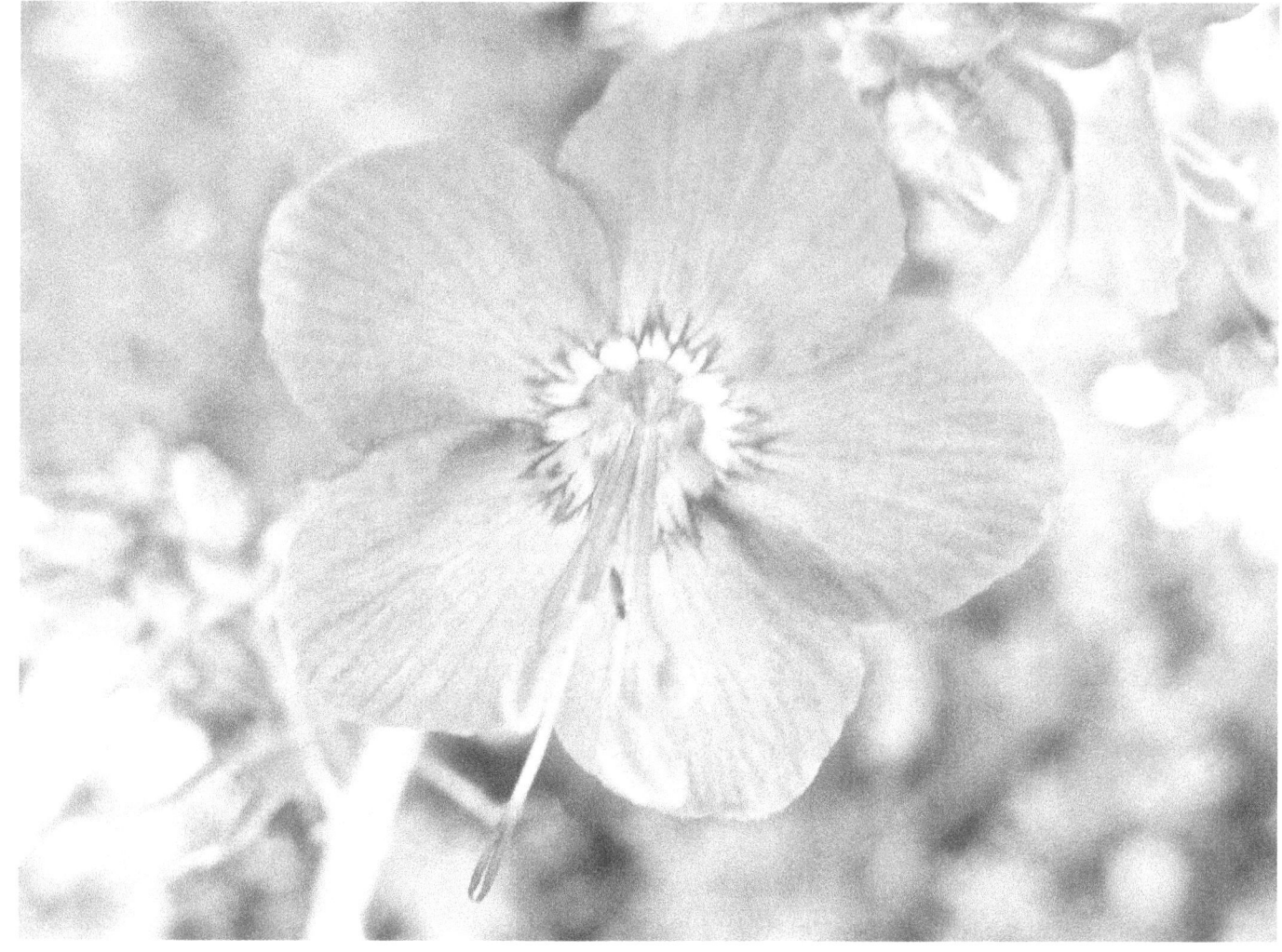

JACOB'S LADDER

Camelliagenin, and related saponins show significant cytotoxic activity against five human cancer cell lines. Zong J et al, *Fitoterapia* 2015 104:7-13.

Isobutyric acid is a branched short chain fatty acid that potentiates insulin stimulated glucose uptake in adipocytes, suggesting improved insulin sensitivity in type two diabetes. Heimann E et al, *Adipocyte* 2016 5(4): 359-68. Healthy gut flora helps produce this important fatty acid. Its absence, or low levels, in human feces may be a sign of irritable bowel and other gastrointestinal inflammatory conditions.

Tiglic acid was originally, in 1819 named sabadillic or cevadic acid, and later found identical to methyl-crotonic acid (1865). Salts and esters of tiglic acid are called tiglates.

Angelic and tiglic acids are also found in horse chestnut seeds.

Note the presence of baicalein in *P. viscosum*. This valuable compound is present in Scullcap, and has a wide range of human health benefits.

Mosloflavone exhibits strong anti-viral activity against enterovirus 71, implicated in neonatal death. It inhibits virus replication during the early stage of infection and inhibits viral capsid protein synthesis. Choi HJ et al, *Biomol Ther* (Seoul) 2016 24(5): 552-8.

The flavonoid also protects against coxsackie virus B3, suggesting the use of this herb and astragalus root in this viral infection. Kwon BE et al, *PLoS One* 2016 11(5).

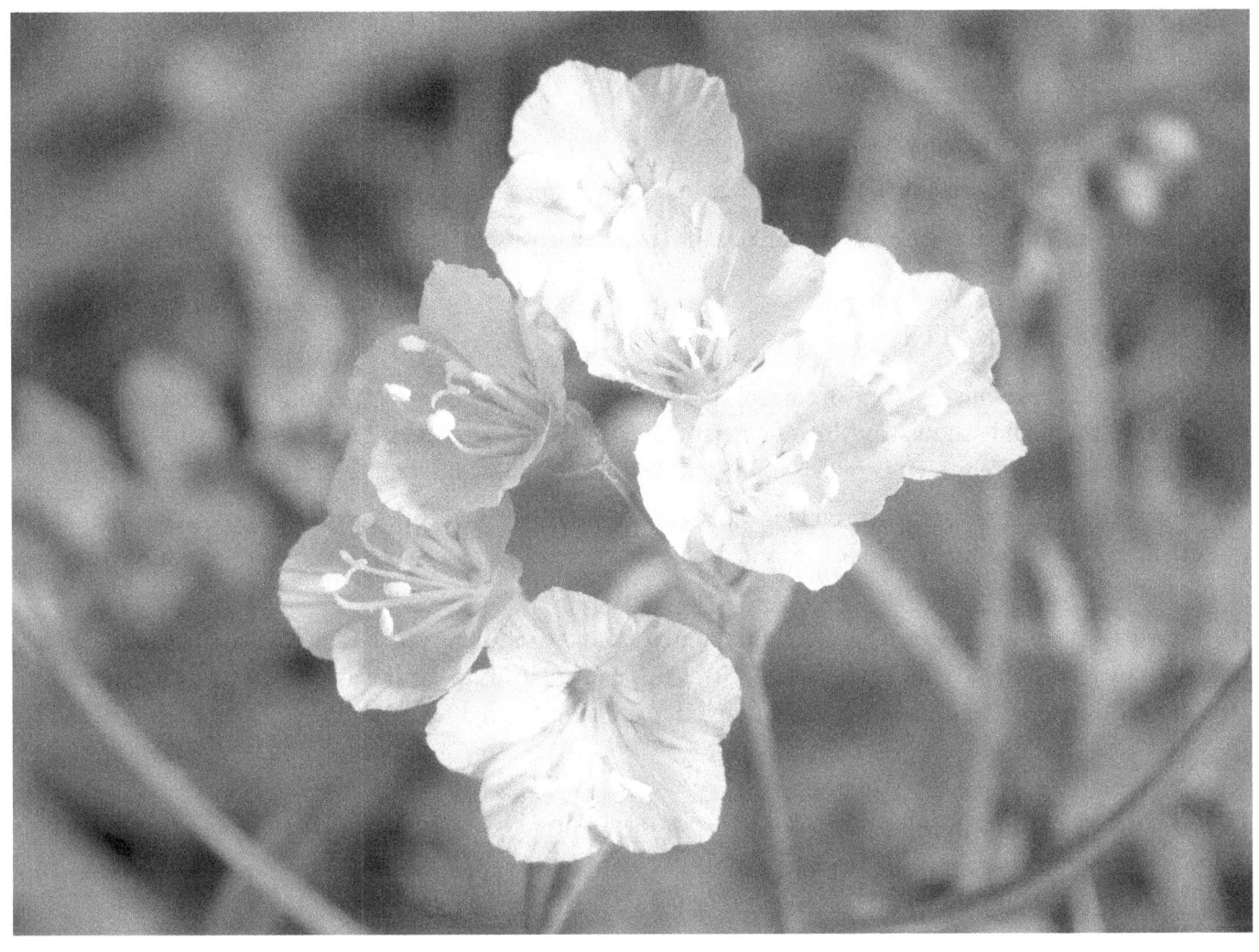

POLEMONIUM REPTANS

It shows anti-inflammatory and immune modulating activity. Singh B et al, *Nat Prod Res* 2013 27(23): 2227-30.

Polygalitol was first isolated and discovered in Senega root (*P. senega*), well-known respiratory herb, native to the Canadian prairies. It is also known as aceritol.

It is a widely used marker of glucose control. The herb may interfere with accurate laboratory results.

Abscess root is diaphoretic, astringent, alterative and expectorant. It is used in cases of febrile inflammatory disease, colds, bronchials, and lung complaints.

## LEAF OIL

Jacob's Ladder aerial parts are simmered in canola oil (1:5) over low heat for an hour. This black oil may be used to dye gray hair jet black. It is a valuable hair-dressing.

## FLOWER ESSENCES

Jacob's Ladder (*P. pulcherrimum*) flower essence is useful for becoming aware of our attempts to control the events of our lives; and allowing mental control to evolve into a disciplined acceptance of spirit.    **ALASKA**

Jacob's Ladder flower essence activates the heart chakra, and may be used where anxiety, and stubbornness create problems in inter-personal relationships and problems in leadership and decision making. It has special use if a child has experienced incest with the father.    **PEGASUS**

Jacob's Ladder flower essence is for individuals ruled by fear. Unlike the Bach Mimulus, which is fear of the known, this essence is associated with fear of loss of control. Appearance and protocol rule over the heart, and decisions are based on etiquette rather than emotion.

It is also a good flower essence for couples that carry conflict into the bedroom. **PRAIRIE DEVA**

Jacob's Ladder is for learning how to ask for, recognize and receive assistance. **HAREBELL**

Jacob's Ladder essence gives ease and confidence. It is particularly useful for firmly rooted and grounded people, helping bring greater creativity. **MIRIANA**

## PERSONALITY TRAITS

The Jacob's Ladder personality is one of control, and keeping a stiff upper lip. It is personified by the rigid, uptight British male, of the old school. Nothing of a personal nature is revealed; and it is no one's business. They tend to be hardest on themselves, and are driven by hard work, hard play, and a sense of duty.

On the positive side, they are remarkably loyal, and once befriended will stick with you no matter what. They will often be able to relax after the battle, and are not ashamed to feel fear or stress under pressure. They feel their exhaustion, and sleep well.

On the negative side, this personality is so tightly controlled and controlling that it is difficult to sleep relaxed. They are driven by fear- of failure, success, rejection, etc. This control leads to cardiovascular risk, and hypertension. They suffer from nerve and muscle spasm and pain, from being so tightly wound. **PRAIRIE DEVA**

## RECIPES

TINCTURE- twenty drops three times daily. Prepare at 1:5 dried root and 40% alcohol.

Cultivation of *P. caeruleum* requires moist soil in sun or partial shade. *P. reptans* likes a rich, humus soil. The former is harvested in summer and dried for infusions.

The root of P. *reptans* is gathered in fall and dried for decoctions or tinctures.

SPOTTED JEWELWEED
SPOTTED TOUCH ME NOT
ORANGE JEWELWEED
(*Impatiens capensis* Meerb.)
(*I. biflora* Walt.) not accepted
(*I. fulva* Nutt.) not accepted
(*I. nortonii* Rydb.) not accepted
WESTERN TOUCH ME NOT
COMMON TOUCH ME NOT
YELLOW BALSAM
(*I. noli-tangere* L.)
(*I. occidentale* Rydb.) not accepted
GARDEN BALSAM

SPOTTED SNAPWEED
(*Impatiens balsamina* L.)
PATIENCE PLANT
BUSY LIZZIE
BUZZY LIZZY
(*I. walleriana* Hook.f.)
(*I. sultanii* Hook.f.) not accepted
SNAPWEED
POLICEMAN'S HELMET
INDIAN BALSAM
(*I. glandulifera* Royle)
(*I. roylei* Walp.) not accepted
PARTS USED- seeds, leaves, flowers

With fierce distracted eye Impatiens stands
Swells her pale cheeks and brandishes her hands,
With rage and hate the astonished groves alarms,
And hurls her infants from her frantic arms.

**ERASMUS DARWIN**

She brooks no condescension
From mortal hand, you know,
For, touch her e'er so gently,
Impatiently she'll throw
Her tiny little jewels,
Concealed in pockets small
Of her dainty, graceful garment,
And o'er the ground they fall.

**RAY LAURENCE**

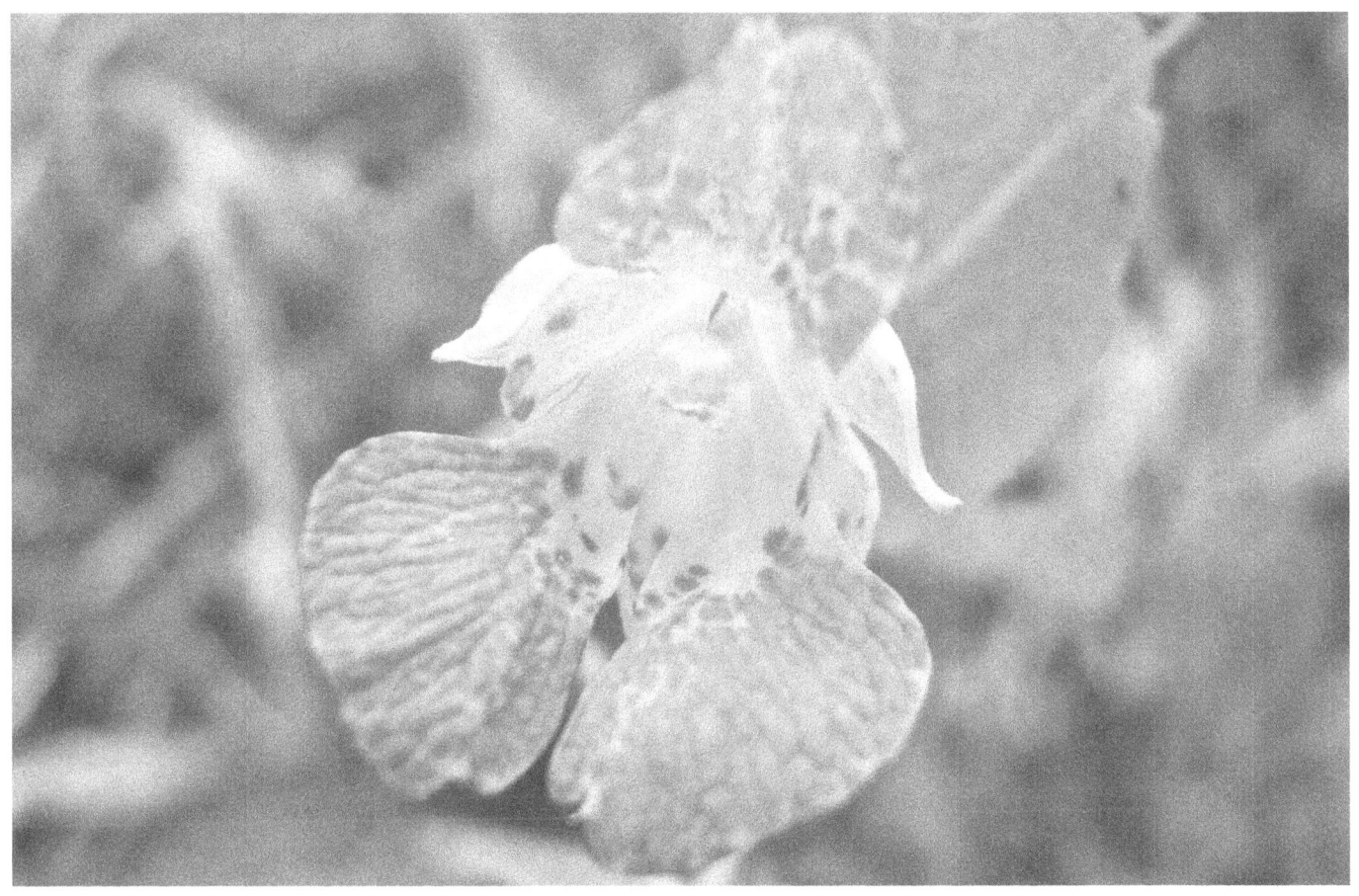

ORANGE JEWELWOOD

Impatiens is from the Latin, meaning impatient, to put up with, to endure. This refers to the seedpods, when ripe, bursting open and scattering seed at the least pressure. Balsamina is related to producing balsam, or balms to soothe.

Jewelweed may refer to the colorful, dangling flowers, the coil fired seeds, or the edge of the leaves, that when wet with dew or rain look like sparkling gems. The flowers are shaped like earrings and the underside of leaves are silver.

Noli-tangere is named for the Eurasian Touch Me Not Balsam from the Latin **NOLI ME TANGERE,** or "I don't touch", or more accurately "a warning without meddling".

These were the words reportedly spoken by Christ to Mary Magdalene after the Resurrection (John 20:17).

Capensis refers to the Cape of Good Hope (a botanical error by Meerburgh, who believed it was introduced from Africa). He named it in 1775, thirteen years before Walter's *I. biflora*, and the mistake has been upheld by the International Code of Botanical Nomenclature ever since.

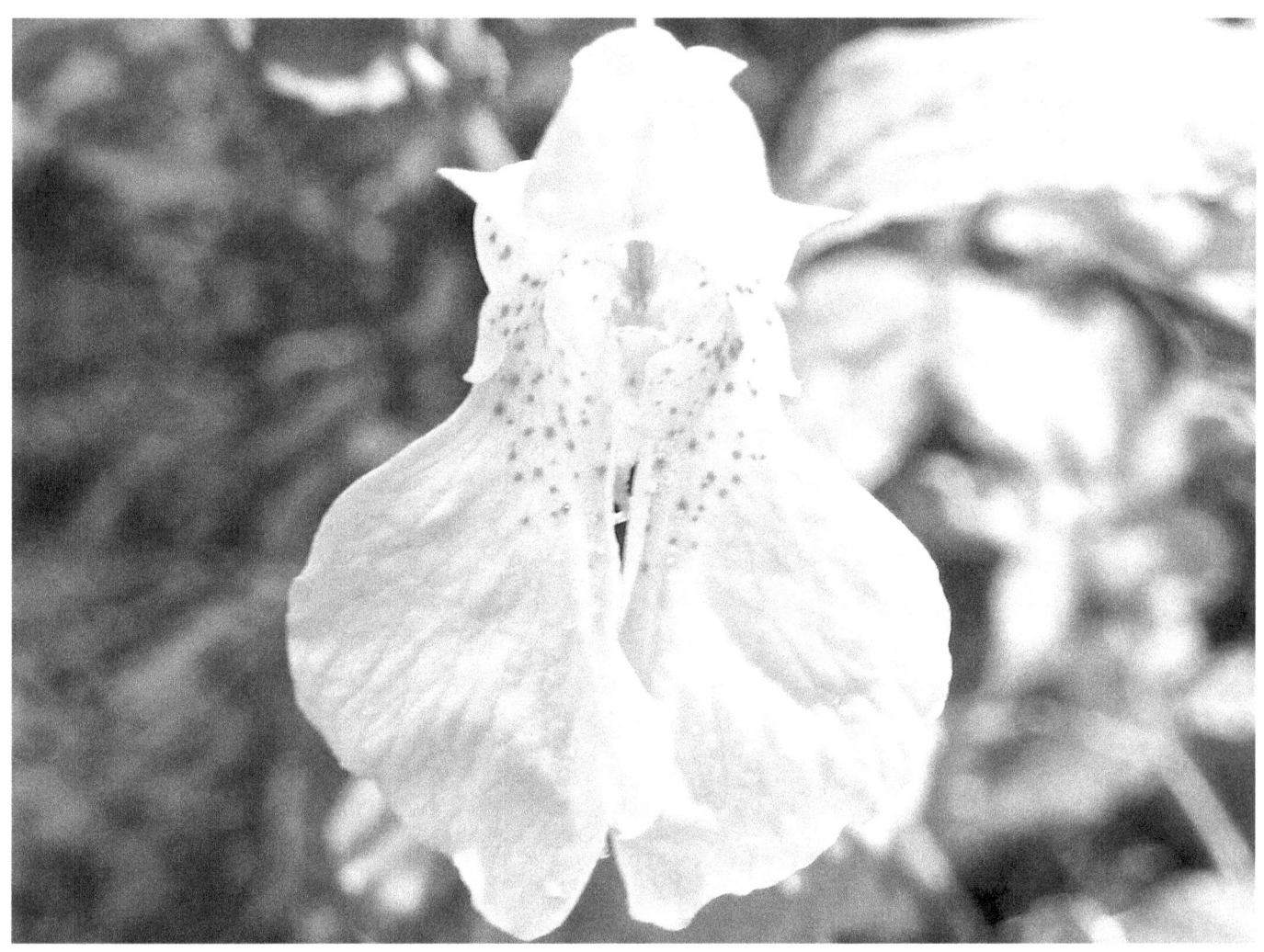

WESTERN TOUCH ME NOT

*Impatiens walleriani* is a garden annual that is named after Horace Waller, an English missionary and plant collector. It was originally called *Impatiens sultani*, after the Sultan of Zanzibar.

Roylei is named after Dr. Royle, a professor of botany who published Illustrations of the Botany of the Himalayan Mountains, in 1839. He introduced the seeds into Britain in the same year. Glandulifera refers to the glands which secrete a spicy tar scent. Policeman's Helmet refers to the bulbous rounded flowers that resemble British police headgear.

The Impatiens family is vast and almost incomprehensible, botanically speaking. Joseph Hooker, famous botanist and curator at Kew Gardens in England, attempted to make sense of the family when he died. He called the family "deceitful above all plants...worse than orchids".

Erasmus Darwin was the scientist grandfather of the more famous Charles.

Spotted Touch-Me-Not is one of my favorite twining wild plants. It is found throughout central and northern Alberta in ravines, and stream banks.

Western Touch-Me-Not grows in the same areas, and is considered a migrated Eurasian plant.

I have seen both in the wild very close to each other; the differences are minor. The former are usually a brighter orange flower, usually spotted with red or purple; the latter is a paler yellow with or without spots.

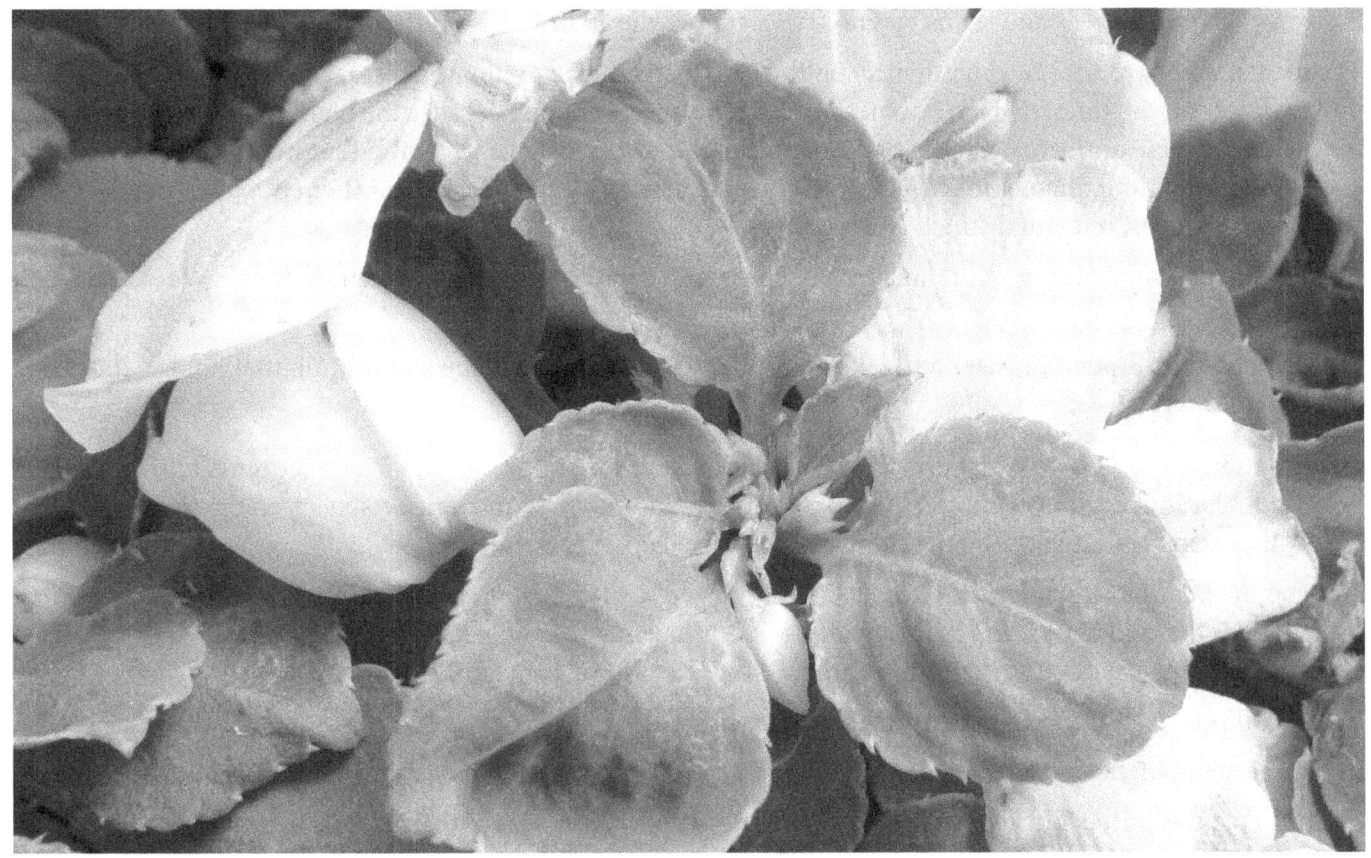

GARDEN BALSAM

The young greens, up to a foot or so, can be cooked as a potherb, with a change of water. Some authors believe that native peoples used the cooking water from jewelweed as a fly repellant.

Kelly Harlton, a noted wilderness instructor, notes that the decocted herb turns the water dark black and quite astringent.

The seeds are edible, but I doubt you could collect enough to sustain yourself.

Some Native American tribes called it crowing cock, due to the flower's form.

Historically, it was used for treating jaundice (called wild celandine).

Spotted Touch Me Not was used by various Native tribes for the relieving juice of the stem in a variety of skin complaints, usually topical in the form of a poultice of flowers, or mashed plant.

The Blackfoot, of the prairie region, rubbed the crushed plant on eczema and other skin rashes.

The Forest Potawatomi call it **TWATUBÎGO-NÎAK**, literally, touch me not, while the Prairie Potawatomi call it **WASAWA'SHIAK** meaning yellow slippery. Infusions were taken internally for chest colds or stomach cramps.

Others, such as the Cherokee, used *I. capensis* leaves as an infusion for measles; the root for babies "bold hives".

The stems were decocted for helping to ease childbirth; an interesting association with the oriental cousin.

The Iroquois infused the roots to help increase urination, and used cold infusions of the whole plant to help reduce fevers. The neighboring Ojibwa call the plant **OZAAWASHKOJIIBIK**.

The Mik'maq used the plant for treating jaundice; while others used the plant for a variety of stomach complaints such as cramps.

A strong tea of the leaves and stems was used as a skin cleanser, or to ease the pain of sunburn.

The plants rarely produce seed on their main flowers. Instead they pollinate cleistogamous "hidden marriage", flowers lower on the stem, that have no nectar, and require less energy. Because the plant is an annual, it ensures the plants survival, until cross-pollination can occur. The seedpods produced by either method are hair trigger, and led to the common name-Touch-Me-Not. On a hot summer day, you can hear them popping, much quieter than caragana peas, but still distinct.

An early French superstition was to make young girls touch the plant, and if not a virgin the flower would recoil and fade away.

The leaves can be dipped in water and take on a silvery sheen, due to some leaf coating that holds a thin layer of air on the surface.

Garden balsam is a well-known annual garden plant, usually started from seed, and set out after frost, for its pretty white, pink and purple flowers. Seed germinates in ten days, and can be separated one foot apart. No yellow flowered version has been developed as yet.

It is a popular garden annual in the Orient, and is used to dye silk. Related species are used in Ethiopia by women to stain their feet and hands, and in Japan to paint their nails. In fact, one name for the flowers is **ZHI JIA HUA**, which means fingernail flower. Another name, **FENG XIAN HUA**, means Phoenix fairy flower.

In the Philippines, it is put in nests to keep eggs from spoiling.

In Fuji, seven to 15 flowers are boiled in water and given to treat whooping cough, spitting or coughing blood.

The fresh plant is juiced and applied to painful inflammation, carbuncles and bruises in Nepal, where it is known as **PADAKE**. The flowers are cooling and mucilage, and applied to stings and bites. The powdered seeds are given during labour to provide strength.

For hand fungus, the fresh flowers are simply crushed and applied directly.

The flowers are quite sweet with white petals the most efficient producers of reducing and non-reducing sugars at a rate of 23-27 mg/gram fresh weight, following by red, pink and purple in descending order.

Work by Dr. T.C.N. Singh, head of the Botany department at Annamalai University in Madras, India, looked at plant growth and music. He asked a friend to play his stringed Veena to a group of *I. balsamina* plants. After one month the plants and controls were set outdoors and given just water. All plants grew at same rate for one week, but in the fifth week, the musical plants shot ahead and in next two weeks had 72% more leaves and were 20% taller.

Himalaya Balsam (*I. glandulifera*) is a native of the Himalayas, but naturalized in northern North America. It is a frost hardy annual with strong self-seeding tendency. When ripe, the seeds shoot with explosive force, up to several metres away. The current record is thirty-six feet.

It can grow to six feet with thick fleshy stems, with lilac, rose, purple and even white flowers. Growth is rapid, at up to 25 mm per day. The scent of flowers varies in description, from lavatory cleaner to the "ripe smell of peaches, like a girl's breath through lipstick", according to Anne Stevenson. She wrote a love poem to the plant that goes:

"Love, it was you who said, 'Murder the killer we have to call life and we'd be a bare planet under a dead sun.' Then I loved you with the usual soft lust of October that says 'yes' to the coming winter and a summoning odor of balsam."

F.S. Smythe wrote in *Valley of Flowers* 1938, that when the plants "get hold of the ground, pastureland is permanently ruined". Like Purple Loosestrife, it clogs the riverbanks and canals of England, with balsam bashing not uncommon in those parts.

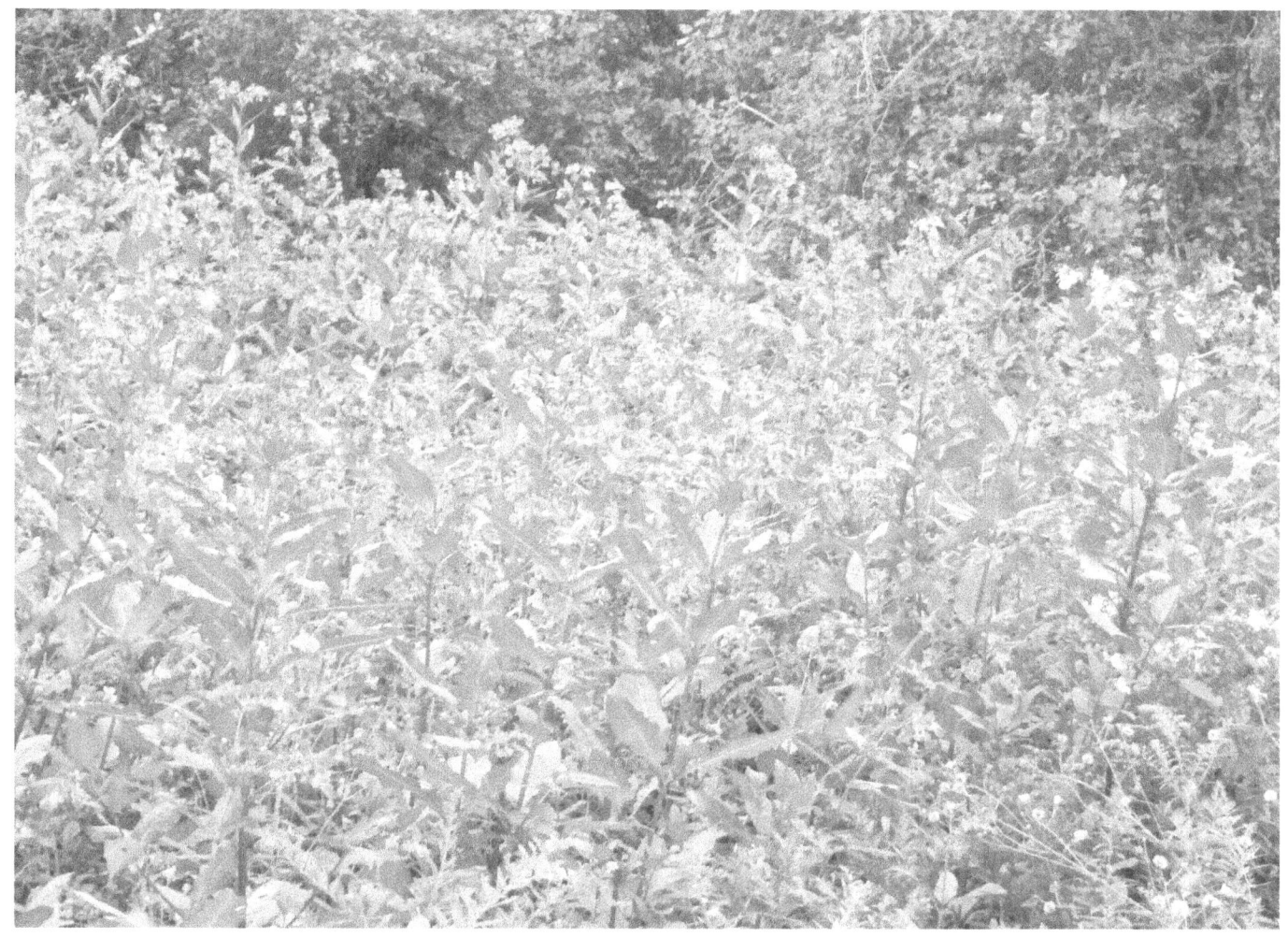

SNAPWEED

Snapweed is easily grown on the prairies, especially from the second generation onward, and is very popular in yards and gardens throughout Edmonton. In fact, escapees are prevalent in Mill Creek Ravine, walking distance from my home. It has recently (2010) been designated a noxious weed in Alberta. Its invasive nature is believed to be due, in part, to the release of a naphthoquinone compound that inhibits growth of native herbs, and ectomycorrhizal fungi. Ruckii R et al, *J Chem Ecol* 2014 40(4): 371-8.

The plant does represent impatience and the birth date of July 24th.

The succulent, juicy thick stems remind one of domestic Impatiens, while the yellow spotted pink/purple flowers also resemble the Patience Plant above. The stems are fleshy and hollow, like a succulent bamboo, and tinged in a copper bronze tone.

The stem sap can be used like the rest of the genus, for its soothing effect.

The seeds of the closely related *I. gigantea* are considered edible.

Patience Plant (I. *wallerana/sultanii*) is the familiar impatiens, usually found indoors; in hanging baskets or on window sills and boxes. It is more sensitive to cold than Garden Balsam, with watery stems that also relieve skin irritations. All the plants are annual, except patience plant that may be considered perennial indoors.

The petals or entire leaf can be used as a garnish for salads. They are crunchy. Patience plant stalks are dipped in boiling water and the sap sucked out for liver pain in Africa. Both the leaves and root are considered abortifacient in decoction.

# MEDICINAL

*I. balsamina* seed–balsaminones, 2-methoxy-1,4-naphthoquinone, saponins, various glycosides including quercitin and kaempferol derivatives, and fixed oils including balsaminasterol and parinaric acid, Ib-AMPs (peptides); numerous baccaharane glycosides called hosenkosides.

Pericarp of fruit- 2-methoxy-1,4-naphthoquinone, balsaminones A and B. flowers- flavonols, flavanoid pigments, naphthoquinones and anthocyanin pigments.

corolla- balsaminolate, impatienolate and other napthoquionone sodium salts.

leaf- 1,2,4-trihydroxy naphthalene-4-glucoside, kaemperferol, kaempferol-3-arabinoside, scopoletin, gentisic acid, p-hydroxybenzoic acid, ferulic acid, lawsone, lawsone methyl ether, methylene-3,3'-bilawsone.

plant- hosenkol A (triterpenoid), impatienol (bisnaphthquinone derivative)

bud- indole-3-acetonitril

stem- various flavonoids including kaempferol-3-glucoside, quercitin-3-glucoside, pelargonidin-3-glucoside, cyanidin-3-glucoside.

root- bisnaphthoquinone, methylene-3,3'-bilawsone, two naphthoquinones (lawsone, and 2-methoxy-1, 4-naphtho-quinone), two coumarin derivatives (scopoletin and isofraxidin) and spinasterol.

The root tips of *I. balsamina, I. capensis,* and *I. sultani* contains anthocyanin pigmentation from cyanidin-3-glycoside.

flowers- anthocyanins, sugars.

White flowers- balsamisides A-D.

*I. capensis*- lawsone (2-methoxy-1,4-naphthoquinone) salicylic acid, gentisic acid, p-hydrobenzoic acid, vanillic acid, ferulic acid, p-coumaric acid, caffeic acid, scopoletin, and 2-hydroxy-1,4-naphthoquinone.

*I. sultani*- scopoletin and trace of ferulic acid

*I. walleriana*- ferulic and caffeic acids

*I. glandulifera*- stems and leaves- p-hydroxybenzoic, vanillic, gentisic, protocatechuic, ferulic, p-coumaric, caffeic acids, as well as scopoletin. This species contains the highest amounts of naphthoquinone derivatives in the genus, including lawsone, and 1,4-naphthoquinones. The stems contain glanuliferins A-B as well alpha spinasterol, and glucopyranosides.

Flowers- ampelopsin, eriodictyl-7-O-glucoside, kaempferol-3-O-glucoside (astragalin), kaempferol-3-O-6"-malonyl-glucoside, and other flavonoids.

Root- 2-hydroxy-1', 4-naphthoquinone.

The Wild Touch Me Not is an important wilderness remedy for rashes, and allergic reactions to aggressive plants like nettle, cow parsnip and poison ivy.

One physician in 1957 treated 115 people with poison ivy rashes over a period of time. He found that 108 (over 95%) cleared up in only two to three days using the fresh juice.

David Winston, noted herbalist, says that jewelweed succus applied 3-4 hours after exposure to poison ivy or oak is 90% effective. The fresh juice can be frozen in ice cubes for longer storage.

The saponin content of *I. capensis* was found to reduce poison ivy dermatitis, in a study by Abrams MV et al, *J Ethnopharm* 2015 162: 163-7. The content of lawsone did not correlate with poison ivy rash prevention.

The extracts were also tested against various human cancer cell lines, and cytotoxicity was noted against MCF-7 breast cancer cells, and cytostatic activity against HT-29 colon cancer cell lines.

The saponins also exhibited a possible positive chronotropic effect on heart rate.

It relieves the pain of insect bites, burns, sprains, and a variety of skin diseases including ringworm. This mild fungicidal action makes it a good choice for athlete's foot, especially on the trail. Work by Thomas Sproston at the University of Vermont in 1950, tested 73 plant extracts for anti-fungal activity and found Wild Touch Me Not, Nasturium and Muskmelon the most active.

It can be made into an ointment for relieving hemorrhoids, warts, corns, and other related conditions.

Jewelweed is a good hair rinse for itchy scalp.

Although lawsone, the active anti-inflammatory, and crystalline substance is found throughout the plant stem and leaves, it is most abundant in the small reddish protuberances near the root.

Lawsone appears to suppress human colon cancer cells, not by apoptosis, but by decreasing NF-kappaB activity that results in suppression of cyclin B1 and cdk1. Wang SB et al, *Biomed Pharmacother* 2017 89: 152-61.

Lawsone makes a superior anti-fungal mouthwash, compared to Listerine, based on a 60 person trial on diabetics wearing dentures. Sujanamulk B et al, *J Clin Diagn Res* 2016 10(6): ZC90-5.

It also ameloriates induced acute pancreatitis. Biradar S et al, *Ind J Exp Biol* 2013 51(3): 256-61.

Lawsone is also found in Garden Balsam flowers and Henna (*Lawsonia inermis*), both used as dyes for nails or hair.

Lawsone is used as UVA sunscreen agent. In one test, panelists with normal skin colour were exposed to UVA/UVB light to determine their minimal erythema dosage. They were then exposed to 1.2-4 times plant extract or water control. When used at 10%, the jewelweed extract, pH 5-7, provided 2.4 SPF units of protection from UV erythema.

In tests on the plant including alcohol, acidic and saline solutions, as well as ether; the plant showed activity against fungi and both Gram positive and negative bacteria.

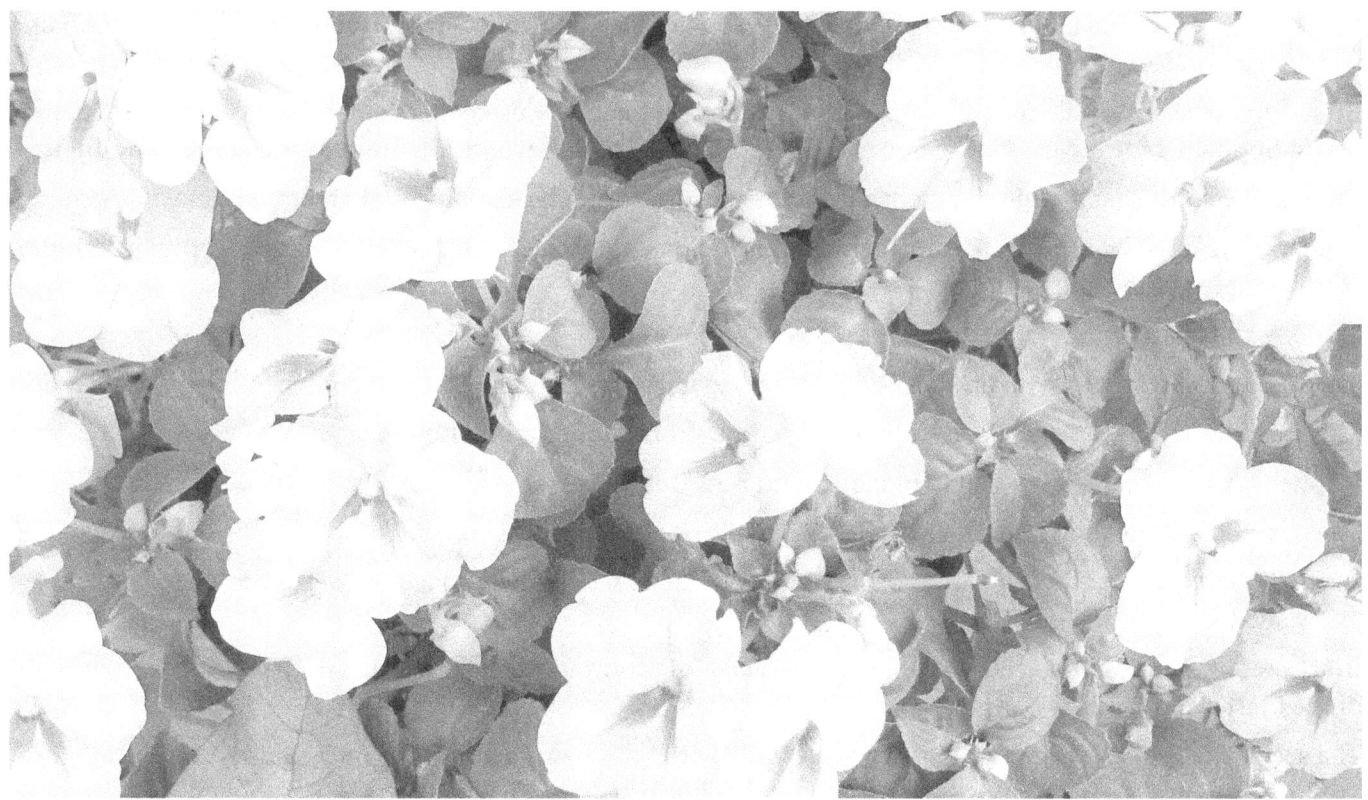

IMPATIENS WALLERIANA

Garden Balsam Touch Me Not stems contain a soothing juice applied to stinging nettle, poison ivy, or inflamed skin of various origins.

In the folk medicine of Japan, the white flower petals were painted topically on the skin for dermatitis, including urticaria. In Japan the plant is known as **HOSENKA**.

The flower is an important part of Traditional Chinese Medicine, and known as **JI XING HUA** (Mandarin), or **JEK CHIN FA** (Cantonese). The flowers are sometimes called **FEN XIAN HUA**, which means Phoenix fairy flower.

Alcohol extractions of the flowers exhibit antinociceptive activity, in both central and peripheral nervous systems. Opioid receptors are involved. Imam et al, *J Ethnopharm* 2012 142(3): 804-10.

The flowers are used for amenorrhea, trauma and injury to tissue such as sprains, arthralgia, furuncles, and ringworm. It is taken as a tea infusion, or washed on affected areas.

From the white petals have been isolated anti-anaphylactic, anti-histaminic and anti-pruritic compounds. Balsamisides A-D show potential for anti-neurodegenerative activity. Kim CS et al, *J Nat Prod* 2017 80(2): 471-8.

In studies by Oku et al *Phytotherapy Research* 1999 13:6 on the phenolic compounds of petals it was found that petal extracts were effective in regulating hypotension caused by platelet activating factor. Later work by the same author in same journal, 15:6 found 35% petal extracts effective in chronic serious pruritis and for treating atopic dermatitis.

In volume 15:8, the same author reported on a 95% ethanol extract of the dry aerial parts effective against 5 gram positive, and two gram negative bacteria. It was also effective against drug resistant fungal infections.

The flowers contain depside derivatives with anti-hepatic fibrosis and anti-diabetic activity. Li Q et al, *Fitoterapia* 2015 105: 234-9.

Work published in *Biol Pharm Bull* 2002 25:5, by same author identified several compounds in the corolla with significant COX-2 inhibition, supporting the traditional use for treating articular rheumatism, pain and swelling.

Work by Fukumoto et al, *Phytotherapy Research* 1995 10:3 showed white petal extracts preventing anaphylactic shock in laboratory studies.

Both Garden balsam and Ground Ivy (*Glechoma hederacea*) plants are used interchangeable by some practitioners of Traditional Chinese Medicine. Known as **TOU KU TSAO,** both plants are used for the above conditions.

But it is the seeds that are most valued; a tradition that was brought from India at an earlier date.

Known as **JI XING ZI**, meaning short temper, in Mandarin, the seed is considered warming, pungent, bitter, stimulating, relaxing and softening.

It affects the heart and liver meridians primarily.

The seeds are used with regularity in formulas for relieving symptoms related to amenorrhea and dysmenorrhea.

This includes scanty, painful or absent menses, and unknown abdominal lumps.

It softens hardness, disperses stagnant blood, and removes toxins.

They exhibit contraceptive effect, as the seeds are inhibitory on ovulation.

As might be expected, the seeds are abortive, and have been used in miscarriage, as well as prolonged pregnancy and stalled labor.

In laboratory studies, oral doses of the seed extract show contraceptive action in mice, and decreased weight of the uterus and ovaries.

The seeds are used as a digestive relaxant, especially with hard painful abdomen or intestinal colic.

The seed tea has been used traditionally for esophageal obstruction, or choking due to the accidental swallowing of bones.

More recently the seeds have been found to contain saponins and fatty acids that act against tumors in esophageal and stomach cancer.

Thirty cases of esophageal cancer and 26 of gastric cancer treated with *I. balsamina* seed and honey, obtained symptomatic improvement with respect to vomiting, and pain of the thorax and epigastrium.

Cis-parinaric acid is selective against malignant glial cells compared to normal astrocytes. Zaheer A et al, *Neurochem Res* 2007 32(1): 115-24. This polyunsaturated fatty acid is fluorescent.

Alcohol extracts of the plant induce apoptosis in human HSC-2 human oral cancer cells. Shin JA et al, *Pharmacogn Mag* 2015 11(41): 136-42; *J Oral Pathol* Med 2015 44(6):420-8.

The whole plant, but particularly the pod, shows very strong activity against *Helicobacter pylori*, even exceeding the drug metronidazole. Wang et al, *Am J Chin Med* 2009 37(4): 713-22.

The compound 2-methoxy-1, 4-naphthoquinone is active against antibiotic resistant *H. pylori,* and equivalent to amoxicillin. Wang YC et al, *Evid Based Complement Alternat Med* 2011:704721.

Wang et al, *Fitoterapia* 2012 83(8): 1336-44 confirmed anti-bacterial activity above, as well as potential against gastric adenocarcinoma necrosis.

Garden Balsam seeds have been found to contain peptides that inhibit a wide range of fungi and bacteria, and yet are not cytotoxic to cultured human cells.

Work carried out by Tailor et al in the United Kingdom, showed the peptides to be 20 amino acids long and the smallest plant derived anti-microbial peptides isolated to date (Sept 1997). They are arginine and cysteine amino acid based.

Continuing work by Patel et al, University College in London, is trying to determine the mode of action of this protein; and possible sites of interaction.

An anti-microbial peptide (ibAMP4) has been found to combine with thymol (Thymus species) against drug resistant *Klebsiella pneumoniae*, and with the antibiotics vancomycin or oxacillin against *Enterococcus faecalis.* Fan X et al, *Pharmazie* 2013 68(7): 628-30.

The leaves and flowers have been examined with ether and water extractions demonstrating activity against fungi, yeasts, gram positive bacteria and mycobacterium.

Water extracts of the flowers inhibit the growth of *Staphylococcus aureus* and *Streptococcus pyogenes,* the latter infamous for causing strep throat. The red and white flowers are considered superior for some reason.

Leaf extracts show anti-microbial activity against various fungi, yeasts, mites and bacteria. Sakunphueak A et al, *Nat Prod Res* 2012 26(12): 1119-24.

Ishiguro et al, *Phytotherapy Research* 2000 14:1 found aerial parts contain impatienol, which exhibits significant testosterone 5alpha-reductase inhibitory activity. That is, it blocks the intracellular metabolism of testosterone and inhibits the growth of the prostate suggesting use in prevention or treatment of prostate cancer.

Several anti-pruritic compounds named balsaminones, have been isolated from the pericarp of garden balsam by Ishiguro et al in Japan. More intensive research is warranted, considering the seeds apparent anti-inflammatory, anti-allergic and antioxidant properties.

The leaves and flowers, when decocted, dissolve out significant amounts of magnesium sulphate, the organic form of epsom salts, perhaps explaining part of their anti-inflammatory and muscle relaxant properties.

A compound, 2-methoxy-1, 4-naphthoquinone, has been found to inhibit Wnt signaling, which is a step in formation of cancer cells. Mori et al, *J Nat Med* 2011 65:1.

This is a powerful medicine, with some degree of toxicity. Dosage is important.

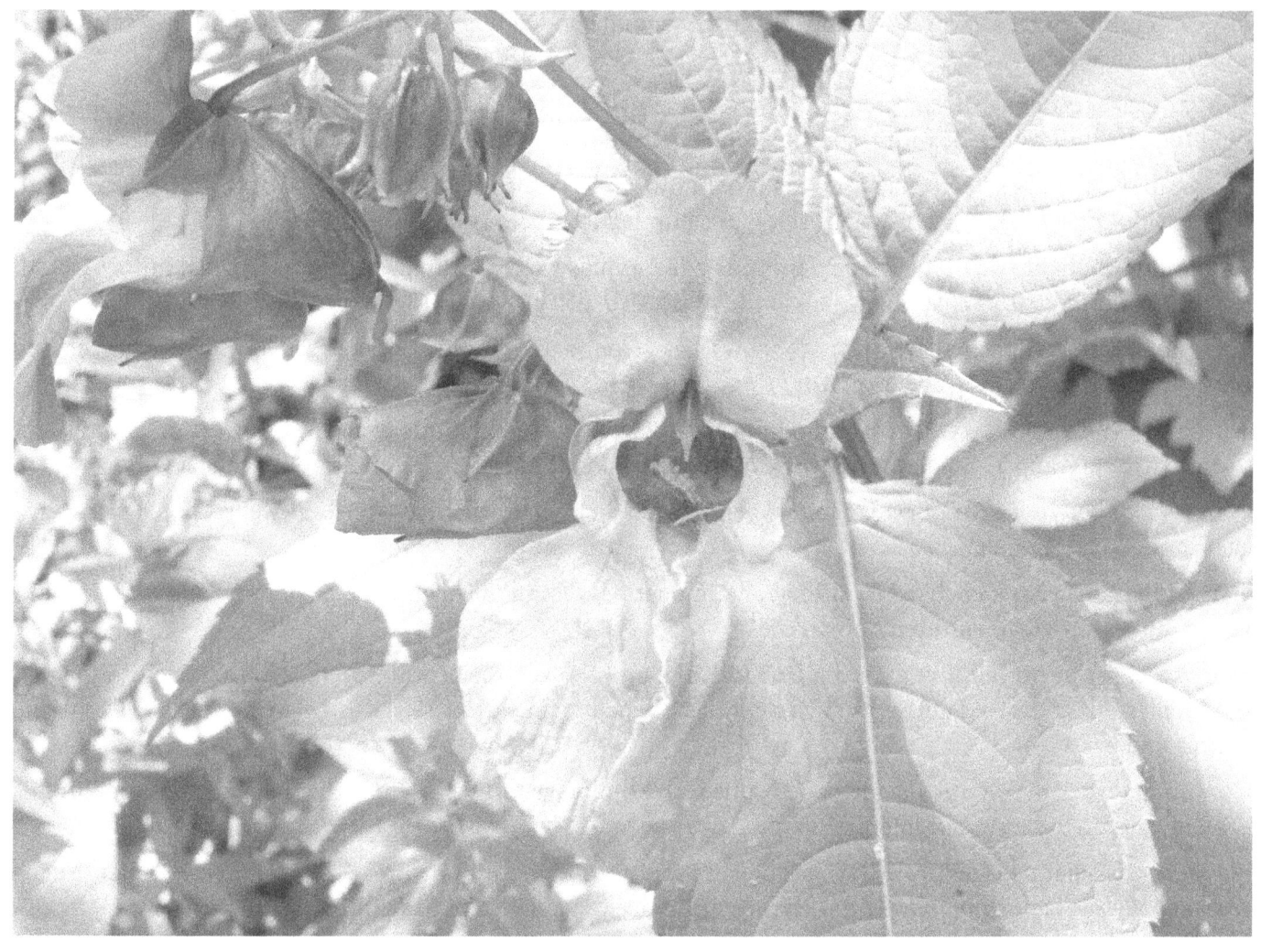

SNAPWEED

The stems of Snapweed (*I. glandulifera*) contain glucosylated steroids that exhibit cytostatic activity on U373 glioblastoma cell lines. Cimmino A et al, *Fitoterapia* 2016 109: 138-45.

The related *I. bicolor* shows inhibition of acetylcholinesterase, a marker for treatment of Alzheimer's disease. Shahwar et al, *J Med Plants Res* 2010 4:3.

The leaves of related *I. parviflora* contain galactolipids that may be useful in conditions associated with the loss of hyaluronic acid. Grabowska K et al, *Nat Prod Res* 2016 30(10): 1219-23.

## HOMEOPATHY

Impatiens (*I. roylei*) is indicated in acute pain of nerve type, and it not only often gives rapid relief, but in many cases apparently effects a cure of the nerve condition. It has also a beneficent action, and patients frequently report, in addition to relief of symptoms, a much improved mental state with loss of depression and fears, a generally brighter outlook being obtained.

Amongst cases successfully treated are intense headaches, sciatica, acute neuralgias, tic douloureux, and acute pain in malignant disease. In some cases it has given relief after morphia has failed.

**DOSE**- The mother tincture was originally prepared by Dr. Bach (see flower essences below), from the mauve flowers only by trituration.

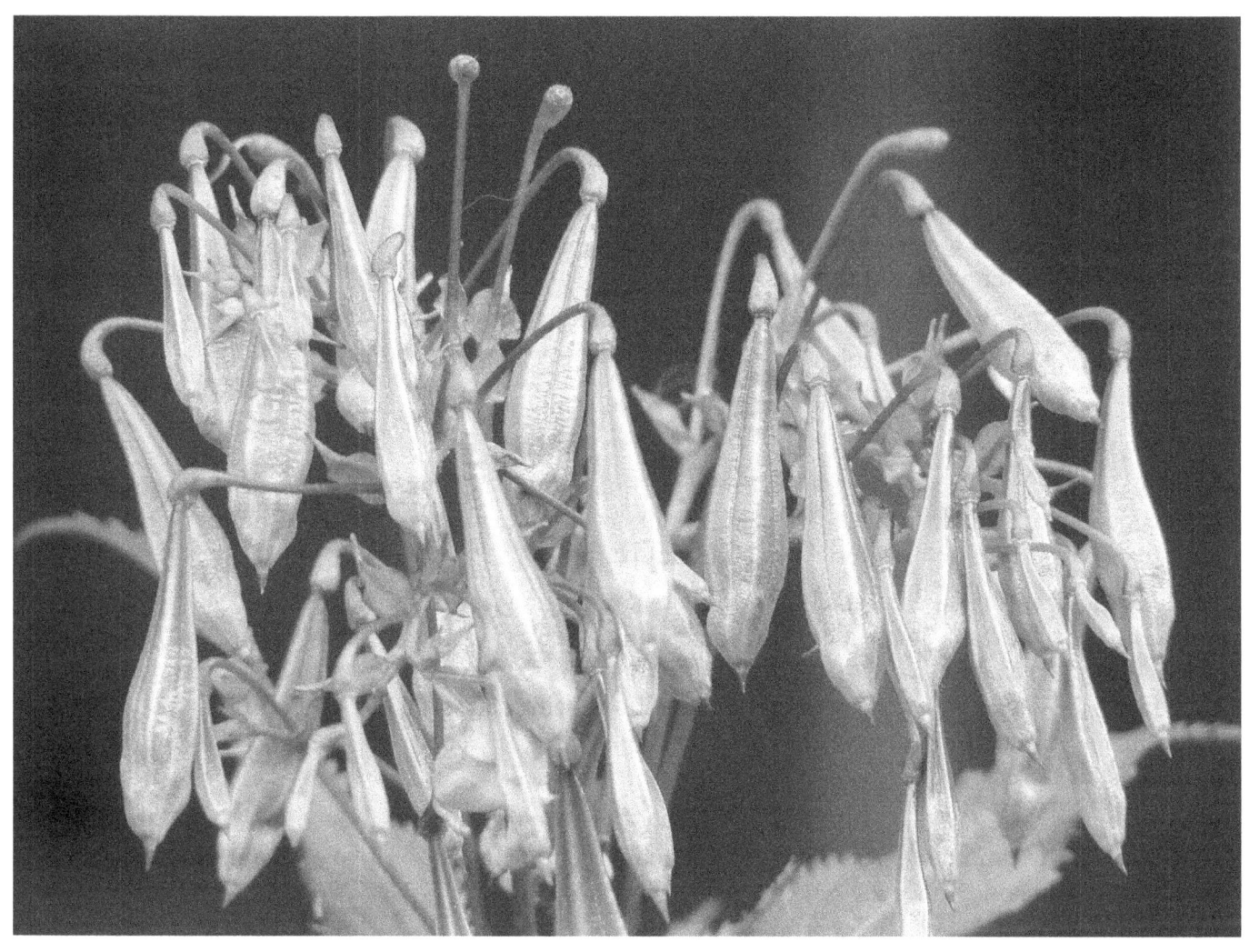

SNAPWEED SEED PODS

## ESSENTIAL OILS

The essential oil derived from I. *glandulifera* herbage is only 0.22%. It contains seventy six compounds dominated by monoterpenes (28.2%) and alpha-terpinyl acetate (16.6% and phellandral (3.8%). Phthalides were characteristic with (Z)-ligustilide (11%) and (Z)-butylidenphthalide (8.5%) with small amounts of their (E)-isomers and butylphthalide. Also includes beta-phellandrene (7.4%), cryptone (5.7%) and many minor compounds.

The root oil is quite different, with linalool (5.3%), borneol (4.9%), bornyl acetate (4.3%), beta-barbatene (5.3%), vulgarone B (14.9%), acorenone (4%), pentadecanal (5.8%), and minor other compounds.

Garden Balsam (I. *balsamina*) aerial parts give an essential oil containing hexahydrofarnesyl acetone (13.4%), myristic acid (3.3%), dodecanoic acid (4.1%), (E)-beta-ionone (5.7%), geranylacetone (2.7%), (E)-beta damascenone (3.6%), and traces of other compounds. Yield is 0.1%.

Western Touch Me Not herbage yields an essential oil rich in (Z)-hex-3-en-1-ol (9.5%), benzaldehyde (4.7%), linalool (6.5%), beta-ionone epoxide (3.7%) and others.

## SEED OIL

The seed oil of I. *balsamina* contains alpha spinasterol, beta ergosterol, balsaminasterol and parinaric acid, the latter of particular interest.

# HYDROSOL

Touch Me Not water is good for skin itching, biting, sores, and scabby breasts.                    **BRUNSCHWIG**

# FLOWER ESSENCES

Impatiens (*I. balsamina*) flower essence is used for those who are irritable, impulsive, impetuous, active and intelligent; though prone to nervous tensions and accidents. They are given to outbursts of temper; and is similar to the Impatiens flower essence of the Bach system.                    **FLORIAS DE MINAS**

Impatiens (*I. glandulifera*) flower essence is for impatience, irritation, tension and intolerance. The essence helps restore patience, acceptance and an ability to flow with the pace of life and others.                    **BACH**

The mother stock is prepared from the pale mauve flowers only, even though the red outnumber them by ten to one.

Research, reported to FES suggests the flower essence may be of benefit in various physical symptoms. Gayle Eversole found oral drops helped relieve phantom pain from spider bite, and Mimi Ellisom the pain associated with osteoporosis with fractured vertebrate and sinus pain.

It is interesting to note that Bach initially gave a different indication for its use; "excruciating and very acute pain, no matter what the cause…It is indicated in acute pain of nerve type and it not only gives rapid relief, but in many cases apparently effect a cure of the nerve condition. It has also a beneficent action and patients frequently report, in depression and tears, a generally brighter outlook being obtained. Amongst cases successfully treated may be mentioned intense headaches, sciaticas, acute neuralgias, tic douloureux and acute pain in malignant disease. In some cases it has given relief after morphine has failed."

Jewelweed essence promotes a gentle, loving, joyous, humble, peaceful state of being-ness. Helps one to face one's fears with this attitude- to feel them without being overwhelmed and let go of them. It allows change to manifest while remaining inwardly centered, feeling love and loved.                    **LIGHT MOUNTAIN**

Indian Balsam essence is for the warrior at inner peace, waiting patiently for the right moment to act.                    **HORUS**

Pink Impatiens is for the idealist, the moralist who compromises through struggling to maintain his or her standards.                    **LIVING ESSENCES**

Impatiens (*I. walleriana*) essence calms anger, encourages patience and tolerance in those who get easily annoyed and aggressive with others.                    **HAWAIIAN GAIA**

# SPIRITUAL PROPERTIES

Red Garden Balsam (*I. balsamina*) represents generosity. It is about giving, and giving itself with bargaining.

It also is about generosity in the physical; as it likes abundance and likes to give abundantly.

White and purple balsam is spontaneously generous, and gives of itself unstintingly.

Pink Garden Balsam contains psychic generosity, of thought and act, and gives for the joy of giving.                    **THE MOTHER**

Patience Plant represents the works of love, the best condition for work.                    **THE MOTHER**

One day, while sitting by the stream and contemplating what felt like a dire financial situation, I asked for a plant to come to assist me…My gaze wandered to Jewelweed…the windless day found one stalk waving energetically at me. I picked one of its leaves and put it in the water, watching as the silvery sheen sparkled…and allowed my consciousness to move into the daydream of Jewelweed.

Suddenly I was walking through silver birch and other silver plants onto the grounds of a silver castle. There was…a large pool with a silver fish [that] stepped out of the pool and became a silver Queen. She said, "I am only silver in my fluidity and so you must stay fluid"…She poured silver fluid into me through the top of my head, reminding me of the abundance in my life…

As I became aware of the leaf in the water, I again felt as fluid as the leaf and realized how stuck I had become in a negative thought pattern about money and how it was binding up my energy. A few days later I received an unexpected check in the mail thanks to the help of Jewelweed. **MONTGOMERY**

## PERSONALITY TRAITS

The Sugar Plant, which goes by the botanical name of *Impatiens sultani*, grows on its branches granules which crystallise and which not only taste like cane sugar but also contain an equal proportion of sucrose and dextrose.

When these crystallised granules are gathered others grow in their place and it does not sound, therefore, such an extravagant idea, especially in times of sugar rationing, to suggest growing a sugar plant in a pot as a centre piece for everyone's dining-room table and reach out to it for granules when wishing to sweeten our tea, coffee, or other beverages! **VICOMTE de MAUDUIT**

Overburdened with the self-imposed pressure of too many things to do and far too little time allocated, irritation and frustration build up inside, until one is dangerously close to bursting. Others are forcefully and selfishly ejected out of the way. There is no room for anyone else.

With hair trigger sensitivity, one slight touch or poke, a glance or comment and one explodes with great force, flinging anger with expulsive dispersion. More than impatience, there is such a lightning fast, sudden, startling, far-flung burst of temper that anyone nearly might just jump out of their skin…As impatience deepens to anger, the anger can deepen to rage, hate, malice and cruelty. The intimidating, malicious manner gives off the clear signal of 'touch-me-not' or else. Their whole life is fiery, forceful, flaring, frantic and frenzied." **VERMEULEN**

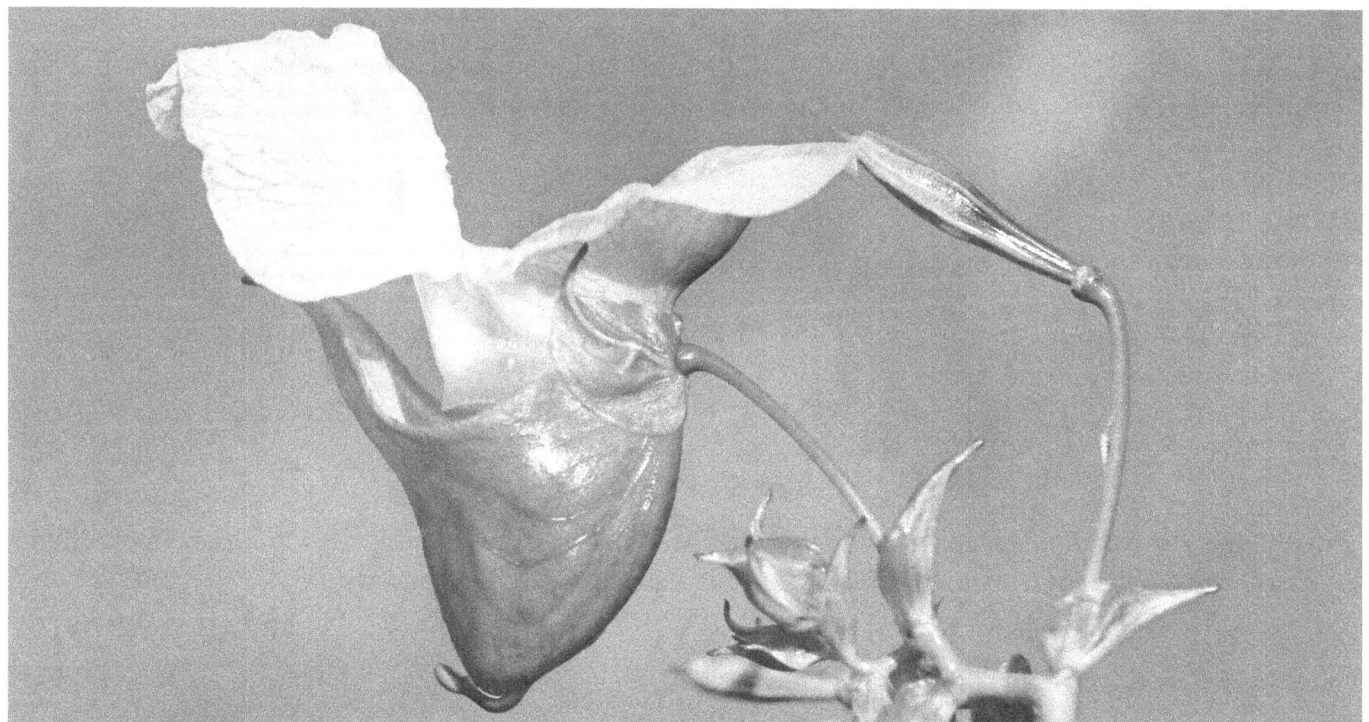

SNAPWEED

55

## DOCTRINE OF SIGNATURES

Snapweed, or Impatiens (*I. roylei*) smoothness of the skin is most striking- being filled with water the stems are cool to touch. Yet for all the boldness of the growth, the plants are rather delicate and crush easily. Impatiens gains protection by growing en masse and lacks the fibre and woody strength of other plants.

The smell of Impatiens grows stronger when it is touched. The scent is unusual: strong and pungent rather than sweet, like a spicy tar, not unpleasant but warding rather than attracting. Again there is a sense of isolation rather than joining as this scent dominates the area.

The jagged edge to the leaves is antagonistic. Saw-toothed edges look as though they would cut- a visual cue to keep away. Crush the stems and they sound like crunching a cane, a hollow pain as the fibres are torn...

The explosive force with which the seeds are propelled...have already been noted.                    **J. BARNARD**

## RECIPES

Wild Touch Me Not, or Jewelweed juice is best preserved in ice cube trays frozen. This is done by pressing or juicing the whole plant stems and flowers.

**TINCTURE**- Make the fresh plant tincture at 1:2 with only 25% alcohol.

Ointments for hemorrhoids, etc. are best made with sun infusion of whole plant using coconut oil. Suppositories can then be shaped easily at later date.

**ICE CUBES**- The best way to store the juice of jewelweed is freeze in ice cubes. I prefer the small cocktail size for this particular plant, as you only need small amounts at a time. Remember to mark and identify your bag of ice cubes.

**GARDEN BALSAM TINCTURE**- 2-4 ml.

**DECOCTION**- 3-12 grams. For cancer 15-60 grams are used

**INFUSION**-flowers- 3-6 grams

**CAUTION**- Being a uterine stimulant, and having some cumulative toxicity, the seeds are contra-indicted during pregnancy and breastfeeding. Do not use continuously for any length of time.

| | |
|---|---|
| **GROUND JUNIPER** | **CREEPING JUNIPER** |
| **DWARF JUNIPER** | (*J. horizontalis* Moench) |
| (*Juniperus communis* L.) | **SABIN/SAVIN** |
| **ALPINE JUNIPER** | (*J. sabina* L.) |
| (*J. sibirica var. montana* Aiton.) | **CHINESE JUNIPER** |
| (*J. alpina* [Sm.] Gray) not accepted | (*J. chinensis* L.) |
| **ROCKY MOUNTAIN JUNIPER** | **PARTS USED**- bark, roots, leaves, and berries (cones). |
| (*J. scopulorum* Sarg.) | |

"And upon earthenware tiles there lay juniper berries, smouldering and exhaling their aromatic smoke, filling the cabin with a bluish haze, through which the awful majesty of death was mistily visible."          **REYMONT**

Fatal sabina, nymph of infamy.                    **ABRAHAM COWLEY**

I never drink anything stronger than gin before breakfast.                    **W. C. FIELDS**

Wine is sweet, and gin is bitter
Drink all you can, but you won't forget her.                    **EVERLEY BROTHERS**

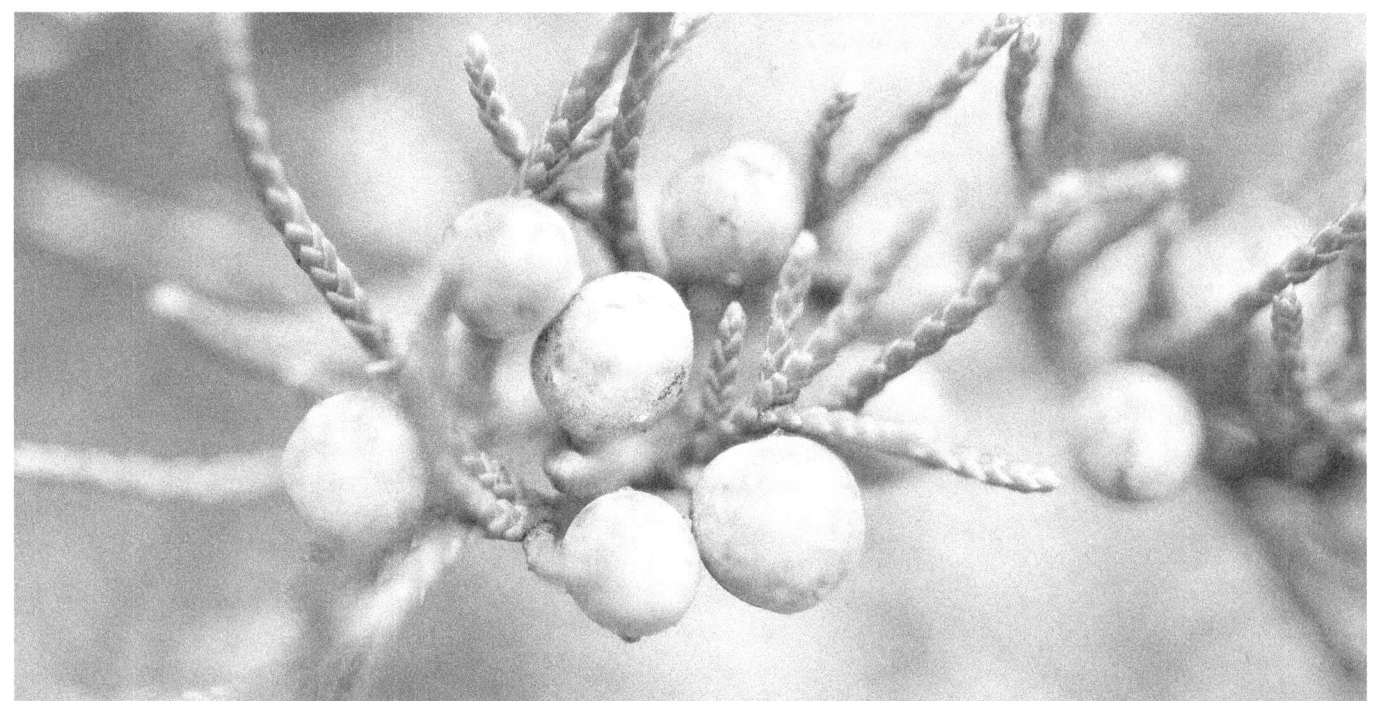

CREEPING JUNIPER BERRIES

Juniper is from the Celtic **JENEPRUS**, meaning acrid, bitter or rough. It may be from the Celtic **GEN** meaning small bush, and **PRUS**, for bitter hot.

Or it may derive from the Dutch **JENEVER**, meaning juniper; or the early French **GENEVE**. The city of Geneva was so named for the juniper forest that once grew there. King Arthur's wife, Guenevere, and the modern Jennifer are from the same root. Juniperus means "youth producing", the mysterious ability to stop time. The appearance of both mature black and immature green cones on the same bush at same time may have led to the Latin **JUNIORES**, in reference to the constant new berries, from junior meaning younger and parere "to appear".

Another possibility is from the Italian word for juniper, **ENEBRO** related to the word for over-consumption or inebriated. Scopulorum is Latin for, "of the rocky cliffs". Horizontalis is obvious.

Juniper is a long-lived shrubby evergreen distributed throughout the world.

It is a hot, and vigorous plant, assigned to Mars and Aries. Ironically, it came in Victorian times to mean delectable.

Symbolically, Juniper means initiative and ingenuity, as well as confidence and protection from enemies. The birth date associated with this plant is September 22nd. The 16th Nordic Rune Sigel is associated with juniper.

Juniper appears on the herald badges of the clans Gunn, MacLeod, Murray and Ross. Its signature is the number three.

Nearly every European culture cites juniper as the symbol of protection. In northern Germany, the juniper spirit helps discover thieves. Madam Juniper (Frau Wacholder) a deva of the Juniper, was invoked to make thieves return stolen good.

In Scandinavia, a needle was pulled off the bush and touched to part of body with pain. The needle is stuck back so to take on the pain.

In Scotland the branches were set on fire and carried throughout the house on New Year's Day to dispel infection and protect from evil. The same was practiced in Italy. To chop down a tree in Wales meant misfortune, or death in the family.

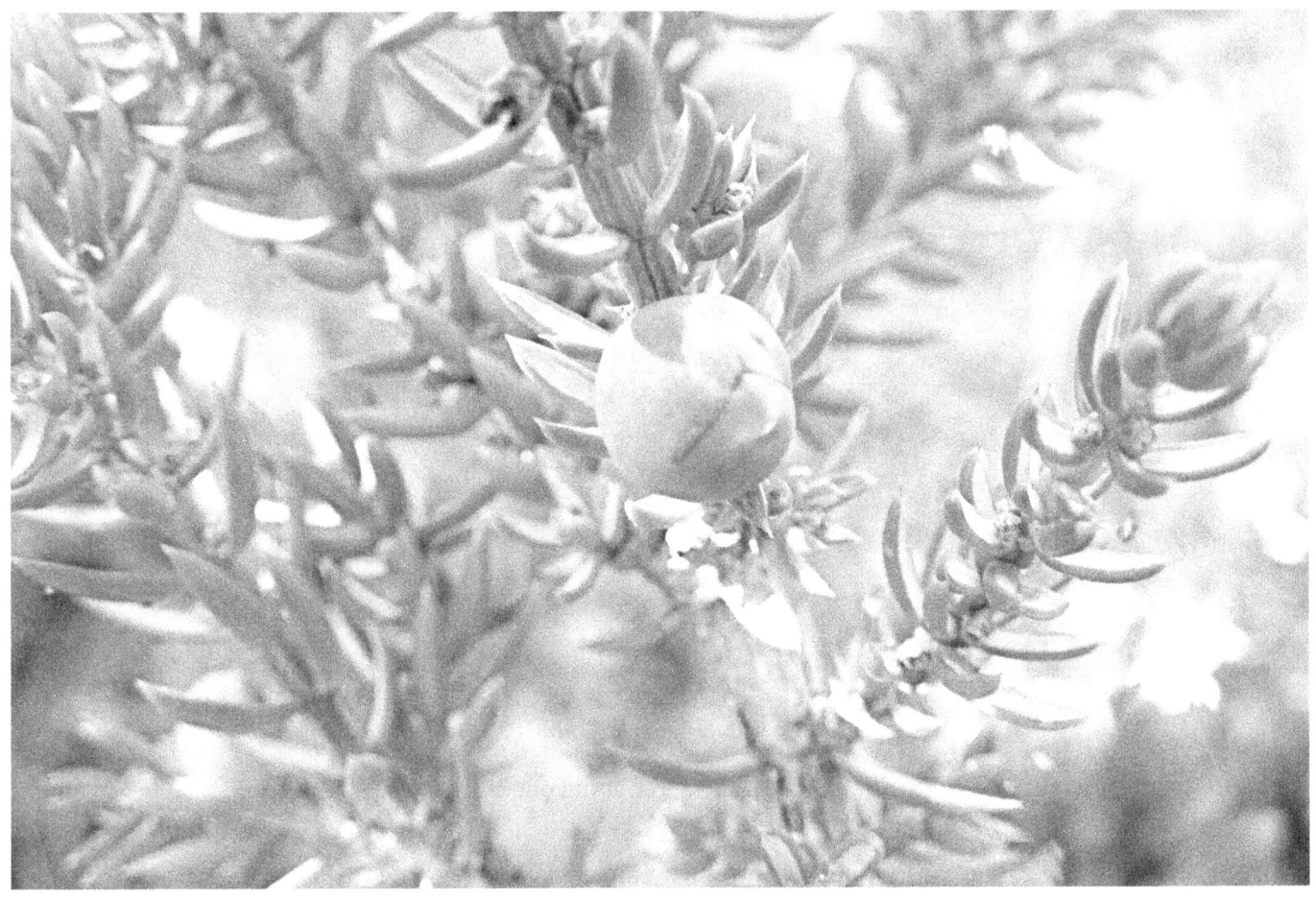

UNRIPE JUNIPER BERRIES (*J. COMMUNIS*)

On Samhain (All Souls Night) when the gates to the dead are believed more open than any other time, the branches were burned on doorsteps to keep unwanted spirits out. Samhain may to related to the Gallic name for juniper, samh.

To dream of juniper signified great honor or the birth of a male child.

The dried wood burns with very little smoke and was used as fuel for illegal whiskey stills in former times. The smoke gives a slight turpentine flavor to hams.

The Cree call Common Juniper **KAHKAKEWAHTIK**, raven wood or **MASAKIYS**. The newly released Cree Dictionary says juniper is known as a medicinal spruce tree, or **MIHKWAPEMAKWAHTIK**.

Decoctions of the branches were gargled for sore throats, as well as anti-dandruff hair rinse. Bark decoctions were applied to wounds for antiseptic purpose, while the inner bark was softened in hot water and applied as a poultice to wounds.

The Blackfoot decocted the root of **SIIKSINOKO** (*J. horizontalis*) with poplar leaves to treat back pains; and an infusion of the root only as a general internal tonic, as well as wash to keep their horse's hair glossy and healthy.

The Thompson of British Columbia used cool leaf infusions to treat hypertension. Gary Raven, a traditional healer from Manitoba suggests the same thing, one glass morning and evening.

The Eastern Cree would boil the bark until the outer bark could be separated. The inner bark was pounded until it formed a jelly; that was then applied to painful boils and wounds. Root decoctions were used for cystitis, Bright's disease or urinary calculi.

The bark is called **WAKIMAKIN** by the Cree living in the Hudson Bay region.

The inner bark is scraped out and applied to skin wounds.

The debarked stems can be made into a tea to treat diarrhea, or chest congestion.

The Chipewyan call it **DATSA"JIE**. This means the raven tree. Green cones were decocted for kidney complaints.

The dried green cones are smoked in pipes to relieve asthma. The Gitksan call it "boughs of the supernatural", or **LAXSA LAXNOK**.

The Dena'ina of Alaska call the plant "brown bear's spruce bough, or **TSUNI ELA**, and the cones "mouse's berry", or **DLIN'A GEGA**.

The fragrant leaves were burned as incense on top of wood stoves. They boiled the branches and cones for colds, sore throats, tuberculosis and difficulty urinating.

The Wet'suwet'en used boughs and berries of **DETSAN** for flu and venereal disease.

Some native tribes used the dried, powdered leaves to dust psoriasis or eczema.

Creeping Juniper (*J. horizontalis*) is called by the Cree **MASEKESK**, or **MASIKESKATIK**, and sometimes **NAPAKASEHTAK**. It has similar use to the Common juniper, with the leafy stems boiled for colds, or teething babies.

The leaves were burned and the smoke inhaled to clear sinuses or added to sweet grass as a prairie incense.

Other tribes like the Zuni used juniper leaf tea to relax uterine muscles following birth, while the Hopi drank it to produce a daughter. In Mongolia, the tea was given to women at the onset of labour.

The branches were used to cover the floor of medicine lodges, and the Blackfoot used the plant on the altar of the Sacred Woman during the Sun Dance ceremony.

The Blackfoot call it **TSEKIE-SINO-KOSA** and use decoctions of the leaves to treat lungs and venereal disease.

The Cheyenne decoct both leaves and cones for coughs, sore throats, tonsillitis, and considered the tea a valuable sedative to calm hyperactive persons. The Montana group performed a special ceremony around a lone juniper to alleviate fear of the Thunder. They believed lightning never struck juniper because a power exists between it and thunder. Flutes carved from wood were used for courting and played at night.

The berries, **SIKSINOUKOO** (black round objects), were strung as necklaces; to which Catholic nuns later tried attaching a crucifix. The berries were dried, greased and held in smoke until blackened; then polished and strung alternately with wolf willow seeds.

The berries decorated ceremonial headdress, for fashion and fumigation. The headpiece has seven berries representing the Bunched Stars (Pleiades); the same stars portrayed on tipi designs.

The berry seeds were used for kidney ailments in tea form.

The Crow name for Creeping Juniper is **BAGE ELI GEE CHI BAGUA**. Alma Snell recommends chewing up four or five berries for headache, as well as sore throat and lung congestion.

Natives of Nevada made beads of juniper berries. The fresh, ripe berries were placed on anthills, so that the ants ate out the sweet part leaving a convenient hole for stringing. The Navaho tied juniper berry bracelets on the wrist of newborns to ward off bad dreams.

The Navaho flavored their food with the ash of juniper needles and branches, and made a tea from the ash to treat muscle injury and diarrhea. Christensen et al, *J Am Diet Assoc* 1998 98 found the ash contributed calcium, iron and magnesium to the diet.

The Tanaina of Alaska boil juniper branches for colds, sore throats, urinary retention, and tuberculosis.

The smoke of the boughs was used to remove curses, and rid dwellings of ghosts and evil spirits. Upon death, the bedding and belongings were washed in juniper. The Hopi men washed in juniper after burying the dead.

The berries were boiled and the wax on top skimmed for its fragrant quality.

Combine this with beeswax for insect bites and wounds that do not heal.

Some tribes roasted and ground the berries as a hot beverage; as well as flavoring and preserving meat.

A wine jar dating back to 3150 BC has been found at the burial site of Scorpion I at Abydos, Egypt. It contained juniper berries, sage, artemesia species, savory and thyme, as well as pine resin.

In medieval Europe, berries were carried by men in their pockets to increase their sexual prowess. The ancient Greeks burned juniper berries and branches to appease the gods of the underworld.

Pliny the Elder wrote "gossip records a miracle that to rub it (crushed juniper berries) all over the male part before coition prevents conception". Dioscorides gave the same message, but suggested they be placed on the vulva prior to insertion.

Tibetan shaman traditionally burned the cones in the Sang Cho, or "smoke offering".

Juniper was burned during childbirth to keep fairies from substituting a changeling for the newborn baby. Father Kneipp reported "our body, our most loyal and precious home, needs juniper fumigation and vapors at certain times".

In the 1600s, a Dutch medical professor, Franciscus Sylvius developed an alcoholic extract from juniper berries as an inexpensive diuretic. It was called Jenever, from the Dutch for Juniper.

Another story says Lucas Bols found a distillery in Amsterdam in 1575 and started making juniper-flavored liquor.

The phrase Dutch Courage comes from the expression 'zich moed indrinken', meaning to drink in courage.

In certain spirits, such as **BRINJEVAC**, the berries contribute not only flavour, but up to 25% fermentable sugars.

Today, juniper berries are used in the production of gin, and flavoring of sauerkraut and pickled fish.

Traditionally, a beer from juniper berries, called **GENIEVRE** was made in France. Today, in Germany, "The Watchman", or **WACHOLDER** beer contains juniper berry extract. I enjoy a beer crafted with juniper berries called Rogue John Ale out of Newport, Oregon. Scandinavian aquavits use the berry extract.

Incidentally, the other herbs used in the manufacture of Dutch gin are angelica stem, coriander seeds and iris (orris) root. One kilogram of berries are used for every 400 litres of gin produced. In England alone, this amounts to about 200 tonnes annually. In the past, the berries were used in parts of Scotland to flavor whiskey.

The phrase bathtub gin came from the Prohibition production of grain alcohol and mixing juniper berry extracts to mask the harsh poor quality spirit.

The mature, black berries or cones are de-seeded and made into jam in Nordic countries. A conserve called Latwerge is eaten with cold meats in Germany.

The dried, roasted berry (250 degrees Fahrenheit) may be put into a pepper mill and used as a tasty condiment; or coffee substitute.

Extracts from juniper are used in frozen dairy, candy, baked goods, chutneys, puddings and meat products; including Italian pastrami. Belgian Ham (Jambon d'Ardennes) is smoked with wood and berries.

Juniper berries are often used in Poland as a seasoning for wild mushroom marinades. Mmmm.

A very effective, natural spray for roses is produced by covering a handful of juniper berries, with warm water overnight. Spray your bushes twice weekly, and throw the old berries around the base.

The gnarled wood is crushed and used as moth repellent like cedar.

Older herbalists say that the eagle lives so long because it feeds on the berries.

Ashes from the burned juniper made into a tea were said to cure dropsy, and an external wash for itchy skin, scabs and sores. The ashes of the wood were considered beneficial to those with scurvy, to rub the gums.

Root decoctions were used in Poland to heal herpes and skin rashes.

Some writers have suggested that the gnarled, hard and knotty appearance of juniper suggests that by the doctrine of signatures, it is useful for arthritis and rheumatism.

Work by Gross et al, *J Biomed Mater Res* 2003 64A:4 looked at the use of juniper wood as a possible implant material. The natural impregnated essential oil gives antiseptic properties. Femoral implants in rabbits showed good acceptance after three years, with bone apposition, abutment into pores, and growth into drilled cavities.

Various Native tribes utilized juniper wood for making bows. It was ideally harvested around February, as it was dry enough to work without having to cure. Wood from the south side was also considered better than that from the north side, for bow making, because the sap runs more on the north side, and the south side was easier to work.

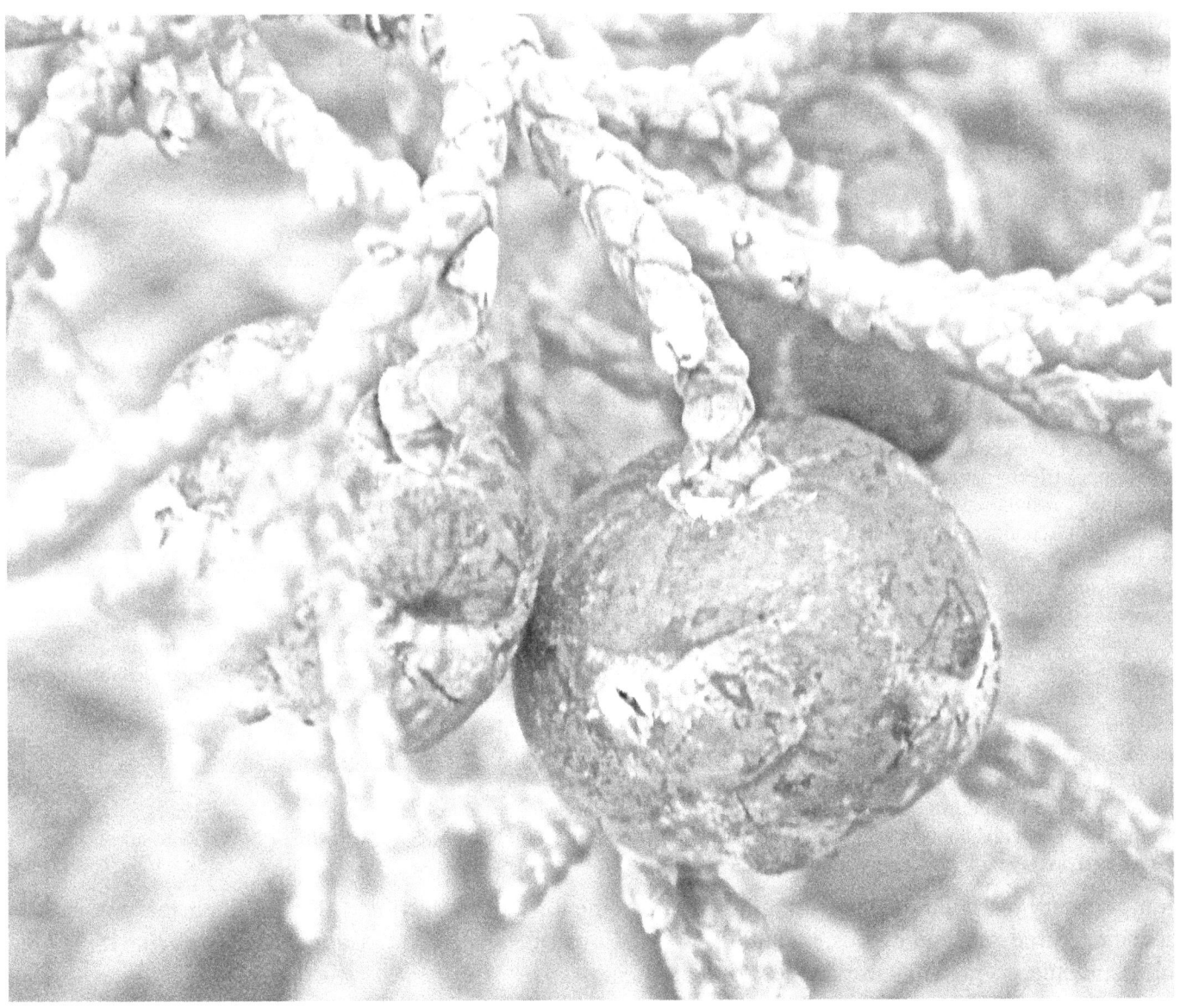

JUNIPERUS HORIZONTALIS BERRY

Jethro Kloss recommended juniper berry, gentian and calamus root be combined for gout, sciatica, and rheumatism.

Juniper berries have been used in veterinary medicine to stimulate flagging appetite in animals. Juniper leaf is abortifacient to pregnant cows due to isocupressic acid.

The Juniper Tree is one of the Brothers Grimm fairy tales, and tells of the death of a pregnant woman after eating the berries. This was Savin.

Savin or Sabin oil was the abortifacient of choice as mentioned by Cato in ancient Rome. Pliny the Elder suggested rubbing crushed berries on the penis before sex to prevent conception.

It was carried north by monks and nuns to parts of northern Europe and planted in their kitchen gardens.

It is named for "saving" young women from shame. It had many names including Kindermord (child murder), abortion tree, lucky herb, bastard killer and plant of the damned.

Linnaeus, a conservative Lutheran, said it was used by "women who are whores, and though they think their sin is secret, God sees it." This is rich coming from a confirmed bachelor who wrote sexually laden letters to women around the world.

Juniper extracts are used in personal care products such as Bath and Body Instant Antibacterial Hand Gel.

Chinese Juniper is fully hardy to -40°C and stay low to the ground, ensuring good snow cover.

Termites forced to eat only juniper sawdust die prematurely, according to Charles Kane. Now you know.

# MEDICINAL

**CONSTITUENTS-** *J. communis* leaf/needle -numerous flavonoids, juniperin (bitter), pentosane, essential oils, tannins, podophyllotoxin and resins.
berry- monoterpenes (50-90%), including alpha and beta pinenes, juniperin (bitter), terpinen-4-ol, lignans and various sesquiterpenes, geijerone, diterpene acids such as imbricatolic, myrceocommunic, communic, sandara-copimaric, isopimaric, and torulosic acids; flavonoids such as iso-scuttelarein and 8-hydroxyluteolin; bioflavonoids like amentoflavone, hypnokiflavone, cupressoflavone and methyl biflavone; various sugars, especially fructose and glucose (up to 30%). The fruit contains over 150 identified constituents, including high concentration of chromium, cobalt and tin.
The dry seed is nearly 31% protein, and 54% fat. Small amount of vitamin C.
wood- unusual diterpenes including communic acid and pimaric acid, sesquiterpenes including thujopsene, widdrol, , juniperol, ferruginol, cuparene, cedrol, and pygmaein; phenols sugiol and xanthoperol in wood, and longifolene and totarol in root and bark; gallocatechins, podophyllotoxin and stigmasterol.
Roots- longifolene, totarol.
*J. horizontalis*- communic acid, cedrol, widdrol, thujopsene, cupressiflavones, savinin, cedrene, cuparene, sciadopitysin, and sitosterols.
*J. sabina*- volatile oils ( 3-5%), lignans including deoxypodorhizone, deoxy-podophyllotoxin,, deoxypicropodo-phyllotoxin, dehydro-podophyllotoxin; hydroxycoumarins: cumarsabine, 8-methoxy-cumarsabine, siderin, 4-methoxy-5-methylcoumarin-propio-phenone; and others including 2-hydroxy-3,4-dime-thoxy-6-methyl-propiophenone; various flavnoids including catechin, quercitin, isoquercitrin, rutin and isoscutellarein 7-O-beta-D-xylopyranoside.
*J. chinensis*- bark- 12-hydroxycupressic acid, cupressic acid
root- 7beta-hydroxy-sandaracopimaric acid
heartwood- cedrol, widdrol, savinin, calocedrin, 10-oxowiddrol, 12-hydroxywiddrol, (+)naringenin, (+)taxifolin, (+) aromadendrin, styraxlignolide, vanillic acid, alpha-methyl artoflavanocoumarin and 5,7,4'-trihydroxy-2-styrylchromone.
leaf- 8-acetyloxyelemol, 8-hydroxyelemol, hinokiic acid.

Juniper berry (*J. communis*) is used in herbal medicine for it's disinfecting action on the urinary tract. It is specific to urethritis and cystitis, including chronic forms, associated with acidic urine. The urine takes on a pleasant violet scent, while working its wonders.

In cases of chronic nephritis, juniper berry may be combined with couch grass, cleavers, uva ursi, goldenrod and aspen poplar bark. The resultant tea or tincture should be taken at body temperature, but never hot.

It is contraindicated due to its mild uterine stimulating effect during pregnancy. Menopausal women with irritation of the bladder and intense desire to urinate, however, may find juniper berry gives quick relief.

The berry is an excellent appetite stimulant; perhaps part of the attraction of a pre-dinner gin martini. The volatile oils in the berry dilate the capillaries of the mucous membranes of the digestive tract.

Blood flow is increased and the stomach responds by producing more hydrochloric acid. You can simply chew a few berries before meals.

Fresh berry juice can be bought commercially, and is used for increasing appetite, relieving gas and bloating and purifying the blood stream.

The oils are fatal to bacteria, as the action is penetrating and destroying.

In asthma conditions, juniper reduces mucous production by the lungs; and cleans out the tar residue after quitting smoking. It combines well with Thyme or Thuja cedar for recurring respiratory infections. William Salmon wrote in 1692 that juniper acts on cold, damp, mucus and spasms of the lungs. "Asthmas, coughs, difficulty breathing, wheezing, shortness of breath, hoarseness, and other the like cold and moist diseases of the lungs."

In arthritic conditions, two or three berries can be taken every day before lunch. Work by Tunon et al, *J of Ethnopharmacology* 1995 48 found that water extracts, in vitro, inhibit prostaglandin biosynthesis, and PAF, or platelet activating factor, and induced exocytosis. This appears to confirm some of the early use of juniper berries for inflammatory conditions.

Mascolo et al, *Phytother Res* 1987 1 found the anti-inflammatory activity of a berry extract, 60% the strength of indomethacin.

In India, the berries are part of Ayurvedic Medicine. **HAPUSA** is a digestive stimulant, with a bitter, pungent, hot, saline and heavy property. It cures aggravated pitta, obstinate abdominal diseases, including ascites, aggravated hemorrhoids, sprue syndrome, colic pain, and phantom tumours.

Juniper leaf tea encourages menstruation delayed by exposure to cold. The berries are soaked in wine, and given for removing retained placenta afterbirth.

It strengthens the brain, memory and optic nerve of the eye.

The hypoglycemic activity of juniper berries can be attributed to an increase of peripheral glucose consumption, making it useful for diabetic conditions, and adrenaline hyperglycemia.

Scientists, led by Sanchez De Medina, at the Universidad de Granada in Spain tested decoctions of the berries on both normal and diabetic rats, and found it lowered blood glucose levels, and reduced mortality. They concluded that juniper berry potentiated the release of insulin from the pancreas. *Planta Medica* 1994 60.

Previous studies by Swanston-Flatt et al, *Diabetologia* 1990, found juniper berries could retard the development of chemical-induced diabetes in lab animals.

Gray & Flatt, *Proc Nutr Soc* 1997 56 however, found no hypoglycemic effect in streptozotocin-induced diabetic mice. This may have been related to the ten-fold lower dosage than above, cited in study by De Medina, according to the authors.

Van Slambrouck et al, *Oncol Rep* 2007 17:6 found juniper berries decrease the growth of MCF-7/AZ breast cancer cell lines.

Inbricatolic acid, found in alcohol extracts of fresh ripe berries, prevents cancer cell cycle through unique pathways. De Marino et al, *Planta Medica* 77:16 1872-8.

Berry extracts induce p53 apoptosis in human SH-SY5Y neuroblastoma cells. Lantto TA et al, *Int J Mol Sci* 2016 17(7).

Amentoflavone, derived from berries, relieved induced arthritis in rat models. Bais S et al, *Biomed Pharmacother* 2017 86: 381-92.

Alcohol/water extracts of berries suppresses melanin synthesis, via tyrosinase inhibition. The active component hypolaetin 7-O-beta-D-xylopyraniside may be useful for treating skin pigmentation disorders. Jegal J et al, *Biosci Biotechnol Biochem* 2016 80(12): 2311-17.

Recent studies indicate juniper has anti-tumor and anti-viral activity in animals; podophyllotoxin being the active principle.

Juniper lignans inhibit herpes simplex virus. Markkanen et al, *Drugs and Experimental Clinical Research* 1981 17.

Deoxypodophyllotoxin, the lignan found in the needles and berries of savin, as well as golden chervil (*Anthriscus sylvestris*) exhibits anti-tumour and anti-viral properties. Podophyllotoxin is also found in *Thuja occidentalis* and used as starting compound for three semi-synthetic cancer drugs.

Etoposide is sometimes used with cisplatin in treatment of numerous difficult carcinomas and sarcomas. Podophyllotoxin gels are used to remove venereal warts.

Feliciano et al, 1993, found five cyclo-lignans in savin, with activity against herpes simplex and vesicular stomatitis virus.

Juniper bark, sapwood, heartwood and leaves are all anti-microbial. Clark et al, *Phytotherapy Research* 1990 4.

McCutcheon et al, at UBC found the branches active against 9 of 11 bacteria tested. They exhibit great inhibition of *Pseudomonas aeruginosa* K99. *J Ethnopharm* 1992 37.

The berry showed anti-fungal activity against *Penicillium notatum*. Hejtmankova et al, *Acta Univ Palacki Olomuc Fac Med* 1973 60.

Isocupressic acid and communic acid from the leaves display activity against *Mycobacterium tuberculosis*, confirming indigenous use for this disease. Carpenter CD et al, *J Ethnopharm* 2012 143(2): 695-700.

The active ingredients of *J. occidentalis* wood appear to be alpha and beta cedrene, which show activity against *Fusobacterium necrophorum, Clostridium perfringens, Actinomyces bovis* and *Candida albicans*. Johnston et al, *Phytother Res* 2001 15:7.

Fungi of the genus *Hormonema*, isolated from juniper leaf are strongly inhibitory of *Candida albicans*, and moderately efficient in mice on disseminated candidiasis.

Activity against *Aspergillus fumigatus* is comparable to pneumoncandin. Pelaez B et al, *System Appl Microbiol* 2000 23:3.

In Germany, juniper wood is used in a few diuretic, rheumatic and blood purifying teas.

Externally, juniper leaves benefit arthritis, gout and rheumatic pain. Sitz baths are great for venous congestion, vaginal discharges, and even chronic constipation.

Extracts show anti-cancer activity. Goun EA et al, *J Ethnopharm* 2002 81 337-342.

The leaves of male *J. communis* sub-species show significant anti-oxidant activity. Emami et al, *Pharm Bio* 45:10. *In vitro* studies suggest anti-microbial activity similar to amphotericin B. Leaf extracts are hepatoprotective, and cytotoxic to HepG2 cancer cells. Ved A et al, *Pharmacogn Mag* 2017 13(49): 108-113.

Aerial parts show cytotoxicity against four human cancer cell lines, A549, MCF-7, TK6 and U937. Pollio Z et al, *Molecules* 2016 21(4): 395.

Juniper leaf tip tea helps promote healthy digestion.

Even juniper root is useful medicinally.

The root is mashed and applied to the gums to strengthen them. The heartwood, in vitro, is comparable to streptomycin against microbes.

The root contains longifolene and tortarol, both most active against tuberculosis, including isoniazid, streptomycin and moxifloxacin-resistant strains. Gordien et al, *J Ethnopharm* 2009 Oct 13.

Totoral is active against a wide range of mycobacterium as well as enterococci, staphylococci, streptococci, pseudomonas and other gram negative bacteria. It is highly synergistic with other constituents of juniper, and is effective against skin problems, like severe acne, and is a strong NorA efflux pump inhibitor, meaning it makes staph bacteria more susceptible to anti-bacterial compounds in the herb.

A study in *Z Phytotherapie* 1994 15 by Schilcher & Heil was a critical review of all the literature on nephrotoxicity of juniper berries from 1844 to present day. They conclude erroneous interpretation and possible contamination of juniper oil with turpentine has led to the impression that juniper berry is contraindicated in acute kidney infection.

Rats given high doses of juniper berry oil (1000 mg/kg body weight) showed absolutely no signs of kidney damage, according to an article by lead author in *Arzneim Forsh* 1997 47. They further speculate that the suggested nephro-toxicity may arise from the fact that in acute kidney infections an increase in pathological protein values in urine may be noted. This is normal, and in no way due to juniper constituents. See berry essential oil below.

An earlier human study conducted by Wegener and Schmidt, *Biologische Medizin* 1995 24 2 on the safe and gentle action of juniper berry preparation on the kidneys. Chloride ion secretion increased 119% in one rat study following ingestion of a water infusion of the berries.

A report in *Fitoterapia* in 1994 suggested, "potent anti-fertility activity" from juniper berry extract. Adult female rats experienced interference with progesterone activity thereby preventing conception. More study is needed, and underway. Leaf and berry tinctures help stimulate uterine contractions. Take 30-45 drops every half hour during active labor.

Cypressiflavones derived from *J. horizontalis* inhibit cyclic nucleotide phosphodiesterases.

The needles contain podophyllotoxin and essential oils. Work by Cantrell CL et al, suggests you can extract both from needles consecutively. *PLoS One* 2014 9(9).

Savin leaf infusion is a remedy for intestinal worms, but use with caution. Research at the National Cancer Institute reveals that *J. sabina* is indeed active against tumors.

In China, the leaves and twigs are used for rheumatoid arthritis. Work by Zhao J et al, *Pharmacogn Mag* 2016 12(47): 178-83 confirmed the marked decrease of synovial inflammation and hyperplasia in joint of treated rats.

Water extracts inhibit HepG-2 and K562 cancer cell lines by apoptosis. Huyan T et al, *J Ethnopharm* 2016 185: 289-99.

Savin has been used in the past to counteract digitalis overdoses. Not sure this is a good idea.

Extracts from J. *chinensis* exhibit anti-angiogenic and anti-hepatocellular carcinoma activity. Kuo ZK et al, *BMC Complement Altern Med* 2016 16: 277.

Widdrol inhibits vessel sprouting and growth, and reduced tumor growth and blood vessel formation in colon tumor xenograft mice. Jin S et al, *Oncol Rep* 2015 34(3):1178-84.

Coumarin type compounds from the heartwood exhibit anti-cholinesterase and beta-site amyloid precursor protein cleaving enzyme, suggestive of benefit in Alzheimer's disease. Jung HJ et al, *Chem Pharm Bull* (Tokyo) 2015 63(11): 955-60.

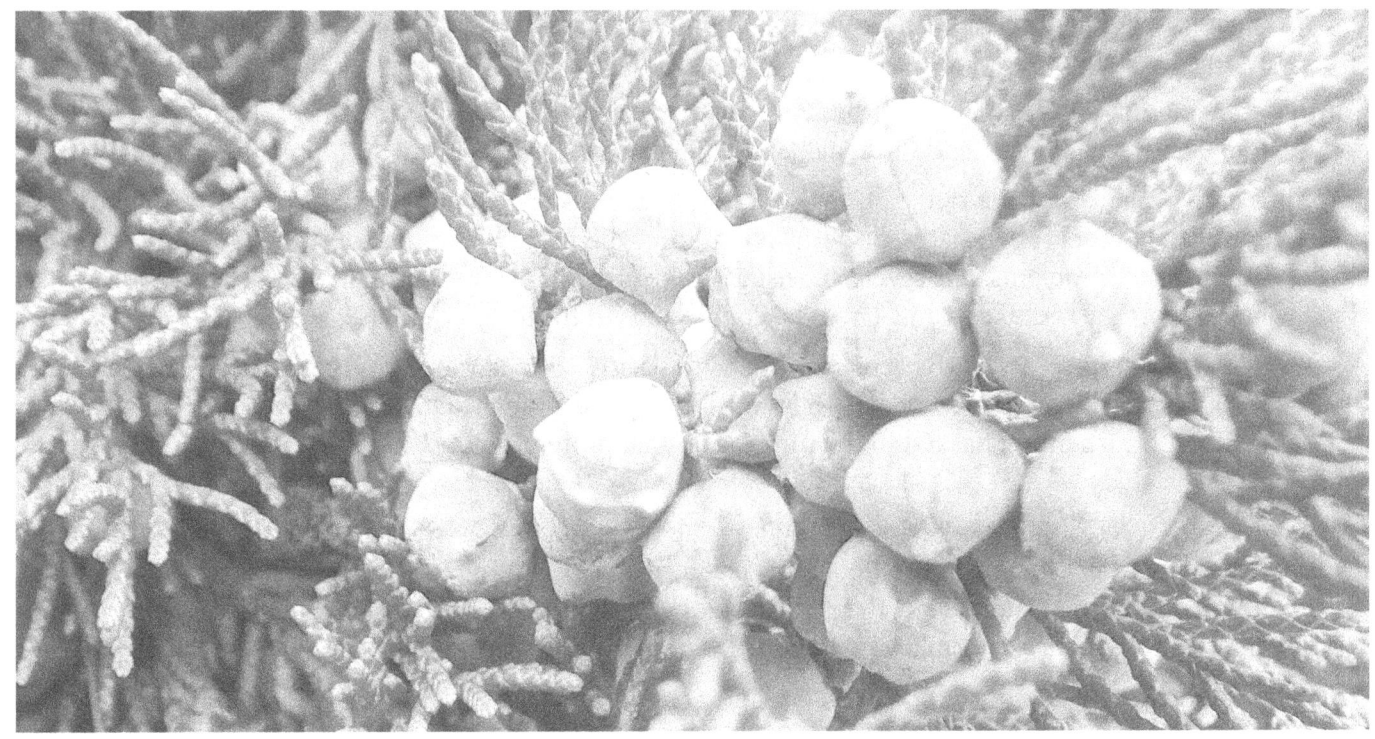

UNRIPE BERRIES ON *JUNIPERUS HORIZONTALIS*

## HOMEOPATHY

Juniper berry is very useful for catarrhal inflammations of the bladder, or in suppression of urine in older people with poor appetite. There may be a burning, cutting pain in the urethra when passing urine. In nephritis or similar kidney inflammation it is best to take the first or second potency.

Confusion of mind, dreams of childbirth, fastidious, careless, loss of memory, desire for spiritual improvement.

**DOSE**- Tincture- one to ten drops up to three times daily in water. The mother tincture is prepared from the fresh ripe berries. There are no provings but above is based on clinical observations by Boericke, Clarke, Hale, Stubler, Krug and Mangialavori.

Sabina (*J. sabina*) has a very special action on the uterus. There may be severe pain from the sacrum to the pubis. If there is a tendency to miscarry, it will be in the third month.

Sabina also helps the after effect of abortion, when anxiety, guilt and other emotions lead to self-doubt and recrimination.

Music is intolerable, especially from piano. Sense of duty and responsibility. Unwilling to talk about inner feelings and more intimate things. Dreams of people falling down dead from a height.

Uterine pains are debilitating during menses and made worse by the least movement. An almost paralytic pain in the small of the back is often present. One of my clients suffered for seventeen years until this remedy changed her life.

There may be blood in the urine or bleeding hemorrhoids. The patient finds music upsetting and produces more nervousness. Warts and fig warts on the skin may itch or burn. Human papillomas (genital warts) also respond to internal and external therapy.

Acne during pregnancy,

It can be useful for uterine and cervical cancers, or simply inflammation of the cervix.

For threatened miscarriage use the 3X potency four times daily until crises has passed.

It relieves chronic articular gout, even when nodosities have begun to form, as well as arthritic pains of the periosteum, chest, head, as well as joints.

Worse from warm room or bed. Allergy to the sun.

**DOSE**- Tincture applied locally for warts. Internally, third to thirtieth potency. The mother tincture is prepared from the fresh tips of the twigs with leaves of the plant. The juice is expressed from the fresh leaves with a mortar, adding half its quantity of alcohol, rubbing the mixture for awhile, then expressing the juice, and adding two-thirds of its weight of alcohol. A clear liquid can be drawn off after a few days. Camphor and Pulsatilla are antidotes. Early provings were collated by Stapf with 14-16 provers using tincture from leaves.

## GEMMOTHERAPY

*Juniper communis* shoots are activators in cases of liver insufficiency. It is specific for a very deficient liver that fails to respond to regeneration in cases of jaundice, and cirrhosis caused by alcoholism.

Juniper's biological action is very deep, and should be taken for no more than six weeks. It eliminates urea and uric acid in retention, and treats nephritis, pyelitis and chronic cystitis.

It also gives good results in cases of air swallowing, by regulating the digestive system.

**DOSE**- 1D of the glycerin macerate. Take twenty to thirty drops daily alone or in small amount of water before meals.

## ESSENTIAL OILS

Juniper plant produces oils from the wood, leaves and berries. Work by Kostylschew et al, in 1931 issue of *Pflanzenphysiologie*, estimated up to 30 grams of terpenoids evaporate daily from a large juniper shrub. Good for a healthy environment.

### CADE
### (*J. oxycedrus*)

**CONSTITUENTS**- cadinol,d-cadinene, sesquiterpenes, dimethyl-naphthalene, quaiacol, cresol.
*J. communis* heartwood- 3.8% yield consisting of 27.2% alpha cedrene, 7.7% beta cedrene, 27.6% thujopsene, 15,8% cedrol, and minor amounts of widdrol, cuparene, and beta-cedrene
*J. scopulorum* heartwood- 3.4% yield consisting of nearly 58% thujopene, and minor amounts of various components listed for *J. communis*.

Cade oil is a dark orange, brown tar like substance produced by dry distilling the woody bark. It is smoky, leathery and used in small amounts in perfumery for leather or pine compositions (0.2%).

It is used by the food and fragrance industry for liquid smoke, and adding smoky flavour to meat and fish. This shrub is named in the bible as "heath".

Medicinally, it is used in salves for treatment of eczema, psoriasis and scalp problems. It was formerly combined with yellow wax to form an ointment called *Unquentum olei cadini.*

It is a common product in dandruff and hair loss shampoos and considerably safer than coal tar derivatives.

It was at one time applied to the penis for contraception, but I cannot vouch for neither the safety nor reliability of this use. It was used historically for corneal opacities, lice, and dental cavities with pain.

Internally, it is used for the removal of parasites, three to five drops in water.

It is used in two to three day intervals in old wounds and ulcers. Veterinarians use 1-5% cade oil ointments for parasitic skin problems.

## JUNIPER WOOD

*J.horizontalis* -10% of the dry weight is produced by an acetone extract of the wood. Petroleum ether extract yields 2.5%. This is similar to cade.

## JUNIPER BERRY

**CONSTITUENTS**- *J. communis* ripe berry- l-terpinen-4-ol, alpha pinene (53%), beta pinene, camphene; sesquiterpenes such as cadinene, and carophyllene. The black, ripe berries are richer in monoterpenes than the green. In unripe berries sabinene is nearly 14%, and myrcene 8%; whereas in ripe berries it is 15% myrcene and 5.5% sabinene.

The unripe green cones or berries contain a large amount of alpha pinene, with mycrene content increasing with ripening and beta phellandrene content decreasing.

The yield is fairly good from steam distillation (0.5 ml per 100 grams of berries).

Juniper berry oil acts on the skin, digestion, urinary tract, blood, nerves and respiration.

It is effective in viral, bacterial and fungal infections of various origins, the former thought due in part to the flavonoid amentoflavone. Extensive anti-microbial activity was found in work by Glisic et al, *J Serb Chem Soc* 2007 72:4 311-320.

The diuretic action of juniper oil is caused by irritating and enhancing the glomerular filtration; with potassium, sodium and chorine being excreted.

Work by Schilcher et al, noted above, found juniper berry oil quite varied in composition. Those oils with a low ratio of irritating terpenes to terpinen-4-ol (3:1) do not exhibit nephrotoxicity; but some oils have a hydrocarbon to alcohol ration as high as 55:1; and these would definitely irritate kidney tubules. *Arzne Forschung* 1997 47:7.

Rats given high doses of juniper oil suffered no kidney damage in above study.

Tacrolimus, used for immune suppression after organ transplants, can cause severe kidney damage. In vivo rat studies found juniper berry oil completely reversed the damage.

The renal cell membranes incorporated vasodilatory prostanoids, elevated PGF2-alpha urinary excretion, and prevented a precipitous fall in inulin clearance caused by the drug.

It is excellent for rheumatism and gout, and may be used externally in 5% dilution for relieving the pain associated with these conditions.

Juniper berry oil has a strengthening and tonic effect on the nerves and is indicated in states of anxiety and stress. It supports the spirit in challenging situations.

Medicinally, it is useful in oily and congested skin; and has anti-herpes properties. It can be used internally or externally for any number of skin problems due to its antiseptic and disinfecting nature.

It penetrates the skin and has a beneficial effect of inhibition of elastase associated with wrinkling, and aging. Mori et al, *J Cosmetic Dermatol* 2002 1.

Juniper berry oil has been found to inhibit bone resorption, suggesting use in the treatment of osteoporosis. Muhlbauer et al, *Bone* 2003:32.

Na et al, *Clinica Chim Acta* 2001:314 found the oil prevents the caspase-3 activation of human astrocyte CCF-STTG1 cells. Astrocytes are the most abundant glial cell types in the brain and their cell programmed death or apoptosis, is implicated in Alzheimer's and a number of central nervous system diseases.

Juniper berry oil is rich in 5, 11, 14-eicosatrienoic acid, a polyunsaturated fatty acid similar to that found in fish oils. Jones et al, *Hepatol* 1998:28 found the oil more effective than fish oil in protection of rat liver from reperfusion injury, a major cause of graft damage in liver transplants, as well as alcohol-induced liver damage.

The oil has been found to prevent organ rejection in test animals with kidney transplants. Butani et al, *Transplantation* 2003 76:2

The essential oil is effective in treatment of recurring or chronic upper respiratory tract infections association with *S. aureus* and *Pseudomonas aeruginosa*. Camporese A, *Infez Med* 2013 21(2).

The oil is used in soaps, detergents, lotions, creams and perfumes in up to 0.8% concentration.

Because the production of gin requires enormous amounts of berries, a poor quality essential oil is produced from the spent berries after fermentation. This oil is common in the market place and inferior for aromatherapy purposes.

Also, most gin distilled in England today, is flavoured with oil of turpentine. When used, only two pounds of berries are involved in production of 100 gallons of gin.

The LD50 of the essential oil in rats equals the equivalent of 375 grams for a 60 kilogram human.

## SABIN OIL

**CONSTITUENTS**- sabinyl acetate (40%), sabinene (20%), limonene, cymol, iso-thujone, cadinene, 1-8-cineole, terpin-4-ol, gamma terpinene, alpha pinene, and beta myrcene.

Sabin oil is a powerful irritant of the mucous membranes; with a strong effect on the nervous system. It should be approached with extreme caution, although the oils on the market are very often not derived from *J. sabina*.

Externally, the oil is useful in liniments for lumbar and sacral regions. Amenorrhea and sterility have been treated using small doses. It is reputed to cure genital and fig warts, presumably in full strength applied to the affected area.

Dr. Penoel mentions its use for various parasites, but it must be used with caution and never during pregnancy.

The oil develops increased toxicity with age, chiefly through the formation of terpene peroxides during storage.

The fresh tips of the branches have little toxicity, according to the PDR for Herbal Medicines; but the oil and alcohol extracts are quite toxic.

## JUNIPER LEAF

**CONSTITUENTS** *J. communis*- Contains from 44-63% alpha pinene, with lesser amounts of beta pinene, 3-carene, mycrene, cadinenes, sabinene, beta-elemene, spathulenol, muurolene, elemen-7-ol. Yield is 0.7-1.3%.
*J. horizontalis*- needle yields 0.9% rich in delta-sabinene (36%), limonene (17%), as well as delta terpinen-4-ol, alpha-cyparone, elemol, and alpha thujene. Distillation time will vary content of limonene, sabinene and alpha pinene.
*J. scopulorum* leaf oil is similar to above, and does not vary with the seasons or sex of the shrub.
*J. sibirica* leaf- alpha thuyene (46%), delta cadinene (6.3%).
*J. sabina*- sabinene (64%).

Juniper leaf oil is produced from various juniper species. The oil is green, fresh, and herbaceous, and blends well in woodsy and balsamic perfume creations.

It does not have the therapeutic properties of the berry oil.

# SEED OIL

The seed oil from *J. communis* yields over 20%; and is rich in linoleic (30%), palmitoleic (25%), stearic (12.5%) acids; as well as smaller amounts of arachidic, oleic and palmitic acid.

# WAX

A crude wax, extracted from the needles of *J. sabina* has a melting point of 73°C, saponification value of 241. It contains juniperic, sabinic and thapsic acids.

# HYDROSOL

**CONSTITUENTS-** terpinen-4-ol 75%, alpha terpineol 5%, linalool 3.6%, and other minor constituents like carone, thujone, p-cymene, eucalyptol, alpha phellandrene, and 2-butanone.

Juniper berry hydrosol tastes sort of like you would expect- a very dry martini! It has a very low pH 3.3 to 3.6, and yet is somewhat unstable and has less than a year of shelf life.

The hydrosol can be used for many of the same purposes as the herb.

Viaud considers the hydrolat diuretic, a kidney cleanser, and helpful in rheumatoid arthritis and skin problems.

Grosjean also suggests the hydrolat for rheumatism and all manner of acidic conditions. Two tablespoons in 1.5 litres of distilled water are taken during the day by individuals with a diabetic tendency.

Suzanne Catty warns to avoid it during the first trimester of pregnancy (prudent) and in cases of kidney disease (probably based on the repeated contraindication in nearly every herb book in print, but this may not be true).

She also recommends it for water retention and cellulite.

The hydrosol can be added to marinades, sauces and gravies according to Catty and Jeanne Rose.

Juniper berry water is distilled from the crushed, ripe black berries. It is for gravel of limbs and bladder, disease of members due to cold, helps one urinate, provokes menses and removes dead children from the womb.
**BRUNSCHWIG**

The leaf hydrolat is an astringent toner for oily and acne skin, according to Len and Shirley Price.

# FLOWER ESSENCES

The cone buds of the juniper are small, the yellowish male and green female on separate bushes. The flower essence made from the cone is for individuals that need psychic protection.

This is not like pink yarrow, but rather a more assertive and forceful approach that is present on the physical as well as psychic level.

The cone energy releases the internal shakiness, and internal fear that accompanies confrontation; whether imagined or not. It is for the individual that needs to surround themselves with positive vibrations, as an antidote to intuited or imagined threats; or fears about the future.

The energy of this cone bud is masculine, and assertive. It is indicated for the occasional shot of courage when personal credibility, or belief systems are challenged by authority figures. Remember, if you do something important, there will always be critics. If you don't like critics, don't do anything important.  **PRAIRIE DEVA**

Rocky Mountain Juniper essence enhances sensitivity and understanding of feminine moods and cycles. For women, this helps to affirm and celebrate their womanhood.

For men, it nourishes their feminine side.

It is for women, or men obsessed with body image, or those who hate their own bodies.        **CAN FOREST**

Juniper essence is for inner peace and contentment, to help focus on our own feelings and life instead of on others. It helps release worry, attachment to being recognized and appreciated.        **ICELANDIC**

Juniper essence is for renunciation of the past; generosity; relaxation; releasing old stresses; ancestral patterns.
**GREEN MAN**

Juniper essence is helpful for learning from one's mistakes and making the mistakes of others more tolerable.
**MIRIANA**

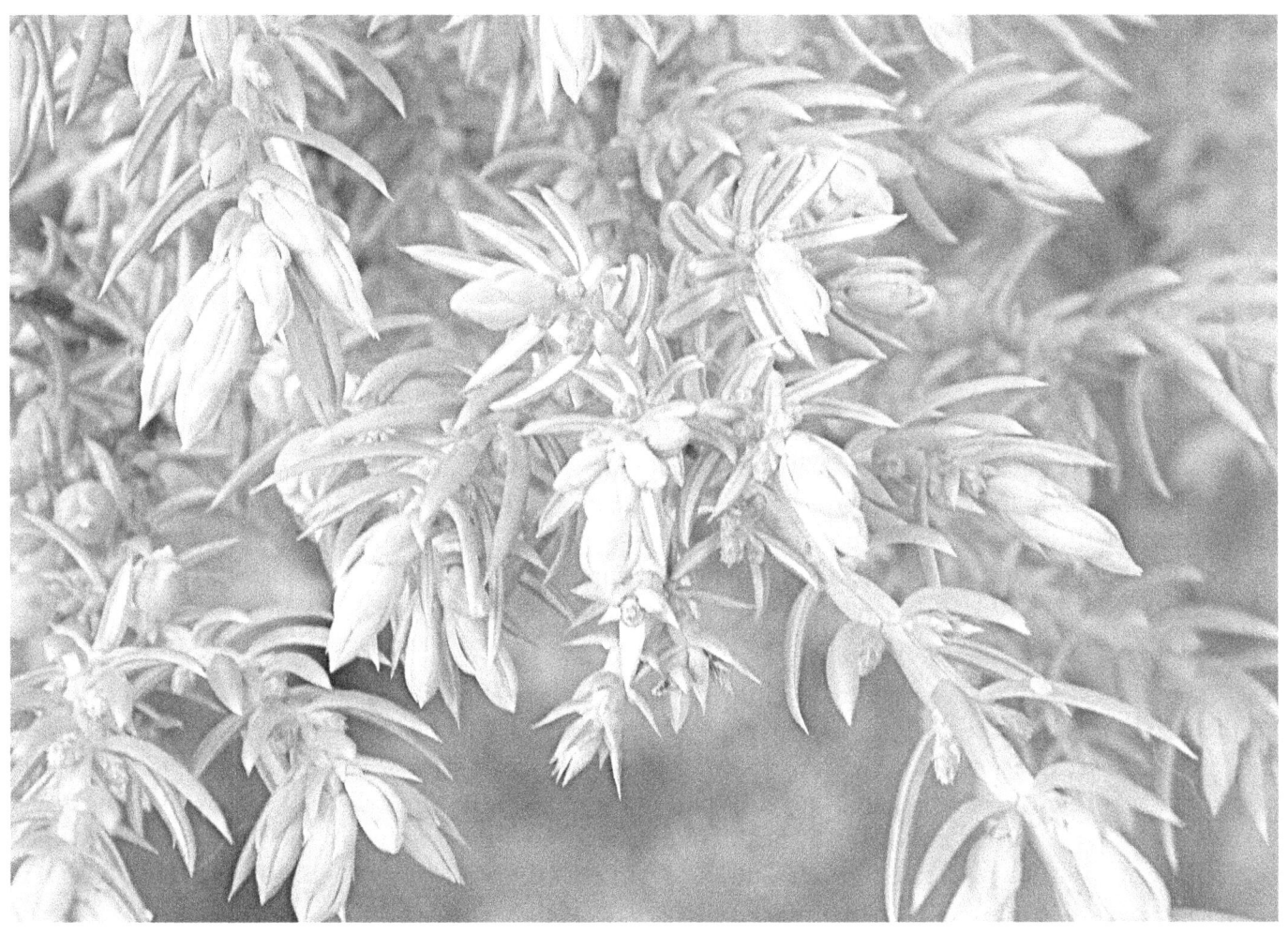

COMMON JUNIPER YOUNG NEEDLES

## PERSONALITY TRAITS

The Juniper person has swollen legs, with feet and ankles having little definition. The fluid retention is obvious in the upper arms, waist, face and under chin.

The negative Juniper fluid retention leads to disturbance of the adrenal glands; and adrenal hormone insufficiency can lead to this body shape and pre-diabetic imbalance.

Juniper berries provide abundant potassium to naturally excrete the excess fluid and stimulate kidneys. Lignin, present in the berries, adheres to the kidney tissue, and removes chalk, gravel and other impurities.

The positive juniper drinks fluid and urinates more; with no fluid retention.

Juniper, Jupiter, jovial and joyful. The personality of Juniper is hearty and fun loving. This is not only in nature but also around the waist. Falstaff, the gin imbibing, red-faced, rotund story-teller was a classic "Juniper".

**DOROTHY HALL**

The [Juniper] patient is...tired, lethargic, mentally dull and slightly depressed. The patient has poor appetite, weak and slow digestion, recurring flatulence and colic, a tendency to chronic phlegmy cough, and repeated respiratory infections. The patient also has chronic edema and a recurring ache and weakness in the lower back. The abdomen and lower back feel cold and damp.

**ROSS**

The Juniper personality is radical in that they have no concern for human authority, preferring to be directed by their intuition or religious belief. They have a reverence for anything sacred and will inevitably take a spiritual path through life…the Juniper personality has a profound spiritual ease that is obvious to all who come into contact with them.

When they're negative, Junipers appear very vulnerable, as if their very soul is being attacked.

Junipers are best suited to professions that allow them freedom of thought and speech…they often wrongly feel that they will never find their soul mate or true love. **WORWOOD**

Juniper Berry's key words are: trust, stalwart and dependable. It transmits surety and helps one to rebuild trust in the face of fear. **E. MULDERS**

The juniper alcoholic tends to non-violent, melancholic, morose and withdrawn. When the juniper type drinks, the alcohol does not fuel rage, but rather, it helps to sustain his need for withdrawal from life's relentless assaults. The juniper alcoholic craves a barroom's sheltering darkness and quietness and is moved by songs of pain and loss coming from the jukebox. Juniper is associated with the sycotic miasm, a keynote of which is secretiveness…The hiding of the juniper type is a strategic retreat, a self-imposed isolation due to the feeling that one is misunderstood and unsupported by others. In concert with his desire to withdraw, a type of aloofness due to acquired skepticism, cynicism, loss of social confidence and an inability to place trust in themselves or others should guide the blender to juniper oil. **BRUCE BERKOWSKY**

The seeds of all the junipers have a mind of their own. They have dormant embryos and impermeable seed coats. They have inhibitors to germination either in the seed coat or in the outer fleshy portion of the berry … they are matched perfectly to the intestinal flora of the large birds that eat them. The seeds will go through the digestive tract of a raven or large game bird and come out smiling in the acid-rich silt and pop up as an epigeal germinator with the plumule, or baby seed head, coming heads-up first. It would appear that the big birds need the juniper in its ecofunction just as much as the juniper needs the birds. **BERESFORD-KROEGER**

If I wished to differentiate between the *J. sabina* and *J. communis*, I should say that the former has a greater affinity for the generative organs, while the latter affected in preference the urinary organs.

Both, however, have similar properties; both affect the uterus and kidneys. It is not so much a difference of mode of action as a difference of degree of action.

I have known cases of dysmenorrheal and uterine haemorrhage cured by the common juniper, and I have treated some kidney and bladder difficulties with Sabina. The popularity of pure gin in dysmenorrheal is owing to the effects of the oil of Juniper berries, which it contains. In domestic practice, an infusion of Juniper leaves and berries is used successfully in amenorrhea and dysmenorrheal, as well as retention, suppression, and other urinary troubles. **HALE**

## SPIRITUAL PROPERTIES

Flutes made from juniper wood were highly regarded by the Cheyenne. Two kinds were made, both for courting, and were played only at night: one was simply for making music; the other was made by men who were believed to possess peculiar powers and were able to charm a girl whom a man loved and to make her love him.

To make a flute, a cylinder of juniper wood about 18 inches long was split. Each half was whittled out to make a shell. Glue and a lashing of sinew or deerskin strings held the two halves together, and six finger holes were made with a hot iron.

In earlier days, flutes were ornamented with porcupine quills wrapped around the instrument near the mouthpiece and between the holes. In recent times, ornamentation was usually of beadwork. Below the mouthpiece, the figure of an animal, often a horse or bear, was carved, or a snake or duck head was made at the end.

The odor of burning juniper is the sweetest fragrance on the face of the earth, in my honest judgment; I doubt if all the smoking censers of Dante's paradise could equal it. One breath of juniper smoke...evokes in magical catalysis, like certain music, the space and light and clarity and piercing strangeness of the American West. Long may it burn.                                                                                                                    **EDWARD ABBEY**

The aromatic properties of all parts of Juniper plants have been used against bad magic, plague, and various negative influences in so many cultures… If unrelated traditions say that Yarrow clots blood, it is easy to accept that it is probably the case; if we say that Juniper clears "bad vibes", many of us back off and start to twitch skeptically. Our mechanistic approach to "primitivism" is too selective, accepting the possibility of drug effect on one hand and nervously rejecting something as subjective as warding off of bad influences on the other.                                                                                                     **MICHAEL MOORE**

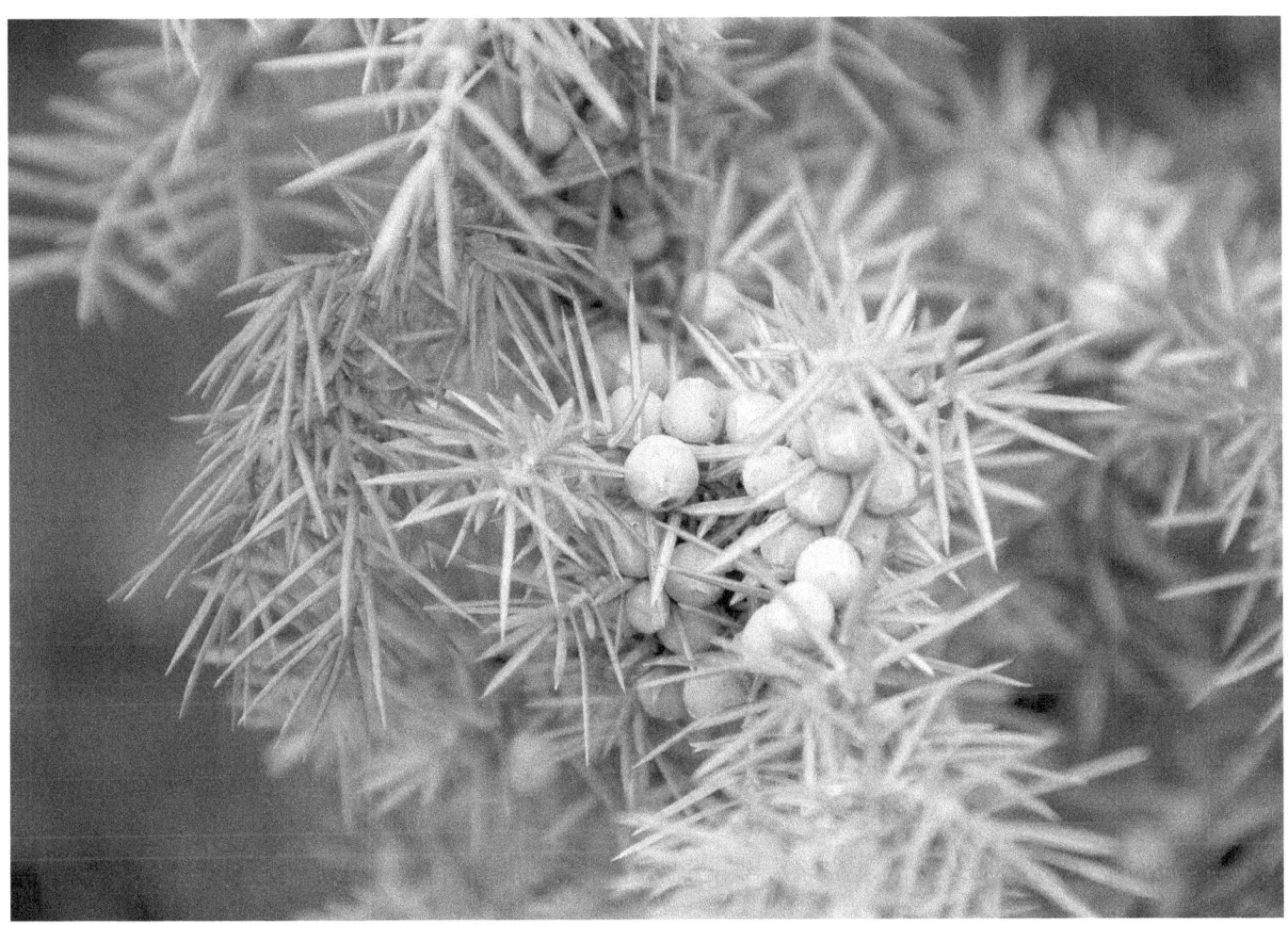

COMMON JUNIPER NEEDLES AND UNRIPE CONES

## DOCTRINE OF SIGNATURES

Juniperus has the number three in its signature, as the botanical features demonstrate. The Furies, associated with the plant, were three in number. There is Tisiphone the Avenger of Blood, Alecto the Implacable and Megaera the Jealous One.

Swedish folklore assigns great significance to this. For making ointments or medicines three twigs were taken on the third day of the week. To treat toothache, three berries were held in the mouth. Beverages made from juniper berries were required to ferment for three days.                                                                                            **VERMEULEN**

# MYTHS AND LEGENDS

In Grimms' Fairy Tale, The Juniper Tree, a pregnant woman eats the berries of the juniper growing in her garden, and as a result becomes ill and lives only until the birth of a son. She is then buried beneath the juniper tree. The father marries a woman with a daughter, who schemes to have all of the father's wealth left to her daughter, rather than her stepson. She beheads the stepson, and feed a stew of his flesh to his father. His half-sister lays her brother's bones under the juniper tree.

The bones are transformed into a bird with magical strength, and he lifts a huge milestone and drops it onto his stepmother, killing her. The bird is transformed back to a child, who lives happily thereafter. **SMALL**

## BOTANICA POETICA

If you need to urinate
Juniper might be for you
The kidneys it will stimulate
It's an antiseptic too
It's not for a pregnant or nursing mom
The volatile oils do not please
Its heavy resins, kidneys harm
Avoid for kidneys in disease
Collect the berries when they're ripe
Crush, infuse, make an extraction
It might improve your appetite
Clears your gas and help digestion
And when you go to Louie's Pub
For booze and lust and other sin
Let it be known that Juniper Berry
Is flavouring your shot of gin!

## SYLVIA CHATROUX MD

# RECIPES

**INFUSION**-Take from 2 to 10 grams of crushed berries to one pint of boiling water. Steep twenty minutes. Drink four ounces up to four times daily. Daily dose is 2-10 grams of the berries.

**TINCTURE**- berries- Fifteen drops three times daily before meals. The dried berries are tinctured at 1:5 in 75% alcohol.

**JUNIPER WINE**- One ounce of berries and one half ounce of leaves. Chop well and add to litre of wine. Steep four days. Take 3-4 ounces before or during meals.

**ESSENTIAL OIL**- berry- The daily dose is 20-100 mg of essential oil of *J. communis*.

**CAUTION**- Sabin oil- very toxic- as little as 6 drops toxic; death can occur from respiratory arrest in from 10 hours to several days.

The oil is used to counteract the overdose of cardiac medications like digitalis/foxglove.

For treatment of suspected poisoning, castor oil, followed by gastric lavage or emesis; followed immediately with a saline cathartic. Treat the symptoms, and then give milk and plenty of fluids.

**JUNIPER BERRY JUICE**- commercially available as directed.

**SAVIN LEAF POWDER**- for the treatment of fig warts, apply twice daily.

**JUNIPER CURE**- from a famous European spa. On the first day, five fully ripe and dried berries are eaten. One the second day six, and so on, up to fifteen berries. Then the order is reduced, until down to five again. The berries are chewed in divided doses, three times daily. Do not ingest fresh berries, as they will strongly stimulate and irritate the gastric mucosa.

**JUNIPER ALE**- There are seven different versions of Juniper Ale used in Norway. Here is a modern version.

Boil two pounds of juniper branches with berries for one hour in seven gallons of water. Remove branches. Mash five pounds of two-rowed malted barley with two gallons of juniper water for 90 minutes.

Sparge with the remaining water, boil the wort until reduced to five gallons. Let cool to 70F, pour into fermenter, and add yeast. Ferment until finished, prime with 1/2 tsp sugar, fill and cap. Ready in one month.   **BUHNER**

**CAUTION**- Do not use any juniper products internally during pregnancy and **severe** kidney inflammation.

## KNOW MOTHER ROOT
## ANT'S EGGS MOTHER
(***Anemarrhena asphodeloides*** Bunge)
**PARTS USED**- rhizome

I learned so much in Laos. I learned that fried silkworm larvae are delicious. I learned how to make ant-egg salad.   **RUTH REICHI**

Know Mother Root is a literal and poor translation from Mandarin. It resembles Asphodel in appearance and is a night flowering plant.

The herb's use was first recorded in an Herbal by Shen Nung around 200 AD.

This hardy perennial (zone 2) looks like a tall grass, but has beautiful yellow-white, and sometimes light purple flowers that are wonderfully fragrant in early evening of late summer/early fall.

The plant is actually a night blooming lily, which after the first year, projects an elongated raceme of flower clusters. They are pollinated by moths, and grow easily from seed. It is now placed in the Asparagaceae family, sub-family Agavoideae.

It was successfully trialed by Alberta Natural Health Agricultural Network members from northern Alberta for hardiness. I suggested we research its viability and it proved to be extremely robust, and could be widely grown for the organic herbal market.

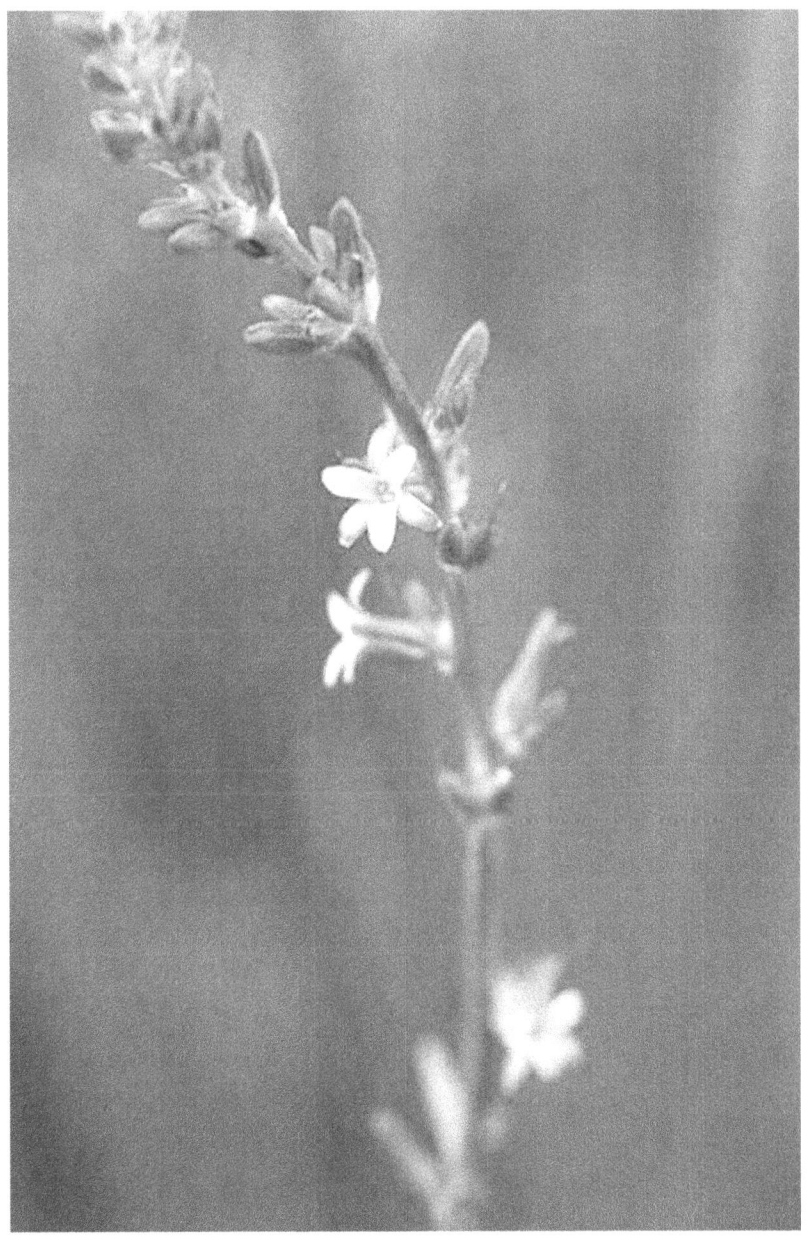

**KNOW MOTHER ROOT FLOWERS**

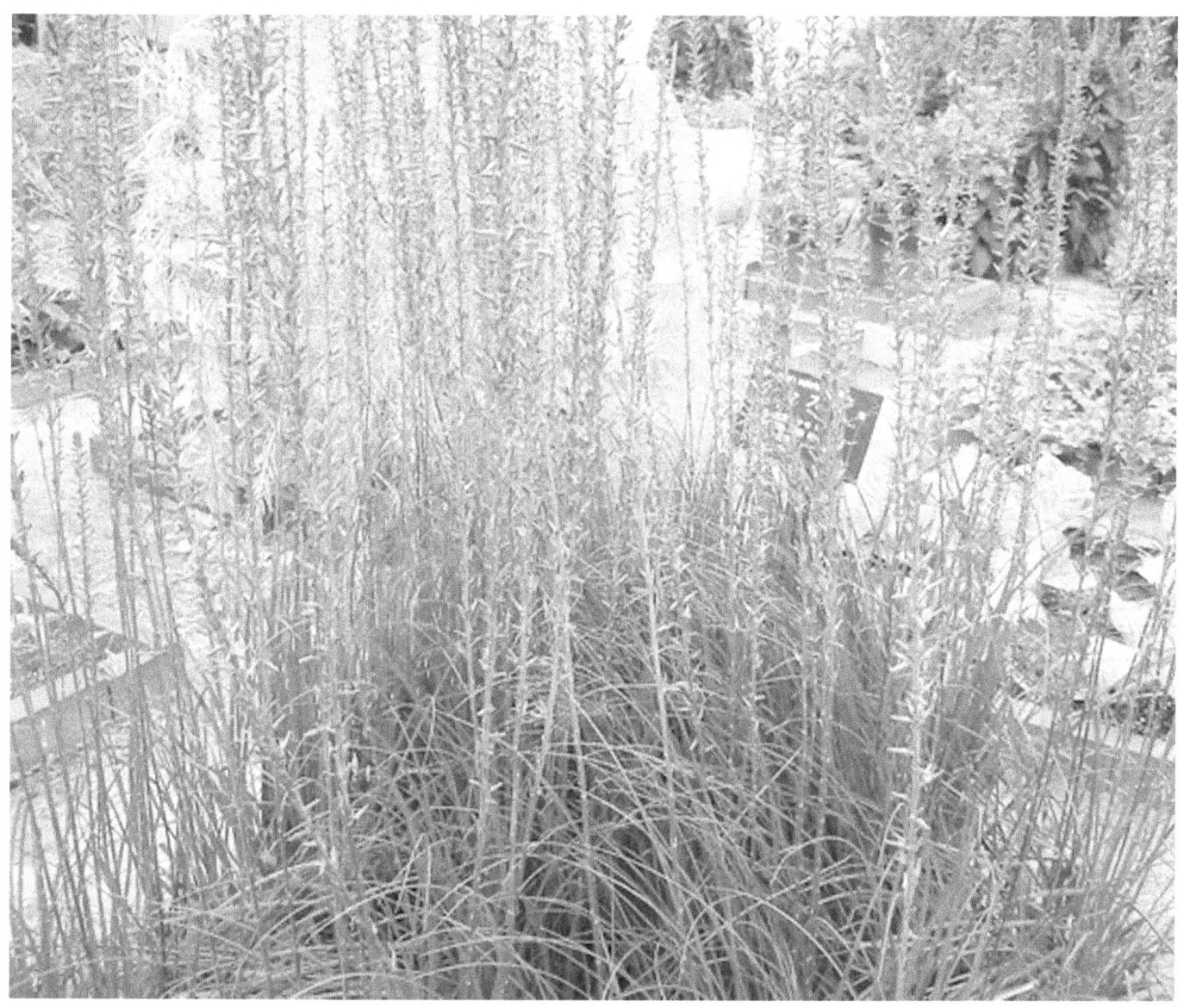

KNOW MOTHER ROOT

# MEDICINAL

**CONSTITUENTS**- rhizome- various steroidal and furostanol saponins (6%), including anemarsaponin B 11 (012-1.48%), timosaponins B1-2, A1-4, D, E1-2, F, X and Y, timopregnane B, anemarrhenasponins I and Ia, hinokiresinol, oxy-hinokiresinol, cis-hinokresinol, 4'-methyl-cis-hinoki-resinol; anemarans A-D, aglycones, sarsapogenin, markogenin, asphonin, and neogitogenin; timbiose, xanthose, isomaniferin; glycans-anemarans A-D, C-glucoside (xanthone), mangiferin (1.3%), tannins, mucilage, fatty acids, vitamins B3 and B5, procathechic acid, (-)-nyasol.

Know Mother Root, and Ant's Eggs Mother are two of several most unusual names for this beautiful medicinal lily.

Zhi Mu has been long used in Traditional Chinese Medicine. It also goes by Chih Mu, meaning Ant Egg Mother, Ti Mu, Cicada Mother, Ku Xin, and Di Shen, meaning Earth Ginseng. In Mandarin it may be found as **HUO MU**, meaning Goods Matrix, or in Cantonese as **JI MOU**.

In Japanese Kampo Medicine, the rhizome is known as **CHIMO**.

Oriental herbalists use it to treat heat in the hands and feet, relieve high fever, and coughs with heat and yellow sputum.

Two forms are available from Chinese herbalists, **MAO CHIH MU** with the root peel intact, and **KUANG CHIH MU** with the brown covering removed.

Both are very useful in dealing with hot and dry conditions, such as bronchitis with insufficient mucous or expectoration.

The root is sweet, bitter and oily, and helps restore through its moist, cool, and calming influence.

In some ways, it is similar to *Lilium brownii*, and combines synergistically for the treatment of depression, possibly due to regulation of noradrenaline and 5-hydroxytryptamine (5-HT). Du H et al, *J Pharm Biomed Anal* 2016 128: 469-79.

It is interesting to note in TCM, that over half of the dozen or so respiratory restoratives are in the lily family, and that most contain mucilage and saponins, in their main biochemical makeup.

Know mother root is combined with *Astragalus* root and American/Canadian Ginseng in helping restore respiratory health. This includes symptoms such as chronic dry cough, acute bronchitis, pneumonia and even tuberculosis.

It is a heat-clearing herb with some Yin moistening properties that combine well with Amur Cork Bark for yin deficiency with heat, or Goldthread for heat and deficient saliva production. Think berberine rich herbs as a substitute.

For the latter condition, also think of Northern Prickly Ash bark.

A combination of Know mother root and goldthread ameliorates colitis and rheumatoid arthritis, by correcting the Th17/Treg imbalance, and inhibiting inflammation by regulating innate immunity. Lim SM et al, *Biomol Ther* (Seoul) 2016 24(6): 638-49.

Mangiferin (and neomangiferin) content may play a role in correcting the Th17/Treg cells in colitis. Lim SM et al, *Int Immunopharmacol* 2016 34: 220-8; Lim SM et al, *Phytomedicine* 2016 23(2): 131-40.

Like astragalus and American ginseng, the root is considered a pituitary and adrenal restorative, particularly in cases of exhaustion, poor stamina, and adrenal weakness.

Ren et al, *Pharmazie* 2007 62(1): 78-9 found evidence of anti-depressant activity.

Therefore, it has a role in night sweats and menopause, combining well with black cohosh or baneberry, and can be combined with borage for adrenal restoration after cortisone therapies.

For dizziness, night sweats, and vertigo, it is often combined with berberine rich herbs; or with figwort in the treatment of mouth ulcers, and bleeding gums.

The root helps arthritis conditions that are warm to the touch and aggravated by the heat of bed at night, especially in the lower limbs.

It combines well with flowers of Japanense Honeysuckle (*Lonicera japonica*) to increase osteogenesis and decrease osteoclastogenesis in stem and bone marrow cells. Seo BK et al, *J Ethnopharm* 2016 193: 227-36.

When the root is stir-fried, **CHAO ZHI MU**, it lessens the cooling nature of the uncooked.

Another form, salt mixed fried root, is often used for evening fever, night sweats, and oliguria or anuria due to kidney yin vacuity accompanied by damp heat of the bladder.

The root contains a high level of steroid saponins that the body can make use of for hormone production. It exhibits cortisone-like effects. The timosaponins appear to inhibit platelet aggregation.

At the same time, it is balancing to urogential excitation, including premature ejaculation, increased sex drive and seminal incontinence in men. As a sexual sedative, it is an excellent cooling and restorative herb when "deficient heat" from adrenal depletion is noted. One constituent of the root inhibits testosterone 5 alpha reductase activity, suggesting its use in preventing benign prostate enlargement. One TCM formula contains the root, amur cork bark and motherwort.

In one study of the herbal combination on 80 patients with benign prostatic hypertrophy, an 86% improvement was noted. *Zhong Xi Yi Jie He Za Zhi* 1988 3:155.

The steroid saponins, in mice studies, exhibit promotion of bone formation but not inhibition of bone resorption, as well as prevention of uterine atrophy. Nian et al, *Acta Pharm Sinica* 27:6.

The root has been shown to retard the catabolism of cortisol by liver cells.

This same damp heat can affect the bladder creating painful and scanty urination, low grade and intermittent fevers and thirst. Lab studies have confirmed the roots anti-pyretic effect. Research on rabbits inoculated with *E. coli* found the water extract decreased their fevered body temperature.

It is helpful in cases where extreme restlessness and thirst are not relieved by drinking cold water.

The rhizome can be used in cases of high blood sugar, or when stomatitis, or pancreatitis is threatening digestive health. In laboratory studies on rabbits, water extracts given orally reduced blood sugar levels aggravated by alloxan.

Ichiki et al, *Bio Pharm Bulletin* 1998 21:12 showed mangiferin and its glucoside lowered blood glucose levels orally in laboratory mice. More recent study by the same author in the *Journal of Natural Medicine* 2007 61:2 found inhibition of a-glucosidase and aldose reductase associated with eye health.

This may be due to the content of mangiferin or a range of bio-chemicals.

Mangiferin appears to moderate IgE responses and pruritis, suggesting usage in topical creams. Lee B et al, *Planta Medica* 75:3.

It had no influence on blood glucose in control mice, and improved hyperinsulinaemia in mice bred for non-insulin dependent diabetes mellitus. It is often combined with goldthread (3:1 ratio) when treating patients. Traditional Chinese Medicine texts suggest it helps increase the metabolism of sugar and increases glycogen synthesis in the liver. It has no effect on insulin release.

Work by Nakashima et al, *Journal of Nat Products* 1993 56:3 showed the herb lowered blood sugar levels by increasing the production of glycogen stored by the liver.

Another pathway is via rhizome steroids that inhibit alpha glucosidase by 4.6 fold compared to drug acarbose. Khang PV et al, *J Asian Nat Prod Res* 2016 23:1-6.

It combines well with schisandra berry for diabetes due to yin deficiency.

Timosaponins are believed responsible, as they act by inhibiting hepatic gluconeogenesis and/or glycogenolysis in a dose dependant manner. Timosaponin B-11 reduced palmitate-induced insulin resistance and inflammation . Yuan YL et al, *Am J Chin Med* 2016 44(4): 755-69.

Timpsaponin B-11 inhibits acetylcholinesterase and prevents oxidative stress, suggesting potential benefit on cognitive and behavioral impairment. Zhao X et al, *Metab Brain Dis* 2016 31(6): 1455-61. The saponin also ameliorates diabetic nephropathy. Yuan YL et al, *Drug Des Devel Ther* 2015 9:6247-58.

The rhizome may be useful in the treatment of acute renal failure, possibly due to content of neomangiferin, mangiferin and isomangiferin. Seo CS et al, *Nat Prod Commun* 2014 9(6): 829-32.

It may also have potential benefit in preventing ischemic heart disease like myocardial infarction, based on a rat study. Deng XY et al, *Chem Biol Interact* 2015 240:22-8.

Nyasol and broussonin A may suppress iNOS as a possible mechanism of reducing inflammation. Jin Lee E et al, *Chem Biodivers* 2014 11(5): 749-59.

Timpsaponin A111 induces apoptosis in HeLa cancer cells, and inhibits the growth of human colorectal cancer cells. It also inhibits migration and invasion of A549 human non-small cell lung cancer cells. Jung O et al, *Bioorg Med Chem Lett* 2016 26(16):3963-7. The steroidal saponin also induces apoptosis in human melanoma A375-S2 cancer cells, without obvious side effects on normal cells. Wang Y et al, *Arch Pharm Res* 2017 40(1): 69-78. It appears to inhibit melanoma cell migration, necessary for metastasis, by inhibiting expression of COX-2, NFkappaB, PGE2 and PGE2 receptors. Kim KM et al, *Cancer Sci* 2016 107(2): 181-8

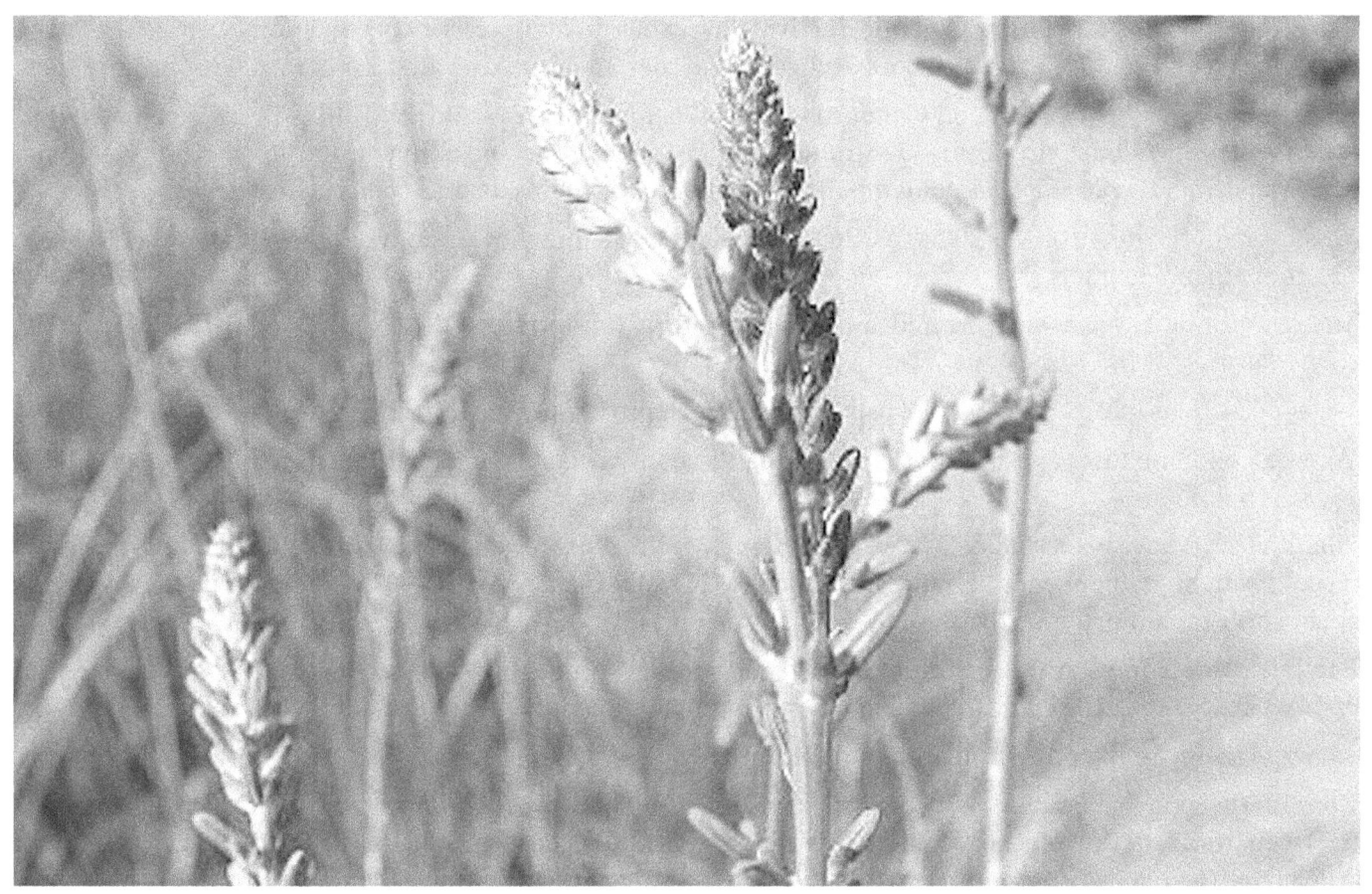

UNOPENED FLOWERS

It also induced multi-drug resistance in human chronic myelogenous leukemia cells, and regained adrimycin sensitivity. Chen JR et al, *Int J Oncol* 48(5): 2063-70.

It probably work by inducing HL-60 apoptosis through JNK1/2 pathways, and may be a useful adjunct for acute myeloid leukemia. Huang HL et al, *Tumour Biol* 2015 36(5): 3489-97.

Timosaponin D displays anti-proliferative activity against HepG2 and SGC7901 cancer cell lines. Yang BY et al, *Molecules* 2016 21(8).

The rhizome contains a wealth of saponins that appear cytotoxic to cancer cells. Three compounds exhibit stronger inhibition against A549, HepG2 and Hep3B cell lines than the drug 5-fluorouracil (5-FU). Sun Y et al, *Bioorg Med Chem Lett* 2016 26(13): 3081-5.

The root shows potent inhibition of adipogenic activity suggestive of benefit in obesity. Youn et al, *J Nat Prod* 2009 72:10.

Kimura et al, *Phytotherapy Research* 1999 13:6 looked at the hypoglycemic effects of water extracts of ginseng, licorice and know mother. All lowered blood glucose levels in diabetic mice, but when combined, the effects were less than as individual herbs.

Hoa et al, *Methods Find Exp Clin Pharmacol* 2009 31:3 found the root to lower blood sugar levels in lab mice. The phenolic fraction may also play a role in reducing insulin resistance in adipocytes via regulation of AMP-kinase activity. Zhao W et al, *Planta Medica* 2014 80(2-3): 146-52.

The root possesses anti-inflammatory activity. Ji-Yeon Kim et al, *Food Chem Tox* 47:7. It also decreased diabetes related beta amyloid inflammation of the brain. Liu et al, *J Ethnopharm* 139:1.

Externally, the rhizome exhibits anti-fungal activity that can be used in a variety of conditions such as ringworm, or athlete's foot. For this purpose, make a decoction and soak affected area with a hot fomentation, or foot soak.

Iida et al, Journal of Ag and Food Chemistry, 1999 47:2 identified nyasol ([Z]-1,3-bis [4-hydroxyphenyl]-1, 4-pentadiene), with activity against 37 strains of fungi and bacteria, including various *Bacillus spp., Shigella, Vibrio cholerae, E. coli, Staphylococcus aureus, Streptococcus hemolyticus,* and *Diplococcus pneumoniae.*

Most were in the range of 100-200 MIC after seven days, but some showed activity at levels as low as 12.5 and 25, from ethanol extracts.

The compound (-)-nyasol is strongly anti-inflammatory, inhibiting COX-2, iNOS and 5-LOX. Lim et al, *Arch Pharm Res* 2009 32:11.

Water decoctions inhibit the growth of pathogenic dermatophytes such as *Achorion schoenleini* and *A. violaceum.*

Water/alcohol mixtures appear active against six anti-enterovirus 71 agents. Liu M et al, J *Chromatogr A* 2014 1368: 116-24.

Hinokresinols have been studied by Lee et al, *Planta Medica* 1999 65:4 and show moderate binding affinity to receptors on human polymorphonuclear leukoctyes (IC value of 5.24 microM). This suggests usefulness in the area of anti-inflammatory activity.

Earlier work shows hinokiresinol and its derivatives possess significant inhibitory activities on cAMP phosphodiesterase in vitro, and potentiate barbital influence. Nikaido et al, *Planta Medica* 1981 43.

Sarasapogenin, on the other hand, inhibits the activity of ATPase.

Jeong, in the same publication, isolated two norlignans (cis hinokresinol and 1,3-di-p-hydroxyphenyl-4-penten-1-one) with hyaluronidase inhibitory activity. This mechanism is present in plants such as Echinacea, and helps prevent cellular destruction by viruses, as well as the breakdown of tissue in auto-immune rheumatic/arthritic conditions.

A close follow-up study in volume 7, by Meng et al, found various new timosaponins stimulated superoxide generation from peripheral human blood cells.

The herb can inhibit platelet aggregation, and of Na, K-ATP-ase and of DNA-polymerase.

Work by Li ZS et al, *Yao Xue Xue Bao* 2003 38:7 suggests the root saponins may have benefit on cardiovascular disease by modulating the function of vein endothelial cells.

A good review of the ethnopharmacology, phytochemistry and pharmacology up to 2013 was written by Wang Y et al, *J Ethnopharm* 2014 153(1): 42-60.

## RECIPES

**DECOCTION**- 6-15 grams. The root is collected in spring or fall and dried in sun. The rhizome is sliced and stir-baked with salt.

**TINCTURE**- 2-4 ml. The tincture is prepared from the fresh root at 1:3 and 60% or dry root 1:5 at 40%.

**FRESH ROOT GLYCERITE**- 4-6 ml.

**CAUTION**- Do not use this root in cases of loose stool associated with digestive deficiency, and yin deficient heat as it helps clear excessive heat.

Do not use in diarrhea or spleen/stomach cold conditions. It is a yin boosting remedy, but should not be taken in large amounts or for too long, as this may actually damage yin.

This remedy is for hot, dry, inflamed conditions, and relies on its cold, oily demulcent properties to work. Large amounts at one time may cause sudden drop in blood pressure. Be aware.

The root should be harvested in August, and dried for a long time at a low temperature for best results, in retaining important constituents.

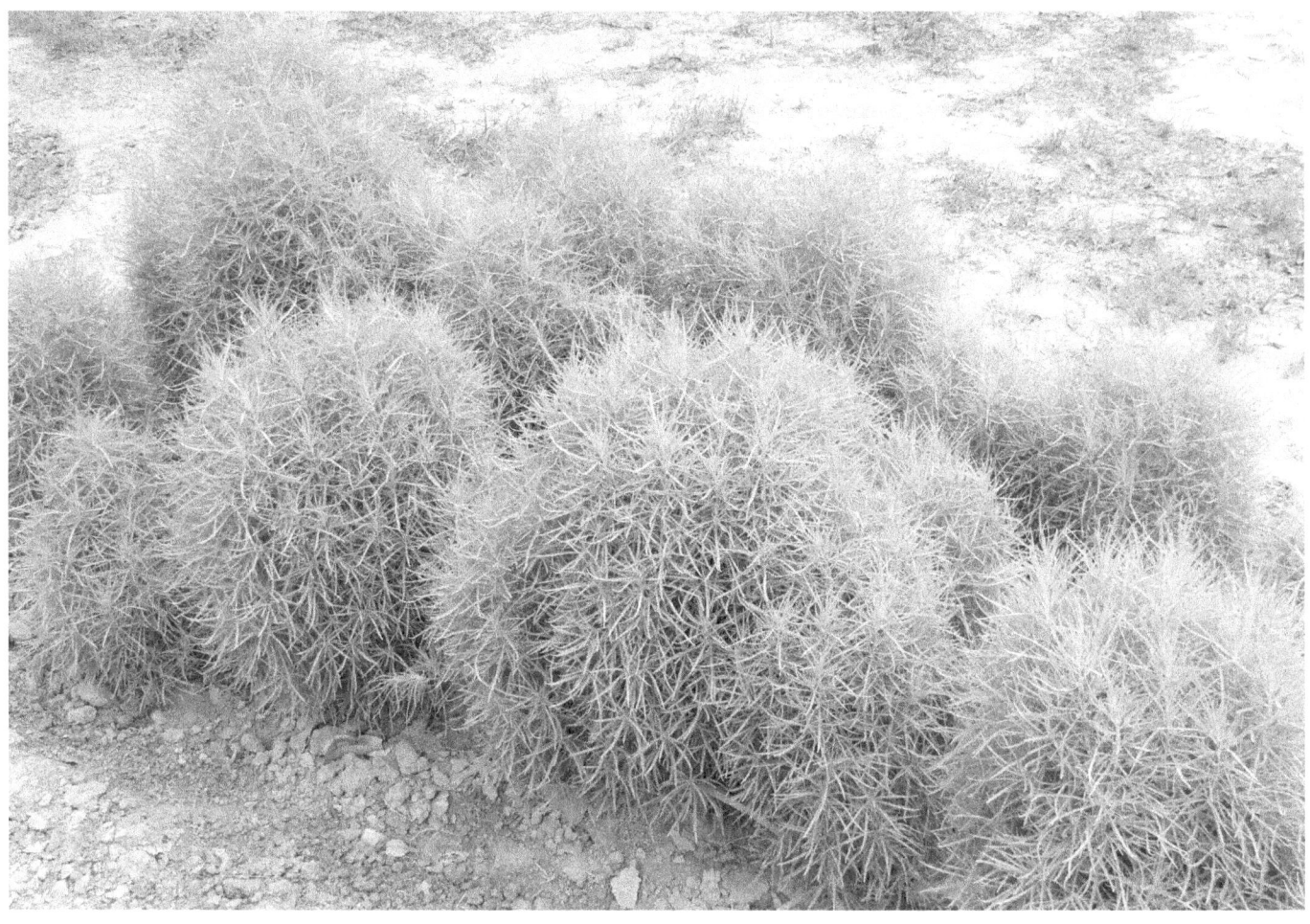

KOCHIA

**KOCHIA**
**BELVEDERE**
(**Kochia scoparia** [L.] Schrad.)
(**Bassia scoparia** [L.] A. J. Scott.) not accepted
(**Chenopodium scoparia**) not accepted
**FIVE HOOK BASSIA**
(**B. hyssopifolia** [Pall.] Kuntze)
**PARTS USED**- seeds, leaves

I've been learning a lot about how to make a martini and all the variation that you can have with a few ingredients with Belvedere.
                                                            **STEPHANIE SIGMAN**

**SCOPARIA** means broom-like, from the Latin, an obvious reference to its look and common usage. **KOCHIA** was named in honour of Dr. Wilhelm Koch, a famous German Botanist at Erlangen University. Belvedere, a name given before 1597, means beautiful view, in reference to the fiery pinks, reds and purple colors. The name was usurped by a cigarette company much later.

Bassia is named after Ferdinando Bassi, an 18th century botanist that first described a related species.

In some older herbals, the plant was assigned *Chenopodium scoparia*. This is interesting because lamb's quarters (*C. album*) is sometimes used medicinally as a substitute in parts of China. Artists in the country use branches and leaves of *Bassia* species for calligraphy brushes.

Kochia is a common annual weed of the plains, preferring the dry, alkaline soils common to southern Alberta and Saskatchewan. It is often found along railway lines.

Plant nurseries often sell Burning Bush, or Red Summer Cypress var. *trichophylla* as an ornamental that turns bright red-violet in fall.

The young shoots make an acceptable potherb. The seeds can be ground up for use as a flour, or cooked whole as a form of porridge.

In Japan, the fruit of *Kochia scoparia* is used as a food garnish, called **TONBURI**.

Studies have shown that it can yield 3-5 tons of fodder per acre- exceptional for the type of soil it favors. It contains very low concentrations of methionine and cystine, but is a boron accumulator.

It grows like tumbleweed, and can be used to make a broom. Recent proposals have suggested using Kochia for artificial firewood, or fuel briquettes.

The Navaho used a species of Kochia for healing external sores. The Cree of Alberta call it, **MACIKWANASA KA TIHTIPIPAYIHK**.

The Chinese combine Kochia seeds with alum as a wash for treating warts, and combine both herb and seeds to treat uro-gential problems. An older Chinese name is **QIAN XIN JINU**, meaning Thousand Minded Prostitute. Other names include **TI FU TZU** meaning ground cover, **DI FU ZI** meaning earth skin seed, and **SAO CHOU TS'AI**, broom grass.

The bush was formerly grown for raising silkworms, which form their cocoons on the twigs.

Five Hook Bassia (*B. hyssopifolia*) is generally found on saline soil in the southern prairies.

**CAUTION**- the use of Kochia for forage should be controlled as excessive intake can intoxicate animals. Canadian researchers have studied it for livestock feed potential. It appears insoluble oxalates are excreted by animals without harm, but soluble oxalates are absorbed into the blood stream.

It can cause serious photosensitization in animals and people under certain circumstances.

Kochia poisoning in cattle has been shown to produce polio encephalomalacia, blindness, gastro-intestinal disorders, liver cirrhosis, and rumen impaction, a condition very similar to Beath's blind staggers.

# MEDICINAL

**CONSTITUENTS**- n-alkanes, and esters, sterols including campestrol, stigmasterol and sitosterol (71%), quercitin, harmane, harmine, betanin, phyllocactin, ferulic, caffeic, cholorogenic and phenolic acids, saponins, and tannins.
fruit-various triterpenoid glycosides including momordin Ic, the 6'-methyl ester of momordin Ic, momordin IIc, 2'-O-beta-D-glucopyranosylmomordin Ic, 2'-O-beta-D-glucopyranosylo-momodin IIc; oleanolic acids; kochianosides 1-IV; fatty acids, and 20% saponins. Also include tectorigenin, pratensein, iriflogenin, fumalic acid, N-transferuloyltyramine, stigmasterol, oleanolic acid, beta-stigmasterol, daucosterol.
*B. hyssopifolia*- betaine- 180 mmol/kg of dry plant material.

Kochia seeds, **DI-FU-ZI** in Mandarin; **DEI FU JI** in Cantonese, are used in Traditional Chinese medicine for dispersing wetness and heat, stopping itching, and promoting urination. Because the seed resembles wheat it is sometimes called **TI MAI** or **DI KUI**, meaning Earth Big Flower.

They are often added to formulas for painful, turbid and difficult urination, or where the patient has a sudden need to urinate. Impotence formulas often contain the seeds, if the symptoms fit. It is used in inflammation or pain of the testicles, and combines well with Yellow Loosestrife and Akebia caulis.

Vaginal discharges, jock itch, eczema, sores, scabies, pruritis and other damp skin afflictions are soothed internally, and topically. A mixture of rose and kochia extracts showed therapeutic activity for photo aging skin. Jeon H et al, *Int J Mol Sci* 2016 17(11).

The seeds have broad-spectrum anti-fungal and anti-bacterial properties. In TCM, kochia seed and amur cork bark are decocted, and a saturated tampon is inserted vaginally for treating yeast infections.

This combination is also effective for carbuncles, sores and eczema taken internally.

For urinary tract infections during pregnancy, use alone; but otherwise combine with licorice root, plantago seed, and umbrella polypore.

Research confirms the anti-pruritic effect of the oleanolic glycosides in Kochia seeds. This is helped by anti-allergic activity in the seeds, probably due to momordin Ic. Matsuda et al, suggest kochia seeds inhibit humoral immunity and influence cellular immunity; and reduce both pain and anti-inflammatory responses. *Biological and Pharmaceutical Bulletin* 1997 20:10. Kochia seed modulates IgG response, which has great importance in allergy and chronic inflammatory conditions.

The seeds show a low LC50 against neuroblastoma cell lines, suggestive of anti-tumor potency. Mazzio et al, *Phytother Res* 2008 Oct 9.

Choi et al, suggests that momordin Ic and its aglycone oleanolic acid, may be of benefit in rheumatoid arthritis. *Arch Pharm Res* 2002 25:3.

Alcohol extracts of Kochia fruit, have been investigated, and found to inhibit the increase in serum glucose-loaded rats. Mormordin Ic and its 2'-0-beta-D-glucopyranoside , which are the principal saponins of this medicinal food, were found to potently inhibit the glucose and ethanol absorption in laboratory studies. A decrease in gastric emptying and interstinal GIc uptake was noted. Matsuda et al, *Chemical and Pharmaceutical Bulletin* 1997 45:8.

Kochia seeds are about 20% saponins, which are believed responsible, in part, for the protective effect on stress-induced ulcers. This is not due to gastric acid reduction, but to activation of mucous membrane protective factors.

The seeds contain cardiotonic properties. The fresh seed juice is used for eye drops when there is heat and pain as in conjunctivitis (pink eye).

The powdered seeds can be combined with warm alcohol, for treating mastitis, by inducing sweating.

As well, the seeds can be fried until fragrant and combined with warm alcohol for treating hernias. Borelli et al, reported on saponins from *K. scoparia* possessing anti-ulcer activity, *Phytotherapy Research* 2000 14:8.

Combine equal parts of radish and Kochia seeds as a wash for relieving the pain and swelling of carbuncles. Combine with mugwort for itchy skin lesions.

The mature seeds induce apoptosis of oral squamous cell carcinoma, and may be suitable for oral mouth rinse. Han HY et al, *Journal of Ethnopharmacology* 2016 192:431-441.

Methanol seed extracts inhibit cell proliferation and induce apoptosis in breast cancer cells. Han HY et al, *Pharmacogn Mag* 2014 10(supp 3):S661-7.

The young stems and leaves of Kochia are called **DI-FU-MIAO** by Mandarin Herbalists. They consider it to have cold and bitter properties; and therefore useful for dispelling heat, detoxifying in cases of dysentery, diarrhea, hot urine, red eyes or skin.

The fresh plant juice is used as a wash or poultice for various inflamed skin problems. The plants are a rich source of betaine, like beets.

The aliphatic, hydrocarbon and sterol constituents of Kochia show activity against various human pathogenic bacteria. Other recent laboratory studies confirm its anti fungal and diuretic effects.

One study looked at tyrosinase activity (oxidation rate of DL-dopa) as a measure of treating vitiligo. Li-Hong Wu et al, *Journal of Clinical Dermatology* 2000 29. They found *Kochia scoparia* was particularly potent at activating tyrosinase, and has potential for treating vitiligo in humans. Puncture Vine (*Tribulus terrestris*) was also particularly potent.

Harmine and harmane are MAO inhibitors found in Buffalo Berry and Puncture Vine. Kochia seed has been found to possess anti-obesity and hyperlipidemia activity, by inhibiting pancreatic lipase activity. Han et al, *Phyto Res* 20:10.

## SEED OIL

Kochia seed oil contains various acids including palmitic (9.4%), 5-hexadecenoic (4.9%), palmitoleic (0.1%), stearic (2.2%), 5-octadecenoic (1.1%), oleic (17%), linoleic (55%), 5, 9,12-octadecatrienoic (1.3%), and linolenic (5.1%).

The oil contains a compound that has been investigated as a mosquito attractant. The compound, (5R, 6S)-6-acetoxy-5-hexadecanolide, has been extracted by Olagbemiro et al, in Nigeria, and found to act as an oviposition pheromone for the female mosquito. Further info can be found in the *Journal of Agriculture and Food Chemistry* 1999 47 3411-3415. Each gram of seed oil contains 0.04 grams of pheromone. My brother David and I researched the possibility of commercialization, many years ago.

Since the plants produces high seed yields, of up to 11,000 kilograms per hectare; nearly 3 kilos of active pheromone per hectare could be produced.

Five Hook Bassia seeds contain similar oil consisting of 57% linoleic acid, 17% oleic, 10% palmitic, 5.2% 5-hexadecenoic acid, 2.2% stearic acid, 2.1% 5-, 5,9- and 5,9,12-C18 acids, 0.2% palmitoleic acid and 1.8% others.

## FLOWER ESSENCE

Kochia flower essence is made from the small stalk-less, petal-less yellow flowers growing at the base of the bracts.

It is a catalyst of movement; the lighting of fire under a complacent, don't rock the boat mental attitude. Gurdjieff, in his various writings, alluded to the need for the individual to give themselves numerous "shocks" to the emotional and spiritual centre; before the universe provides a much needed shakeup to the psyche.

Kochia flower essence provides the spark and zest that is lacking in certain personality types; and provides new opportunities for soul integration. **PRAIRIE DEVA**

## RECIPES

**DECOCTION**- Leaf- 30-60 grams in one litre of water for twenty minutes.

**SEED**- 4-14 grams

**TINCTURE**- 2-4 ml. The tincture is best made from the mature seed, freshly ground, at 1:4 and 60% alcohol.

**LAMB'S QUARTERS**
(*Chenopodium album* L.)
**STRAWBERRY BLITE**
(*C. capitatum* [L.] Ambrosi)
(*Blitum capitatum*)
**RED GOOSEFOOT**
(*C. rubrum* L.)
**QUINOA**
(*C. quinoa* Willld.)
**NARROW-LEAVED GOOSEFOOT**
(*C. leptophyllum* [Moq.] Nutt. ex S. Watson)

**MAPLE-LEAVED GOOSEFOOT**
(*C. gigantospermum* Aellen) not accepted
(*C. hybridum* auct. non L.)
(*C. simplex* [Torr.] Raf.)
**OAK-LEAVED GOOSEFOOT**
**ROCKY MOUNTAIN GOOSEFOOT**
(*C. glaucum* **var.** *salinum* [Standl.] B. Boivin)
**NETSEED LAMBSQUARTERS**
(*C. berlandieri* Moq.)
**GOOD KING HENRY**
**FAT HEN**
(*C. bonus-henricus* L.)
**AMBROSIA**
**JERUSALEM OAK**
**FEATHER GERANIUM**
(*C. botrys*) not accepted
(*Dysphania botrys* [L.] Mosyakin & Clemants)
**PARTS USED**- leaves, seeds, flowers and roots

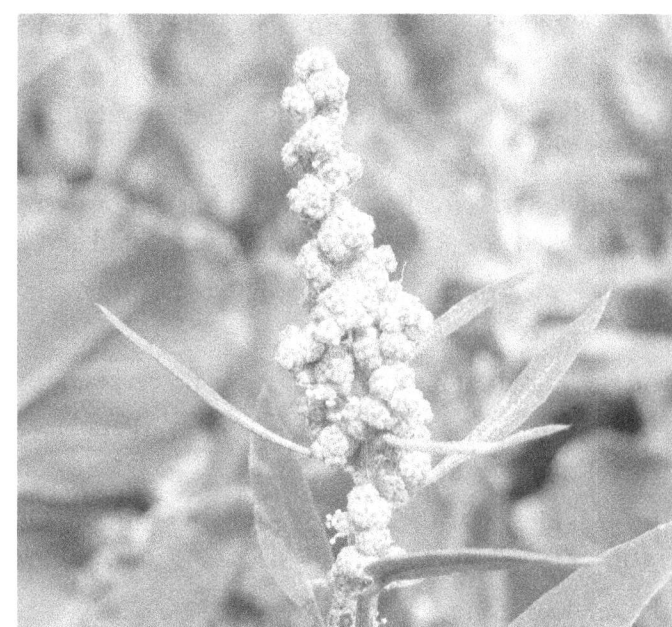

LAMB'S QUARTERS SEED HEAD

Civilization is the lamb's skin in which barbarism masquerades. **T. B. ALDRICH**

The quinoa struck me as being a crop from which a choice breakfast food could be made. It was starchy with just enough tang from its pigweed blood to produce a good flavour. **H. V. HARLAN**

I love quinoa. It's great, it cooks like rice and is better than caviar. **CLOTILDE HESME**

Chenopodium is from the Greek **CHEN** meaning goose, and **POUS** for foot. Its other common name goosefoot is from the German **GANSEFUSS** and remotely from the botanist's Latin **PES ANSERINUS**.

Blite is from the Greek **BLITON**, referring to the insipid taste and not blight as in rust suggested in some books.

Botrys means a bunch of grapes. Album means white, rubrum is red. Berlandieri is named in honor of Jean Louis Berlandier, the French physician who collected plants in Texas and Mexico.

Good King Henry is an adaptation of Guter Henrich, which in Germany refers to a Teutonic elf or goblin, who after helping housemaids with their work, asked for a saucer of cream. The plant habitually grows near houses and barns. In some ways, he resembled the Robin Goodfellow of English lore.

Some books allude that the name refers to King Henry IV of Navarre, who decreed that all peasants should have weekly fowl to eat.

Lesley Bremness claims the name distinguishes it from the similar looking Malus Henricus or Bad Henry, which is poisonous. And hence Good Henry, to which future generations added King, at least in England.

Ambrosia is from the Greek **AMBROTOS** meaning immortal. See Ragweed (*Ambrosia* genus) for more information. Jerusalem Oak refers to the leaf shape.

Lammas quarter was a traditional harvest festival held at the beginning of August in the 9th century English church; and one of the quarter days for marking off the year.

Lammas, in turn, was a slur of "Loaf Mass", or the grain harvest, and it was noticed that the plant bloomed at this time.

Lamb's quarters is related to the common spinach found in gardens, and can be used for food in the same manner. Like spinach, it contains oxalic acid that eaten raw or in large quantities can irritate or cause kidney stone formation.

The steamed vegetable is both safer, and actually better tasting.

A cultivar called Magenta has been developed in California for the restaurant trade. The presence of this herb is an indication of good soil fertility and condition.

Up to seventy thousand seeds are produced by a single plant. And they are hardy! Seeds found at archeology sites in western North America and buried for over 1700 years germinated. They are dried and ground into flour, cooked as a whole grain cereal, or roasted and used as a coffee substitute.

They are a warm chi tonic, according to Susun Weed, and after roasting can be added to enrich flour or flavor tomato sauce.

The seeds are best harvested when the flowers turn pink to orange.

The plant produces non-dormant seeds early in the year and dormant ones as its main crop, giving an extra generation per year.

The Ross site, near the Oldman River in southern Alberta, contained a cache of seeds from a site occupied by the Blackfoot from 1500-1600 AD.

The Anglo-Saxons called it Melde, from the Old Norse **MELDR**, the Viking word for a certain quantity of ground meal, and referring to the texture of the undersides of the leaves. In parts of Ireland, the stem is decocted and drunk for rheumatism.

Napoleon had his cooks use the poppy-like seeds to make "black bread" for his troops. The sprouted seeds are also edible like buckwheat. The protein composition is very balanced with respect to the essential amino acids.

The seeds are excellent food for domestic birds, with the added benefit of de-worming them at the same time.

In Mexico, the flower heads are battered in egg and fried. It is interesting to note that the Aztec name for the plant, **QUILITL**, is very similar to its name by the ancient Moors of Spain, **QLIQL**.

The Japanese also enjoy it as a vegetable, and call it **SHIROZA**.

The Cree call it **WITHINIWPAKWATIK**, and used decoctions of the whole plant for painful limbs- as a tea internally, and to wash affected areas. The Fox tribe infused the root, and drank the tea to halt urethral itch.

In India, the plant is known as Bacon Weed, or Bathwa. The powdered leaves are used as an antiseptic dusting powder around the genitalia of children. Like the Cree, decoctions of aerial parts are rubbed on the body for arthritis and rheumatism.

The plant powder (25-50%) is mixed with normal food to suppress the estrus cycle.

In *Atharva Veda* it is used for hemorrhoids and worms, while *Sushruta Samhita* suggests it is pungent, enhances memory, appetite, digestive power, strengthens the body and destroys all worms.

In British Columbia, the plant is used in veterinary medicine for treating internal and external parasites, particularly in the organic rabbit and poultry industry. Lans C & Nancy Turner, *J Ethnobiol Ethnomed* 2011 7:21.

Among the Zulu, an infusion of leaves is used as an enema for curing intestinal ulcers; and is said to be useful in piles. They also use the dry powdered leaf of lamb's quarters to soothe irritated external genitalia of children.

Like nettles, the presence of lamb's quarters usually indicates excellent soil.

Even the stems are useful, and used for making paper, like hemp and nettles.

In China, the fresh root is used to treat joint rheumatism, like the Cree, as well as insect bites and sunstroke. In India, the plant is used for its laxative and anthelmintic action.

Work by Jabbar et al, *J Ethnopharm* 2007 114:1 found sheep fed 3 grams/kg in body weight of seeds, eliminated 82.2% of nematode eggs, compared to levamisole at 7.5 mg/kg eliminating 95% of eggs.

Methanol extracts of the flower heads show significant anti-fungal activity against *Macrophomina phaseolina*. Javaid et al, *Nat Prod Res* 2009 23:12.

The root juice (about 6 tsp. three times daily) is given in Nepal to treat bloody dysentery. The plant juice of **BATHU** is used to relieve eye troubles. The seeds are chewed for urinary troubles, and for semen discharge in the urine. In neighboring Kashmir, the plant is known as **NEMU** and is used to protect clothing from insects.

In Hungary, studies have shown that 25-50% of the herb mixed with food suppressed the estrogen cycle. Watt et al, *The Medicinal and poisonous plant of southern and eastern Africa* 2nd Ed, 1962.

Various b-ecdysones and related compounds have been extracted from Lamb's Quarters, as well as Catchfly. An ecdysone derived from Lamb's Quarters has been shown by a single injection (50 g/kg), to enhance the weight gain of rats.

The plant fiber cell walls have a pectin containing surface with a unique ability. Permselect is a purified plant cell wall made from *C. album*. A package containing one dry gram of Permselect eliminates 99-100% of leukocytes from 80 ml of fresh, preserved or red blood cell concentrates. This is much higher efficiency than commercial filter materials such as cotton, etc.

Lamb's quarters has been investigated for the optical and magnetic properties of copper in plastocyanin, in studies conducted by Blumberg and Peisach.

Linda Kershaw, in her excellent book, *Edible and Medicinal Plants of the Rockies*, suggests the crushed roots can be used as a mild substitute for soap. Lamb's quarters, planted near Zinnia, Marigold, Peony or Pansy, helps make them more vigorous.

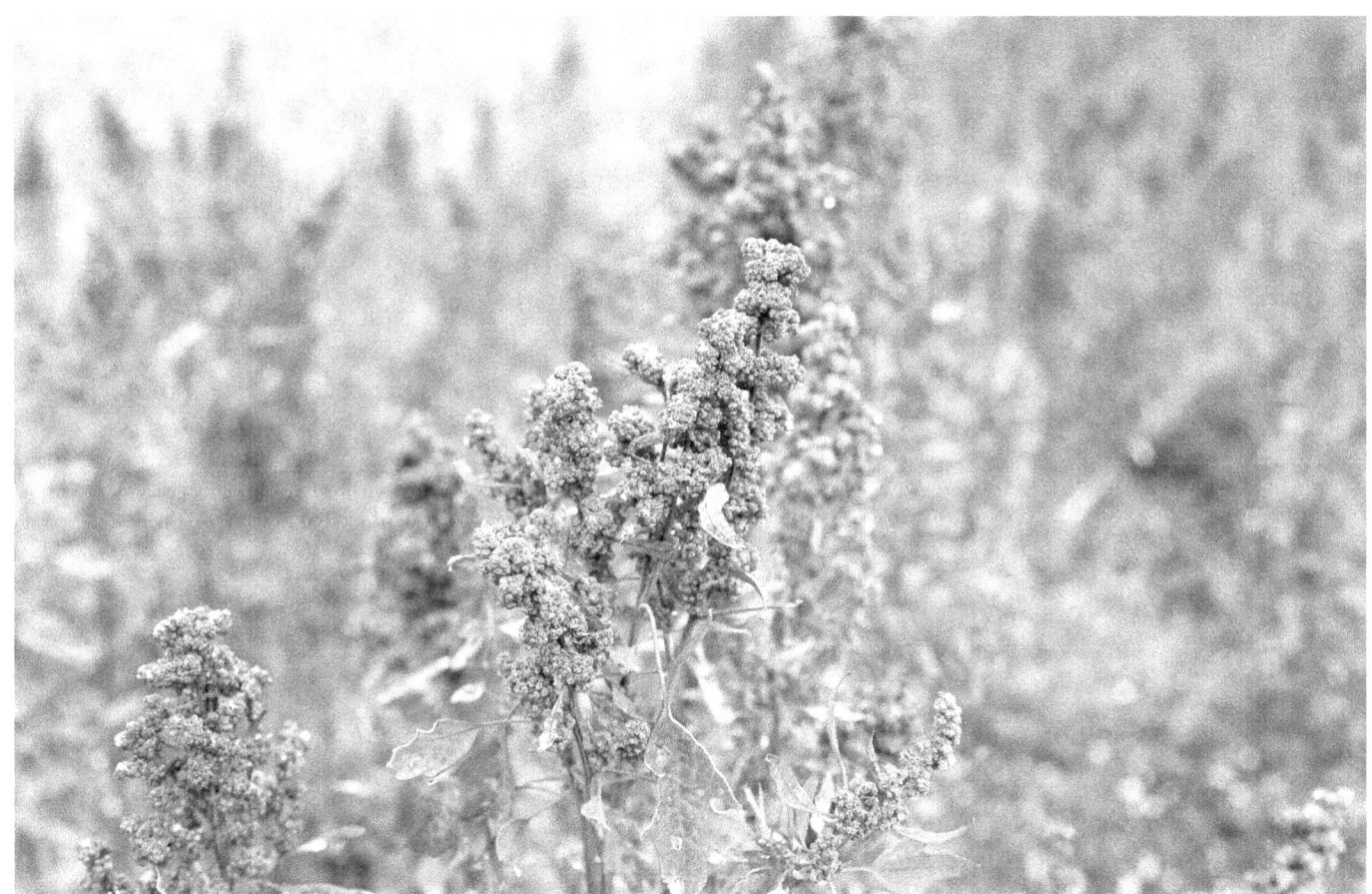

QUINOA

While living in Peru, I discovered Quinoa (pronounced keenwa), a pseudo-cereal, high in protein (16.2%), and low in gluten, that grows well in parts of the prairies. I brought some back from Peru in 1982, and grew it successfully around Lesser Slave Lake in northern Alberta.

There is now a small amount of organic quinoa production on the prairies.

Quinoa has been cultivated for over 5000 years, probably originating in the region of the alto-plano near Lake Titicaca. It was called the mother grain and believed brought from heaven by the bird, **KULLKU**.

The Inca combined the grain with animal blood and pressed them into the shape of their Gods. These were eaten during Holy Days and represented the eating of body and blood of their Gods. The Roman Catholic Spanish invaders, who consumed wafers and wine, representing the body of Christ, saw this as idolatry and symbolic cannibalism, outlawed the practice and destroyed the quinoa fields.

It has the advantage of minimal allergic response, and is in much demand as an alternative crop. The fatty acids from the seed oil appear to be very similar to soybean. Our former foster child, Melchorita, who lives in the Andes of Peru, ate quinoa as a regular part of her diet.

Quinoa is rich in methionine, cystine and lysine, and has a protein rating of 4.6 as compared to soybean at 2.8. Unlike most grains, it contains all nine essential amino acids, and is 16.2% protein. It has a high proportion of D-xylose (120 mg/100g), and maltose (101 mg/100g), with low glucose and fructose, suggesting it may be useful in malted drink formulations.

It is extremely rich in calcium (141 mg/100 grams), iron (6.6), phosphorus (449), and magnesium. In fact it contains three times more magnesium than calcium.

Quinoa has a high water absorption capacity at 147%, with low foaming, 9% and stability 2%. The flour has a least gelation concentration of 16% w/volume.

It thrives in low rainfall, high altitudes, thin, cold air, hot sun, subfreezing temperatures and even poor, sandy, alkaline soil. Sounds like it is pretty suited to the prairies!

When sprouted, it forms a root one-quarter inch long in 24 hours, and in 2-3 days is a beautiful red and white shoot with hint of green. It becomes bitter with age so eat right away.

The young leaves make a good potherb, and the ashes from old stems, or root, is used to make a paste that is chewed with coca leaves in the Andes. When buying coca leaves in the markets, they will also sell you a small amount of "lime" or "ash" that is needed to combine with the leaves to release the active ingredients.

Believe me, when you are hiking and sleeping at 16000 feet, as I have, you require coca leaf chew, to slow down your heart and increase your oxygen intake.

In Peru, the stalks are burned for fuel, while the saponins removed from the grain (fruit) are used as a shampoo. Seed banks in Peru and Bolivia have over 1800 ecotype samples of quinoa in storage.

It is sometimes used, like corn, to make Chicha, a popular fermented beer-like beverage.

The stems and leaves contain up to 22% protein, 52% carbohydrate and low ash. They are used in the Andes as animal fodder, and a green pellet from the quinoa plant is estimated to cost 1/3 to 1/2 the cost of producing grass or alfalfa.

Starch granules are complex conglomerates of 4-6 microgranules; ten times smaller than starch granules from corn or wheat.

Small starch granules produce smooth, creamy texture and make excellent carbohydrate based fat replacers. The smooth mouth feel lends to applications in baked and frozen desserts, and food bars.

Biodegradable films for grocery and garbage bags are another application of small granule starches.

These starches can be sprayed with bonding agents and used for the food or cosmetic industry, releasing flavor and scent over time. Chewing gum is an example of this type of application.

Work by Tom Li, at the *Summerland Agriculture Research Centre*, found that the powdered leaves of Quinoa were superior to nettle, dandelion, yarrow and comfrey, in not just nitrogen, potassium and phosphorus levels, but also in providing the best growth of Rosemary. Perhaps there is another previously overlooked use of the leaf for Quinoa farmers.

The removal of the anti-nutritional saponins can be accomplished by treating in an industrial tumbler drier at 200° C. Feeding experiments on rats in Denmark, show no toxic effect after heat treatment.

The saponins in white Quinoa can be used to produce pharmaceutical steroids, whereas other colors have application for beer, shampoos, detergents, soaps, cosmetics and synthetic hormones.

Netseed lambsquarter is a tetraploid native plant that interbreeds with quinoa, resulting in offspring with partial male fertility restoration. Repeated cycles of the introduced quinoa interbreeding with the local "weed" needs closer attention.

The seed coat thickness has decreased by up to 75% through domestic breeding.

In Mexico, there are three sub varieties, or cultivars of this plant grown for food. The most important is **HUAUZONTLE**, of which the flower containing the small fruit is eaten. They are dipped in batter before cooking, and then eaten by pulling a section through the teeth so that the fruit and tough stringy stalk are left.

It is often served in Mexico City, in some of the better restaurants.

Netseed Lambsquarter is believed to have been cultivated throughout much of North America for the last 3500 years.

Red Goosefoot is a rather neglected annual, common to dried slough beds and lakeshores. The fruit turns red in fall, but not in bright strawberry-like bunches like *C. capitatum*. The production of betacyanins can be greatly increased by feedings of tyrosine.

It contains melatonin that helps synchronize circadian rhythms. Other natural sources are sunflower seeds, sour cherries, St. John's wort and Feverfew.

Strawberry blite is loaded with bright red flower/seed heads. They readily stain red, and were used by native peoples for decorating baskets, porcupine quills, marking beadwork patterns on moose hide, and rubbing on the body for ceremonial purpose. The Thompson, of the interior of British Columbia call it Smeared Blood Top Plant, an apt description of its staining ability.

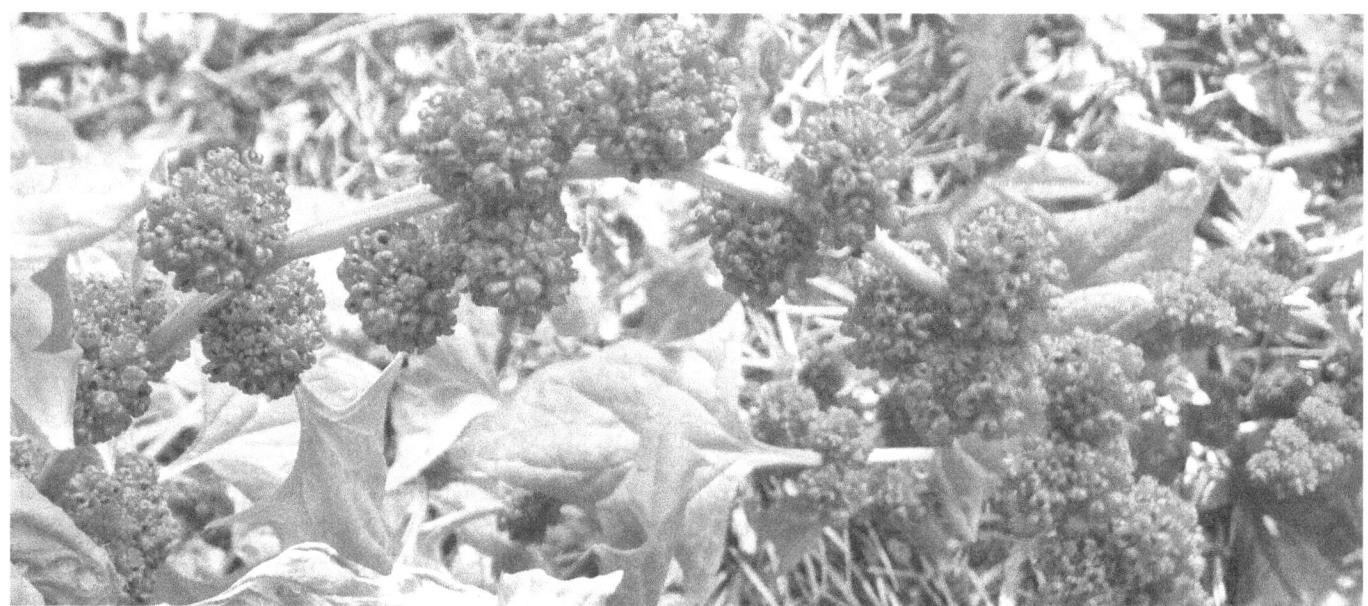

STRAWBERRY BLITE

Spruce roots, used for baskets were also dyed red when the fruits were ripe.

The Alaska natives thought the plant was bad luck and called it dog's nosebleed. The Slave name is Beaver Berry, or **TSA DZHI**.

The Potawatomi name is **MÊNA'-KWOSKÛK** meaning, "stinking or scent weed". The ripened red heads were used to paint the cheeks of maidens, before the dream dance, or applied to the chest for lung congestion, combined with a tea of the same.

The plant was introduced to Europe in the early 1800s, as an ornamental food plant, exactly what it is.

Good King Henry was used in Europe as a cleanser for skin sores, and in ointments for joint pain. It has mild laxative and diuretic effects, rich in iron and vitamin C.

My great grandfather was the blacksmith for the village of Chester Basin, on the south shore of Nova Scotia. Good King Henry has an affinity for the blacksmith's forge or smithy, and was called Smiddy Leaves. No doubt, my great grandfather used the fresh plant on the many sores, cuts and burns common to his trade.

The German settlers further south also used it for pain of hemorrhoids, pulping the fresh leaves in a little butter and milk and swabbing on affected area.

The leaves were also plastered on the pain of gout, with good results.

The roots were given traditionally to sheep as a cough remedy; while the seeds were used to manufacture cloths with rough surface for polishing such as shagreen or artificially grained leather.

Fat Hen is from the German **FETTE HENNE**, for the use of the plant for fattening poultry. In the Middle Ages, Fat Hen, known as **MELDE** in Old English, was a staple food. Various towns and cities in England derive from the name, such as Melbourn, and Milden. In 1970, citizens of the latter erected a cast iron statue of the plant at edge of village.

The plant grows well on the prairies, a good example being found at the George Pegg Botanic Garden near Glenevis, Alberta.

Ambrosia (*C. botrys*) is naturalized to North America. It was grown in Germany to control moths, and for medicinal purpose. One cultivar, Green Magic, has been developed in the Netherlands, and has a delicious, nutty flavour. The Bantu of South Africa use it as a potherb.

In the Dutch East Indies, the plant was used for treating intestinal parasites.

The herb is also known as Jerusalem Oak, which according to Dioscorides, is because the leaves have oak-like lobes, and "like unto Cicorie, many, all of it is of a wonderful scent, wherefore it is also laid amongst clothes".

In France, the herb was used to preserve clothing and bedding, because the pleasant odor also repels moths.

In various Mediterranean countries, the herb has been used to relieve spasms such as asthma and other inflammations of the nose and respiratory system; as well as migraine headaches.

According to Grieve, the oil is used as an expectorant for congested lungs.

After its introduction to the New World, the Cherokee used infusions for colds and headaches, both internal and externally.

They used root decoctions for fever, and as part of anthelmintic mixtures.

In the American Southwest, the introduced plant is now an escapee, and called **YERBA DEL CHIVATITO**. It is steeped as a tea for "cold in the stomach", or to help stop bedwetting in children. Two small branches are soaked in a gallon of cold water until it turns a wine colour. This is taken daily until success.

In Alabama, a seed syrup was used traditionally as a vermifuge, as would be expected. The inner bark was also boiled and mixed with molasses to make a candy for the same purpose.

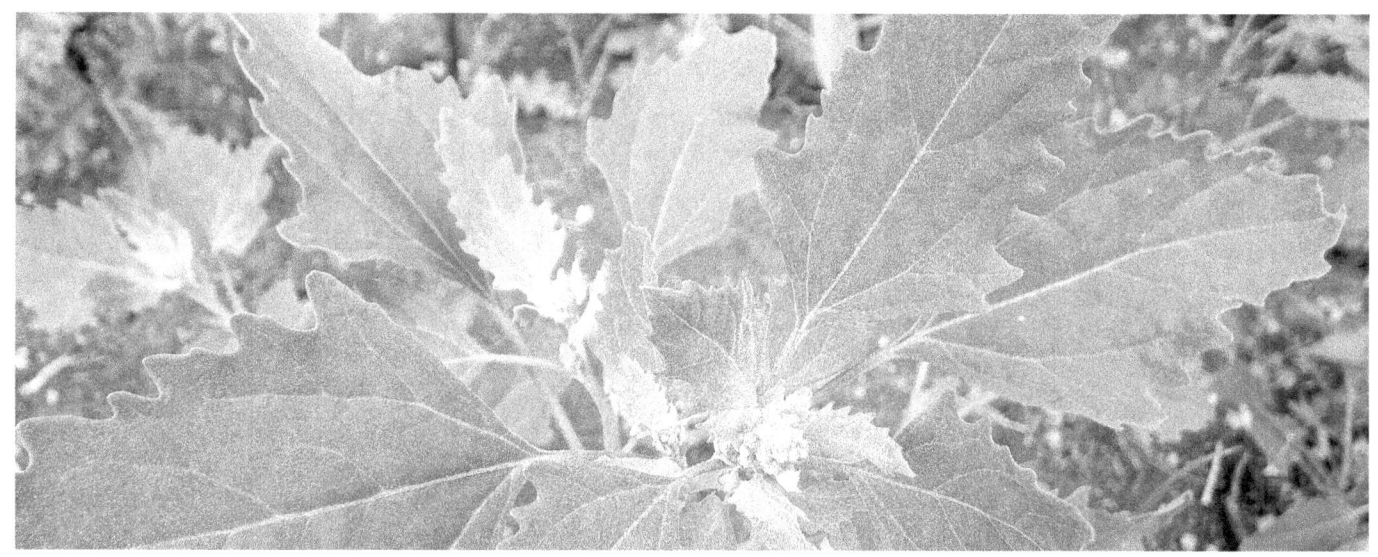

**YOUNG LAMB'S QUARTERS**

The Thompson tribe of British Columbia also recognized its benefits, and called it "good plant". James Teit, in his anthropological report of early 1900's had this to say. "This common plant is glandular pubescent and viscid throughout, making it strongly scented, and is used in great quantities as scent. It is wound in necklaces and stuffed in pillows, bags, pouches and baskets. The Indians often tie it on their clothes and in their hair, or wear it in little skin bags tied to parts of their clothing".

Paul LaFlamme, a plant research specialist, grew Ambrosia successfully in the Grande Prairie region of Alberta for a number of years.

Maple and Oak leaved Goosefoot are introduced plants, the former in waste areas and the latter in wet, salty soil throughout the Peace Country and southern Alberta.

Stinking Goosefoot (*C. vulvaria*) has a distinct vaginal odor. Note the species name as well.

# MEDICINAL

**CONSTITUENTS**- *C. album* herb- betaine, cholesterol, spinasterol , beta-sitosterol, cryptomeridiol; ferulic, vanillic, syringic, cinnamic, sinapic, gallic and oleanic acid, iron, calcium (309 mg/100g) boron (44 ppm), manganese (138 ppm), ammonia and amines, hydrocyanic acid, kaempferitrin, apocarotenoids, Vitamin A (11600 I.U.), vitamin C (155mg/100g), volatile oils (1-2%), various ecdysteroids, rubemamine, saponins, chenoalbicin. The leaves contain high protein (4.2%) with a balanced amino acid profile, with high lysine and methionine content.
root- three saponins, one secoglycoside, various ecdysterones, including 20-hydroxyecdysone, phenolic amide
Ascorbic and +dehydroascorbic acid content is a high 155 mg/100 grams when fresh. Topoisomerase (type I). Protein content is 31.7%. Oxalic acid is from 360-2000mg/100g dry weight.
Nineteen flavonoids compounds have been isolated so far from the leaves of *C. album*; various alkaloids, chinoalbicin, apocortinoid, xyloside, phenols and lignans, including pinoresinol, syringaresinol and lariciresinol.
Fruit- gallic and protocatechuric acids, arginine, gluctamic acid, lysine, desgalactotigonin.
*C. leptophyllum*- various sterols, including sitosterol, avenasterol, stigmasterol, 2,2-dihydrospinasterol, and 24-methylcholesterol.
*C. rubrum*- seed- betaine- 167mmol/kg of dry weight.
leaf- (+)-tubocurarine, invertase, vits A, thiamine, riboflavin, B6, and C.
*C. quinoa* seed- high in histidine and lysine, which are deficient in most grains. Also three groups of saponins (12 triterpenoids, oleanolic acid, hederagenin, and phytolaccagenic acid; as well as 5 ecdysteroids; five kaempferol and quercitin glycosides and well as vanillic glucoside, lunasin, various polysaccharides, betalains, glycine betaine
Aerial- aklylresorcinols, branched chain alkylresorcinols and methylalkylresorcinols.
*C. botrys*- sinensetin, hispidulin, salvigenin, 5-methylsalvigenin, 7-methyleupatulin.
*C. bonus-henricus*- aerial parts- flavonoid glycosides such as patuletin, spinacetin and 6-methoxykaempferol,

91

Lamb's quarter is used successfully by those who are constipated, with a weak liver and auto-intoxicated body. It is good for iron deficient individuals, and helps boost their energy levels. Yadav et al, *J Food Sci Tech* 2002 39:1.

Rubemamine elicits a strong intrinsic umami taste, and modulates the response to MSG by 1.8 fold. Replacement would be best, but this is a start. Backes M et al, *J Agric Food Chem* 63(39): 8694-704.

Studies conducted at the University of Exeter by Dinan 1992, showed very high levels of ecdysteroids in flowering lamb's quarter. This could lead to some exciting new product developments. The seeds contain 0.45-1.3 mg/g dry weight, the aerial parts 0.3 mg, growing tips 0.6 mg, immature flowers 1.9 mg, open flowers 1.1 mg, green fruit 1.4 mg per gram. These compounds are an insect molting hormone, but are used for anabolic, muscle building by athletes and the elderly suffering catabolic wasting.

The roots, leaves, flowers and seeds all contain ecdysterones that have potential to increase muscle mass and protein synthesis.

In Ayurvedic medicine, the plant is known as **CILI**, and considered useful for curing parasitic infections, promoting intellect, power of digestion and strength. It is alkalizing and laxative, cooling and drying.

The leaves are used as poultices, and applied to areas of inflammation, or as Terry Willard suggests, bruise the leaves and apply to relieve headache and body heat from too much sun. Work by Arora SK et al, *J Ethnopharm* 2014 155(1): 222-9 found the anti-rheumatic activity of aerial parts due to inhibition of NFkappaB.

Internally or topically, the herb has been used for vitiligo.

The water from steamed greens can be used for mouth and throat inflammation.

The roots are decocted and used to treat mouth sores; and externally a wash for rheumatism. The leaves possess laxative, aperient, and tonic properties. Infusions can be given in biliousness, hepatic disorders, and splenic enlargement.

Research by Tahara et al, conducted at Hokkaido University in Japan, found that *C. album* leaves exude mucondialdehyde, a novel fungitoxic metabolite, in response to stress.

Kaempferitrin is a flavonoid fraction found in various *Chenopodium* species, including *C. album*.

The carotenoids include retinol precursors and biologically active lutein for eye health. Sangeetha et al, *Food Chem* 2010 119:4.

The rich source of iron and carotene in dehydrated leaves suggest use in food supplementation. Singh et al, *Nat Prod Rad* 2007 6:1.

In laboratory studies by Gohar et al, *Phytotherapy Research* 1997 11:8 kaempferitrin produced hypotension in genetically prone hypertensive rabbits, but did not block alpha or beta 1 adrenoceptors.

The herb reversed IgG2/IgG1 ratios and increased IFNgamma and IL10 production in asthma models. Mousavi et al, *Iran J Allergy Asthma Immunol* 2008 7:1.

Further work by Ueda et al, at Joshi Eiyo University, found that water extracts of Shiroza exhibited anti-mutagenic activity.

Methanol extracts of the leaf show activity against MCF-7 breast cancer cell lines. Khoobchandani et al, *Ovid Med Cell Longevity* 2009 2(3): 160-5.

Extract of the plant prevent cell growth and induce apoptosis in human lung cancer A549 cells. Zhao T et al, *Exp Ther Med* 2016 12(5): 3301-7.

Water extracts of the leaf are active against *Staphylococcus aureus*, while methanol extracts strongly inhibit *Pseudomonas aeruginosa*. Singh, KP et al, *Int J Appl Biol Pharm Tech* 2011 2:3. Ethanol extracts of the leaf show activity against *Bacillus subtilis*. Elif KS et al, *Chemosphere* 2013 90(2): 374-9.

Dai et al, *Journal of Ethnopharm* 2002 81:2 found ethanol seed extracts possess significant anti-pruritic and anti-inflammatory activity, suggesting a use in itchy, skin conditions. It inhibits scratching behavior induced by 5-hydroxytryptamine (5-HT) that not only facilitates inflammatory pain by itself, but potentiates pain from noradrenaline and prostaglandin E.

The leaves have been used traditionally for kidney disease and urinary stones. Recent work found both alcohol and water extracts exhibit anti-lithiatic effect, and induced urine levels of calcium, phosphorus, urea, uric acid and creatinine, as well as decreased urine volume, pH and oxalates. Effect is similar to cystone, for inhibiting crystallization and stone dissolution. Sikarwar I et al, *J Ethnopharm* 2017 195: 275-282.

The seeds help reduce spleen enlargement associated with lymphatic congestion or stagnation.

The seeds and aerial parts of this plant and *C. hybridum* show significant anti-proliferative effect on ovarian carcinoma (TOV-112D) cell lines. Nowak R et al, *Saudi J Biol Sci* 2016 23(1): 15-23.

Water extracts of the seeds show appreciable spermicidal potential as a vaginal contraceptive. Kumar et al, *Contraception* 2007 75:1. A more recent study identified the compound desgalactotigonin, which is $2 \times 10^{(4)}$ times more potent than nonoxynol-9, and 80 times more potent than decoction of seed. Chakraborty D et al, *PLoS One* 2014 9(9).

The pollen is a major allergen for some individuals; more common in females.

Red Goosefoot contains tubocurarine, an acetylcholine antagonist and channel blocker. Research started by Weiser and Bentrup, *FEBS Lett* 1990 277(1): 220-2, could lead to more interesting possibilities for human use of this plant. Nowak (2016) above, noted *C. rubrum* herb extracts exhibit high anti-oxidant activity

Strawberry blite is useful in cases of nutritional deficiencies. When decocted, the whole plant is used for healing mouth and throat ulcers; or cooled and used as vaginal douche for infections; and a retention enema for internal hemorrhoids.

Good King Henry is a good potherb for iron deficient anemia, due to high iron and vitamin C content.

Medicinally, it is useful for its anodyne, anti-spasmodic and expectorant properties.

In Gloucestershire, the fresh leaves are infused for bladder troubles.

Various flavonoid glycosides, derived from aerial parts, are safe hepatoprotective agents, comparable to the silybin, derived from milk thistle seeds. Kokanova-Nedialkova Z et al, *Fitoterapia* 2017 118:13-20. Various methylflavonol glycosides, derived from the root, were found to protect liver health as well.

Quinoa contains five ecdysteroids, the most abundant of which is 20-hydroxyecdysterone (20HE). What is most interesting is there are few sources of ecdysteroids, from seeds and functional foods.

Phytoecdysteroids can regulate gene activity, the metabolism of nucleic acids, protein synthesis, as well as development and reproduction in insects.

Concentration of 20-hydroxyecdysone can be accomplished by leaching seeds during initial seed germination. See recipes below.

Cryptomeridiol, isolated from the seeds, shows significant growth-promoting activity. Bera et al, *Fitoterapia* 1991 62.

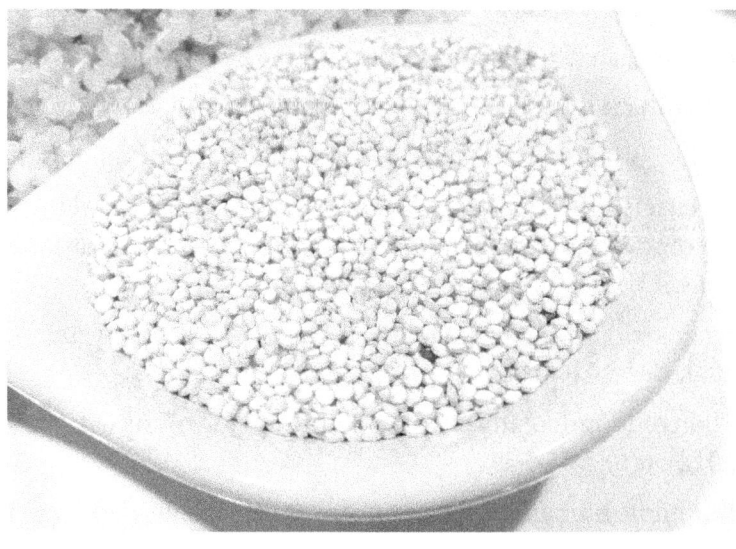

QUINOA

They have been shown to inhibit high blood sugar and cholesterol levels in rats. This may be due in part to bran and hull fractions inhibiting alpha-amylase and alpha-glucosidase. Hemalatha P et al, *Food Chem* 2016 199: 330-8.

Work by Berti et al, *Eur J Nutr* 2004:43 found quinoa showed low glycemic index and hypoglycemic potential.

The saponins suppress adipogenesis and thus effective in modulating adipose tissue mass. Yao Y et al, *Food Funct* 2015 6(10): 3282-90.

At least four clinical studies have demonstrated quinoa supplementation exerts significant positive effect on metabolic, cardiovascular and gastrointestinal health in humans. Graf BL et al, *Compr Rev Food Sci Food Saf* 2015 14(4): 431-45.

Work by Pasko et al, *Plant Foods for Human Nutrition* 2010 March 31, found quinoa moderately protective against fructose-induced changes in rats.

The hulls contain 5-10% saponins with potential to increase mucosal immune response. Dr. Alberto Estrada, at the University of Saskatchewan found that when mice were orally immunized with 50 mg of ovalbumin, with 20 mg of quinoa saponins, both IgG and IgA anti-ovalbumin responses in the intestine were favorable. More work is needed, but this could lead to new approaches in immune response. *Com Immun Microbiol Infect Dis* 1998:21.

Quinoa saponins appear to change intestinal permeability, with a number of medical applications.

The flowers and seeds contain at least 20 triterpene saponins. Those with triterpene groupings have been found to induce apoptosis and exhibit cytotoxicity against cancer cell lines. Kuljanabhagavad et al, *Phytochem* 2008 69:9.

Polysaccharides in the seeds are immune regulating and exhibit anti-cancer activity against human liver cancer SMMC 7721 and breast cancer MCF-7 cells. Hu Y et al, *Int J Biol Macromol* 2017 99: 622-9.

The protein content has been found to help lower cholesterol. Takao et al, *Food Sci Tech Res* 11:2.

Saponin fractions from the seeds inhibit growth of *Candida albicans*. Woldemichael & Wink, *J Ag Food Chem* 2001 49.

The peptide, lunasin, possesses anti-oxidant and anti-inflammatory activity. Ren G et al, *J Sci Food Agric* 2017 Feb 20.

The hulls of red quinoa contain a bitter principle, that was used by the Eclectic physicians as an anti-periodic and emetic.

Ambrosia (*C. botrys*) has been used traditionally as a stimulant, and to relieve migraines, bronchitis, asthma and spasms.

Both alcohol and water extracts exhibit significant pain relief in animal studies. Uddin G et al, *Pak J Pharm Sci* 2016 29(3): 929-33.

Dr. King, an Eclectic physician, used the herb in both catarrhal and humoral asthma, and as a useful expectorant.

In China it is used to treat insect and spider bites, while in Pakistan the herb is used for hypertension.

Unlike other members of the genus, the essential oil does not contain ascaridol.

Sinensetin, one constituent of the plant has been found to possess anti-fungal activity. This flavone is also found in some citrus fruit. It enhances adipogenesis and lipolysis by increasing cAMP levels in adipocytes, suggesting benefit in weight loss and obesity.

Sinensetin inhibits alpha glucosidase and alpha amylase, suggesting benefit in type 2 diabetes. Mohamed EA et al, *BMC Complement Altern Med* 2012 12:176.

The compound exhibits potent anti-angiogenesis activity and low toxicity. Lam IK et al, *Mol Nutr Food Res* 2012 56(6): 945-56.

It inhibits human AGS gastric cancer cell proliferation and induces apoptosis, probably due to up regulation of p53 and p21 mechanisms. Dong Y et al, *Zhongguo Zhong Yao Za Zhi* 2011 36(6): 790-4.

It may also inhibit MDA-MB-468 human breast adenocarcinoma, without affecting normal breast cell lines. Androutsopoulos VP et al, *Toxicology* 2009 264(3): 162-70.

*In vitro* studies suggest it may influence CYP1A2 liver enzyme activity. Maybe.

Hispidulin protects premature skin aging from UVA irradiation. Chaiprasongsuk A et al, *J Pharmacol Exp Ther* 2017 360(3): 388-398.

The compound, as well as salvigenin, inhibits xanthine oxidase, a measure of benefit in gout and rheumatic conditions associated with uric acid. Tuzun BS et al, *Med Chem* 2016 Dec 9.

It plays a role in lipid metabolism, via activation of PPAR alpha as an agonist, comparable to fenofibrate. Wu X et al, *Lipids* 2016 51(11): 1249-57.

Hispidulin induces apoptosis in acute myeloid leukemia cells. Gao H et al, *Am J Transl Res* 2016 8(2): 1115-32.

A good review of the many benefits of hispidulin is published by Atif M et al, *Acta Pol Pharm* 2015 72(5): 829-42.

Salvigenin is also found in White Sage (*S. apiana*), an herb that shows moderate cannabinoid receptor activity.

It also exhibits anti-tumor and immune-modulating effect on tumor tissue in mice models of breast cancer. Noori S et al, *Cell Immunol* 2013 286(1-2):16-21. And induces apoptosis in human neuroblastoma SH-SY5Y cells. Rafatian G et al, *Mol Cell Biochem* 2012 371(1-2): 9-22.

Yadav et al, *Nat Prod Rad* 2007 6:2, is a good review of the medicinal properties of *Chenopodium* genera.

## HOMEOPATHY

*Chenopodium glaucum aphis* is used for cracking noises in ear, relieved from blowing nose, chewing, sneezing and swallowing. Toothaches extend to ear, temple and cheekbone and aggravated from warm perspiration. Burning rectum pain during diarrhea, and pain in dorsal region below left scapula.

**DOSE**- 6th to 30th potency. The mother tincture is prepared from plant lice on Chenopodium spcies.

## ESSENTIAL OIL

The plant and seed heads of Lamb's Quarter contain up to 2% essential oils, with ascaridole (45-70%), cymene (15%) and terpenes (10%) the main constituents.

Lamb's quarters leaves contain ascaridole, useful for treating parasites, according to a report by Boche and Runquist, *Journal of Organic Chemistry* 33.

Like several southern and European relatives, the Chenopodium oils are used to rid the body of roundworms, hookworms, and other parasites.

In Peru, the closely related Paico (*C. ambrosioides*) was a traditional medicine used for its nervine, anti-rheumatic and anthelminthic activity.

The oil has an antiseptic action, with sedative effect, in small amounts, on the central nervous system, and various spasmodic nervous disorders. It will also lower blood pressure, but only in those suffering hypertension.

I have been able to obtain essential oil of Good King Henry (*C. bonus-henricus*) from Europe, where it is used in aromatic medicine for parasites.

The essential oil of *C. botrys* possesses both anti-fungal and anti-bacterial activity. Maksimovic et al, *Fitoterapia* 2005 76(1):112-4.

It is composed of 16.3% elemol acetate, 14% elemol, 11% botrydiol, and 9.5% alpha chenopodiol. *J Herb Spice Med Plants* May/June 2007.

## HYDROSOL

The distilled water of Fat Hen (*C. album*) is used to help in cases of intestinal problems with tapeworm infection.

**VIAUD**

## SEED OIL

Lamb's quarter seeds can be also cold pressed, and yield about 7% of an oil rich in oleic and linoleic acids (over 61%).

Red Goosefoot seed oil yields 2%.

Quinoa contains seed oil with acid value of 0.50, iodine number of 54, peroxide value of 2.44%, and saponification of 192. Yields range from 1.8 to 9.5%, with an average of 5.8%, higher than corn. It also contains more linolenic acid, linoleic acid and sterols than corn oil.

The press cake contains 40% protein of high quality, comparable to casein from milk. This press cake has significant application for both human and animal protein supplementation.

## FLOWER ESSENCES

Lamb's quarter flower essence is for accessing information through the heart, before it is allowed to be processed through the mind.

**ALASKA**

Strawberry blite flower essence is for those individuals that have trouble with the duality of life. Expressions such as " accepting the bitter with the sweet", or the yin/yang of nature, are difficult to integrate into the belief system. Somehow the psyche has difficulty accepting the seeming injustice of nature.

This flower essence is for those who continually feel that the activities on the planet are somehow not perfect.

**PRAIRIE DEVA**

## MYTHS AND LEGENDS

In legend, the sun sent Manco Capac and his wife Mama Ocllo, the first Incan couple, to the world. They emerged from Lake Titicaca and followed the sun's instructions for building their empire…The sun gave Manco Capac a golden planting stick and told him to find a place he could sink the golden planting stick into the earth with one thrust. He should build the empire there, the sun said. Then he taught Manco Capac the cycle of seasons and how to plant. Manco Capac found the place the sun had told him about, named it Cuzco, and built the sun a great temple.

The Inca worshipped quinoa as they did the sun that gave them the grain and the divine king who sowed the seeds.

**TAMRA ANDREWS**

## RECIPES

**SEED TINCTURE**- Lamb's quarter seeds are tinctured at 1:4 and 40% alcohol. Take 10 drops up to three times daily.

**ECDYSTERONES**- Germinate quinoa seed in water, then use 70% ethanol, at 80 degrees Celsius for four hours with a solvent ratio of 5ml/g seed. This leachate contains 0.865 20HE, 1.0% phytoecdysteroids and over 20% protein and 12% oil.

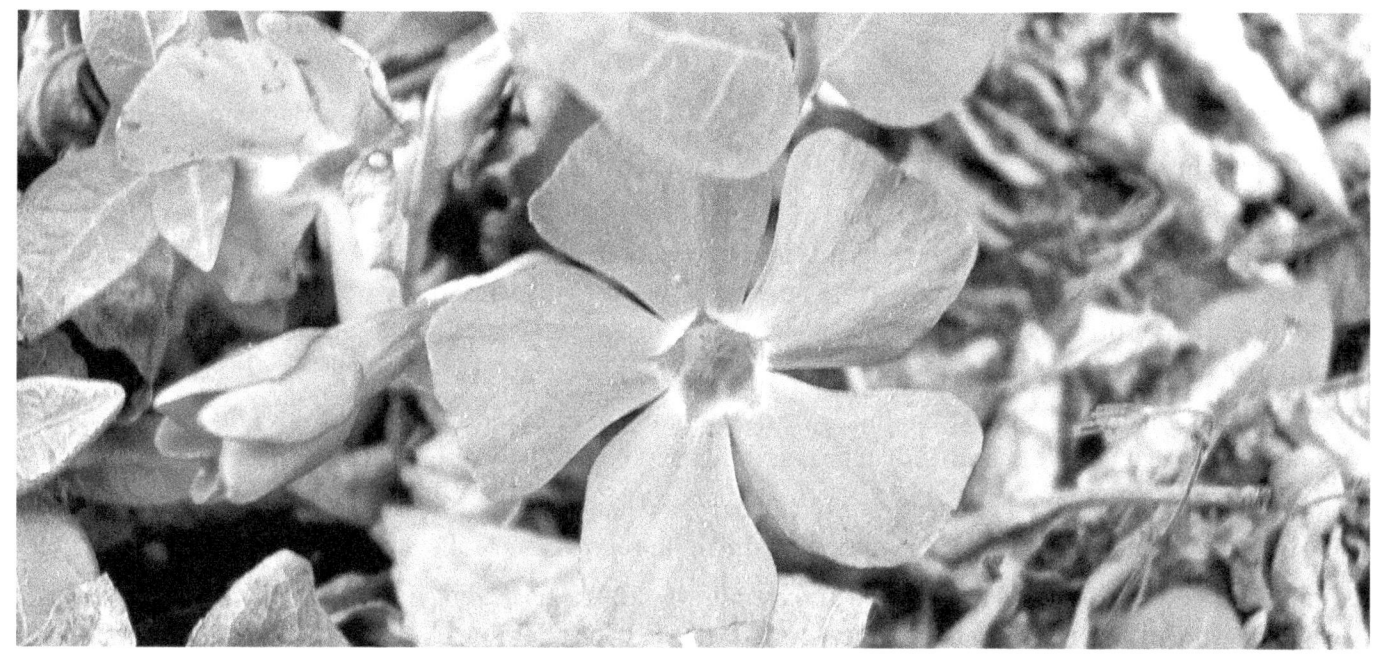

PERIWINKLE IN FLOWER

**LESSER PERIWINKLE**
**DWARF PERIWINKLE**
(*Vinca minor* L.)
**HERBACEOUS PERIWINKLE**
(*V. herbacea* Waldst. & Kit.)
**PARTS USED**-whole plant above ground

"Through primrose tufts in that sweet bower, the fair periwinkle trailed its wreaths."        **WORDSWORTH**

Vinca is from the Latin **VINICO** meaning "to bind", and refers to the strong, sprawling stems that bind and stunt competing plants. Vinca is the past tense of the verb **VINCERE**, meaning to conquer, overcome or overpower. **PER** means through; and **PERVINCA** was the name given the plant by Pliny the Elder. It may derive from the Russian **PERVI** meaning first, in reference to early spring.

So the name, either to bind closely, or to overcome, is still up in the air, scholastically speaking.

An early translation of *Book of Secrets* attributes Albertus Magnus expressing the following statement.

"Periwinkle when it is bcatc to a poudr with worms of ye earth wrapped about it and with an herbe called houselyke, induces love between a man and his wife if it be used in their meals."

Periwinkle was, at one time, believed to help those suffering nightmares.

About 25 years ago, my wife, Laurie, and I bought a home in the southern burbs of Edmonton. We moved in October, with the ground covered in white snow.

The following spring, as the snow was melting, I noticed our neighbor's ground cover with shiny dark green leaves moving into our yard.

And it soon blossomed with beautiful sky-blue flowers. The plant is an evergreen perennial that flowers, but rarely ripens to seed on the prairies.

When my neighbor told me he thought it was periwinkle, I didn't really believe him. But I scurried back to my herbal books. Sure enough!

It was introduced to our zone two region by early Ukrainian settlers; and is known as Barvenok.

In the rhyme for new bride's apparel, the something blue may be blue periwinkle, for in parts of England, it is worn in the garter for fertility.

Periwinkle is often planted in newly weds yards to ensure a lucky and happy marriage. Other magical properties have been associated with periwinkle. It was believed that if a husband and wife ate the leaves together, it would bind them more closely. It has come to symbolize pleasant recollections, and associated with birth date of March 28.

European peasants used the herb to both dry up over-abundant milk production, or to dry off in late stages of pregnancy. It is also used for chronic diarrhea, and to arrest bleeding wounds, and internal hemorrhage.

According to Grieve, it as a familiar flower in the days of Chaucer, who called it "fresh Pervinke rich of hue." Bacon says that bands of periwinkle stem tied around a limb prevent or relieve cramp.

An older name was "Sorcerer's Violet", as it was believed to exorcise evil. In parts of England, garlands of periwinkle were place on prisoner's heads before execution. Vinca pervinca became periwinke. Another name Saint Candida's Eyes, from western Dorset, refers to a medieval healer.

In France it is sometimes referred to as "the violet of witches".

In Italy, it was known as **FIORE DI MORTE**, or flower of death, for its use as decoration on the funeral pyres of deceased children.

Herbarium, written by the 2nd century AD writer Apuleius, described vinca minor virtues "against the devil sickness and demonical possessions and against snakes and wild beasts". For snakebites, it was steeped in vinegar, and taken internally to neutralize the venom.

Vinca minor is a great protector, and is gathered when the moon is 9 nights old, according to tradition. That is, nine lunar months into the new year.

The Italians call it **CENTOCCHIO** or hundred eyes, to the Germans it is the "Flower of Immortality" and to the French it is an emblem of friendship.

The Cree of Alberta named the introduced plant, **KA PAPAMIKIHK WAPIKWANE**, a trailing evergreen flower.

An old recipe for inducing love between a man and wife was a mixture of periwinkle, houseleek, and earthworm, somehow disguised in a meal. Children enjoy the small fairy-like paintbrush left over after all the petals have been removed.

Culpepper said it was good for bleeding of the mouth and nose when chewed; and useful in hysteria and fits. "It is good in nervous disorders, the young tops made into a conserve is good for the nightmare."

In Somerset, decoctions of the stem were taking to prevent cramps.

Medieval herbalists prescribed *Vinca minor* for headaches, vertigo and memory loss.

For whitlows, or other skin growths associated with poor circulation, a bath decoction is used to bathe the affected area with excellent results. Another name, Cutfinger, refers to its healing properties of skin.

The root is used in sub-Saharan Africa to treat hypertension, while in Norway the fresh leaf is given for internal hemorrhage, especially after injury.

Herbaceous periwinkle looks similar but is only of medium hardiness.

*Vinca major*, a variegated perennial, is sold on the prairie regions as an annual that flowers the first year from seed. It is not very hardy, but in milder climates is used as a perennial ground cover.

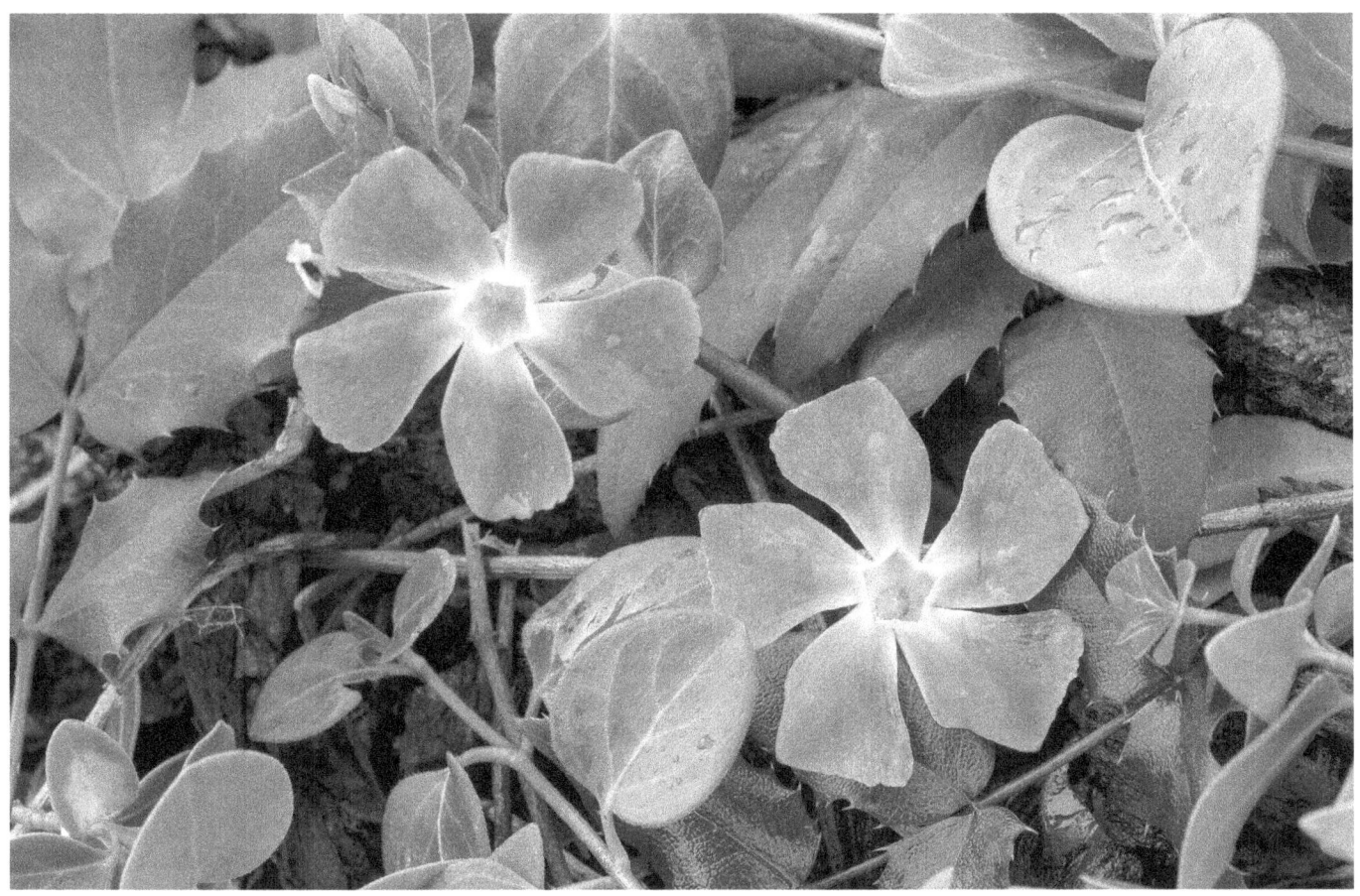

LESSER PERIWINKLE

# MEDICINAL

**CONSTITUENTS-** *V. minor-* over 70 carboline, dimeric imidazolidino-carbazole and quaternary alkaloids (0.58-0.85%) including vincamine (200-17,500 ppm), vincarubine, vicarine, vincine, vincaminorine, vincaminoreine, apovincamine, and vincadifformine; 30 indole alkaoids of the eburnan type; 1-norvincorine; 4-methyl-raucubainum chloride, 4-methylstrictaminium choride, and 4-methyl-akummicinium chloride; akumnicine, akuammine, akuammine N-oxide, ervine, isomajdine, majdinine, reserpinine, resperine, robinin; and various uncharacterized alkaloids including minoveinceine, vincareine, vincoridine, vinerine, tombozine, vincamajine, vincorine, vinomine, vallesiachotamine, isovallesiachotiamine, and vinoxine.
*V. herbacea-* vincanine, majdine, isomajdine, norfluoro-curarine, hervin, akuammicine, dl-vincadifformnine, akuammine, carapanaubine, ervine, vincaherbinine, herboksine, isomajdine, isoresperpinine, majdine, 11-methoxy-vincadifformine, vincarine (0.064% dry weight), herbadinc ( 0.081%), herbamine (0.077%), reserpinine, skimmianine, tabersonine, venalstonine, vincamajine, N-oxide, vincalines,and tabersonine.

Lesser Periwinkle (*V. minor*) has long been used in herbal medicine for its purgative effect. The fresh leaves are an excellent gentle laxative for young children, and for chronic constipation in the elderly, but used with care. It can also be used for the milk crust on scalp common to young children.

The fresh flowers can be made into a laxative syrup, by simmering them in honey or maple/birch syrup for about ten minutes. James Duke reports that the flowers "are said to be poisonous", but I have eaten them with no ill effect.

The leaves possess stomachic and bitter properties, useful in chronic stomach belching, intestinal inflammation and flatulence; combining well with *Agrimony*.

It possesses astringent and tonic properties useful in uterine hemorrhage; in between period bleeding and excessive menstrual flow during menopause.

Lesser Periwinkle will also help decrease the flow and quantity of breast milk, when applied as a heated poultice externally.

It clears mucous from the lungs, and intestinal tract; and as an astringent gargle will relieve sore throats, tonsillitis, canker sores, and the irritating crust formation with the nasal septa.

For bleeding hemorrhoids and internal hemorrhage it may be taken internally, as well as applied externally, or taken as a retention enema.

Michael Moore used the closely related *Vinca major* for migraine headaches that occur after adrenaline stress from circumstance or rebound reaction of low blood sugar from skipping meals. He suggests it be used for short-term acute use, as this is a complex alkaloid plant.

Chewing the fresh leaf will give quick relief to toothache.

It combines well with gingko to stimulate vascular and cerebral circulation.

It is good for cerebral insufficiency, "yin" migraines, for impaired memory and cognitive function, behaviour disorders, irritability, restlessness, and speech disorders.

It is very useful for poor circulation to peripheral areas of the body- hands, feet and brain, in cases associated with diabetes and atherosclerosis.

Lesser, or Dwarf Periwinkle may treat Parkinson's disease at the cellular level, by decreasing microglia activation, attenuating damage from radical oxygen species, supporting correct protein folding, chelating iron, increasing the substantia nigra blood flow, and promoting dopaminergic cell growth. Morgan LA et al, *J Diet Suppl* 2017 14(4): 453-66.

Water extracts of leaves and ethanol extracts of flowers exhibit strong anti-tumor activity. Yildirim AB et al, *Asian Pac J Trop Med* 2013 6:8 616-24.

Vincamine was extracted from the leaves industrially in 1955, and has been used for treating cerebrovascular problems since 1959. It is recommended for tinnitus and Meniere's disease. Vincamine is a muscle relaxant.

One team of researchers summarized their findings as follows: "The trends discovered with ECG monitoring show that vincamine undoubtedly improves the diffuse changes in electrical activity in the brain.

This improvement in the whole cerebral vascular system is all the more interesting if one considers how difficult it is to interpret changes in human cerebral metabolism."

Vincamine has been used for insufficient flow of blood to the brain, difficulty sleeping, mood changes, depression, hearing problems and high blood pressure.

It ameliorates amyloid-beta 25-35 peptides induced cytotoxicity in PC12 cells, possibly through up-regulation of SOD and activation of the P13K/Akkt pathway. Han J et al, *Pharmacogn Mag* 2017 13(49): 123-8.

One problem is the poor solubility of vincamine. Research has found the standardized leaf dry extract is seven times more orally bioavailable, than the pure indole alkaloid, vincamine. Hasa D et al, *Eur J Pharm Biopharm* 2013 84(1): 138-44.

Vinpocetine is produced by transforming the chemical structure of vincamine. It is a cis(3S,16S)-derivative of vincamine with anti-anoxic, anti-ischemic and neuro-protective properties.

Vinpocetine has been widely studied for the treatment of tinnitus. Konope et al, *Otol Pol* 1997 51; Ordogh et al, *Ther Hungarica* 1978 26; Ribari et al, *Arzn Forsch* 1976 10.

It also inhibits *Streptococcus pneumoniae* up-regulation of mucin associated with over production, leading to catarrhal deafness. Lee JY et al, *J Immunol* 2015 194(12): 5990-8. For this condition, combine with fresh plantain leaf juice (*Plantago major*).

Vincopetine prevents the accumulation of sodium in brain cells, lowering their overall charge and preventing tissue destruction reactions of sodium and oxygen when circulation is restored after stroke. It also possesses calcium channel blocking activity and phosphodiesterase inhibition.

Phosphodiesterase is the enzyme responsible for breaking down ATP, or adenosine triphosphate, which is the primary energy of all cells. The inhibition is specific to the brain, resulting in localized increase in energy to neurons.

Manganese excess in the brain is known to be associated with excitotoxicity and neuroinflammation. Vinpocetine may protect the brain by modulating oxidative stress in manganese-induced neurodegeneration. Bora S et al, *Biol Trace Elem Res* 2016 174(2): 410-18.

Vinpocetine is not only a cerebral vasodilator, but selectively enhances circulation and oxygen use with increasing systemic circulation.

It also inhibits platelet aggregation and decreases deformity of red blood cells. Kuzuya, *Therapia Hungarica* 1985 33.

Vinpocetine enhances both glycolytic and oxidative reactions of glucose breakdown in brain. Vamosi et al, *Arzn Forsch* 1976 28.

It also prevents vascular calcification (hardening of the arteries). Ma YY et al, *PLoS One* 2016 11(9).

It does all this without significantly affecting systemic blood pressure and without serious side effects.

The herb can be of use in treating brain trauma, and disorders of blood flow to the retina.

Clinical studies have shown vinpocetine helps maintain healthy microcirculation to the eyes and inner ear. One study of patients with mild burn trauma to eyes showed enhanced healing, due to increased blood flow to damaged tissue.

It is approved for use in 47 countries, and has been in clinical practice since 1978. The Hungarian company Gedeon Richter markets vinpocetine under the drug name Cavinton for the treatment of various cerebral insufficiency conditions. In one study with Cavinton on cerebral glucose metabolism in chronic stroke patients, the drug shows significant improvement in transport of glucose to the brain tissue damaged by stroke.

Periwinkle can be used to dry up an overly abundant milk flow in animals, or to dry off when in later stages of pregnancy.

The root is hypotensive, and used for high blood pressure. It acts on the central nervous system as a sedative. It is adrenolytic and lowers the peripheral resistance.

Lesser Periwinkle show not be confused with *Vinca rosea* from Madagascar, from which alkaloids have been isolated and used successfully in various childhood leukemia.

However, Sturdikova ct al, *Pharmazie* 1986 41:4 have shown three alkaloids from *Vinca minor* to possess cytotoxic and anti-tumour activity. They had considerable inhibitory effect on leukemia P388 cells, with vincadifformine the most active, stopping cell proliferation in vitro at 50 mcg/litre concentration even after twelve hours. The activity was greater than vinblastine, derived from unrelated Madagascar Periwinkle.

The plant is cytotoxic to HT29, Caco2 and T47D cancer cell lines. Khanavi et al, *Pharm Biol* 2010 48:1.

Eburnamonine is converted from vincamine. This compound is cytotoxic against acute and chronic lymphocytic leukemias and acute myelogenous leukemia. Gunasekara DC et al, *ChemMedChem* 2016 Sept 28.

The alkaloid content of leaves is highest during flowering and fruiting; and should be collected at this time. Water extracts of the leaves show activity against gram-positive bacteria.

In France, the extract vincamine is prescribed at 40-60 mg/day for a variety of cerebral senility problems. It is contra-indicated in cerebral tumours with intracranial hypertension, and in pregnant women.

One study of the elderly, involved 30 mg for 12 weeks for primary degenerative and vascular dementia on 152 patients aged fifty to eight-five. Therapeutic efficacy was shown in this study.

Dr. Weiss reports very good results with *V. minor* in cases of Meniere's disease and tinnitus. In one study of treating hearing loss after acoustic trauma, improved hearing was found in 79% of patients, and improved conditions of tinnitus in 66%.

Robinin, a flavonol 0-glycoside, is an HIV-I protease inhibitor.

Vinpocetine has been the subject of over 300 studies published in medical journals. Vinpocetine is a vincamine derivative, and a synthetic ethyl ester of apovincamine. It is also known as Intelectol, Calan and simply Vinpocetine as a brand name.

Vinpocetine has been shown to increase production of the neurotransmitters norepinephrine and dopamine, and increase the release of serotonin. It is considered a pro-acetylcholine as it increases concentration and may help alleviate depression via the increase in serotonin levels.

It inhibits acetylcholine release provoked by glutamine (MSG) and other neuro-excitory amino acids.

More importantly, it is a powerful vasodilator that relaxes the smooth muscles of the vessels leading to the brain, making more oxygen and glucose available to the brain. Combining with a source of rutin, such as buckwheat or violet leaf is even better.

It inhibits cyclic GMP phosphodiesterase, and speculated to enhance cyclic GMP levels in vascular smooth muscle. This is probably the route of increasing blood flow to the brain.

It inhibits platelet aggregation and increases the deformability of red blood cells of erythrocytes, reducing blood viscosity and enhancing mircro-circulation. Schmid-Schonbein et al, *Drug Dev Res* 1988 14.

Vinpocetine may be useful in alleviating migraine headaches, including those associated with PMS.

It may help in the prevention of gastric ulcers, inhibiting the development of lesions. Nosalova et al, *Arzn Forsh* 1993 43.

Interesting work by Miyata et al at the Taisho Pharmaceutical Company in Japan found blood levels of alkaline phosphatase and bone osteocalcin decreased after ingesting vinpocetine. The study looked at kidney dialysis patients, with administration of 15 mg daily for 3-12 months leading to complete elimination of calcinosis in all eight patients.

Some herbalists find it useful in treating retinitis, combining well with pulsatilla. It may be tried in retinopathy, which is a more chronic condition, characterized by congested blood flow, combining well with bilberry or blueberry fruit.

Work by Kaham et al, *Arzn Forsch* 1976 28, found vinpocetine helped inhibit platelet aggregation to blood vessels of the eye in a study of 100 patients.

Wollschlaegger, *J Am Nat Assoc* 2001 4:2 looked at 39 articles written on vinpocetine over the years.

One of three met proper methodology, according to the author leaving a total of 327 patients with the drug or placebo in selected clinical trials. Statistically significant improvement in cognitive function and memory was noted.

Vinpocetine may be useful in the phase between mild cognitive impairment and the development of senile dementia or Alzheimer's disease; at least slowing the disease process and decreasing the incidence. Vinpocetine is, however, ineffective in improving cognitive function in those patients suffering the disease.

Studies have shown antioxidant activity equivalent to vitamin E.

Vinpocetine may be of help in protecting from the after effects of ischemic stroke, at least in one randomized clinical trial.

In a multi-centre, double-blind, placebo-controlled study of 203 patients suffering mild to moderate psycho-syndromes, including primary dementia, significant improvement was noted after 16 weeks.

In Russia, vincamine is prepared with methanol to produce a drug called Metvin. This product possesses a ganglion-blocking action, accompanied by a dilatation of the blood vessels, and a fall in arterial pressure. It is recommended for medical practice in that country.

Vintoperol is another derivative of vincamine that enhances blood flow to the lower extremities, but has toxic side effects.

Vasicine possesses cerebral stimulating properties.

The leaves and stems of *V. minor* and *V. variegata* have been studied in Iran, for their inhibitory effect on *Leishmania major*.

Studies have shown plants fed tryptophan, tryptamine or lysine contain many more alkaloids (vincamin, vincin, vinaminin, vincinin), especially in young shoots.

Tryptophan and lysine together, however, caused an unexpected drop in alkaloid content.

The LD 50 for vincamine in mice is 1000 mg/kg, about one-third the toxicity of caffeine.

The plant contains the indoles, resperine and reserpinine. The former is a monamine transporter, and vesicular monamine transporter to the brain and adrenals, with anti-hypertensive, anti-psychotic, tranquilizing, neuroleptic CNS anti-depressant activity.

Reserpinine is a VMT transporter as well. Both names are commonly associated with the medicinal herb *Rauwolfia serpentina,* or Indian Snakeroot, long prized for anti-depressant and hypotensive activity.

Herbaceous periwinkle (*V. herbacea*) contains majdine and isomajdine, compounds which exhibit apoptosis, anti-oxidant and anti- free radical effects. Gulcin I et al, *J Enzyme Inhib Med Chem* 2012 27(4): 587-94.

## HOMEOPATHY

*Vinca Minor* (Lesser Periwinkle) is considered a useful remedy for various skin conditions like eczema of the head and face.

There is a great sensitivity of the skin, with redness and soreness from slight rubbing (corrosive itching).

The scalp can have itching, or bald spots; with oozing moisture that mats the hair.

The individual may suffer whirling vertigo, and have a ringing or whistling in the ears.

The nose is red on tip, with sores and stoppage in one nostril. Seborrhea on the upper lip and base of nose is common. Weeping inflammations of the upper respiratory passages, as well as nasal polyps indicate this remedy.

Passive, uterine hemorrhage between periods, or continuous, heavy and excessive menstruation; and hemorrhage from fibroids are all symptoms of its use.

Symptoms are worse after swallowing.

Mentally, the patient is cross, with quick temper but repentant soon afterward.

They may dream of being threatened and cursed by a patient that has been treated unsuccessfully.

There may be the sensation of insects or spider webs on face.

**DOSE**- First to third potency. The mother tincture is made from the fresh plant, gathered when coming into flower.

The original proving was down by Rosenberg on five provers with mother tincture in 1838. In 1893 a proving was conducted by Schier, on two females and six males with tincture, 2x, 6c, and 10c potencies.

## GEMMOTHERAPY

*Vinca minor* is hypotensive and helps thin blood. It is useful for increasing circulation to the brain and relieving migraines associated with spasmodic conditions.

**DOSE**- 10-30 drops three times daily of glycerine macerate.

## HYDROSOL

Periwinkle herb is distilled in May and the water is used for women with a cold womb or stomach.

**BRUNSCHWIG**

## FLOWER ESSENCES

Periwinkle (*V. minor*) flower essence helps one integrate personal philosophy and ideals with higher spiritual concepts.

The conscious, subconscious, and super conscious minds are linked; and some subconscious impulses may conflict with ideals. The person may be restless with their current status and are looking for a deeper meaning to life.

**PEGASUS**

Periwinkle flower essence aids in clearing past life experiences which block the flower of energy to a particular organ.

**PETITE FLEUR**

Periwinkle essence has a calming and balancing effect. It promotes "nerves of steel".

**KORTE**

At the physical level, Periwinkle affects hypertension, hemorrhaging and nervous disorders especially anxiety states. It calms the mind. It is also used for SAD, which is a type of depression caused by insufficient sunlight to stimulate the production of a hormone called melatonin during the winter months.

Periwinkle lifts the dark cloud of depression regardless of what apparently caused it. It moves us to the place of inner knowing, our place of deepest wisdom, where we remember who we are.

**PACIFIC**

*Vinca minor* flower essence helps create strong nerves and lets us keep track under chaos.

**MIRIANA**

## PERSONALITY TRAITS

Perry Winkle's Paint Brush

The first Spring descended upon the earth, and…the view from the hilltop across mile after mile of wildflowers with all different blossom and leaf shapes revealed one startling, glaringly obvious thing. Somehow, the finishing touch had been overlooked! All the flowers were one color-White!

The very last flower to have been created was the humble periwinkle. Thus, he was the one called upon to solve the problem of coloring all of the flowers.

"Goodness, gracious" said Perry in a small, blue voice. "I am depressed. There is just no way a little flower like me could color all the flowers in the world."

"Perry," a deep, soft voice resounded, "what you need is a little faith! In this world everyone has a job and is expected to work. The job for you and your family will be to paint all the flowers every color to be found on our earth and in our sky."

"But how can I do such a thing? There are not enough brushes or paint in the world to color the millions of flowers you have strewn on this planet." Perry said in a defeated tone.

"The rainbow will be your never-ending supply of colors. And listen closely: Slip your petals off, and you will see that I have given every periwinkle in my kingdom its very own paintbrush."

**LOVEJOY**

# RECIPES

**TINCTURE- LEAF AND ROOT-** six drops up to three times daily. One part plant to five parts 45% alcohol for dry plant; 1:2 of fresh herb at 60%.

**INFUSION-** One ounce dried herb to one pint of boiling water. Infuse 15 minutes. Drink one-half cup as needed.

**VINCAMINE-** 10-20 mg 3 times daily. It takes from 3-6 weeks before subjective and objective improvements are noted.

**VINPOCETINE-** 10 mg three times daily. Bioavailability is improved 60-100% when taken with food, mainly absorbed via the small intestine. Absorption is as low as 7% on empty stomach.

**CAUTION-** Periwinkle is contra-indicated in low blood pressure. In excess, it can produce granulocytopenia and bone marrow depression. Do not use with brain tumours or acute brain injury, and due to a reduction in ability to clot, should be avoided by hemophiliacs and those taking anti-coagulants. Do not use during pregnancy.

**PROPAGATION-** By root divisions in the spring or fall. Propagation from cuttings, using a rooting hormone, works very well.

Space plants 15-20 inches apart. Prefers partial shade, but will do well in full sun.

**HARVESTING-** Microwave technology appears to be quite useful in drying medicinal herbs, with the majority of cases showing no negative effect to the pharmacological compounds. However, in one study by Kartnig et al, *Pharmazie* 1996 51:12 vincamine was the only substance altered by microwave (300-1200 watts) energy. In many cases, the microwaved herbs contained higher concentrations of determined constituents than the air-dried herbs. Odd but true.

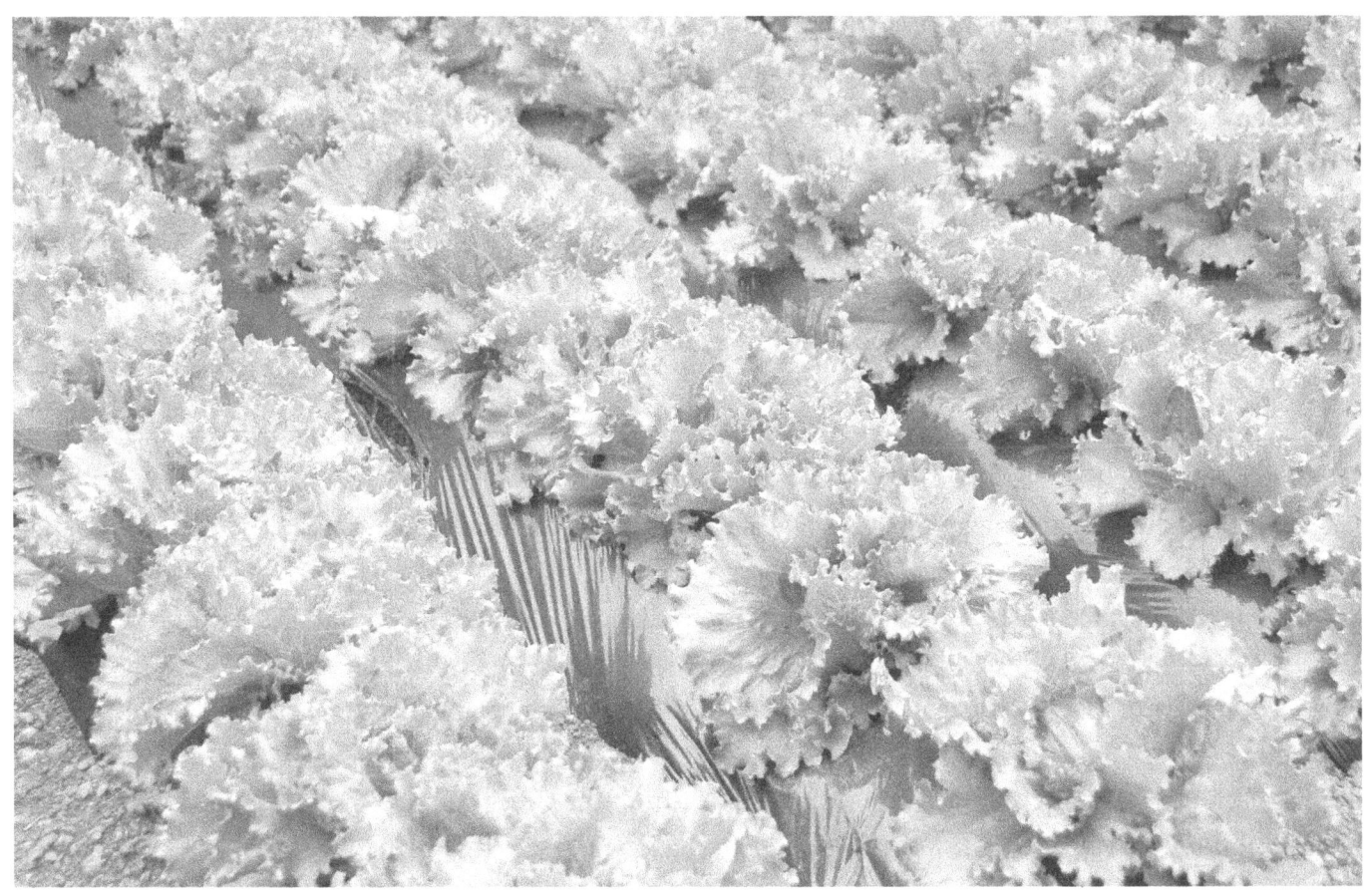

LETTUCE FIELD

**PRICKLY LETTUCE**
**WILD LETTUCE**
**COMPASS PLANT**
(*Lactuca serriola* L.)
(*L. scariola* L.) not accepted
**BITTER LETTUCE**
**POISON LETTUCE**
(*L. virosa* L.)
**WILD BLUE LETTUCE**
(*Mulgedium oblongifolium* [Nutt.] Reveal)
(*L. pulchella* [Pursh] DC) not accepted
(*L. tatarica* [L.] C. A. Mey) not accepted
**TALL BLUE LETTUCE**
**BIENNIAL LETTUCE**
(*L. biennis* [Moench] Fern.)
(*L. spicata* auct. non [Lam] Hitch) not accepted
**TALL YELLOW LETTUCE**
**HORSEWEED**
(*L. canadensis* L.)
(*L. elongata* Muhl. ex Willd.) not accepted

**CULTIVATED LETTUCE**
(*L. sativa* L.)
(*L. sativa var. crispa* Res.)
**WESTERN LETTUCE**
(*L. ludoviciana* [Nutt] Riddell)
**WHITE LETTUCE**
**RATTLESNAKE ROOT**
**LION'S FOOT**
**GALL OF THE EARTH**
(*Nabalus albus* [L.] Hook.) not accepted
(*Prenanthes alba* L.)
(*P. alba* **var.** *serpentaria*) not accepted
**WESTERN RATTLESNAKE ROOT**
(*P. alata* [Hook] D. Dietrich)
(*P. alata* **var.** *sagittata* A. Gray) not accepted
**GLAUCOUS WHITE LETTUCE**
**PURPLE RATTLESNAKE ROOT**
(*P. racemosa* Michx.)
**PARTS USED**- stems, leaves, resin

Among these inebriants the insipissated milky juice of the common garden lettuce is considered as powerful in its operation as opium itself. **W. T. MARCHANT 1888**

I am no worshipper of Hygeia, who was the daughter of that old herb-doctor Aesculapius, and who is represented on monuments holding a serpent in one hand, and in the other a cup out of which the serpent sometimes drinks; but rather of Hebe, cupbearer to Jupiter, who was the daughter of Juno and wild lettuce, and who had the power of restoring gods and men to the vigor of youth. **THOREAU**

The salad or lettuce increases the milk of sucklers and lessens the fire of love. The sharp eye of the eagle is said to be due to the fact that it eats lettuce from time to time. **K. RITTER VON PERGER**

Its juice is of use to those who have wet dreams and it distracts a man from the subject of love-making. **DIOSCORIDES**

Look at this vigorous plant that lifts its head from the meadow; See how its leaves are turned to the north, as true as the magnet; This is the Compass flower... **LONGFELLOW**

Lactuca is from the Latin meaning Milk plant, and alluding to the juice from the stem. The Old French **LAITUES**, from which lettuce was derived, also means milk.

Serriola comes from Skariole, an English name for this particular lettuce since 1400 AD. Escarole is another variation. Scariola refers to the thin, membranous leaves; while prickly refers to the stem and midrib.

Horseweed refers to a large, coarse plant, as in Horseradish, Horse Chestnut and not necessarily useful or good for equines.

Prenanthes means drooping, or face downward flowers, from the Greek, **PRENES**, and **ANTHOS**.

Alba is white, while Alata means winged with protruding ridges that are wider than thick, referring to the winged leaf stalks. Serpentaria relates to the root shape, and hence the common name Rattlesnake Root.

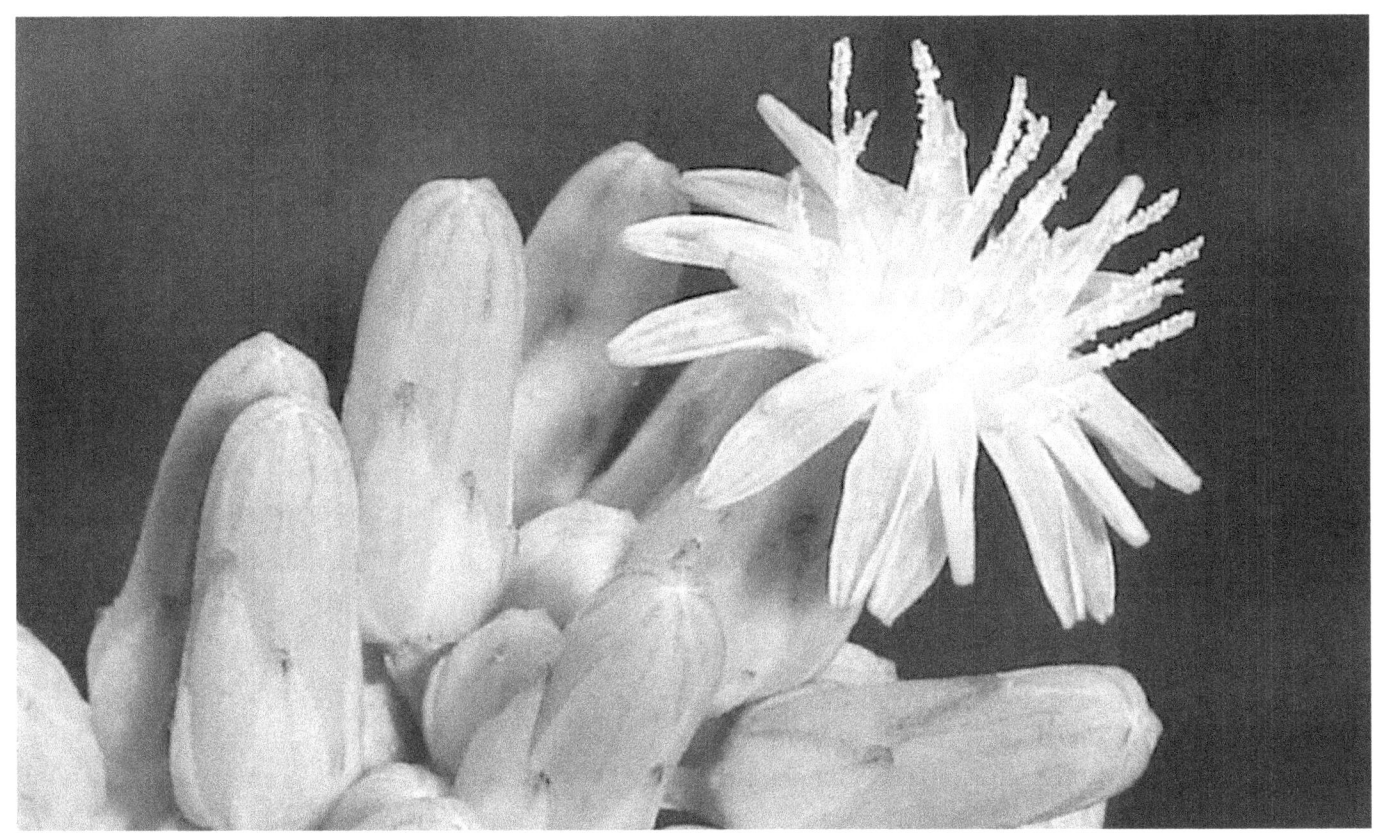

CANADIAN WILD LETTUCE

Wild Lettuce has been long used in herbal medicine. The Assyrians used lettuce and cumin seeds as a poultice for the eyes; the latex as a cough mixture. The first record of lettuce dates from 4500 BC.

The Egyptians cultivated lettuce, which was held sacred to Min, the God of fertility, probably due to the resemblance of milky juice to semen. Temple priests were forbidden to eat the plant.

This is surprising as the Greeks called it the "Eunuch plant" and considered it an an-aphrodisiac. One of the Pythagoran poets, Ibykos called lettuce **EUNUCH** suggesting impotence.

One Greek legend says that after the death of Adonis, Venus used a bed of lettuce leaves to calm her mind and soothe her grieving. Some scholars believe this is an allegory for the impotence associated with the plant.

Ancient Egyptians used wild lettuce, peppermint flowers and the resin from the Acanthus plant to exterminate worms.

Dioscorides noted that the effect of the plant was similar to opium poppy. Comedy poets of the time wrote of the disadvantages of lettuce.

"Two cheers for the lettuces, a plague on them. If a man, even of less than sixty years, eats them and then takes a woman to him he will toss and turn all night long without managing to do what he wants to, even with a helping hand to rub the offending part".

And in the first century AD, Rufus of Ephesos said that eating lettuce fogged the memory and prevented swift thought.

Galen, a century later, ate it late at night, to stop his ever-churning mind.

But to dream of lettuce is said to portend trouble!

Hildegard de Bingen recommended wild lettuce for "anyone with uncontrollable lust". And Gerard asserted the juice "cooleth and quencheth the naturall seed if it be too much used."

A lettuce tea was drunk at bedtime to prevent lustful dreams in young soldiers and monks. It was known as the Eunuch's plant.

Lettuce gained a reputation as an anaphrodisiac to the point where women in England would count the number of heads in their gardens for fear of sterility.

Wild Lettuce seeds exposed to only a brief flash of light will have a high germination rate, even over a wide temperature range.

But, the same seeds, if kept in the dark, will have very poor germination. If, after a flash of light, the wild lettuce seed dries up again, it somehow stores the memory, and when next wet, will begin to grow.

Biennial lettuce is only common around the North Saskatchewan River valley and near Lesser Slave Lake, or at least, that is where I have found it in my part of the world. It has blue to white flowers, sometimes yellowish.

The Bella Coola of British Columbia used decoctions of the root for vomiting or diarrhea, hemorrhages, body pain and heart trouble.

The Ojibwa used plant infusions of **DADOCA'BO** to relieve caked breasts and ease lactation.

Prickly or Wild Lettuce, an introduced annual, has yellow flowers and can be up to four feet tall, distinguished by its row of prickles on the leaf midrib and milky sap. It gives the strongest plant sap in our region. It has somewhat of a reputation as a Compass Plant. In sunny areas, the leaves twist at the base and face east to west, with the edges pointing due north and south.

Work by Werk et al, *Plant Cell Environ* 1985:8 manipulated stem orientation in the plant and showed vertical leaf orientation in a north south plane reduces water loss significantly.

It was traditionally used in Europe, with apple cider vinegar and honey to help relieve edema, by increasing urination.

While living around Lesser Slave Lake, in northern Alberta, I began to experiment with culinary and medicinal herbs. I ordered dozen of species from seed catalogues, including Wild Lettuce.

It grew well. Too well! Before I knew, it had spread itself to adjacent fields and remains well entrenched some 40 years later.

I cut the tops, harvested the dried resin and made tinctures. It is quite a potent hypnotic.

The Fox tribe was quick to integrate this plant into their repertory. They infused the leaves and gave the tea to new mothers to hasten the flow of milk.

The Navaho-Ramah included the herb in ceremonial emetics.

Blue lettuce is smaller, perhaps up to two feet with blue or blue purple flowers, and is perennial.

Gum, from the root of *L. pulchella* was chewed by various Native tribes. The Iroquois made a poultice of the plant and applied it to hemorrhoids.

As Millspaugh says, "one who searches through the domestic literature of medicinal plants, wonders why the bite of snakes ever has a chance to prove fatal. As an alexiteric, the milky juice of the plant is recommended to be taken internally, while the leaves, steeped in water, are frequently applied to the wound, or a decoction of the root is taken...and found useful in dysentery, anemic diarrhea and as a stomachic tonic."

He rates the different species according to yield of latex, with *L. virosa* the richest source followed by *L. scariola*, *L. canadensis* and then common lettuce.

Wild Lettuce juice, when diluted, can be applied to acne or weather damaged skin to both soften and reduce soreness. The extracts will often be found in soaps, lotions and bath products.

Wild Lettuce is an important genetic resource for improved cultivated lettuce. A gene for resistance to downy mildew and leaf miner has been incorporated.

Tall Yellow Lettuce (*L. canadensis*) is a native annual/biennial found in Eastern Canada, and somewhat rare on the prairies.

The Cherokee used infusions for calming nerves and sleep, while the Chippewa used the milky sap on warts, and the Menominee on poison ivy.

The Iroquois used the herb in compound infusions for back and kidney pain; and poulticed the root for bleeding wounds.

Western Lettuce is a biennial, native to Manitoba. The flowers are a washed yellow, the plant uncommon, but found alongside waterways.

Tall Blue Lettuce (*L. biennis*) roots were decocted for heart problems, internal bleeding, chest pains, vomiting and diarrhea by various native tribes.

The Ojibwa, according to Smith, brewed, "this plant to make a tea given to women with caked breasts to render lactation easier.

A dog whisker hair is used to pierce the teat...(They) use this plant to make a hunting lure and say that they cut off the roots and nibble at them when hunting.

The roots are milky like the stem and the hunter wanting a doe will pretend he is a fawn trying to suckle and thus attract a doe close enough to shoot with a bow and arrow."

The Potawatomi know it as Teat Weed, or **NONA'GONAWÛCK**.

The Ojibwa used the crushed leaves and flowers for bee and wasp stings, and made a decoction for colds.

Tall Blue Lettuce (*L. biennis*) and its odour were not appreciated by the Gitksan of British Columbia, who named it **SGANKW'ATS**, meaning excrement plant.

Common Lettuce (*L. sativa*) seed is used in Egyptian folk medicine to treat coughs, rhinitis, asthma, pertussis, insomnia, rheumatism and insanity. Most of the bitterness, and medicinal virtues have been bred out, but can still have benefit. In the Yucatan, leaf decoctions are taken several times daily for constipation. The well-strained water is also used as eye drops in cases of inflammation. Both leaves and stems are a sedative for insomnia and heart palpitations, taken last thing at night.

Lettuce seed is quite emollient, and when blended in water produces an emulsion that is almond-like in odour and taste.

It is useful for soothing irritated and inflamed membranes. Lettuce leaf and seed oil are used in Aussie Hair Salad Conditioner and similar personal care products.

In Guatemala, the latex is added to Blessed Thistle and Valerian root decoctions to relieve hypertension and nervous conditions.

Lettuce can be companion planted with Chervil and Dill to protect against aphids.

Around 18 million metric tons of lettuce is produced annually around the world. Large amounts of waste are associated with the industry, and other uses for leftover parts would be good.

The base of commercial lettuce drips latex after cutting. Place it on an empty glass to collect the slow dripping juice that can be dried for later use.

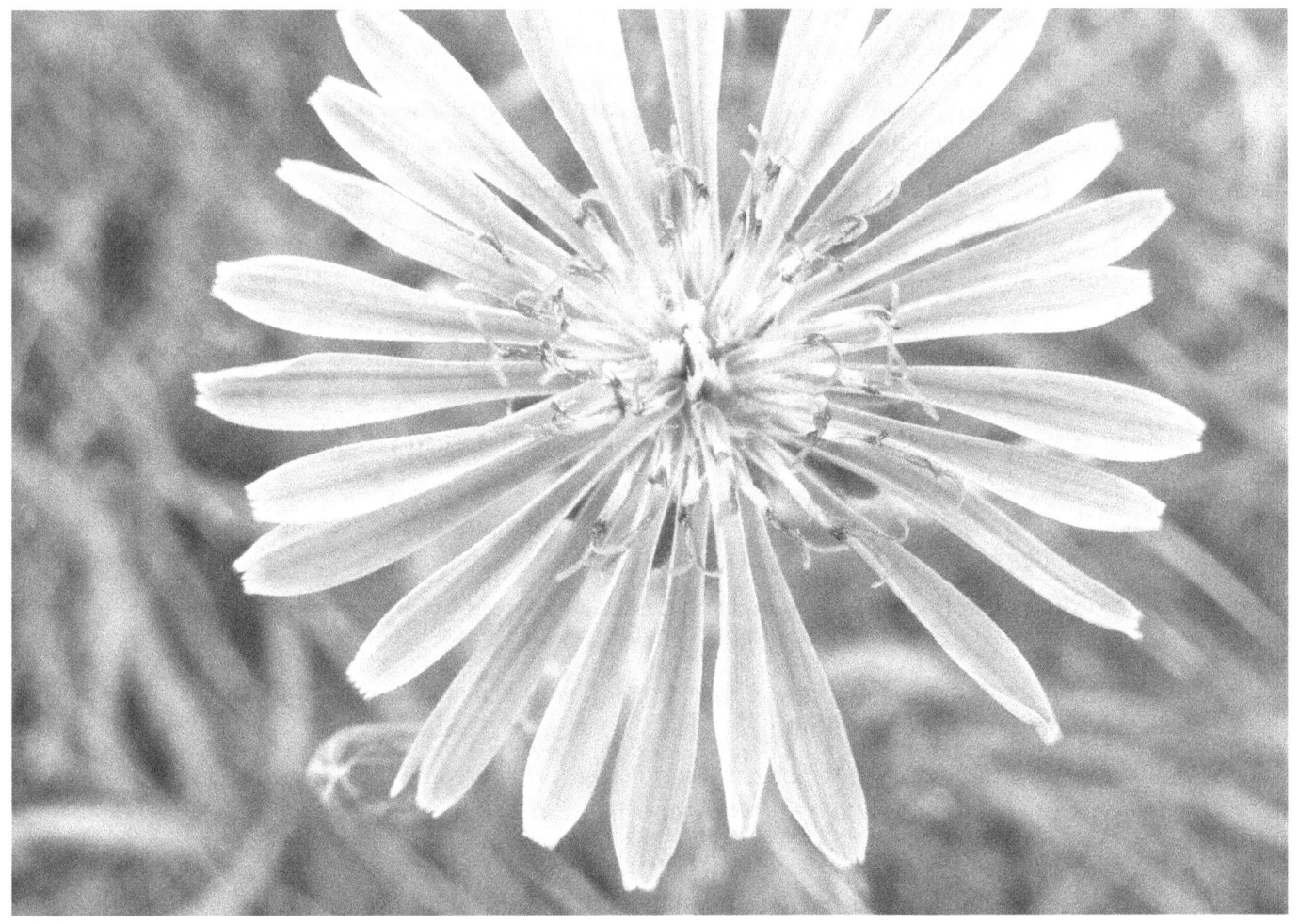

BLUE LETTUCE FLOWER

Dr. John Vederas, a chemistry professor at the University of Alberta, is studying the possibility of producing industrial quality rubber from Sunflowers and Lettuce.

He has already identified a brand of Canadian lettuce that naturally produces rubber of high quality with a long rubber molecule. A very exciting and innovative project!

Celtuce (*L. sativa var. augustana*), or Chinese Lettuce, is an "oriental vegetable", that is excellent both raw and cooked. It is more heat resistant than lettuce, but will still bolt in hot temperatures. The stems can be eaten like celery. Very versatile!

Western Rattlesnake Root (*P. alata*) was decocted by the Bella Coola and taken for colds, with small doses for babies. They also poulticed the roots or chewed them and applied it to burns or other painful parts of the body.

White Lettuce is found in open woods throughout the prairies.

White Lettuce, or Rattlesnake Root was dried and powdered and added to food of new mothers by the Chippewa to produce breast milk. It is known as Milk root, or **DADO'CABODJI'BIK**.

The Iroquois poulticed the roots for rattlesnake and dog bites, and hence the common name. An infusion of the roots was used as a wash for weakness.

The Ojibwa used the milk from the lettuce as a diuretic, particularly for women. The root was used as an unspecified female remedy.

Glaucous White Lettuce flowers are greenish or yellowish white but enclosed in purplish bracts.

110

# MEDICINAL

**CONSTITUENTS-** *L. virosa*-sesquiterpene lactones including lactucpicrin (lactupictin, intybin), lactucin, 8-desoxy-11b, 13-dihydrolactin, jaquinelin and lactucerin; glucoside lactuside A, germanicol, lactucone, flavonoids and coumarins, such as cichoriin and aesculin; flavones including agigenin and lactupicrin, lactucin (0.2%), lactucone (50-60%), lactucic and pectic acids, citric, malic, oxalic and cichoric acids, catachou, essential oils including camphor, mannitol, gum, lactucerol (triterpene), potassium nitrate, polyacetylenes, taraxasterol (beta lactucerol) and beta amyrin.
root- sesquiterpene lactones including jacquinelin, jacquinelin glucoside and lactuside A.
*L. serriola*- roots- sesquiterpenoids, glucozaluzanin, 11,13-dihydro-glucozaluzanin, 9-hydroxy-zaluzanin, and 9-hydroxy-11,13-dihydro-zaluzanin
tops- lactulide, lactucopicriside, macroclinoside, lactuasides, and di-hydrosantamarin.
leaves- lactucin, lactucerin, lactupicrin, hyoscyamine, beta amyrin, lactucerols, quercitin-3-0-beta-D-glycopyranoside, luteolin-7-0-beta-D-glucopyranoside, luteolin, querctin, kaempferol, 1beta,13-dihydrolactucin
seed- arachidic, caproic, linoleic (20%), oleic, stearic, palmitic acid, as well as squalene.
*L. sativa*- Romaine lettuce is rich in folic acid; 100 grams providing 75% of RDA; lettucine.
Red leaf lettuce- various phenolic acids including quercitin 3-malonylglucoside.
*L. canadensis*- lactucrin, lactuopicrin
*L. indica*- latucain A-C, lactucaside, 11beta, 13-dihydrolactucin, cichoriosides B, quercitin, quercitin 3-O-glucoside, rutin, apigenin, luteolin and chlorogenic acid.
Root- 19 sesquiterpene lactones, including three pairs of zaluzanin C-type guaianolides, and eudesmanolides.
*P. alba*- resins, tannin, extractive, gum and wax.

Prickly or Wild Lettuce is the source of lactucarium, or lettuce opium. This dry, brown, milky sap looks and smells like opium and was once listed in the United States Pharmacopoeia.

To collect the milky sap, wait until just flowering and then take your scythe or hedge clippers to the tops.

Allow the sap to gather at top and dry a bit. Scrape into bowl. Snip again, dry a bit, and scrape again.

The alternative method is to absorb the latex from the broken stems with a sponge, squeeze into a cup and let harden.

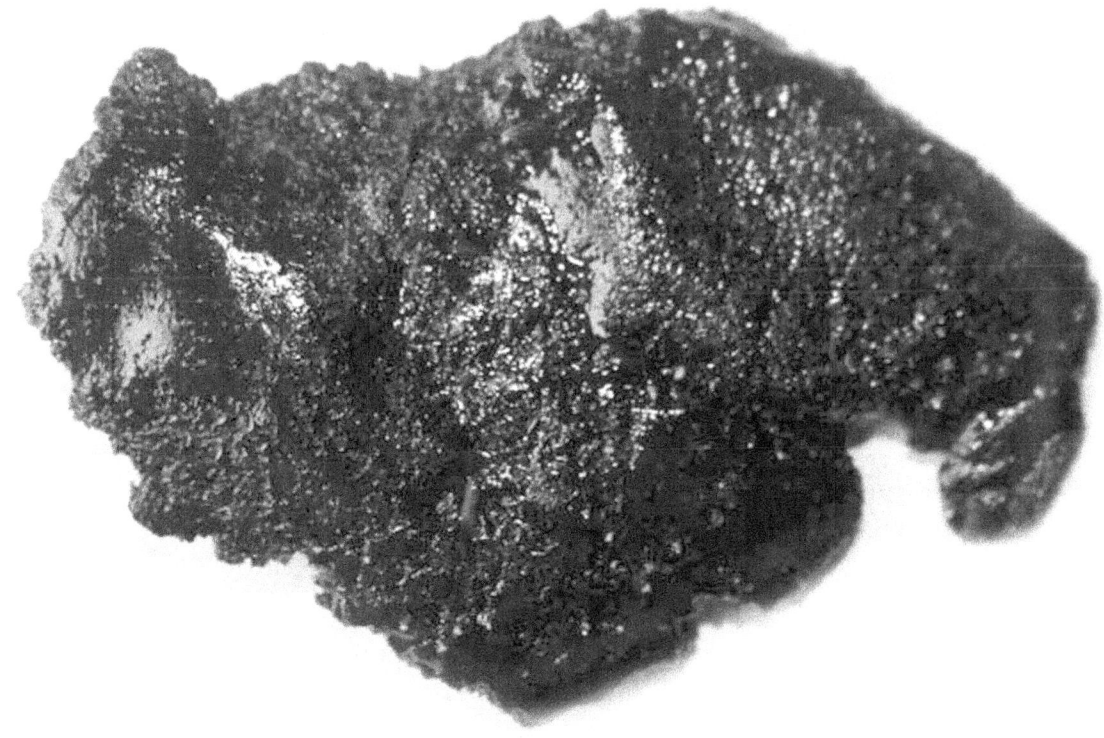

WILD LETTUCE RESIN

Some herbalists believe the flower seeds are every bit as strong. That has never been my observation. Traditionally, the resin has been used as a calmative, hypnotic, sedative and analgesic. The whole plant is bitter, sweet and cooling.

It relieves insomnia in both the young and old, when the nervous system has been over stimulated. Lactucin, for example is both a bitter tonic and sedative.

An analgesic effect is produced by the extract that inhibits the activity of a neutral endopeptidase, which plays a role in the breaking down of encephalins. Funke et al, *Z Phytother* 2002 23:1.

It helps irritable, excitable conditions where there is poor digestion, anxiety and manic states. This includes sexual overstimulation or a constant erection not always related to sexual desire.

If Wild Lettuce does not give relief, see a trained health professional as priapism is some times associated with acute leukemia. It may be of benefit in middle-aged males taking Viagra or Cialis with persistent erections that become painful.

Matthew Wood has an interesting theory regarding the benefit of wild lettuce in hyper-androgenic conditions.

"Androgen is hard for the liver to break down and is one of the causes of 'bad blood' and skin eruptions. High levels occur in teenagers, both boys and girls, as they enter sexual maturity and their bones grow—androgen stimulates bone growth.

Lactuca is one of the great remedies for teenagers.

One would associate high androgen levels with a high sex drive—we certainly see this in teens—but high levels do not translate automatically to a successful sex life. Indeed, they are often associated with frustration and the need to make changes in life."

Young women with painful menstrual cramps may benefit.

It quiets the chronic dry, irritated coughs of children, alleviating sleeplessness and general irritability, the resin combined with a pleasant taste in syrup.

Although it is limited in strength, the herb does, nonetheless, exert an influence on the spinal cord, by depressing pain, and sedates the sympathetic ganglia of the thoracic. It is still listed in the *Edinburgh Pharmacopoeia* as a cough suppressant, and is used especially for whooping cough. Gumprecht T, *Med Chir Trans* 1815(6): 608-17.

It combines well with Valerian for insomnia, with Black Cohosh for joint or muscular pain, and with Skullcap for those shaking addictions.

For nervous, irritating coughs, it combines well with mullein, marshmallow root, and even wild cherry bark when the picture suits. Do not use for acute severe coughs unless modified as part of formula.

Work by Eskander, *Egyptian Journal of Pharmaceutical Sciences* 1995 36:1-6, and 253-70 looked at a herbal formula containing *L. virosa*, Coriander (*C. sativum*), Black Cumin (*Nigella sativa*) and Garden Cress (*Lepidium sativum*) for anti-diabetic activity. After ten days of the water extract, all lab animals exhibited normal blood glucose levels. The therapy also increased serum insulin levels, restored SGOT, SGPT and alkaline phosphatase to normal range.

Lactucopicrin, for example, has been shown to possess hypoglycemic activity. It is also found in chicory.

Lactucopicrin may be a promising neurotrophin-mediated neuroprotective compound for neurodegenerative conditions. It inhibits acetylcholineasterase and promotes neurite growth. Venkatesan R et al, *J Ethnopharmacology* 2017 198: 174-83.

Wild Lettuce contains sedatives like lactucin, as well as an alkaloid similar to hyoscamine (see Henbane), with activity as a parasympathetic nerve depressant. All Lactuca species contain nanograms of morphine.

These two activities appear to give Wild Lettuce its neuromuscular sedative and relaxing properties, combined with anti-spasmodic, anti-inflammatory and analgesic action.

Animal studies found alcohol extracts reduce spasms of the intestine, bronchioles and vasculature, comparable to dicylomine, a muscarinic antagonist, as well as a possible Ca(++) channel blocker. Janbaz KH et al, *Evid Based Complement Alternat Med* 2013:304394.

Germanicol, derived from wild lettuce, induces apoptosis of human colon cancer cell lines HCT-116 and HT29. Hu YL et al, *J BUON* 2016 21(3): 626-32.

Matthew Wood contributes a great deal more to our knowledge of this plant.

"Lactuca relaxes tight muscles and settles insomnia. It is indicated for stiff, sore persons with painful muscles, especially in the lower back. The pulse is slow and hard…it indicates 'cold blockage' or 'internal cold' as it would be termed in Chinese herbalism. This is cold that has invaded the body, causing hardness, stiffness, and pain. It is the opposite of 'deficient cold' which arises from a lack of internal heat; the pulse is slow and deep.

Wild Lettuce is one of the bitter/acrid remedies that disperse tension caused by penetration of cold. Cold often constricts the pores of the skin. However, in this case the cold goes to a deeper level, anchoring in the muscles and articulations, resulting in stiff, sore muscles, lack of bendability, soreness in the lower back, and shallow respiration from tight muscles across the chest."

He continues. "Lactuca is one of the best remedies in existence for teenage acne, or any acne where the face is involved and there is a rough, cystic form with deep cysts slowly coming to the surface; the whole causing unsightly roughness and scar tissue. It will clean this up from the inside, reducing the acne on the face for several weeks. Then, a new crop—the cysts from below—boil up at about the third week and cause a new outbreak.

After that the face clears up and even old scars seemingly disappear because the heat, swelling and waste products in what appear to be scars are dissipated. Meanwhile, the hard, slow pulse softens."

Wild Lettuce may be used in treating hyperactive thyroid, combining well with Melissa, or Bugleweed. Wild Lettuce lowers libido, like Hops, acting as an anaphrodisiac.

Prickly lettuce, and chicory both contain 8-deoxylactucin that in lab studies has shown to have cytotoxic and anti-tumor activity.

Extracts of Wild Lettuce show activity against *Candida albicans*. Work by Kim, *Arch Pharm Res* 2001 24:5 found methanol extract of the aerial parts to possess antioxidant activity. Wild Lettuce was originally listed in the *US Pharmacopoeia* from 1820-1951, under the name *L. elongata*.

During the Second World War, codeine from opium was difficult to obtain. Extracts of lettuce juice were given to soldiers for its analgesic, sedative and cough-suppressing effects with some effect. It is not powerful like opium, but it was all they had.

Wild lettuce protects against oxidative stress-induced cardiomyocytes damage from doxorubicin. Hosseini A & D. Mahdian, *Acta Pol Pharm* 2016 73(3): 659-66.

Water extracts of *L. scariola* flowers show activity against gram-positive bacteria.

The seeds of *L. sativa* are used in Hopei province of China as a substitute for the dried fruit of Chinese Teasel (*Dipsacus chinensis*); known as **CHU SHENG TZU**.

The seed decoction enters the kidney and liver meridians and helps to strengthen tendons and muscles, pain due to lacerated tendons or muscles, carbuncles, incised wounds, vaginal bleeding during pregnancy, lumbago and involuntary seminal emissions.

In Western Herbal medicine, the seeds are used for asthma, bronchitis, spasmodic coughs, and, of course, insomnia.

Common lettuce, especially the Iceberg variety so common in supermarkets, also contains small amounts of opium like alkaloids. These slow down digestion, leading to the observation that eating salads after the meal, as is common in Europe, is better than before, especially if it is cold and slows down digestion.

Early Greeks and Romans served lettuce at the end of meals due to its sleep inducing properties. When Domitian became emperor in 81 AD, he insisted lettuce be served at beginning of meal as he believed it stimulated the appetite. He was and is still wrong.

Work by Gonzalex-Lima, isolated a compound from common lettuce with pharmacologically depressant property. *Int Journal Crude Drug Res* 1986 24.

Lettuce juice does have its uses, however. It is a relatively rich source of iron, particularly Romaine, with higher levels than grapes, spinach or raisins.

Magnesium in lettuce juice is revitalizing to muscle fibre, nerves, brain cells and lung tissue. It also assists normal fluidity of the blood; and is known to increase breast milk in lactating women.

Lettuce juice contains good iodine and five vitamins. As a tonic, it helps in anemia, nervousness, acidosis, insomnia, headaches, obesity, urinary disorders, goiter, dropsy and tuberculosis.

It is more palatable, combined with carrot juice in a ratio of 1:2.

Recent work by Piero et al, *J Agric Food Chem* 2002 50 found a lettuce serine-like protease, called lettucine that substitutes well as a rennet substitute for making cheese.

An article in the same journal by Carvalho 2003 51:3 found inorganic selenium retained in the edible portion of lettuce plants, suggesting its possible use in supplementing dietary needs.

An alcoholic extract of Garden Lettuce was found to exhibit a sedative effect on toads, suggesting caution when you feed your pet amphibians! Alcohol extracts also protect mice against anxiety. Harsha SN et al, *J Biomed Res* 2013 27(1): 37-42.

The effects of n-butanol extracts of common lettuce are comparable to those induced by diazepam. Ghorbani A et al, *Iran J Pharm Res* 2013 12(2): 401-6.

Red Leaf lettuce contains various phenolic acids with free radical scavenging activity. Caldwell, *J Ag Food Chem* 2003 51:16. Follow up by Llorach et al, in same journal 2004 2 found lettuce byproducts rich in antioxidant polyphenols that could be used in dietary or functional food applications.

Nicolle et al, *Clin Nutr* 2004 4 looked at lettuce ingestion effect on lipid metabolism and antioxidant effect in rats. Fed 20% of their diet as lettuce for three weeks, decreased cholesterol levels by 41%. It increased plasma levels of vitamin C and E, suggesting benefit as an antioxidant and in cholesterol metabolism, at least in rats!

Work by Deshmukh et al, *J Herb Med Tox* 2007 1:1 found ethanol extracts of *L. sativa* protective of oxidative stress and lipofuscin accumulation in mice.

Lettuce is undergoing genetic manipulation. Work by Daniell et al, *Plant Biotech Journal* July 2007 placed a subunit of cholera toxin with human pro-insulin in lettuce, to produce insulin suitable for humans. Transgenic lettuce has been used to create a vaccine against pig edema bacterial disease. Matsui et al, *Biosci Biotech Biochem* 2009 73:7.

An exciting, or possibly scary development, depending upon your point of view.

Indian Lettuce (*L. indica*) is an edible, wild vegetable used traditionally for anti-inflammatory activity, is anti-bacterial and used to treat intestinal disorders. A recent study by Sheng Yang Wang et al, in *J Agric Food Chem* 2003 51 found six phenolic compounds with anti-oxidant properties in the plant.

Work by Yi-Hsuan Chen et al, in same journal 2007:55 found Indian Lettuce induced apoptosis in human leukemia cell lines. Chia Chung Hou, *J Nat Prod* 66:5 found significant anti-diabetic activity associated with the herb. Latucain and lactucaside show significant anti-diabetic action. Hou CC et al, *J Nat Prod* 2003 66(5): 625-9.

Alcohol extracts protect the liver against hepatitis B virus replication. Various quinic acid derivates and flavonoids are believed responsible. Kim KH et al, *Bioorg Med Chem Lett* 2007 17(24): 6739-43.

Leaf decoctions appear to help reduce bacterial adhesion to epithelial cells of the urinary tract. Luthje et al, *J Ethnopharmacology* 135:3.

The Oregon Poison Center reported the story of three young adults who prepared a crude water extract of *L. virosa* and injected it intravenously. All three rapidly became ill with fevers, chills, abdominal pain, flank and back pain, neck stiffness, headache, leukocytosis and mild liver function abnormalities. All recovered within three days.

Rattlesnake root (*P. alba*) is a bitter astringent that helps relieve dysentery and diarrhea.

The fresh leaves have been used as a poultice on skin wounds.

# HOMEOPATHY

Acrid Lettuce (*Lactuca virosa*) acts principally upon the brain and circulatory system. It is useful for delirium tremens with sleeplessness, coldness and tremor.

It is useful for coldness and numbness of the legs and feet, tremors of the hands and arms, or cramps in the shin bones, extending to the toes and side of leg involving calves.

It is a true galactagogue, increasing the milk flow in breasts.

It aids difficulty in breathing, with suffocative breathing from dropsy of the chest. Constant, tickling coughs, or incessant, spasmodic coughs also respond to Lettuce.

Sensations of fullness and colic in the abdomen, with sensations of weight are relieved.

Forsaken feeling, dreams of flying, desire for yogurt.

**DOSE-** Tincture. 5-10 drops as needed. The mother tincture is made the whole fresh plant in flower. Original 16 provers by Seidel from juice, extract and tincture in 1846. Additional clinical observations by Hering and Mangialavori.

Nabalus or Rattle Snake Root (*P. serpentaria*) is similar to above with a few variations. It is for chronic diarrhea, made worse by eating, at night and towards morning. There is pain in the abdomen and rectum, with emaciation, dyspepsia and acid burning eructations. There may be a craving for acid foods.

Vaginal discharge with a throbbing in the uterus is another symptom.

Depression of spirits in evening, vague foreboding in morning.

**DOSE-** lower potencies. In all likelihood this is actually *Nabalus albus*, now known as *Prenanthes alba*. See Vermeulen & Johnston, *Plants* volume 1 page 762.

Original proving by Lazarus, at first and third dilutions in 1855.

# SEED OIL

The seed of *L. serriola* contains 35-41% oil, mainly composed (20-63%) of linoleic and 5% palmitic acid; as well as 10% epoxy acids such as coronaric and vernolic acids.

The seed oil is used for treating atherosclerosis, and at one time was used as a substitute for wheat germ oil.

Common Lettuce seeds contain 27.4% of the same epoxy acids.

These are of potential interest as replacements for synthetic epoxy compounds used as stabilizers for plastic materials.

The seeds of common lettuce contain oleic acid (61%), stearic acid (20.4%), palmitic acid (9.7%), myristic (2.8%) cis-palmitoleic acid (1.2%), behenic acid (0.5%) and lignoseric acid (0.3%). Both beta sitosterol and beta amyrin are also present.

In Fitoterapia 1996 67: 3, work by Said et al, found the oil showed sedative effective, potentiation of the hypnotic effect of barbiturates, as well as analgesic and anti-convulsant activity. The LD50 of mice was 19.8 ml/kg.

## ESSENTIAL OIL

Common lettuce leaf, both fresh and dry, has been steam distilled. Results of analysis show respectively alpha pinene (5.11% and 4.05%), y-cymene (2-07% and 1.92%), durenol (52% and 50%), alpha-terpinene (1.66% and 1.34%), thymol acetate (0.99% and 0.67%), caryophyllene (2.11% and 1.98%), spathulenol 3.09% and 2.98%), camphene (4.11% and 3.65%), limonene (1.28% and 1.11%) as major compounds. Lesser amounts of beta pinene, alpha terpinolene, linalool, 4-terpineol, alpha-terpineol, o-methylthymol, L-alloaromadendrene and viridiflorene are also present.

The essential oil of *L. sativa* has been found strongly insecticidal and destructive of blowfly larvae. Khater et al, *Int J Dermatol* 2011 50:2.

The seed of *L. sativa* has also been steam distilled. The essential oil has been studied for its diuretic action.

## HYDROSOL

Lettuce water cools the blood when it is over-heated, for when it is not, it needs no cooling: it cools the head and liver, stays hot vapours ascending to the head and hinders sleep; it quenches immoderate thirst and breeds milk in nurses, distil it in May.
**CULPEPPER**

Lettuce water, the hydrosol left over from distillation was very popular in France at one time for treating insomnia. Two to four ounces of the water were taken before bed, known as Eau de Laitre.

Lettuce water comforts the liver, and is good for inflamed and hot blood. It is good for dizziness, trembling in limbs, dysentery, women sucking a child and having little milk; a hot dry cough, sore throat or diarrhea.
**BRUNSCHWIG**

## FLOWER ESSENCES

Lettuce (*L. crispa*) flower essence is indicated in times of restlessness, the inability to make decisions or concentrate, with agitation, and anger.

The essence helps develop clear communication skills, unblock creative expression, and the ability to speak one's truth.
**MASTER**

Lettuce (*L. sativa*) flower essence is for those who tend to escape from perceptive reality whenever a new situation is present. These new emotional states are rejected by the individual leading to the loss of consciousness, hysteria, sexual deviations. The individual need to be grounded and needs "maternal" protection to face the new reality.
**FLORIAS DE MINAS**

## PERSONALITY TRAITS

Lettuce is like conversation; it must be fresh and crisp, so sparkling that you scarcely notice the bitter in it. Lettuce, like most talkers, is however, apt to run quickly to seed. Blessed is that sort which comes to a head, and so remains, like a few people I know; growing more solid and satisfactory and tender at the same time, and whiter at the center, and crisper in their maturity.

Lettuce, like conversation, requires a good deal of oil, to avoid friction, and keep the company smooth; a pinch of attic salt; a dash of pepper; a quantity of mustard and vinegar, by all means, but so mixed that you will notice no sharp contrasts; and a trifle of sugar. You can put anything, and the more things the better, into salad, as into conversation; but everything depends upon the skill of mixing. I feel that I am in the best society when I am with lettuce. It is in the select circle of vegetables.
**CHARLES D. WARNER**

The positive Lettuce state is a joy to behold. Here we see the sailboat personality forging "full speed ahead" into creative projects such as writing, painting, woodworking or calligraphy.

In the performing arts, one in the positive Lettuce state breezes across that fine transition line between the actual creative process and its presentation before an audience.

In the positive Lettuce state, we are able to speak up for ourselves instead of "stuffing it" when we feel mistreated. All too often, repression creates resentment and anger that can later manifest as emotional outbursts.

The negative Lettuce state manifests much like a stampede of horses—a mind running wild with thoughts shooting out in several directions at once—or with emotions that do us harm, anger in particular. Of all the human emotions, anger is probably the most destructive.

It is actually known to destroy brain cells, not to mention causing deep agitation in each and every bodily system…In the negative Lettuce state marked with agitation thoughts or emotions, success is virtually impossible. Attainment of even minor goals remains an illusive dream without the necessary ingredient of concentration; and concentration is the fruit of calmness.                                                                    **LILA DEVI**

I call it the "street person remedy". It is for people with a complete lack of motivation. Before this stage is reached, however, it is a remedy for negative thinking. This came out in the homeopathic provings. Lactuca people sit and think about the worst possible scenarios that could happen, and that keeps them home, brooding over imaginary problems and injustices.                                                                              **WOOD**

## BOTANICAL POETICA

I know you don't want to be eaten anymore than a cow or a pig or a chicken does but
they're the vicious vegetarians
& they say you do
Gobbling up the innocent green beings who gladden any reasonable person's heart
I'll tell you little lettuce you'll see them in cowskin shoes and belts & nobody can make
sense of that those virtuous vegetarians they'll look at you with prim distaste while
you enjoy your bacon.
Makes me want to buy some cowboy movie blood capsules. Imagine an introduction
I'd like you to meet Lily, she's a non-smoking, non-drinking vegetarian separatist
Pisces with choco-phobia
& I smile while secretly biting down on the capsules concealed in my cheeks then
shake her hand drooling blood I whisper
Hi I'm a flaming carnivorous double Scorpio who'll eat anything & as she wilts in
dismay trembles with trepidation
Hisses with disgust. Ah then little lettuces we'll have our moment of laughing revenge.

### CHRYSTOS

# MYTHS AND LEGENDS

The Greek legends tell of when the Gods became enraged with Adonis and his mother Aphrodite hid him in a field of lettuce. Under their leaves, he remained for a number of years protected from the wrath of other Gods.

Lettuce was sacred to the popular Egyptian god Min. The Greeks saw Min as a form of their lusty god Pan, and portrayed with an erect penis. He was the god of the desert, the lightning, and the sandstorm as well as the god of fertility and procreation. He wore a headdress made of ostrich feathers. His symbols were the phallus and the lettuce.                                                                                              **RÄTSCH**

Lechuga is used to guard against evil. In the mysteries of Adonis the lettuce was considered a sacred plant.

It is alluded Emperor Diocletian, after his abdication, that a friend attempted to lure him back to the throne by promises of giving him the finest lettuce growing in his garden. It supposedly exerts a sedative action on the sexual drive. However, this must be only in the form of when taken as the extracted latex, as it has been said that hermits use the extraction to subdue the sex drive. It induces sleep.

Suetonius reports that a statue was raised to Musa, Physician to August, for having cured the emperor of a melancholy by making him eat lettuce. **ANDOH**

The ancient Egyptians depicted Min with an erect phallus and a black body symbolizing the fertile soil. At the annual harvest festival, the pharaoh arranged for Min's statues to be removed from their shrines and for offerings of lettuce to be made to the god; then the god's statues were replaced in their sacred homes.

People marched in possession at Min's festival, carrying heads of lettuce and representations of checkerboard gardens of lettuce, in celebration of fruitful harvests. **TAMRA ANDREWS**

## RECIPES

**TINCTURE-** Take your collected latex and dissolve it in 95% alcohol at 1:2 ratio. The fresh budding tops of wild lettuce are prepared with same recipe.

Take one half to one teaspoon as needed.

For fresh leaves, make a 1:1 ratio in 45% alcohol. This is much weaker product.

**INFUSION-** The dried leaf can be made into a tea; one heaping Tbsp per pint of hot water. Steep and take 2-8 ounces as needed.

**SEED DECOCTION-** 9-15 grams.

**LACTUCARIUM-** 5-20 grains (0.3 -1.0 grams) three times daily.

**WILD LETTUCE ALE-** Simmer 12 ounces of molasses, 8 ounces brown sugar in four litres of water. Cool to 70° Fahrenheit, and pour into fermenter. Chop one ounce prepared sap into small pieces and add both this and yeast. Ferment. **BUHNER**

**CAUTION-** Do not use at maximum doses for extended periods of time, due to cumulative toxicity, unless part of an herbal combination.

One report out of northern Iran, cited eight people with wild lettuce (*L. virosa*) toxicity. Besharat S et al, *BMJ Case Rep* 2009.

Also, do not use if glaucoma or prostate enlargement is present, according to Christopher Hobbs. Avoid during pregnancy.

An interesting site is www.wildlettuce.com .

## LICHENS

Or to swamps where the usnea lichen hangs in festoons from the white-spruce trees. **THOREAU**

Did you hear the one about the fungus and the algae…they took a lichen to each other.

Freddy Fungus met Anne Algae, they fell in love, got married & now their marriage is on the rocks.

Thou for frozen lands wast meant, Ere the winter's frost was sent;
And in love he sped thee forth, To thy home, the frozen north,
"Where he bade the rocks produce, bitter lichens for thy use." **MARY HOWITT**

Lichen is from the Greek **LEIKO** to lick or lick up a habit of the plant to lap its tongues all over the host.

Lichen may also come from the Greek for "leprous, wart or eruption", as Dioscorides thought they resembled the skin of afflicted people, and used the Doctrine of Signatures as an attempted cure. The French scientist, Tournefort named them back in 1700 AD.

Usnea is from the Arabic **USHNA** for moss. Bryoria is derived from Bryopogon and Alectoria, two classifications to which lichens were formerly assigned.

Lichens are a slow growing symbiotic combination of fungi and algae. As such, they do not completely resemble either group, but have their own beautiful and distinctive look. One lichenologist called lichens "fungi that have discovered agriculture" in reference to their symbiotic relationship.

There are 42% lichenized, and 58% non-lichenized fungal species within Ascomycota. Lutzoni et al, *Nature* 2001 411.

Lichen fossils have been discovered dating back to the Devonian period some 400 million years ago.

For a long time, it was believed that the relationship was symbiotic. Many scientists now believe, following laboratory study, that the fungus is really a parasite. When lichens were experimentally separated in labs and grown apart, the algae grew more quickly and the fungus more slowly. However, when the two join forces, they can survive where neither would make it one its own. In fact, scientists could get them to rejoin only when conditions would not support them separately. Strange bedfellows indeed!

When this idea of two organisms living together was first proposed, it was considered quite radical.

Mordecai Cooke denounced this dualism as "unqualified romance, which a future generation will contemplate as fairy tales".

The German, Simon Schwendener wrote in 1869, "This fungus…slaves are green algae, which it has sought out or indeed caught hold of, and compelled into its service. It surrounds them, as a spider its prey, with a fibrous net of narrow meshes, which is gradually converted into an impenetrable covering, but while the spider sucks its prey and leaves it dead, the fungus incites the algae found in its net to more rapid activity, even to more vigorous increase."

The term helotism, suggesting a master slave relationship, may best describe lichens, according to this ancient dictum. They are what they are, and we need to see them as whole organisms instead of reductionist redundancy.

They have the ability to grow in the coldest, snow-free alpine and boreal forest, often growing less than a millimeter a year. Lichens have been found growing on rocks just 264 miles from the South Pole!

It is estimated that from 13,000 to 14,000 lichen species inhabit our planet.

Lichenographs, or printed illustrations were first published in 1480. Linnaeus was not keen on lichens, and called them *Rustici pauperrimi*, or the poor trash of vegetation.

Lichens have been used for natural dyes, including the tartans of Scotland. A few crofters still produce Harris Tweed using the lichen *Parmelia omphalodes*. An added advantage over synthetic dye was that bitter lichen acids repel moths. The related *P. chlorochroa*, which grows on calcareous rocks on the prairie grassland, was used by the Navaho to produce nice warm brown dyes to their wools and blankets.

Brilliant blues, pinks and purples are possible, something highly unusual in the plant kingdom, by using the ammonia of urine, and fermenting for several weeks.

It is said the smell of urine disappears in time and finally exudes a violet-like scent. If not fixed by mordant, the colours quickly dull to a pale brown in sunlight.

*Ochrolechia oregonensis*, which grows with little pink discs on the rough bark of conifers, gives a violet, purple dye, and is somewhat plentiful.

The Cree of northern Canada used *Dicranum* lichen for lamp wicks, and various *Umbilicaria* species for food.

Other lichens, such as the Snow Bed Iceland, were simply used as hot burning tinder.

Throughout the years, there have been used for medicine, food and beer making. Medicinal use of *Evernia furfuracea* has been traced back to 1800 BC.

A thriving brandy-making industry in Sweden and Russia when bankrupt in the 19th century when the lichen supply was exhausted. One kilogram of lichen was needed to produce one-half litre of alcohol.

In France, today, lichens are used in the production of chocolates, using the lichen as a filler and substitute for starch.

After all, lichen fibre is composed mainly of mannose, galactose and glucose, with each species having different make-ups. *Cetraria* and *Alectoria* species, for example, contain significantly more glucose than *Cladina* and *Stereocaulon* species that in turn contain much more mannose and galactose.

This higher glucose level is reflected in higher lichenan content, making these species more than 50% soluble in water, while *Cladina* fiber is less than 5% soluble.

*Aspicilia esculenta*, which is closely related to *A. cinerea* and *A. caesiocinerea*, is believed by some scholars to be the manna mentioned in Exodus 16:31 of the Bible. The lichen forms small round pebble growths that are easily disturbed and blow around by the wind. They swell in morning dew, and are edible.

The lichens were often assigned medicinal properties based on the doctrine of signatures.

A lichen resembling lungs was used for respiratory complaints, for example.

Unidentified black lichen known to the Paiute as **KAWA SIIN**, or Packrat Urine, was scraped off rocks and boiled as liquor for treating venereal disease.

Highly prized in medieval Europe were lichens that grew on bare skulls, for epilepsy. The demand was so heavy and profitable for this "heady" medicine (*mucus cranii humani*) that collectors devised methods to paste the skull and cultivate lichens.

Natives of northern Canada incorporated both *Alectoria* and *Bryoria* into clothing. It was interwoven with cedar or silverberry bark to make vests, leggings and moccasins. Although not very durable in wet weather, it was used by those who could not obtain furs, or as part of ceremonies.

Tanning, perfumery, and even powdered wigs relied on lichens. Architects and model railroad buffs use glycerin soaked lichens for model trees.

Lichens are used for "sizing" in bookbinding for applying gold leaf and colour; and fabric industries for filling pores in the surface of paper and fibre. Lichens are used in funeral decorations, as they will last for several weeks at the grave.

The great mystery in the chemistry of lichens is their " secondary compounds", which are not by-products of normal plant metabolism. Because of the energy required to produce them, scientists speculate they must have important value. Lichens produce over 500 biochemicals that helps control UV exposure, repel herbivores, attack microbes and discourage competition, according to Vermeulen.

During World War II, both the Germans and Americans investigated lichens for antibiotic potential, and found over 50% of species tested showing activity. Over 700 secondary lichen substances have been identified, with new compounds all the time.

Aromatic compounds such as depsides, depsidones and carotenoids are unique to the lichens.

Studies out of India have shown species of *Lepraria* to exhibit hypotensive, analgesic, anti-inflammatory, anti-spasmodic and neuro-muscular-junction-blocking activity. Further studies could be carried out on *Lepraria* species in our region of the world.

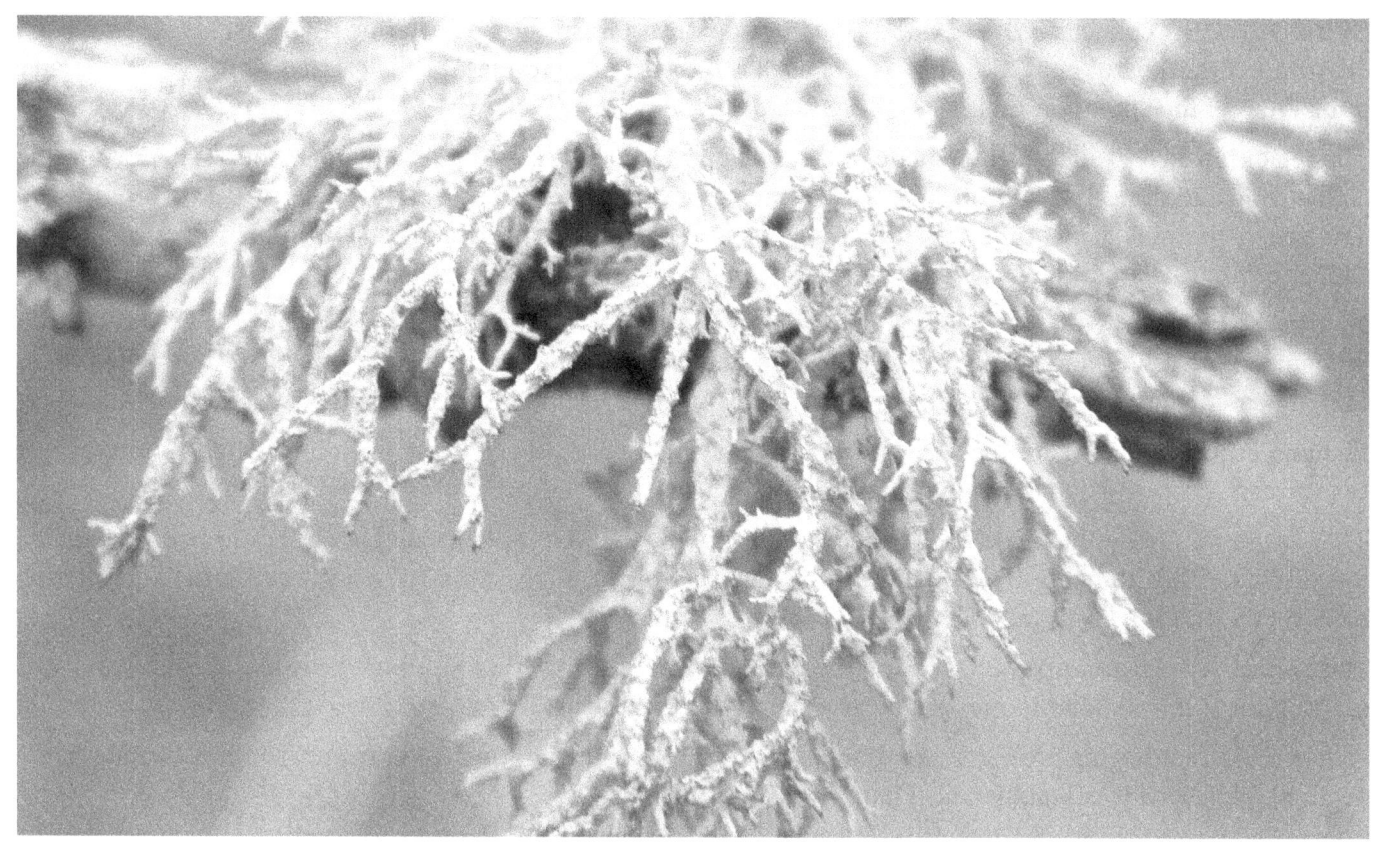

WOLF LICHEN

With two notable exceptions, the lichens of my part of the world are not poisonous.

You must be wary of the big, bad Wolf Lichen (*Letharia vulpina*) a bright yellow lichen, and Powdered Sunshine (*Vulpicida penastri*), a lemon-yellow lichen.

They contain pinastric and vulpinic acid, both extremely poisonous; and previously mixed with ground glass, nails and *Nux vomica* to kill wolves. There is no record in North America of using these lichens for this purpose.

However, the Achomawai of northern California soaked their arrowheads in the wet lichen for an entire year, sometimes combined with rattlesnake venom, to make the tips poisonous to game.

Both these lichens, and *Vulpicida canadensis*. have been used for brilliant yellow dyes they produce; the coastal Tlingit and Haida trading fish oils for the lichen to color their spruce root baskets and dancing blankets.

It should be noted that *L. vulpina* extracts compromise and disrupt cell division in methicillin-resistant *Staphylococcus aureus*. Shrestha G et al, *Pharm Biol* 2016 54(3): 412-8. Both *L. vulpina* and *Vulpicida canadensis* show activity against *E. coli*. Shrestha G et al, *Pharm Biol* 2014 52(10): 1262-6.

Emmons, in his *Chilkat Blanket* of 1907, wrote the moss [lichen] was boiled in the fresh urine of children. Interior people boiled the lichen in water and then soaked their buckskins, horsehair, porcupine quills or mountain goat's wool. The Cheyenne of Montana used the yellow dye for quills as well. The Apache used the lichen to paint crosses on their feet to pass through enemy territory unseen.

The Huna of northern California used it to dye Bear Grass (*Xerophyllum tenax*).

The Okanagan Colville boiled it on occasions with Oregon grape bark as a yellow dye. Both they and neighboring Blackfoot used it externally to treat skin problems; the latter for warts and eczema after blackened in fire.

Be careful when collecting *L. vulpina* as it can cause severe respiratory irritation and nosebleeds in closed environments. The Yuki of California used it as part of bedding, and the Apache carried some with them and put a cross of the colour on their feet to let them pass enemies unseen.

The related Brown Eyed Sunshine Lichen (*V. canadensis*) is used to dye mountain goat wool (hair?). Vulpinic acid is mild antibiotic, but caution is advised. Lauterwein et al, *Antimicro Agents and Chemotherapy* 1995 39:11. The lichen contains usnic, pinastric and vulpinic acids. It shows cytotoxic effects on human liver and breast cancer cell lines. Fernandez-Moriano C et al, *Phytomedicine* 2015 22(9): 847-55.

Natives of the southwest used Physcia mixed with pine resin for a yellow paint. The Paiute of western Nevada recognized the yellow and orange lichens for their anti-bacterial and anti-fungal properties. They called them Lizard Semen, derived from the little pushups that western fence lizards do on rocks.

Lichens, especially usnea are an indicator of pure air. And the bacteria on lichens can live in herbarium storage for 80 years, probably due to polysaccharides.

They are more susceptible to damage from sulphur dioxide that other plants, and good monitors of air quality. Researchers from Italy, in a 1997 article published in *Nature*, suggest a strong correlation between lichen biodiversity and lung cancer.

The lichen, *Hypogymnia physodes*, is the most tolerant macro-lichen to sulphur dioxide pollution, and will incorporate it into cellular tissue, as a measure of toxicity in the area.

A lichen bio-monitoring project in the Athabasca Oil Sands was abandoned after twenty some years, due to the death of all lichens in research zone. Oops!

Lichens are resistant to radiation, and in one experiment they survived 1000 rads a day for nearly two years from a distance of eight metres and continued to grow. A single exposure of 400 rads will kill a human, to put things in context. The potential use of lichens as bio-indicators of radionuclides is very high.

Two of the very few organic chlorine containing substances occurring in nature- gangaleoidin and diploiein- have been isolated from lichens.

One, as yet unidentified lichen growing like thick, yellow-green paint on boulders of the Rockies, is used by Natives as a narcotic. Wild Bighorn sheep, especially young ewes also enjoy a nibble, grinding their teeth to the gums to scrape it off the rocks. It is slow growing, taking over a century to spread over one square inch of rock.

It is a pioneer plant, growing where other plants offer no competition. I suspect it is a *Lecanora* species. Sheep in the deserts of Libya chew the lichen *L. esculenta* to the point of tooth loss from abrasion.

The Pima and Maricopa of the southwestern United States used gray colored lichen on rocks and dead wood with a strong violet odor. They call it Earth Flower, and mixed it with tobacco as a hallucinogen, and attract women, luck and such. It is also sprinkled on cuts and sores, such as rattlesnake bites, that will not heal.

The Waorani of Ecuador utilize a species of *Dictyonema* as a hallucinogen. Davis and Yost, *Botanical leaflet* 29:3 Harvard University.

Natives throughout Canada produced rock pictures, pictographs, of real and grotesque animals by scraping the lichen off large vertical rock faces. These have lasted centuries, due to the slow growth of lichens.

The novel, Trouble with Lichen, by John Wyndham, is a sci-fi novel about their long life span, as it relates to humans.

One species, *Acarospora chlorophana*, a bright yellow crustose lichen found in western Alberta grows so slowly on rocks its growth is almost unmeasurable.

Lichens are being genetically engineered in Japan to produce compounds. Oh yes!

It is widely assumed that lichen acids will act synergistically with a number of antibiotics. This is not always true, as some compounds are actually antagnostic. Bellio P et al, *Phytomedicine* 2015 22(2): 223-30.

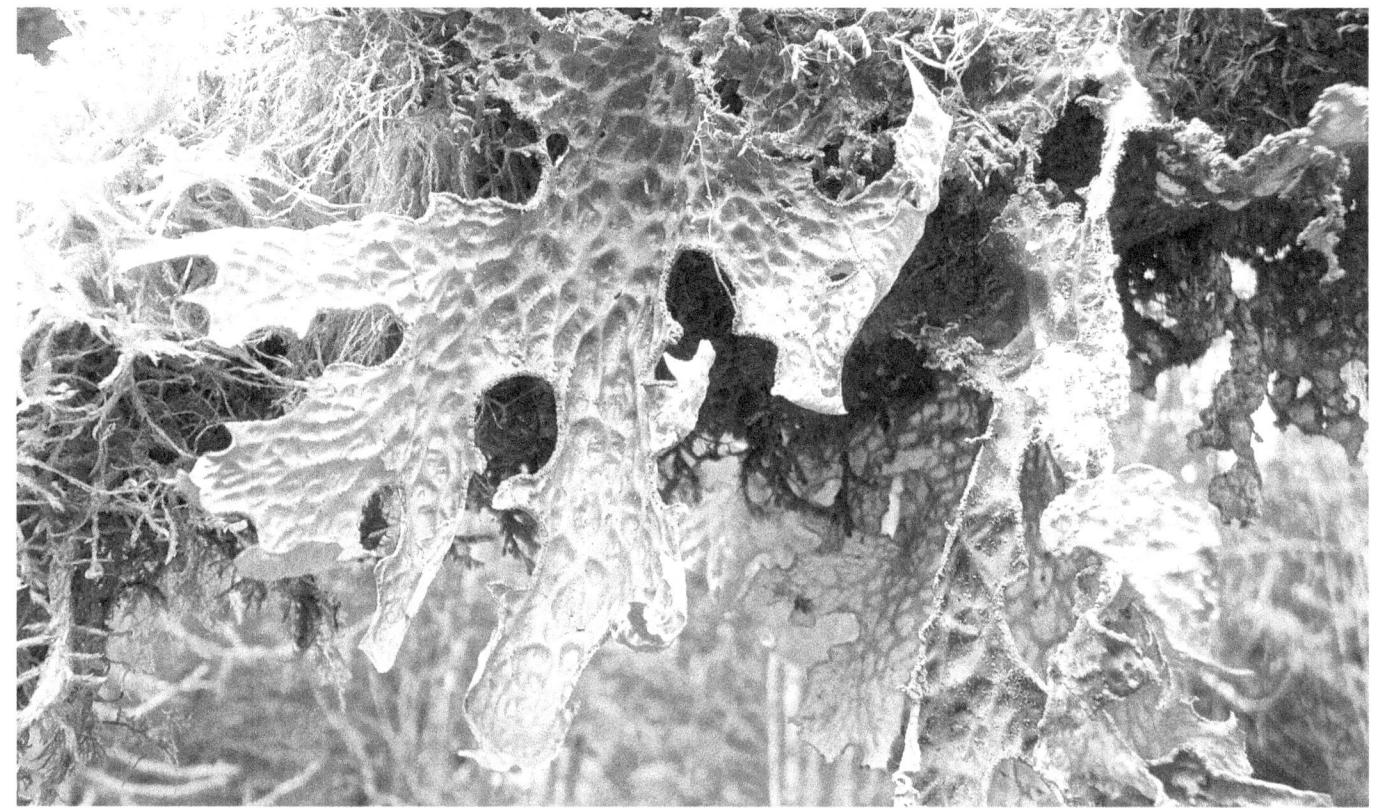

LUNGWORT

**LUNGWORT**
**LUNGMOSS**
**HAZELCROTTLE**
**HAZELRAW**
(*Lobaria pulmonaria* [L.] Hoffm.)
(*Sticta pulmonaria*) not accepted

Note how *Lobaria pulmonaria* is a rhyming couplet, a taxonomic rarity. Another two are *Chrysanthemum leucanthemum*, the Ox-eye Daisy; and *Humulus lupulus*, or Hops.

Sticta is from the Greek **STIKTOS** meaning spotted.

Lungwort grows in the old growth boreal forests, where it's nitrogen fixing is very important. It can be distinguished by large thalli that cover branches and trunks of spruce, poplar and fallen logs. It looks like flaccid lungs, and was used for this purpose by native tribes. As lichens grow, it is fairly luxuriant, with an average annual increase of 4.8 millimeters.

Lungwort was boiled traditionally in milk to make a "cough tea" or "lichen chocolate".

It was also used before hops for beer making in European and Siberian monasteries during the 17th and 18th century, as well as in India and Sikkim; where it was also used as a cleansing hair powder, and to tan hides and woolens an orange brown color.

Lungwort was used in France for perfume, but not plentiful and more rare than other lichens. In Germany it was used for perfume as well and called **LUNGENFLETCHE.**

The Gitksan and other First Nations of British Columbia associate this lichen with frogs. Frog Dress or **NAGAGANAW** was decocted for sore throats. The Hesquiat used it for sunburned faces.

The WSANEC living on Saanich peninsula call it **SMEXDALES**. It was believed that drinking about a gallon of tea made from this lichen would mean she would never have another baby. The same name was applied to the Waxpaper Lichen (*Parmelia sulcata*) found below, so could refer to that species.

The closely related Lettuce Lichen, *Lobaria oregana* is most commonly found in the mountains, on the top of one hundred year old Douglas fir. Here, the lichen capture nitrogen, fall to the ground and decompose, releasing the nutrient to nitrogen deficient soils.

Textured Lungwort (*L. scrobiculata*) is found west of the continental divide, as well as from northern Saskatchewan to Great Slave and Great Bear Lake. It is edible, and can be eaten right from the tree. The Yup'ik of Alaska call it **QELQUAQ.** In Scotland, it was used to dye wool a brown color.

The Haida refer to it as tree blanket, forest cloud, or cloud leaves/medicine, alluding to health properties.

## MEDICINAL

**CONSTITUENTS-***L. pulmonaria*- mucilage (including 30-40% lichenin), lichen acids including stictic, norstictic, sticinic, constictic, peristictic, cryptostictic, methyl stictic, thelophoric, and gyrophoric acid; fumaric and oxalic acids, rhizonaldehyde, rhizonyl alcohol, fatty acids such as palmitic, oleic and linolenic, trace minerals, ergosterol, fucosterol, protein and tannins.
*L. oregana*- stictic, constitic, cryptostictic and norstictic acids.
*L. scrobiculata* [Scop] P. Gaertn.–stictic, constitic, norstitic and usnic acid, scrobiculin. Meta-scrobiculin is five times more concentrated in reproductive parts of lichen.

Lungwort is very useful for all sorts of upper respiratory complaints, including what was formerly called lymphatic tuberculosis.

It is useful in formulas for hay fever, head colds, and flu; as well as intermittent fevers or night sweats.

It's nourishing and blood-building nutrients are useful for those suffering chronic internal dryness. It also restores moisture to the tissue that produces breast milk.

It combines well with borage or herbal lungwort for gastric ulcers, and should be given consideration in treating ulcerative colitis and allergies associated with the gastrointestinal tract. Tannins, quercetin, mucilage and other constituents help repair and regenerate mucosal membranes, and calm mast cell reactivity. This may be due in part to rhizonyl alcohol which suppresses neutrophil infiltration into gastric tissue. Atalay F et al, *Chem Biodivers* 2015 12(11): 1756-67.

The traditional use in Ireland for treating hemorrhoids probably has basis in fact.

It acts on the base of the brain and the vagus nerve, relieving fevers and irritative coughs, both acute and chronic.

The lungwort cough is wheezing, rasping dry and persistent, often worse in the dry dusty months of summer.

Lungwort possesses anti-rheumatic and analgesic activity, useful in pain occurring between the scapula, shoulders and occipital bone of the head.

Sometimes the pain extends into the chest and shoulders. Myalgia and arthralgia of the small joints may also benefit.

Studies conducted by Liu, at the Institute of Radiation Medicine in Tianjin has shown lungwort to be protective of bone marrow stromal and hematopoietic stem cells when exposed to radiation. This may be due, in part, to the anti-oxidant properties reported by Odabasoglu et al, *Phyto Res* 18:11.

Stictic, constictic and norstictic acid from this lichen show significant inhibition of *Salmonella gallinarum*. Crockett et al, *Botany 465 Lichenology* at Oregon State University.

Lungwort shows moderate activity against *Staphylococcus aureus*. Stoll et al, *Experientia* 1947 3.

A depsidone derived from lungwort shows moderate acetylcholinesterase activity. Pejin B et al, *J Enzyme Inhib Med Chem* 2013 28(4): 876-8.

Acetone extracts of lungwort, as well as *Cladonia rangiferina* and *Parmelia sulcata*, degrade prion protein from spongiform encelphalopathy in hamsters, mice and deer. Johnson CJ et al, *PLoS One* 2011 6(5). Chronic wasting disease is an increasingly difficult condition to control, especially in domesticated elk and cattle.

Several constituents of *L. scrobiculata* exhibit cytotoxicity against HL-60 cancer cell lines. Schinkovitz A et al, *J Nat Prod* 2014 77(4): 1069-73.

The related Peppered Moon Lichen (*S. fuliginosa* [Hoffm.] Ach.) contains trimethylamine.

Cabbage Lungwort (*L. linita*) contains tenuiorin. It is common on green alder.

Polyporic acid, derived from *Sticta coronata* was shown to double the life expectancy of mice infected with acute leukemia, as well as other cancers.

Melanic acid compounds in lungwort are induced by UVB radiation.

## ESSENTIAL OIL

An essential oil is steam distilled from this lichen, and used in perfumery. Commonly called Lungwort, it is known in Europe as Hazelcrottle, hazelraw and rage.

## HOMEOPATHY

Lungwort is for a general feeling of dullness and malaise, when a cold is coming on. The patient may feel as if floating in air, and have a great desire to talk.

This is accompanied by dull pressure in the forehead and root of nose, with an un-successful, constant desire to blow.

There may be a dry, hacking cough during the night that is worse on inhalation. The extremities may be red and inflamed. Changes of weather affect the symptoms.

**DOSE**- Tincture to sixth potency. The mother tincture is prepared from the fresh thallus of the lichen.

**BOERICKE**

### ICELAND MOSS
(*Cetraria islandica* [L.] Ach.)

Although called a moss, this brown lichen attaches to rocks in open sub-alpine forests. It is best collected when green and fully-grown between May and September. An average yield of 700 kilos per acre of air-dried Iceland moss could be expected if solidly covered, the exception rather than the rule.

The lichen is symbolic of health, and associated with the birth date January 16. Other lichen, such as *Ramalina*, and *Cladonia* species symbolize dejection, and January 14th.

It is associated with the second Rune, UR.

In Iceland, it is called **FJALLAGROS** and as far back at 1280 AD, the first written laws of that country banned people picking it on another's land. It is a common food item, found in every grocery store in the country.

The Chipewyan used **TSANJU** as a source of both food and medicine.

Iceland moss is used as a source of glycerol in the soap industry, and because of its lack of odour, in cold cream manufacture.

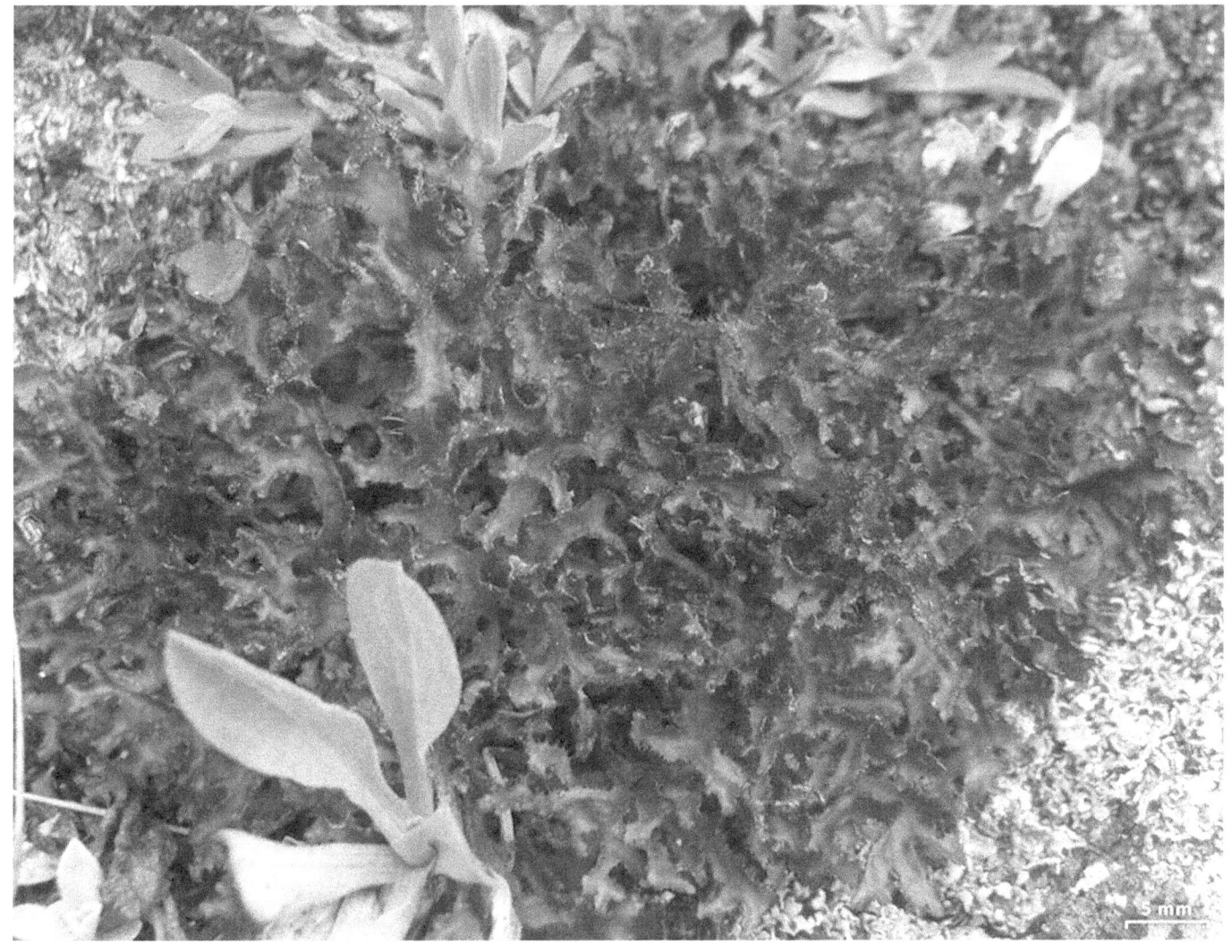

ICELAND MOSS (Courtesy of Jason Hollinger)

In Russia, during World War II, Iceland Moss, *Alectoria ochroleuca* and various *Cladina* species were used to make a type of molasses, with the glucose yield from Iceland Moss at 78% of dry weight.

Bread Moss, or **BRODMOSE**, is a Scandinavian name due to its use in extending wheat flour or potatoes in times of famine. It is also known as **MATMASA** or food moss, and **SVINMASA** meaning swine moss.

In Europe, it was traditionally soaked in birch ash (2%) to decrease the lichen acids before ingestion. The flour was used for porridge, jellies and bread. It was mixed with mashed potatoes or rye or oatmeal at about 25%.

Work by Airaksinen et al, *Arch Toxicol* 1986 9 (Suppl) suggests this is a good thing. When untreated lichen was fed to mice as 50% of diet, they died in 4-5 days. When ash soaked and boiled, survival times increased to 20-22 days, and when only 25% of diet it was well tolerated for six weeks. Enough with the mice studies!

A patent issued in 1951, suggested the use of Iceland moss as a preservative for luncheon meats, or cream filled pastries. It is both antibiotic and heat stable, and safe for human consumption.

It was used for tanning hides and dyeing wool.

Europe's best selling natural tooth whitener, BlanX contains silica and Arctic moss.

Water extracts of the lichen have been found to inhibit development of the tobacco mosaic virus. Even at 1:500, it reduced the number of brown lesions on leaves by 80%, due to an enzyme called ribonuclease.

The lichenin, a hot water soluble polysaccharide, causes the formation of a gel when cooled down.

The closely related Iceland Lichen (*C. ericetorum* Opiz.) is also common, and although similar, does not contain fumarprotocetraric acid, but lichenesterinic acid. Yup'ik of Alaska used it to flavor and thicken soups.

Striped Iceland Lichen (*C. laevigata*) in the extreme north contains fumarprotocetraric, protolichesterinic and lichesterinic acids.

Crinkled Snow Lichen (formerly *C. nivalis*), and now *Flavocetraria nivalis*, is found near the tree line or tundra. It is brewed into a tea in parts of the high Andes as a tonic for heart conditions and to relieve altitude sickness.

Early work by Burkholder et al, *Bull Torrey Bot Club* 1945 72:2 found activity against *Bacillus subtilis, B. mycoides,* and *Sarcina lutea*. Stoll et al, *Experientia* 1947 3 found strong activity against *S. aureus*.

The related *C. palustris* is a bright yellow species that favors Buffalo Berry (*Shepherdia canadensis*), Alder (*A. crispus*), Willow and Labrador Tea (*Ledum groenlandicum*), as well as the base of Pine. It contains + l-usnic acid and vulpinic acid, and shows strong activity against *S. aureus* in work by Stoll, mentioned above.

Curled Snow Lichen (formerly *C. cucullata*) and now *F. cucullata,* is found at higher elevations of coniferous woods and on tundra. Natives of Alaska use it to flavour their fish or duck soups.

Burkholder et al, mentioned above, found activity against all above as well as *Streptococcus species,* such as *S. pneumoniae, S. pyogenes, S. viridans* and *Staphylococcus aureus* and *S. albus* (hemolytic).

## MEDICINAL

**CONSTITUENTS**- *C. islandica*- lobaric acid, glucans lichenin (polysaccharides 30-40%) isolichenin (10%), lichenan (17%), galactomannan (7.6%), various usnic (?), salicylic, cetraric, physodalic and fumaric acids, estrosterol peroxide, protolichesterinic acid (0.1-0.5%), lichesterinic, protocetraric acid (0.2-0.3%) and fumarprotocetraric acids (2-11%), aromatic lichen acids (2-3%), aliphatic lichen acids (1-1.5%), cetrarin, picrolichenin, islandoquinone, oxalic acid, furan derivatives, iodine, Vit A, trace minerals including iron, iodide and calcium salts, fatty acid lactones, terpenes, mucilage, fibre and gums.

Historically, Iceland moss has been used to manufacture antibiotics to inhibit tuberculosis, one kg of antibiotics from 40 kg of plant material.

In Finland, an anti-fungal cream called USNO is made, for treating athlete's foot and ringworm. The lichen entered the Finnish Pharmacopoeia in 1915.

In Switzerland, Iceland moss is used for sore throat pastilles, and as an additive to luncheon meats and pastries to retard spoilage.

Iceland moss is a nutritious and soothing tonic, with slight laxative effect. It helps improve the appetite and digestion of the elderly and those recovering from a debilitating illness. The bitter principles benefit the stomach in both tincture and infusion form, stimulating a poor appetite, through stimulating the production of saliva and gastric juices.

It therefore, can be used, like Queen of the Meadow, for both hyper and hypo-acidic stomach conditions.

Decoctions are used for chronic diarrhea and respiratory problems. Like lungwort, it increases the flow of breast milk, but not with inflamed or sore breasts. Low thyroid and anemia is helped by the trace levels of iodine and iron, and other nutritive properties.

Dr. King's *American Dispensatory* is a classic of Eclectic herbal medicine. He writes the lichen is, "used as a demulcent in chronic catarrhs, chronic dysentery, and diarrhea, and as a tonic in dyspepsia, convalescence and exhausting diseases. Boiled with milk it forms an excellent nutritive and tonic in phthisis and general debility. It relieves the cough of chronic bronchitis."

Lichenin is soluble in hot water, and upon cooling forms a gel; while isolichenin, present in smaller amounts is soluble in cold water.

Lichenan is a polysaccharide similar to beta glucan, found in oats and barley. Work by Stubler et al, *J Phytopathol* 1996 144 found lichenan exhibits strong anti-viral activity.

It soothes nausea from gastritis and vomiting, and combines well with borage and chickweed for peptic ulcers, hiatus hernia and esophageal reflux. In fact, for those individuals with a Yin or fluid deficiency, it would work better than a straight astringent herb.

In an open clinical trial, 100 patients with pharyngitis, laryngitis or bronchial ailments were given lozenges containing 160 mg of an aqueous extract of the lichen. There was an 86% positive response with good gastric tolerance and lack of side effects.

Perhaps it should be considered in cases of diverticulitis and even cystic fibrosis in children.

Mild infusions of Iceland moss can be used as a vaginal douche for its soothing, demulcent properties.

Tincture form is best for whooping cough, asthma, TB, and kidney/bladder complaints; especially those related to a dry, irritating condition. Here, the sweet, moist and astringent nature of Iceland moss helps address the underlying concern.

It may be used for night sweats or fevers, but is taken during the day to prevent recurrence. Do not use Iceland moss when a fever is present.

Protolichesterinic acid has been found to exhibit anti-tumor activity in mice.

More recent in vitro studies have shown protolichesterinic acid to be a potent inhibitor of HIV, the virus associated with AIDS; as well as 5-lipoxygenase. Pengsuparp et al, *J Nat Prod* 1995 58.

It also shows significant activity against *Trypanosoma brucei brucei*. Igoli JO et al, *Curr Top Med Chem* 2014 14(8): 1014-21.

Protolichesterinic acid shows inhibition against twelve cancer cell lines. Lobaric acid was weaker but still showed activity at higher levels. Haraldsdottir S et al, *Planta Medica* 2004 70(11): 1098-100.

Other components, such as polysaccharides have been found to stimulate the immune system, in studies by Ingolfsdottir et al, *Planta Medica* 1997 60:6. Earlier, the author found the polysaccharides comparable to the fungal polysaccharide lentinan (*Shiitake*) used for clinical cancer therapy in Japan.

The author found extracts of Iceland moss to suppress the growth of *Helicobacter pylori* that contribute to gastric and duodenal ulcers. *Antimicrob Agents Chemotherapy* 1997 41.

Protolicheresterinic acid has been found by Ogmundsdottir et al, *J Pharm Pharmacol* 1998 50:1 to be significantly anti-carcinogenic with regards to two breast carcinoma and erythro-leukemia cell lines as well as anti-inflammatory properties. The ED50 for lobaric acid is between 14 and 44 ug/ml for these three cancer cell lines.

Haraldsdottir et al, *Planta Med* 2004 70 found lobaric acid very effective against a number of human cancer cell lines *in vitro*.

Both lobaric acid and protolichesterinic acid inhibit 12(S)-HETE production in human platelets. Bucar F et al, *Phytomedicine* 2004 11(7-8): 602-6.

Lichen extracts show activity against human melanoma and human colon carcinoma cell lines. Grujicic D et al, *Cytotechnology* 2014 66(5): 803-13.

Fumarprotocetraric acid protects neurons from oxidative stress, and may be useful in neurodegenerative disorders. Fernandez-Moriano C et al, *Toxicol Appl Pharmacol* 2017 316: 83-94. Earlier work by same authors, Phytomedicine 2015 22(9): 847-55 found neuroprotective activity and cytotoxicity against human liver and breast cancer cells.

The lichen may be useful in early intervention of risk associated with type 1 diabetes. Colak S et al, *Toxicol Ind Heath* 2016 32(8): 1495-1504.

Work by Gulcin et al, *J of Ethnopharm* 2002 79:3, determined Iceland Moss contains significant potential as a natural antioxidant. Just 50 micrograms of water extract showed higher anti-oxidant activity than 500 mcg of alpha tocopherol.

Eight secondary compounds in *C. islandica* decreased by 52% when screened of natural UVA and UVB radiation. Bachereau et al, *Symbiosis* 1997 23.

Protocetraric acid shows significant activity against *Salmonella typhi* and the fungi *Trichophyton rubrum*, significantly better than standard anti-fungals. Nishanth KS et al, *Nat Prod Res* 2015 29(6): 574-7.

The compound, found in various lichens, is cytotoxic to UACC-62 human melanoma cancer cells. Brandao LF et al, *Chem Pharm Bull* (Tokyo) 2013 61(2): 176-83.

The closely related Snow Bed Iceland lichen (*C. delisei* [Bory ex Schaerer] Nyl) shows significant activity on estrogen through inhibition of aromatase. Extracts at a concentration of 40 ug/ml showed 82% inhibition. Aromatase inhibition is one approach to preventing overgrowth of hormone sensitive cancer cells. It also contains gyrophoric acid.

Ragbag, or Varied Rag Lichen (*Platismatia glauca*) was formerly classified as *Cetraria glauca*. It has been used in the past for yielding a chamois colored dye for wool.

The species contains caperatic acid, atraric acid, chloroatranorin and atranorin. Acetone and ethylene extracts show anti-biofilm activity against *S. aureus* and *Proteus mirabilis*. Miltrovic T et al, *EXCLI J* 2014 13: 938-53.

Activity against various human cancer cell lines was noted by Bezivin C et al, *Phytomedicine* 2003 10(6-7): 499-503.

The related *C. halei* contains alectoronic acid.

The common Spiny Heath Lichen (*C. aculeata*), also known as *Coelocaulon aculeatum*, has significant effect on various bacterial systems, including *Salmonella typhimurium*, but not mammalian cells. It showed cytotoxic effect on various mammal cancer cell lines. Zeytinoglu et al, *Phytother Res* 2008 22:1.

The lichen extract and its active constituent, protolichesterinic acid exhibits activity against *Aeromonas hydrophilia, Proteus vulgaris, Streptococcus faecalis, Bacillus cereus, B. subtilis, Pseudomonas aeruginosa,* and *Listeria monocytogenes*. Turk et al, *Zeit Naturforschung* 2003 58:11-12.

## HOMEOPATHY

Iceland Moss (*Cetraria islandica*) is used for acute and chronic bronchitis, asthma, and pains in the chest while coughing.

**DOSE**- 10-20 drops of tincture as needed. The mother tincture is prepared from the dried lichen.

## ESSENTIAL OIL

Iceland moss is steam distilled, and yields brownish oil (0.051%). It has a saponification value of 98 and acid value of 72.

The bulk of aliphatic acids are saturated (66.8%), composed mainly of palmitic, stearic and behenic acid. Unsaturated composed the rest with oleic acid and linoleic acid most common.

## SPIRITUAL PROPERTIES

Iceland moss and its spiritual properties are related to the signature of this lichen. Individuals struggling with their personal evolving of spiritual issues, or those in difficult environments, physically and emotionally, will benefit from this plant.

When an individual comes close to achieving deeper awareness of God, there is often great fear, and unwillingness to continue. This is often related to the incorrect belief that nothing will remain to be done on earth.

Those working towards spiritual goals based in Eastern philosophies will also be helped. In the martial arts, one seeks to let go of the mind, and yet be ready for full physical response. Iceland moss will help develop this trust, as well as help an individual discover and feel comfortable with their own level of spiritual purpose.

**GURUDAS**

## PERSONALITY TRAITS

The moistened *Cetraria* gives off an aroma that suggests still other mammals or things mammalian- a blended whiff of suede worn by an equestrian, and of the horse, sweating.

It is a good-bad-intriguing scent, probably with pheromonal powers, and of the sort that is used as ballast in the making of a perfume.

I would not be at all surprised if an essence of this plant is eventually stirred into some concoction with a name like The Devil's Dew, to be dabbed on by would be Dionysians.

**GEORGE SCHENK**

**USNEA**
**SHAGGY OLD MAN'S BEARD**
**SUGARY BEARD**
(***Usnea hirta*** [L.] F. H. Wigg)
**POWDERY BEARD**
(***U. lapponica*** Vainio)
**PITTED BEARD**
(***U. cavernosa*** Tuck)
**SCRUFFY BEARD**
**STRAW BEARD**
(***U. scabrata*** Nyl.)
**FISHBONE BEARD LICHEN**
(***U. filipendula*** Striton)
(***U. dasypoga*** acut non [Ach] Shirley)
**METHUSALA'S BEARD LICHEN**
(***U. longissima*** Ach)
(***Dolichousnea longissima*** [Ach.] Articus)

Usnea, or Old Man's Beard, hangs in grey-green strands from larch and spruce of the boreal forest. Look for the central white, elastic thread inside Usnea for correct identification.

Usnea was recommended in the Formulary of Al-Kindi around 850 AD. It was suggested for a swollen spleen, a part of the immune system. Earlier in ancient Greece, both Hippocrates and Dioscorides recommended *Usnea barbata* for uterine problems.

The Chinese have used various usnea species, (Sung-Luo) for thousands of years. It is prized for its broad-spectrum antibacterial and immune stimulating properties in various respiratory and urinary infections. *Usnea diffracta* has been called Lao Tzu's beard.

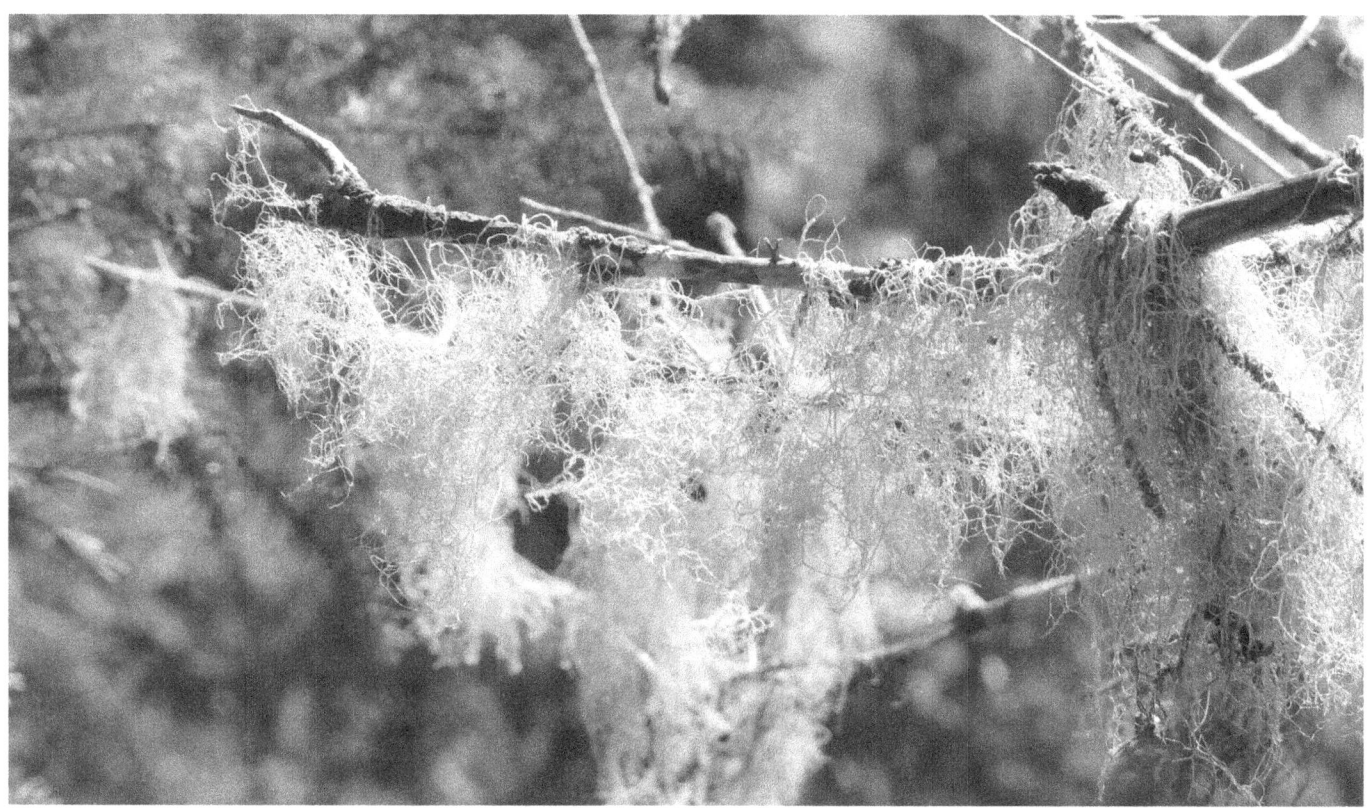

USNEA

He wrote the *Tao Te Ching* some 2600 years ago. Chinese herbalist will only gather this lichen during the fifth lunar month for maximum benefit.

Usnea is very effective in trichomoniasis, giardia, and candida infections; and particularly effective in cervical erosion, or dysplasia, as a douche.

The Malaysians use *Usnea* species as a general tonic and tea for colds; and the neighboring Indonesians used *U. thallus*, or **KAYU ANGIN**, meaning "windy wood" as an astringent and anti-spasmodic for intestinal problems.

It was traditionally burned in homes to combat evil spirits and wind borne diseases.

Usnea species are used in Peru to produce a dark blue dye.

In the Sudan, the closely related *U. molliuscula* is known as **SHEIBA**, and used in perfumery, as an aphrodisiac.

In local medicine, it is used as a bitter stomachic, for coughs, and to relieve menstrual pain.

Usnea has been fed to cows in the alpine regions of Europe to help them get through cold winters and fight mastitis. Sodium usnate is used as a spray for fighting mildew and other plant diseases.

The Blackfoot call it **E-SIMATCH-SIS**, and the Cree by **MITHAPAKWAN**. Both used usnea species for stopping nosebleeds and bleeding wounds. A decoction was also used to wash sore or infected eyes.

The Dakota call it **CHAN WIZIYE**, translating as either "on the north side of the tree", or "Spirit of the North Wind". The northern Chipewyan know it as **K'I TSAJU**, while the Dena'ina call it Spruce Hair, or **CH'VALA ANDAZI**.

The Nitinaht call it **P'U7UP** and used *Usnea* species for diapers, sanitary napkins, and dressing wounds.

Usnea species are used as catalysts, for making fermented corn beverages by the Tarahumara of northern Mexico.

131

It was an emergency food that required more boiling to remove the usnic acid; the more yellow the lichen, the more medicinal, but less edible.

Pitted Beard Lichen (*U. cavernosa*) was used by the Wylackie of California to tan leather. Animal brains were wrapped in the lichen to hold together, and then rubbed vigorously into the hide.

Fishbone Beard Lichen (*U. filipendula*) has been used on Sakhalin Island, now belonging to Russia, as a powder to treat wounds. Modern research indicates it has anti-bacterial activity.

It also induces apoptosis and DNA cell damage in human lung cancer (A549, PC3), liver cancer (Hep3B) and rat glioma (C6) cell lines. Ari F et al, *Cell Prolif* 2014 47(5):457-64.

Sodium usnate has been found effective against the tomato canker (*Corynebacterium michiganensis*); and usnic acid shows a moderate degree of inhibition of the blue staining wood fungus *Trichosporium*, and tobacco mosaic virus.

It is used in a spray at 100-500 ppm for bean rusts, and mildews, as well as brown rot on some stone fruits.

Recent work has found usnic acid strongly inhibits the mould *Neurospora crassa*.

The related *U. subfloridana*, is a boreal forest lichen that was mixed with tobacco and butter, and then boiled and cooled as a lotion for skin in Europe.

Recent work suggests that lichens may produce more usnic acid when levels of UV-B are high.

This suggests a biomonitor for increased radiation levels, and potential for development of more effective sunscreens.

Warty Beard Lichen (*U. ceratina*) was known, by the Pomo of California, as **KÔCHIH**. The lichen was used for diapers and toilet paper. It contains diffractaic acids.

The lichen *U. longissima* is found on the West Coast as well as Eastern North America. It has long been used in Ayurvedic and Unani medicine for arthritis, edema, eczema, cardiac tonics and massage oils for rheumatism, gout and sciatica.

*Usnea longissima* has been used in China and India as an expectorant, while First Nations used it for feminine hygiene products, and bedding.

As noted, lichens are quite slow growing, but this species has been found to double in length annually, in work by Rolstad et al, *Can J Botany* 86:10.

Ayurvedic scholars equate its medicinal use with *Parmelia perlata*.

Tree fellers in western Canada are susceptible to skin rashes and usnic acid has been identified as a potential photo-sensitizer, and respiratory irritant.

Kahlee Keane, or Root Woman, in her enjoyable new book, The Standing People, suggests usnea as a heartworm medicine for wolves. Interesting!

## MEDICINAL

**CONSTITUENTS**- *U. hirta*- (+) usnic acid (3%), alectoric, hirtic, thamnolic, defractic (rare), hertillic and usnaric acids, anthraquinones, hirtusneanoside, and various fatty acids. Usnic acid is also known as 2,6-diacetyl-7, 9-dihydroxy-8, 9b-dimethyl-1, 3(2H, 9bH)-dibenzo-furandione.
*U. filipendula*- salazinic acid, usnaric acid, barbatic acid, d-usinic acid, as well as emulsin.
*U. cavernosa*- salazinic acid, and/or usnic acid.
*U. lapponica*- usnic and/or salazinic acid; and sometimes barbatic acid.
*U. scabrata*- inland only usnic acid.
*D. longissima*- various B-orcinol depsides including usnic acid derivatives including usemanimes A-F, usone, isousone and (-)-usnic acid, evernic, barbatic and diffractaic acids; glutinol, longissimione A and B, arabitol, ethyl everninate, friedelin, dibutyl phthalate, diisobutyl phthalate, beta amyrin, beta sitosterol, barbantinic acid, zeorin, ethyl orsellinate, oleanolic acid, (+)-usnic acid, methylorsellinate, longiusnine, longissimausnone.

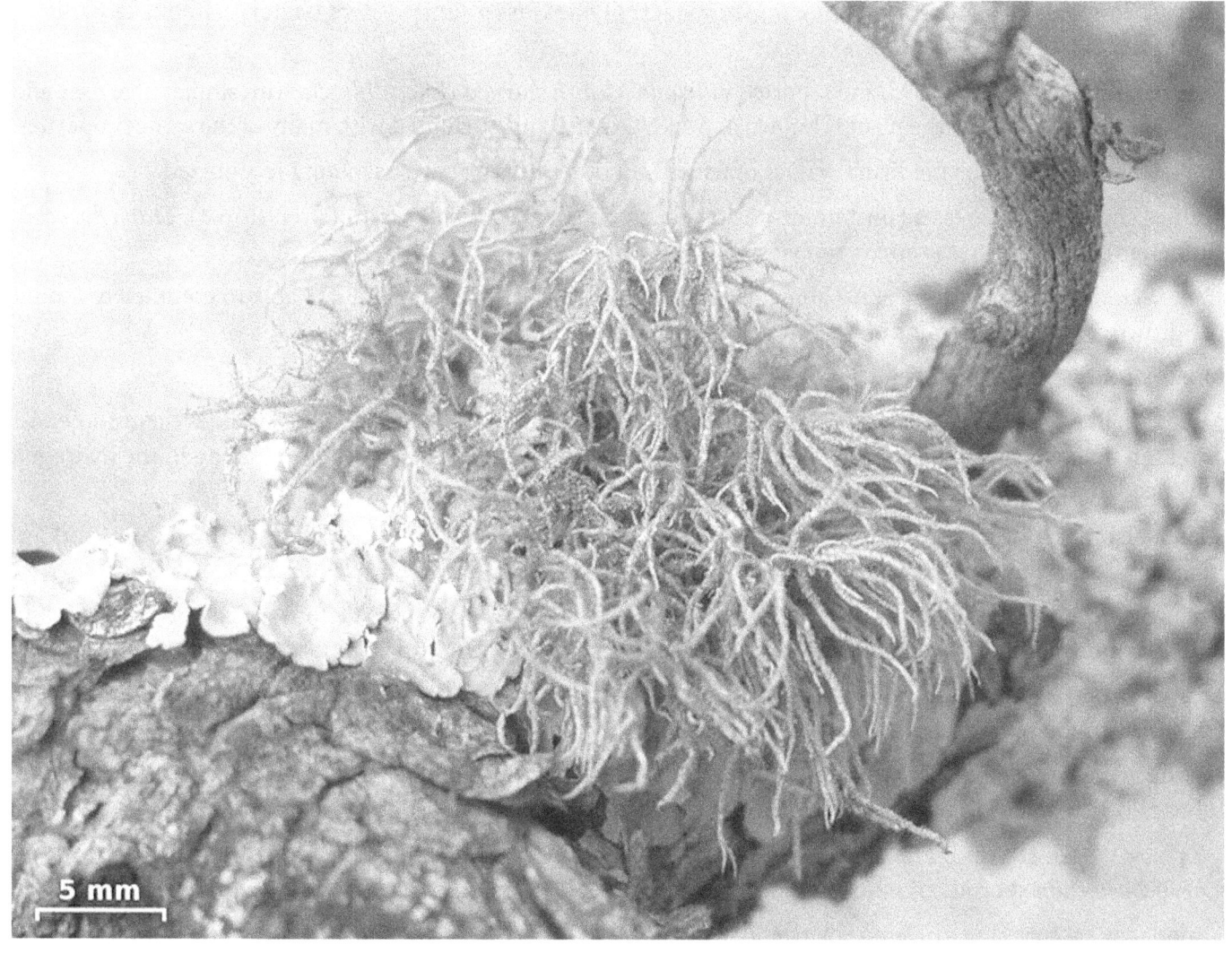

*USNEA HIRTA* (Courtesy of Jason Hollinger)

The outer, green grey cortex contains the antibiotic substance, while the white inner core contains immune stimulating polysaccharides.

Recently, the polysaccharides have been found to possess anti-tumour activity, confirming their traditional use for cancer.

For example, in the case of sarcoma-180 in mice, daily injections for ten days after implantation led to complete regression of tumors compared to controls.

Although not certain of the mechanism, it is thought that an outpouring of lymphoid and plasma cells, as well as macrophages to the area of the grafted tumor is responsible. Similar active constituents are also found in *Umbilicaria, Lobaria* and *Sticta* species.

Other constituents have been found to be nonsteroidal and anti-inflammatory.

In a 1993 Romanian study of *Usnea hirta*, it was demonstrated that the anti-inflammatory activity was comparable, or superior to phenylbutazone and hydrocortisone. The analgesic activity is close to noraminophenazone, and the antipyretic activity equal or superior to aminophenazone.

Work by Vijayakumar et al, *Fitoterapia* 71:5 found usnic acid significantly reduced inflammation in both acute and chronic conditions.

Hirtusneanoside, isolated from *U. hirta*, shows activity against gram-positive bacteria. Renzaka & Sigler *J Nat Prod* 2007 70:9.

Similar studies in Japan in 1995, and reported in *Planta Medica* showed *Usnea diffracta* with similar analgesic and anti-pyretic effect. There, the plant is known as **SARUOGASE** and attributed with many of the same properties.

In Northern Europe, the medicinal values of usnea and other lichens have been long recognized.

Studies show effectiveness against gram-positive bacteria such as *Streptococcus* (strep throat), *Staphylococcus* (impetigo), and *Mycobacterium tuberculosis*.

Usnic acid is more effective against some bacterial strains than penicillin. And it is able to completely inhibit the growth of different strains of human tuberculosis in dilutions of 1:20,000.

Other studies cite its effectiveness at 1 part per million, similar to streptomycin.

Microbes like the tubercle bacterium form heavily waxed coats and stiff cell walls that allow them to persist and even divide inside macrophages. They are able to prevent the host's lyosomes from taking in the hydrogen ions needed to create an acidic environment, and thus neutralizing their effect.

Usnea also has a different mode of action. Synthetic antibiotics resemble the cell wall of bacteria, and are incorporated in the cell. This results in a weak cell structure as the bacteria swell and burst.

Scientists believe usnic acid disrupts cellular metabolism, either by preventing ATP formation, or by un-coupling oxidative phosphorization. Thus, the cells run out of energy and die.

Drug resistant TB is presently undergoing a worldwide resurgence that one WHO health official described as "the most frightening situation I have ever encountered".

Honda et al, *Phytomedicine* 2010 17(5): 328-32 looked at a variety of lichen constituents and activity against tuberculosis. Usnic acid ranked third, behind norstictic acid and the most powerful, diffractaic acid.

Work by Weckesser et al, *Phytomed* 2007 14:7-8 found *Usnea* species active against *Propionibacterium acnes*, *Corynebacterium* species, and most importantly, against MRSA, methicillin resistant *Staphylococcus aureus*.

Usnea may be superior to Flagyl (metronidazole) against *Trichomonas*, a parasite that causes serious uterine and cervical infection, and tissue destruction.

It has good effect in candidiasis, and giardiasis, or beaver fever as it is known, as well as bowel inflammation in general. Usnea is a relaxant of the smooth muscles of the body, including the colon and lungs.

In Russia, a sodium salt of usnic acid called Binan is used for second and third degree burns to prevent infection; and for varicose ulcers, furuncolosis, impetigo, trichomonas, and lupus erythematosus. Binan is a vigorous antibiotic, effective against microbes and protozoa in concentrations of 1:300,000 to 1: 1,000,000 when applied externally.

In Germany, a product called Evosin, a mixture of usnic and evernic acids is used for impetigo, furunculosis and lupus vulgaris, as well as mastitis in cows. Usniplant, containing 0.2% usnic acid, is used for skin conditions.

Likewise, sodium usnate is used in China for pulmonary tuberculosis. In 30 cases treated, 24 were cured, and 6 were improved, after 71 days.

Mastitis in cows, athlete's foot, ringworm, and acute bacterial infections can be treated internally and externally. Usnic acid has been formulated into toothpaste, mouthwash, deodorants and sunscreens, as well as creams and ointments.

Usnic acid shows activity against *Streptococcus mutans*, which creates dental plaque and caries, without disrupting normal oral flora.

Usnic acid is not only anti-fungal and anti-bacterial, but also effective against viruses, and protozoa. It was found effective against the promastigote forms of leishmaniasis, a infectious parasitic disease. Da Luz JS et al, *Scientific World Journal* 2015:617401.

A pretty thorough review of usnic acid was produced by Araujo AA et al, *Nat Prod Res* 2015 29(23): 2167-80.

In Argentina, usnea is used for washing warts. It is a constituent of the Chinese drug **SHI-KOA**, and the Japanese medicinal drug **SEKI-KA**. The Maori of New Zealand utilize usnea to increase resistance to infection and stimulate the appetite.

This led to the unfortunate marketing of a weight loss product, LipoKinetix, which contained sodium usniate. Said to help the body burn fat, it was found to result in one death, two liver transplants and seven cases of non-fatal liver failure. Holy lawsuit!

Usnic acid was tested in one study in Saudi Arabia for the possibility of use for cancer and leprosy. It was found to have no adverse effect on testicular nucleic acids or epididymis spermatozoa in laboratory mice, unlike most anti-cancer drugs.

Usnic acid has been found to inhibit Ehrlich ascitic cells in laboratory studies. It has a vaso-dilating effect, and helps relax the muscles of the uterus, bronchi and intestine.

Other studies indicate usnic acid has anti-proliferative, anti-inflammatory, analgesic, anti-growth, anti-herbivore and anti-insect properties.

Both (+)-usnic acid and (-)-usnic acid, especially the former, show high cytotoxic activity against cancerous cells. Koparal et al, *Nat Prod Chem* 20:14.

Nine usnic acid amine conjugates were tested for cancer on L1210 cell lines. Work by Bazin et al, *Bioorg Med Chem* 2008 16:15 found significant toxicity and induction of apoptosis.

Recent work found (+)-usnic acid inhibits metastasis of non-small cell lung cancer. Yang Y et al, *PLoS One* 2016 11(1). The compound has a distinct mechanism of action.

Usnic acid inhibits both HIV-1 and 2 integrase and mamallian topoisomerases I.

Dr. William Mitchell, Jr. considered usnea a valuable diuretic that combines well with parsley. He recommended up to 90 drops of tincture three times daily.

It combines well with Oregon grape root, dandelion root and Uva ursi for damp heat strangury; and with Scullcap and Elecampane root for phlegm heat in the lungs.

For giardia infection, or amoebic dysentery, combine with Oregon grape root and elecampane root.

The active parts of Usnea are poorly water soluble, slightly better in alcohol and most soluble in oil.

Usnic acid is influenced by the solvent used, pH value, and with what powders or ointments it is mixed.

Usnic acid absorbs UV light and may be used in sunscreen products with good results.

*Usnea hirta* has an LD50 21.02g vegetal material/kg of body weight; according to studies conducted by Dobrescu et al, in Romania, 1993.

Energetically, usnea clears heat and resolves toxins due to its bitter and cold nature.

This makes it very valuable in TCM theory for damp heat in the lower burner, as well as lung conditions when Qi is disrupted due to dampness, phlegm or heat.

The compound (+)-usnic acid shows protection against hyper proliferative skin wound healing, and when combined with gyrophoric acid increased wound closure most effectively.

Hirtuseanoside shows activity against gram-positive bacteria. Renzaka & Sigler, *J Nat Prod* 2007 70:9.

The coastal species *Usnea longissima* has been studied by Lee and Kim, *Phytotherapy* 2005 19:12 for its anti-platelet and anti-thrombotic activity.

Diffractaic acid in this species has been found to enhance the antioxidant defense system as well as reduce effects on neutrophil infiltration. Bayr et al, *Journal Phytomed* 13:8.

This lichen has been investigated for anti-platelet and anti-thrombotic activity. Alcohol extracts showed inhibitory effect on ADP-induced platelet aggregation.

Oral administration of the extract prior to intravenous injection of collagen and epinephrine in mouse thrombotic models, showed significant inhibition of thrombotic death or paralysis. Asprin, a representative anti-platelet drug, showed significant anti-thrombotic death inhibition at one-tenth the amount.

On the other hand, the extract did not show any fibrinolytic activity or alter coagulation parameters, suggesting the anti-thrombotic activity is due to anti-platelet rather than anti-coagulant activity. Lee KA & MS Kim, *Phytotherapy Research* 2005 19(12): 1061-4.

Choudhary et al, *Phytochem* 66:19 identified anti-inflammatory compounds.

Methanol extracts show in vitro melanogenesis inhibition. Tyrosinase glycosylation is believed to be involved. Kim et al, *J Microbiol* 2007 45:6.

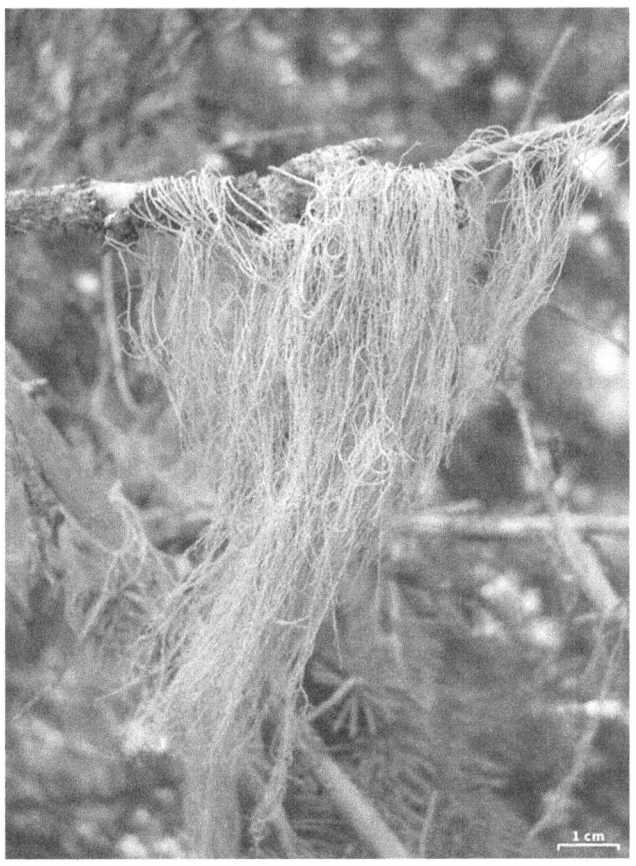

*USNEA CAVERNOSA* (Courtesy of Jason Hollinger)

Work by Odabasoglu et al, *J Ethnopharm* 103:1 found usnic acid from this species both anti-oxidant and protective of indomethacin-induced gastric ulcers. Both Christopher Hobbs and Chanchal Cabrera, noted herbalists, mention its use to treat tuberculosis lymphadenitis.

Usnic acid, derived from Rock Beard Lichen (*U. amblyoclada*) exhibits significant biofilm inhibition against azole-resistant (71%) and azole-senstive (88%) strains of *Candida albicans*. It is found on rocks, rarely bark, from Arizona to South Carolina.

Other lichens are richer in usnic acid. One Haematomma species (*H. coccineum*) is nearly 20% content. The closely-related Blood Spot Lichen (*H. lapponicum*) has no work conducted as yet.

Usnic acid inhibits *Helicobacter pylori*, and is synergistic with clarithromycin for treatment of gastric ulcers, associated with this bacterium. Safak B et al, *Phytotherapy Research* 2009 23(7): 955-7.

Both (+)-usnic and and a liposome inhibit *Toxoplasma gondii*, a nasty pathogen. There are very few high efficiency, low toxicity drugs for toxoplasmosis. Si K et al, *Exp Parasitol* 2016 166:68-74.

A fungal strain, *Corynespora* species, has been found on *Usnea cavernosa*. Work by Paranagama et al, *J Nat Prod* 70:11 found extracts of this strain cytotoxic to breast and prostate cancer cell lines.

Usnic and salazinic acid from *U. filipendula* show activity against *Serratia marcescens*.

Fishbone Beard Lichen (*U. filipendula*) alcohol extracts induce apoptosis in human lung, liver and rat glioma cancer cell lines. Ari F et al, *Cell Prolif* 2014 47(5): 457-64.

Usnic acid, evernic acid and vulpinic acid inhibit the growth of gram positive bacteria such as *Staphylococcus aureus, Bacillus subtilis* and *B. megaterium*, but no affect on gram negative bacteria such as *Escherichia coli* and *Pseudomonas aeruginosa*. Lawrey et al, *The Bryologist* 1986 89.

Usnic acid and atranorin exhibit activity against MRSA, derived from cystic fibrosis patients. Pompilio et al, *Future Microbiol* 2013 8:2.

These two compounds are cytostatic against human prostate and melanoma cancer cell lines. Galanty A et al, *Toxicol In Vitro* 2017 40:161-9.

It may reduce pulmonary fibrosis in cases of patients taking bleomycin for malignant ascites, as well enhance function and reduce toxicity of the drug. Su ZQ et al, *Int Immunopharmacol* 2017 46:146-55.

# HOMEOPATHY

*Usnea barbata* is the remedy to remember for all forms of congestive headaches, especially sunstroke. The head can feel ready to burst at the temples, or the eyes feel like bursting from their sockets. The face is reddish.

**DOSE**- Tincture in drop doses. The 1X dilution is used for elimination of heavy metals.

# ESSENTIAL OIL

*Usnea barbata* and others are extracted with ethanol to produce a Tree moss concrete and absolute.

The semi-solid mass is greenish-brown, and contains methyl beta-orcinol carboxylate, and olivetonide. It is used largely in soap perfumery, although it does supply the requisite "mossy" notes in Fougere and related perfumes.

It should be restricted to 3% of any fragrance compound for best effect.

# LICHEN OIL

Stuff a glass jar tightly full of Usnea and cover with canola or olive oil. Cover with cheesecloth and set in warm, sunny window for several months.

This may be used internally, by filling gelatin capsules, or used externally as a healing salve with beeswax for infected boils, carbuncles, impetigo and even vaginal boluses for trichomonas. Usnic acid is most soluble in oils.

# LICHEN ESSENCE

Usnea lichen essence is useful for individuals in the helping or healing professions. At times, due to the desperate, life threatening situations and energies of the patients, there is danger of empathizing or identifying too strongly patients and beginning to take on their "illness".

It is useful for those working in hospice, and witnessing another journey of the soul.

Usnea essence helps retain boundaries, so that effective work can be carried out without endangering their own health and well-being. This can be subtle, but once observed it can be recognized and easily dealt with.

Usnea essence is for restless discontent, those that are dissatisfied with life and tend to lack tolerance for others. They may be harmful to others, as well as themselves. They may have a short temper and energetically burn the candle at both ends, leading to cravings that are harmful.

Sunstroke damage may have changed personality and this essence may bring back balance. One example of this is the use of food to stuff down emotions. An excellent book by Jack Schwarz (1988) addresses the issue of body-mind connection with nutrition and vitality.

As might be expected, the lungs are most often affected. Traditionally, the lungs were associated with crying and the grieving process. Usnea essence helps protects those suffering from the tuberculinum miasm, recognized in homeopathic medicine.

This makes sense when one considers the mycobacterium nature of this serious disease, and the treatment of patients with antibiotics and anti-fungal medications.

The miasmic taint, or trait is more subtle, and exists on a cellular or predisposed genetic level. It should be noted Usnea essence may temporarily increase skin irritations, particularly those with dry or weeping eczema. Caution is advised, and reducing the standard dosage by one half will often help allay this acute bodily response.

**PRAIRIE DEVA**

## SPIRITUAL PROPERTIES

Usnea represents the north, the place of gray hairs. It maintains the lung system of the planet. When Usnea came to me, personified as a young man, and spoke to me of its uses, it told me that its healing qualities are specific for the lung system of the planet- the trees.

Its use for people was secondary to its primary function. This was the first time I realized that the plants provided medicinal actions with the ecosystem, that they evolved and developed to help the Earth ecosystem, Gaia, maintain a healthy balance within itself.

I realized at that time that it was only because we are a part of the ecosystem that the plants also work for us as healing agents.

There is an ancient compact between Usnea and the trees, and coming into contact with the deeper spiritual aspects of Usnea, one makes contact with ancient powers that existed long before humans.

**STEPHEN HARROD BUHNER**

**DOSE**- Tincture- 20-30 drops as needed. For serious infection like trichomonas and tuberculosis, it is taken long term up to six times daily. When collecting and making tinctures use only living lichens. Use 1:1 at 95% alcohol.

Animal studies suggest possible teratogenic effects from usnic acid in the period of organogenesis, suggesting limited internal use in early pregnancy. Maybe. Silva CR et al, *Biomed Res Int* 2017:5948936.

**GRAY REINDEER LICHEN**
**TRUE REINDEER LICHEN**
(***Cladina rangiferina*** [L.] Nyl.)
**GREEN REINDEER LICHEN**
(***C. mitis*** [Sandst] Hustich)
**TREE REINDEER LICHEN**
(***C. arbuscula*** [Wallr] Hale & Culb.)
**REINDEER LICHEN**
**STAR TIPPED REINDEER LICHEN**
**NORTHERN REINDEER LICHEN**
**CAULIFLOWER LICHEN**
**CARIBOU LICHEN**
(***C. alpestris***)
(***C. stellaris*** [Opiz] Brodo)
(***C. aberrans***)
**BLACK FOOTED REINDEER LICHEN**
(***C. stygia*** [Fr.] Ahti)
**PARTS USED**- thallus

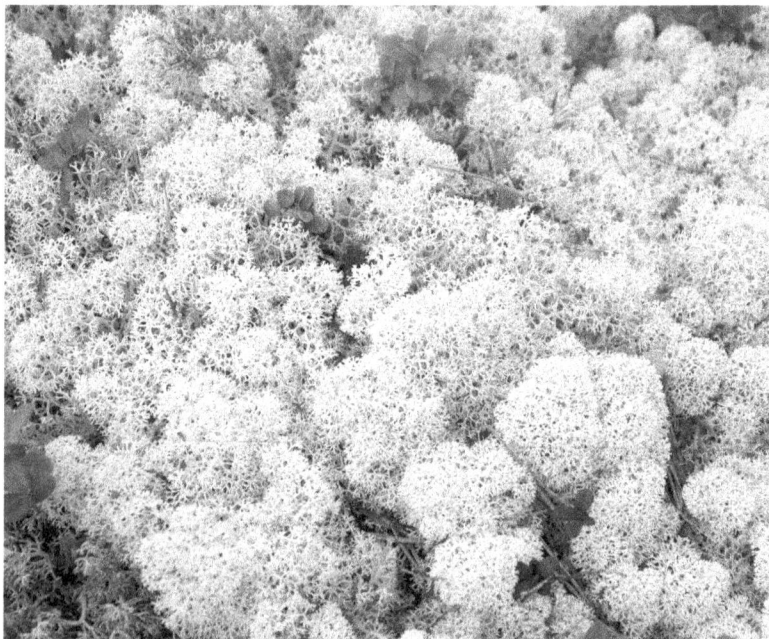

REINDEER LICHEN

Rangifer is the scientific grouping for both reindeer and caribou mammals.

True Reindeer lichen is very common across northern Canada, where it is used as a food source by caribou. It is very fragile and slow growing; averaging 3.4 mm per year.

After grazing by caribou, it takes up to 15 years to recover. Although *C. rangifera* is the true reindeer lichen, the star-tipped lichen is a more important food, and preferred by caribou. Both are slow growing, averaging 3.4-4.1 mm per year.

Caribou, and reindeer produce lichenase in their stomach, which along with bacteria and protozoa in the rumen, help them survive extreme conditions. The enzyme, lichenase, is also found in snail livers.

The Woods Cree of Saskatchewan call it **WAPISKASTASKAMIH** or sometimes **ATIKOMICIWIN**. Decoctions or the dried powder were taken to rid the body of intestinal worms.

Inuit ate the undigested stomach contents of caribou as a source of Vitamin C. They also fashioned wicks from reindeer moss, for blubber oil lamps.

The Aleuts of Alaska used infusions of this lichen for chest pains while the Tanaina boiled and ate it for diarrhea. *Cladina* species, separated from grass in caribou stomachs was stirred with oil, and stirred while the word **TENIYASH**, meaning increase was sung so the mixture would rise and become light.

The Ojibwa decocted *C. rangiferina* to bath newborns, and give them strength. They call the lichen **ASA'GUNINK**.

The Chipewyan call it **TSANJU**. The use of partially digested reindeer lichen from caribou digestive tracts has long been a traditional part of their diet. The contents of the rumen, **EBURTI**, were boiled by placing heated rocks into the cut out rumen or large intestine, with added meat, fat and blood. This is known to the Chipewyan as **EBIE HECHELH**, or bowel soup. The winter feast was preferred due to the fine white *Cladina* being present almost exclusively, whereas in summer you might get blueberries, leaves, grass, mushrooms, etc. It makes a stimulating tea.

The Gwich'in of the Mackenzie delta, call it White Moss, or **UHDEEZHU**. When boiled, the tea is good for stomach and chest pain. It can also be boiled for an hour, and then fried, for a crispy treat.

When taken from the caribou rumen, it is known as **IT'RIK**. It is eaten in soup, or placed on other meat to tenderize and enhance flavour. It is sometimes hung for up to a week to age, and then mixed with fat, marrow, and berries, for a real treat.

In Europe, true Reindeer Lichen has been used to produce an iron red dye for wool. The Inuit of Baffin Island make a broth of **NIRIAT** (*C. stellaris*) for sickness and eye infections. Black et al, *Botany* 2008 86:2.

Reindeer were fed *C. stellaris* containing usnic acid for three weeks, and yet no trace of usnic acid or conjugates were found in the fresh rumen fluid, urine or feces, suggesting its quick breakdown by rumen microbes. Sundset MA et al, *Naturwissenschaften* 2010 97(3): 273-8.

S-(-)usnic acid from this lichen exhibited a strong effect against *Trichomonas vaginalis, in vitro*. It efficacy was equal to metronidazole. Wu J et al, *Zhongguo Ji Sheng Chong Xue Yu Ji Sheng Chong Bing Za Zhi* 1995 13(2): 126-9.

Star-tipped Reindeer Lichen is harvested commercially for flower arrangements, architects and model railway hobbyists for miniature trees and shrubs. In Finland and Sweden, this is a million dollar export business, with some 3000 tonnes harvested per year for Christmas and graveyard wreaths and models above.

Traditionally, the lichen was used in Russia in the form of powder on treating wounds. The Wood Cree decocted it to expel intestinal worms.

Black-footed Reindeer Lichen has a pinkish jelly; as opposed to the clear, colour-less jelly from the true reindeer lichen.

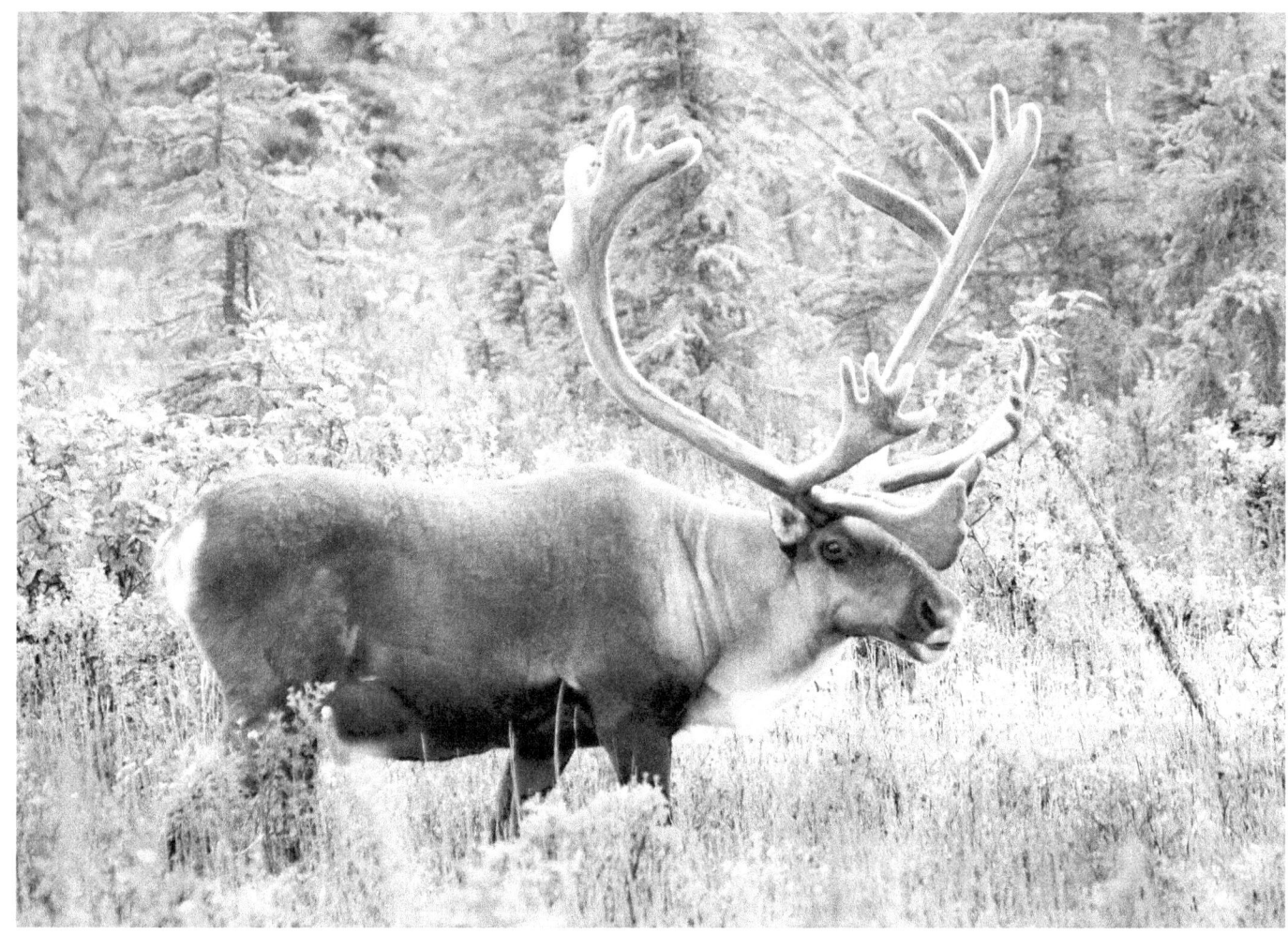

CARIBOU

## MEDICINAL

**CONSTITUENTS-** *C. stellaris-* usnic acid, fumarprotocetraric acid, atronorin, perlatolic acid; various polysaccharides including nigeran, galactomannan, arabinitol and mannitol; and small amounts of rangiformic acid, psoromic acid, pseudonor-rangiformic acid, ventoric acid, proteins and sterols.
*C. rangiferina-* fumaroprotocetraric acid, atranorin, trace of vit D, some ergosterol, arabitol, mannitol, volemitol, alpha trehalose, sucrose, umbilicin; 54-63% lichenin acid
*C. arbuscula-* fumarprotocetraric and usnic acid
*C. mitis-* usnic, rangiformic acid
*C. squamosa-* squamatic acid
Usnic acid is significantly higher in young lichen tissue, with the first few millimetres containing up to 12 times the older growth just 4-8 mm. back.
*Cladina* species are 94% carbohydrate, 2.7% protein, 2% fat, and 1.3% minerals.

Medicinally, reindeer lichen is dried and powdered, and decocted for intestinal parasites.

In Finland, the lichen was traditionally boiled in water as a laxative, or boiled in milk for respiratory affections.

In Denmark, a popular whisky made from the caribou or reindeer moss, so endangered the plant that production was shut down by the government. A similar brandy venture in Sweden also closed down in 1883.

In Russia, *C. mitis* syrup was too bitter for human consumption, and used to produce alcohol, or medium for food yeast, with a glucose yield of 75% dry wt.

Studies conducted by Wu et al, 1995 showed *C. alpestris* water extracts to have strong effect against *Trichomonas vaginalis* in vitro. This would be welcomed by the large number of women affected by this irritation; in the form of a warm water douche. The article, in *Chinese Journal of Parasitology and Parasitic Disease* 13:2 found no significant difference between the effect of usnic acid and metronidazole at concentrations of 0.4 and 0.6 mg/ml.

Reindeer Lichen (*C. rangiferina*) has been shown more effective in chronic inflammation rather than acute conditions, in a study by Surleyman et al, *Bio Pharm Bull* 2002 25:1. Compared to indomethacin, the lichen extract showed 43% inhibition, as compared to the drug at 72%.

Atranorin appears to be stimulated by UVA sunlight.

Recent work identified new compounds, hangokenols A and B. These and other previously identified compounds were tested for activity against MRSA (methicillin resistant *Staphylococcus aureus*) and VRE, vancomycin resistant *Enterococci* species. Yoshikawa et al, *Chem Pharm Bulletin* (Tokyo) 2008 56:1.

Many tons of *C. stellaris* are used by the pharmaceutical industry for its usnic acid.

Both *C. mitis* and *C. stellaris* show activity against *Staphylococcus aureus* and *Bacillus subtilis*, in studies conducted by Harmala et al, *Fitoterapia* 1992 63:3.

Early work by Stoll et al, *Experientia* 1947 3 showed strong activity against *S. aureus* by d-usnic acid in the former species.

Early work by Burkholder et al, *Bull Torrey Bot Club* 1945 72:2 indicated *C. mitis* inhibited activity against *S. albus*, *Diplococcus pneumoniae*, *Streptococcus hemolyticus*, *S. viridans*, *Bacillus mycoides*, and *Sarcina lutea*.

*Cladina alpestris* shows activity against *Bacillus subtilis*.

The latter, known as Caribou Lichen, or **NIRNAIT** to the Inuit, was used to cure eye infections, or boiled until the tea turned black and drunk cold by the sick. In Alaska, the lichen is added for flavouring to duck or fish soup.

Tree Reindeer lichen (*C. arbuscula*) shows activity against *Mycobacterium tuberculosis*. Gordien et al, *Phytother Res* 2009 Oct 13. This follows earlier work that found usnic acid from this lichen exhibited high activity against *M. aurum*, a non-pathogenic organism with similar sensitivity. Ingolfsdottir K et al, *Eur J Pharm Sci* 1998 6(2): 141-4.

## HOMEOPATHY

Reindeer Lichen (*C. rangiferina*) was proved at the 30th potency by Misha Norland in 2002.

Mental symptoms include jealousy, suspicion and delusion. Dreams of crime, evil, guns, murder, war, fights and robbery are prevalent.

Physically, there is vertigo, throat huskiness or loss of voice, head and eye pain. Nasal congestion, burning tongue, stomach nausea, and abdominal flatulence are present. A dry cough, thick expectoration and stitching pain in chest, cold extremities and itching skin are also common. More complete description in book *Fungi* by Frans Vermeulen.

## LICHEN ESSENCE

Reindeer Lichen (*C. mitis*) is for transformation. It revitalizes the lifeblood congestion or over stimulation of the etheric heart that impedes the free circulation of life force. **FINDHORN**

Reindeer Moss (*C. rangiferina*) essence is for those individuals who feel disassociated, fragmented and scattered.

There may be feelings of being trapped, used or coerced by others. In some cases, the individual has begun to take on the persona of those around them, leading to further alienation from their own self-identity.

Individuals that may be helped with this lichen essence may note they are easily swayed by the opinions of others. Tastes in music, film, food and clothing will vary widely, depending upon whom they are presently associated. They may well be aware of this loss of identity, but there is little will or energy to assert oneself.

Associated with these feelings is an overwhelming tiredness, especially in the afternoon.

Issues of jealousy may be present, even though there is no rational basis for the negative feeling. There may be suspicion of other people's motives. Consider combining or using Yellow Witch's Butter or Shaggy Mane, if the picture pattern fits.

On a physical level, there may be blocked nostrils and sinuses, with sensation of cold. Or there may be a constant postnasal drip that has persisted for years.

What has led to such a state of inertia or resignation?

The Platonic doctrine of anamnesia is the idea that we are born possessing all knowledge and our soul once lived in "reality" but was trapped in our body. It once knew everything but forgot. Reindeer Moss may help us "remember".

In many ways the state is reminiscent of the phrase "resistance is futile" from the science fiction series Star Trek. There is a certain resignation associated with this indifference. The client may say things like "whatever", or "who cares" when asked about their lives.

Reindeer Moss essence is like a whiff of oxygen to the weak embers of will, helping rebuild a sense of hope and self-sufficiency.

Again, where did this state begin? Often this condition follows a serious illness, particularly of the nervous system, but may also be present due to emotional trauma in first years of life. Bill Plotkin (2003) suggests trauma at age 2-3 may result in the "loyal soldier" syndrome. These individuals will, throughout their lives, remain constantly vigil to the early wound and react from this perspective. The Reindeer Moss essence helps one to reconnect and nurture this young soul fragment towards integration.

Think back to any events at a young age that excited you. This may be part of your soul path or soul purpose that has become buried under years of responsibility and duty. Feeling trapped today may have its roots based upon inappropriate comments from parents or teachers, giving rise to issues of self-esteem. In turn, the striving to become the best you can, is thwarted leading to loss of self-identity, confusion and resignation.

If nothing is good enough, the psyche may translate this as, "you" are not good enough.

Stuttering is one example of this state that may be helped by Reindeer Moss essence, combining well with Panellus mushroom essence, if the picture pattern fits.                                            **PRAIRIE DEVA**

## CLADONIA

Numerous texts have mixed up *Cladina* and *Cladonia*, but unlike the former it has a squamulose primary thallose that makes for accurate identification. *Cladonia* now refers to Pixie Cup Lichens and their relatives, but previously represented all reindeer lichens.

*Cladonia* species contain usnic and isusnic acids, especially in the cortex, as well as beta-orcinol depsides and depsidones such as barbatic acid, and squamatic acid; atranorin, fumarprotocetraric and proto-cetraric acids, as well as norstitic, psoromic, rhodocladonic and thamnolic acids. They also contain ursolic acid, found in apples and various medicinal herb species.

Usnic acid from *Cladonia* species has shown high cytotoxic activity against cancer cells.

Various *Cladonia* species have been found effective in the treatment of tuberculosis, in studies by Vartia et al, *Antibiotics in Lichens from The Lichens* (eds Ahmadjan & Hale) Academic Press in 1973. This confirms the traditional use in Finland of hot water lichen infusions for this dreadful disease. Didymic acid, found in many *Cladonia* species, inhibits the mycobacterium at 25 mcg/ml. Strepsilin is in several *Cladonia* species and shows antibiotic activity.

Species inhibiting *Bacillus subtilis* include *C. gracilis, C. deformis C. amaurocraea, C. bacillaris, C. coniocrae, C. fimbriata, C. pleurota,* and *C. uncialis.*

Species inhibiting *Staphylococcus aureus* are *C. gonechu,* also known as *C. sulphurina,* as well as *C. deformis* and *C. amaurocraea* that show strong inhibition. Stoll et al, *Experientia* 1947 3.

## BLACK FOOT CLADONIA
## SMOOTH CLADONIA
(***Cladonia gracilis*** [L.] Willd)

Gracilis means slender, referring to the slender cup shape. It may be the most common lichen in dry lodge pole pine forests, growing in huge mats in places.

The lichen has been used to produce an ash green dye for wool.

This lichen shows significant inhibitory effect on estrogen formation from the estrogen precursor, sulfatase. Extracts at a concentration of 40 ug/ml showed an 83% inhibition.

Ingolfsdottir K et al, *Pharm Biol* 2000 38(4): 313-7.

It contains fumarprotocetraric acid, and shows activity against *B. subtilis.*

## LESSER SULPHUR CUP
(***Cladonia deformis*** [L.] Hoffm.)

*Cladonia deformis* has been investigated for an unusual iron substance. Work by Alagna et al in Italy, indicates the iron is present as high-spin Fe(III), and coordinates in an oxygen containing environment arising graciliformin ligands. It also contains zeorin.

It is strongly inhibitory against *S. aureus.* Stoll et al, *Experientia* 1947 3.

## MANY-FORKED CLADONIA
(***Cladonia furcata*** [Huds.] Schrad.)
(***C. subrangiformis***)

*C. furcata* has been shown to weakly inhibit the *Staphylococcus aureus* bacteria, and contains fumarprotocetraric acid.

Work by Liu et al, *Acta Pharmacol Sin* 2001 22:8 identified a polysaccharide in the lichen that induced apoptosis in human leukemia K562 cells.

It also is a powerful anti-microbial, and showed activity against FemX (human melanoma) and LS174 (human colon carcinoma) cell lines. Rankovic BR et al, *BMC Complement Altern Med* 2011 11:97.

A novel, water-soluble lichenin, CFP-2, isolated from this species induces apoptosis and telomerase inhibition; suggesting possible cancer therapeutic potential. Lin X et al, *Biochim Biophys Acta* 2003 1622(2): 99-108.

A previous studied identified CFP-1 that induced apoptosis in human leukemia K562 cells. Lin X et al, *Acta Pharmacol Sin* 2001 22(8): 16-20.

**TRUMPET LICHEN**
(*C. fimbriata* L.)
(*C. major*)

Trumpet Lichen (*C. fimbriata*) contains only 12.9 ug/g of carotenoids, while some *Caloplaca* ssp. contain up to 151 ug/g of various carotenoids.

Work by Czeczuga et al, from Poland, published a list of carotenoids from 34 lichen species in *Feddes Repertorium* 1999 110:7-8.

The lichen also contains atranoric acid, fimbriatic acid, and fumaroprotocetraric acid. It has been used in the past as a red dye for wool.

**BROWN PIXIE CUP**
**CUP MOSS**
**CHIN CUPS**
(*C. pyxidata* [L.] Hoffm.)

**CONSTITUENTS-** Abundant atranorin and fumaroprotocetraric acid, barbatic acid and psoromic acid; mucilage; as well as parellic acid, protofumarcetraric acid and an enzyme emulsin.

Pyxidata is from the Latin **PYXIS**, meaning a box. A pyx is now a term applied at the government mint, for a box containing sample coins. Chin Cup comes from its former use in whooping cough or chin cough, as it was known.

It shows activity against both *S. aureus* and *B. subtilis*. Stoll et al, *Experientia* 1947 3.

Activity against both bacteria was exhibited by *C. pyrixata*. Burkholder et al, *Bulletin Torrey Botanical Club* 1945 72:2.

This lichen is fairly widespread throughout the area; and exhibits demulcent, anti-tussive and expectorant properties.

The lichen has been shown effective against bronchitis, and coughs including whooping cough; combining well with coltsfoot and sundew. It grows mainly on high mineral soil, contributing needed trace minerals to formulas.

Their cup-like shape can identify them.

As well as medicinally, it was used traditionally in Europe to dye wool either red/purple or ash green.

## HOMEOPATHY

Symptoms include hurried feeling, but less anxious and nervous; bloated abdomen, disorientation, uncertainty, dryness of tongue, lips, throat, skin and rectum.

Tired and yet sleeplessness, desire for open air; difficulty breathing in hot room.

**DOSE-** Six to 30th potency. Proving by Izzie Azgad and Rosalind Floyd on 9 provers in 1994. See Vermeulen's excellent book *Fungi* for greater detail.

**BRITISH SOLDIERS**
(*C. cristatella* Tuck.)

This lichen is so named due to its green body and red head, reminiscent of the early British red coats.

The lichen contains usnic, didymic, barbatic and rhodocladonic acid.

Early work by Burkholder et al, Bull Torrey Bot Club 1945 72:2 found activity against *Staphylococcus albus, Diplococcus pneumoniae, Bacillus subtilis, B. mycoides,* and *Sarcina lutea.*

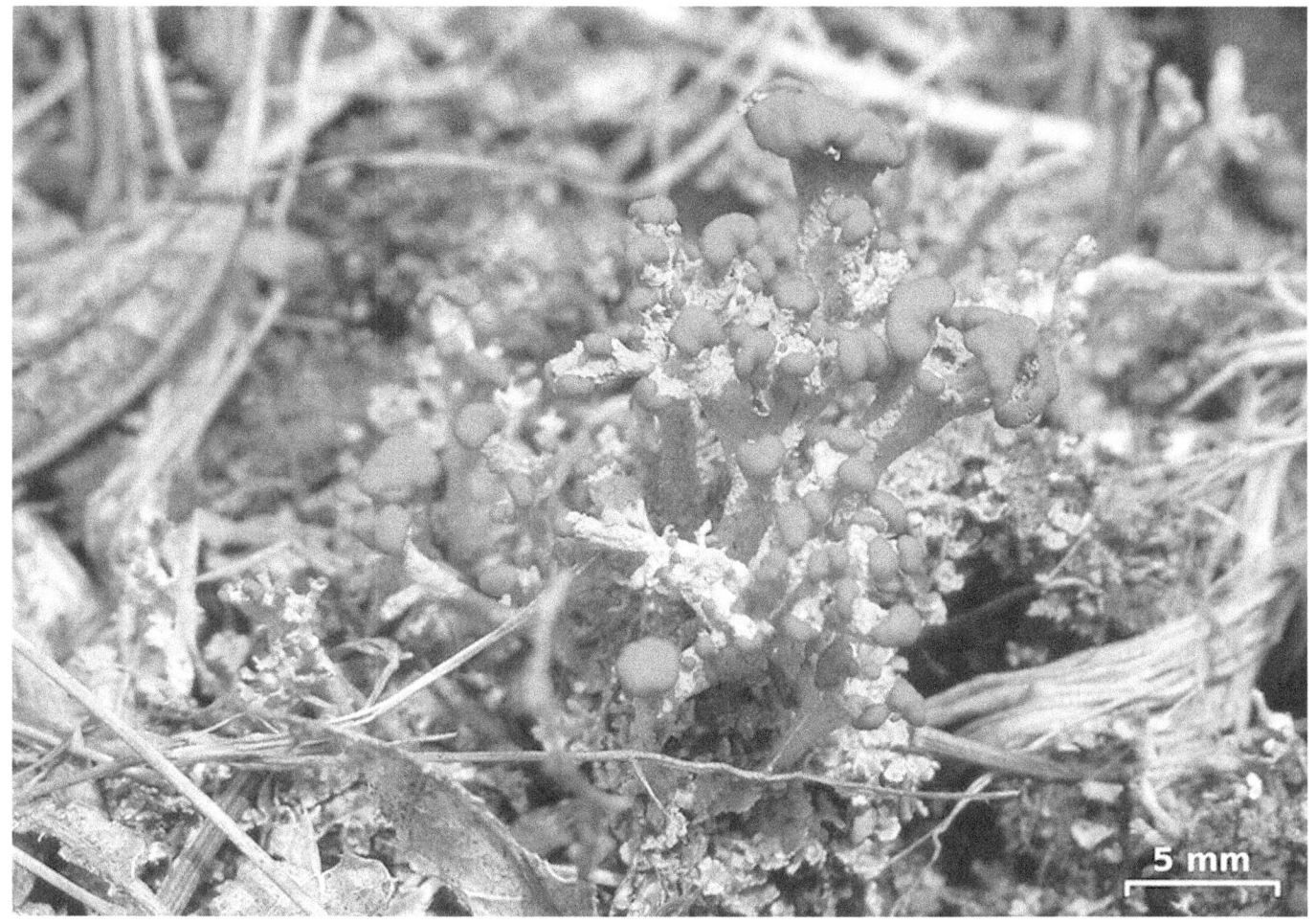

CLADONIA CRISTATELLA (Courtesy of Jason Hollinger)

The same authors found both *C. pleurota* and *C. uncialis* active against the above bacteria as well as several *Streptococcus* species, including *S. pneumoniae, S. pyogenes* and *S. viridans*. The latter contains usnic acid and sometimes, squamatic acid.

The related Powder Foot British Soldiers (*C. incrassata*) is found on the eastern seaboard, from Nova Scotia to Florida. It contains (-)-usnic acid, didymic acid, condidymic acid, squamatic acid, thamnolic acid, prasinic acid and 1,5-dihydroxy-2, 4, 6-trichlor-7-methylxanthone.

Didymic, condidymic and (-)-usnic acid all are active against *Staphylococcus aureus*. Dieu A et al, *Planta Medica* 2014 80(11): 931-5.

Mealy Pixie Cup (*C. chlorophaea*) was boiled by the Okanagan-Colville of British Columbia and used to wash sores slow to heal. It is known as Liver on Rock or **PEN'PEN'EMEKXIXXN'**.

It contains fumar-protocetraric acids. This lichen is an old whooping cough remedy mentioned in early European herbals. It is boiled in milk and used today in Wales under the name **CWPANAU PAS.**

Research in Michigan found four different chemical populations of this species with each race occupying a different habitat, leading to significant difference in constituents, from grayanic acid to cryptochlorophaeic acid to merochlorophaeic acid, to the more common fumar-procetraric acid strain.

Thorn Cladonia (*C. uncialis*) is widespread, ranging from Alaska, and southeast to Georgia. A potent enediyne, isolated from *Streptomyces* species, associated with this lichen shows promise for medicinal applications. Parrot D et al, *Planta Medica* 2016 82(13): 1143-52.

The lichen contains (-)-usnic acid and squamatic acid. Acetone extracts show potent anti-microbial activity against MRSA, methicillin-resistant *S. aureus*. Studzinska-Sroka E et al, *Nat Prod Res* 2015 29(24): 2302-7.

The red-tipped *C. bellidiflora* is common. The Haida dipped the red tip into human breast milk and applied it to sore eyes.

Other *Cladonia* species worth mentioning are Gritty British Soldiers (*C. floerkeana*) containing cocellic acid; and *C. macilenta* with thamnolic acid. Both are eastern species.

Dragon *Cladonia*, or Dragon Funnel (*C. squamosa*) contains atranorin.

*C. bacillaris* contains barbatic acid, which possesses anti-tuberculin activity. It also produces hemolysis.

Arctic Alpine Lichen (*C. coccifera*) has red apothecia, and contains zeorin and usnic acid.

Lipstick Powderhorn, or Pin Lichen (*C. macilenta*), synonym *C. bacillaris*, is widespread and has red tips. It contains a number of compounds found in other Cladonia species, but also contains biruloquinone. Not only does it protect injured PC12 cells, but it is a mixed-II inhibitor of acetylcholinesterase. This suggests benefit in brain health due to anti-oxidant activity but also improving cognitive improvement. Luo H et al, *J Microbiol Biotechnol* 2013 23(2): 161-6.

The European *C. convoluta* contains usnic acid, fumarprotocetraric acid and 9'-(O-methyl) protocetraric acid, the latter of which has been shown to induce apoptosis of murine leukemia cells. Bezivin et al, *Planta Med* 2004 70.

It also inhibits proliferation of human breast cancer MCF-7 cells and induces apoptosis. Coskun ZM et al, *Folia Biol* (Praha) 2015 61(3): 97-103. The related *C. rangiformis* showed similar results.

## LICHEN ESSENCES

Smooth *Cladonia* lichen essence is the mirror- for helping open new doors into consciousness. It is like a spotlight focusing deep within, reflecting up into awareness, an unacknowledged part of oneself.

It helps to discover and understand the patterns developed and enacted today. It allows one to reclaim power through awareness.                                                                      **CANADIAN FOREST**

Arctic Alpine *Cladonia* lichen releases deep-seated patterns and worn-out old issues by transmuting negative karma, which is ripe for resolution. Destructive emotions are then purified, self-punishment, anger and low self-esteem relinquished.                                                               **FINDHORN**

**STUDDED LEATHER LICHEN**
**FAIRY PELT**
**LEMON LICHEN**
**FRECKLE PELT**
**SEA GREEN LICHEN**
(***Peltigera aphthosa*** [L.] Willd.)

Peltigera is from the Greek and Latin, meaning "shield bearing". Pelta means a light shield.

Aphthosa is from the Latin meaning thrush, referring to the disease of the throat, for which it was once a specific. Or perhaps, originally, it is from the Greek **APHTHAI**, meaning pustule or eruption.

When moist, this lichen turns a brilliant green, later dulling to a grey green. It is commonly found growing over true mosses in coniferous forest.

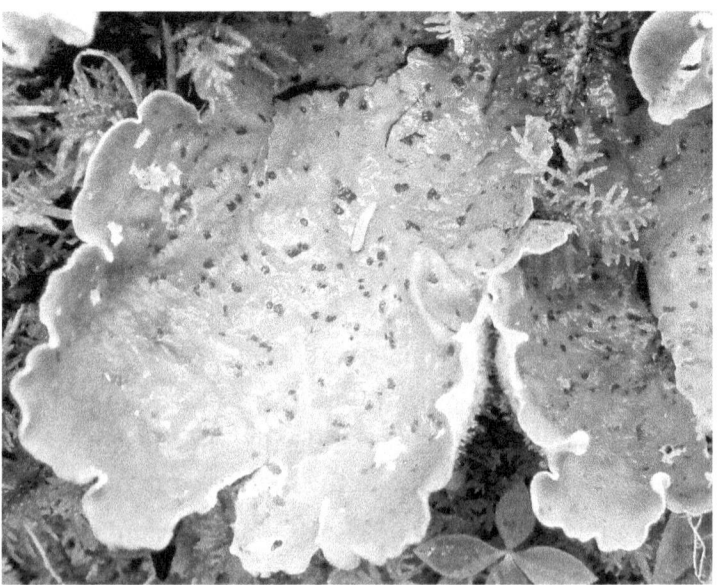

LEMON LICHEN

All Peltigera are used for boiling water dyes, usually brown in nature.

It is a strong purgative and anthelmintic, the combines well with other plants for cleansing worms and other parasites.

The Swedes boil the lichen in milk for treating thrush in their children. Back in the 1800's, it was believed that white spots on the cheeks of feverish children was caused by elves, and used Fairy Pelt to help the cure. This is another example of plant signature, where the cephaloida was thought to be similar to thrush eruptions in children's mouths.

Given the prevalence of chronic thrush and yeast infections today, it is a plant worthy of further attention.

When cooked, the lichen becomes thick and glue like. This is a great remedy for diaper rash, or chapped skin, applied and left to dry. Repeat as needed.

The Nitinaht of Vancouver Island chewed both *P. aphthosa* and closely related *P. britannica* for tuberculosis The Tlingit sprinkled the dry, powdered lichen on scalds and burns, and the Nitinaht used the fresh poultice on leg sores.

## MEDICINAL

**CONSTITUENTS-** *P. aphthosa-* various phenolics, including aphtosin and tenuiorin; methyl gyrophorate, gyrophoric acid, and triterpenoids, phlebic acid A and B.
*P. polydactylon-* 2-3% peltigerin, a derivative of orcinol; as well as tenuiorin, methyl gyrophorate, gyrophoric acid, triterpenes.
*P. membranacea-* lec-2

Fairy Pelt or Lemon Lichen contains a mixture of methyl and ethyl orsellinates that have been shown to be superior to commonly used preservative agents like methyl and proply p-hydroxybenzoates.

The anti-microbial active compounds were found to be effective against fungi and both gram positive and negative bacteria.

It contains several laccases that may have application in biological reactions.

The closely related Ruffled Freckle Pelt (*P. leucophlebia*) was at one time considered the same species, but now distinct. Both are extremely widespread and common.

Studies by Ingolfsdottir et al, in *Pharmaceutical Biology* 2000 38; 4 showed the lichen possessing moderate inhibition of HL-60, human leukemia cells. Early work by same author found petroleum and chloroform extracts show activity against *Pseudomonas aeruginosa*.

Tenuiorin showed weak activity against pancreatic and colon cancer cells. Ingolfsdottir K et al, *Phytomedicine* 2002 9(7): 654-8.

The phycobiont of this lichen, *Coccomyxa* sp., excretes 16 times more biotin in a culture medium than free-living *Chlorella*.

The related Frog Pelt, or Many-Fruited Pelt (*P. polydactylon*) is used medicinally in Sikkim as a paste to stop bleeding and as an antiseptic. It contains 2-3% peltigerin, a derivative of orcinol; as well as tenuiorin, methyl gyrophorate, gyrophoric acid, triterpenes.

Water extracts show activity against various bacteria including *Bacillus subtilis, E. coli* and *Staphylococcus aureus*. Karagoz et al, *J Med Plant Res* 2009 3:12.

Studies in Wales indicate the lichen inhibits the germination of grass seeds, as well as root production and elongation in grass seeds.

This suggests the use of this and other lichens in organic farming and weed control. Water extracts of Dog Pelt, mentioned below, inhibit various bent, meadow and rye grasses as well as fescue.

Membranacous Dog Lichen (*P. membranacea*) was used by the Kwakiutl, of British Columbia as a love charm in an unspecified manner, as well as by Nitinaht men who could not easily urinate. I noted in my clinical practice that difficulty with urination sometimes followed the persistant use of love charms, if you know what I mean.

*Peltigera rufescens* shows remarkably high anti-oxidant activity despite low levels of phenolics. Odabasoglu et al, *Fitoterapia* 76:2. It also exhibits anti-inflammatory activity against chronic conditions in 63% of cases. Tanas et al, *J Nat Med* 2010 64(1): 42-9.

It may reduce toxicity associated with agricultural or clinical use of the fungicide Imazalil, protecting human lymphocytes from genetic damage. Turkez H et al, *Toxicol Ind Health* 2012 28(6): 492-8.

Scaly Dog Lichen, or Born Again Pelt (*P. praetextata*) is common and widespread. Activity against *Bacillus subtilis, E. coli,* and *S. aureus* has been observed. Karagoz et al, *J Med Plant Res* 2009 3:12.

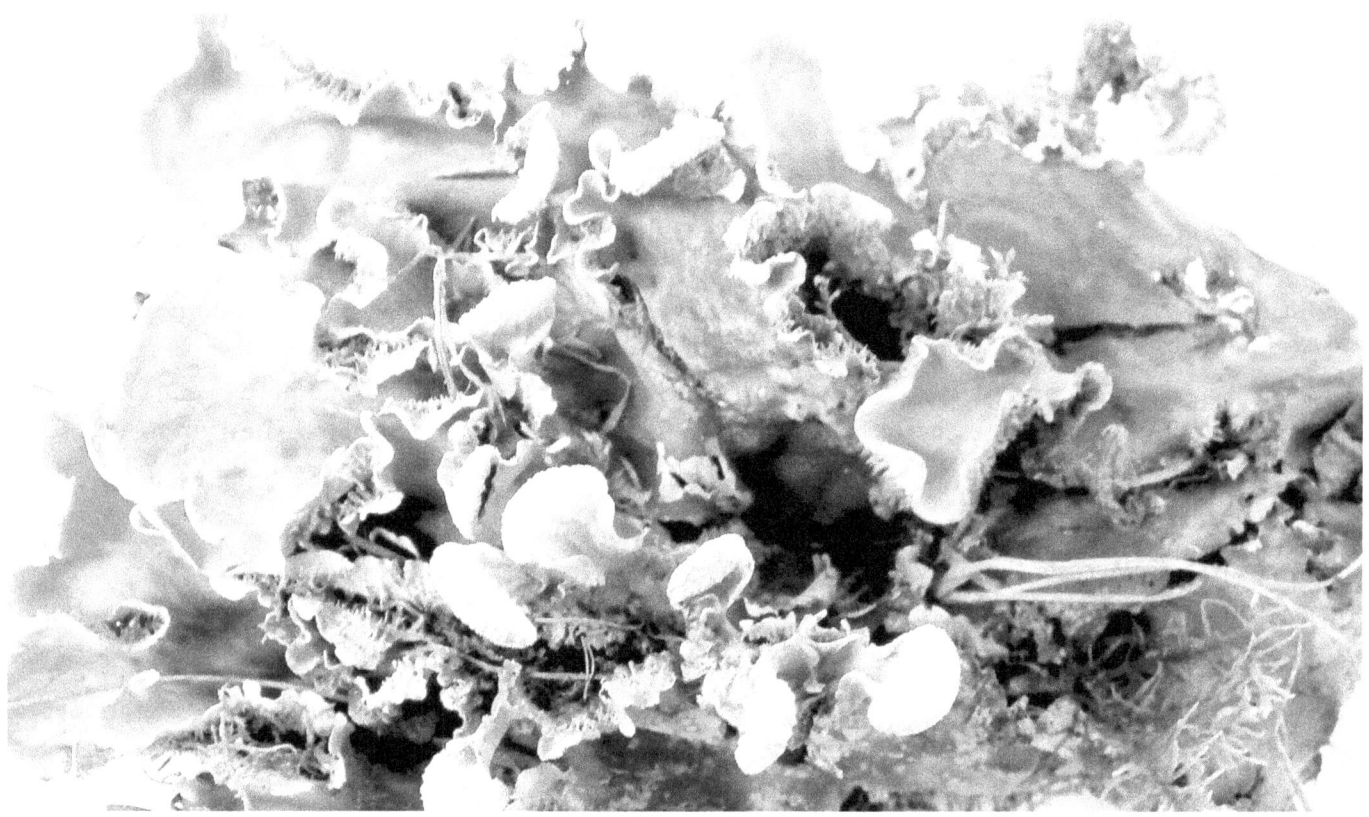

DOG PELT LICHEN

## GROUND LIVERWORT
## DOG PELT
(***Peltigera canina***[L.] Willd.)

The species name canine was based on its former value in protection from dog bites, and the plant signature of the fruiting bodies resembling dogteeth or ears.

Today, it is known as a safe, reliable laxative, if used in moderate amounts, and a mild effective liver tonic.

Early German settlers to North America used the plant for strengthening a weak liver, or cooling one that was inflamed. When ground into a powder and put in white wine, it was given to little boys suffering hernia. In parts of 19th century Wales, it was powdered and mixed with black pepper for dog bites.

The Nitanaht of Vancouver Island used *P. canina* (or *P. aphthosa*) as an infusion for those suffering anuria, or inability to urinate.

The Kwakiult call it **TL'EXTL'EKW'ES** meaning "seaweed of the ground" and used it as a love charm.

The plant has the symbolic meaning of confidence. It was a dye source in Europe as an iron red colour for wool.

# MEDICINAL

**CONSTITUENTS**- ergosterol, emulsin, mannitol-like substances, free methionine. It contains all the essential amino acids save histidine.

Boiled in water, and gargled, the lichen soothes the swelling of tonsils and the uvula.

The distilled water is excellent for an inflamed liver or for treating jaundice, a few tablespoons taken several times daily. The high concentration of methionine may be responsible, in part, for its high curative rate.

Polysaccharides from the lichen influence both the innate and adaptive immune systems. Omarsdottir S et al, *Phytomedicine* 2005 12(6-7):461-7.

Concentric Pelt (*P. elisabethae*), Ruffled Freckle Pelt (*P. leucophlebia*), Veinless Pelt (*P. malacea*) Black Saddle Lichen (*P. neckeri*) Carpet Pelt (*P. neopolydactyla*) and Flat Fruited Pelt (*P. horizontalis*) contain tenuiorin, methyl gyrophorate, gyrophoric acid, peltigerin, and various triterpenes.

Many of the others in our region contain no lichen substances, so you cannot just speculate. Ruffled Freckle Pelt contains methyl orsellinate and tenuiorin. The latter compound showed moderate activity against human breast, pancreatic and colon cancer cell lines. Ingolfsdottir et al, *Phytomedicine* 2002 9:7.

Fan Lichen (*P. venosa*) for example contains zeorin and tenuiorin.

Tenuiorin has been tested against human breast, pancreas and colon cancer cell lines, and showed moderate activity. Ingolfsdottir et al, *Phytomed* 2002 9:7.

Flaky Freckle Pelt (*P. britannica*) was chewed by the Nitinaht of British Columbia to treat tuberculosis. It contains tenuiorin, methyl gyrophate, gyrophoric acid, and triterpenes.

Various Peltigera species contain mycotoxins. A study by Burkin AA & GP Kononenko, *Izv Akad Nauk Ser Biol* 2015 6:573-80 found three mycotoxins in *P. canina, P. didactyla, P. praetextata* and *P. rufescens*; and seven in *P. aphthosa*.

# HOMEOPATHY

Ground liverwort is used whenever there is lots of throat congestion, with profuse expectoration and hoarseness. The throat is tickling and irritating, with a scraping and rough sensation.

Liverwort induces free and easy expectoration; relieving that continual feeling of something caught in the epiglottis.

**DOSE**- Second potency.                                                                                      **BOERICKE**

# PERSONALITY TRAITS

The noble liverwort does not appear,
Without a speck, like the unclouded air,
A plant of noble use and endless fame,
The liver's great preserver, hence its name.                                      **ABRAHAM COWLEY**

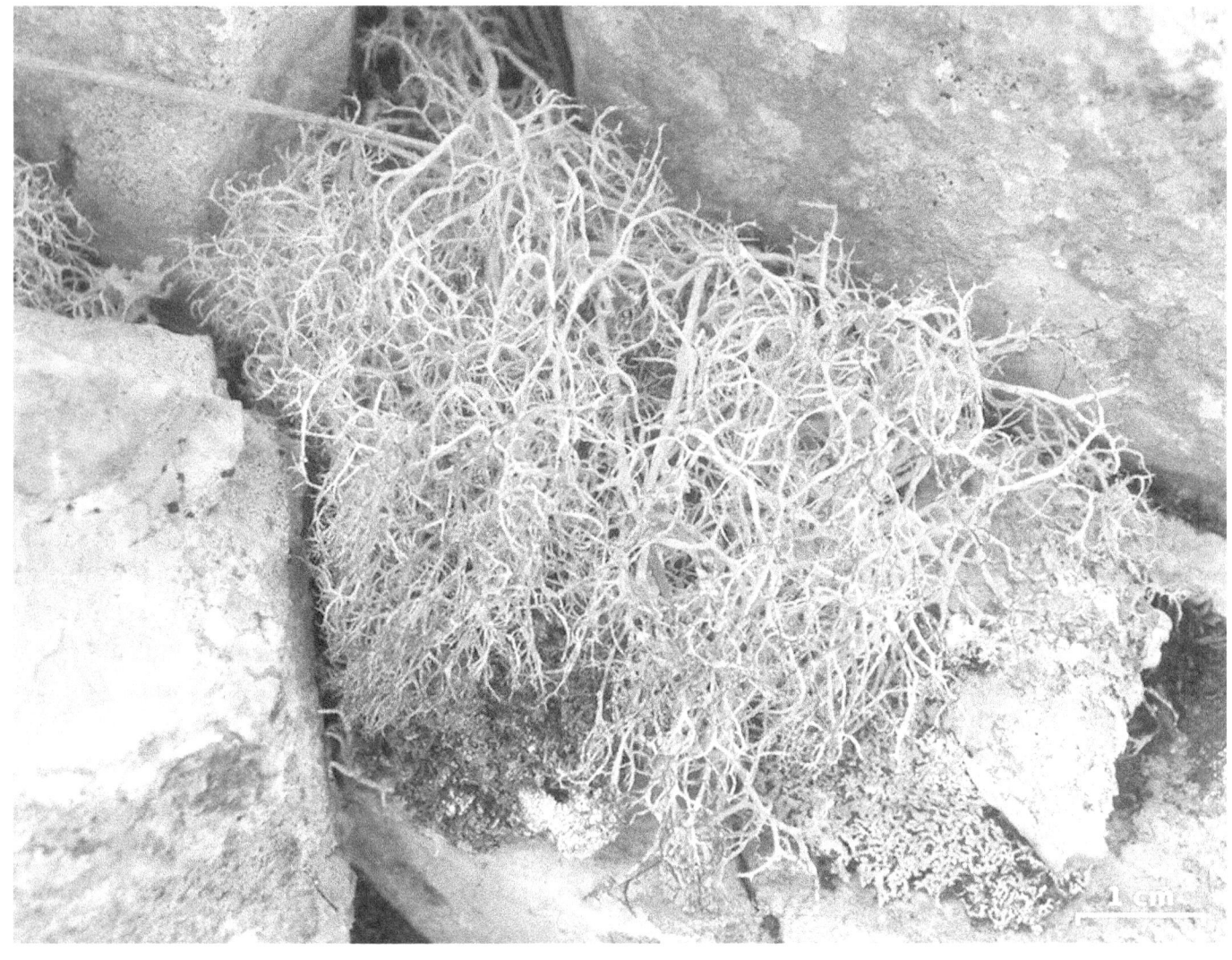

GREEN WITCH'S HAIR (Courtesy of Jason Hollinger)

## WITCH'S HAIR
(***Alectoria sarmentosa*** [Ach.] Ach)
## GREEN WITCH'S HAIR
(***A. ochroleuca*** Hoff.)

This lichen looks at first glance like usnea, but it lacks the central cord. It is found in the same boreal forests, hanging from conifers that are at least a century old.

The Bella Coola of BC used the long hair for their dance masks. They call it limb moss or **IPTS-AAK**. When found on alder, it was used as a poultice for sores and boils.

In Scandinavia, different colored *Alectoria* and *Usnea* lichens are used to make trolls, to warn children to be good and kind to other people. Legends told of deformed children driven into the woods, and dwarves carrying off naughty children.

In Western Canada, it was mainly used as a fibre for mattresses, baby diapers, and sanitary napkins. It was woven with *Bryoria fremontii*, below, for poor quality clothing, when skins were unavailable. It was often interwoven with wolf willow bark to make it more durable.

The Haida call it Crow's Mountain Goat Wool or Crow's Blanket.

150

It was used traditionally to make false whiskers and hair for decorative dance masks by variety of coastal natives.

Green Witch's Hair (*A. ochroleuca*) was used during the 1930s in Russia to make a type of molasses. It yielded 82% of its dry weight to glucose, and produced light yellow syrup. It contains diffractaic acid. Llano, *G.A. Econ Botany* 1956 10:4.

The Inuit call it Greenbeard, Caribou Moss, or **TINQAUJAIT** meaning, "what looks like pubic hair". It is a handy fire starter.

## MEDICINAL

**CONSTITUENTS-** *A. sarmentosa-* dibenzo-furanoid lactol, (-)-usnic acid, physodic acid, 8'-0-ethyl-beta-alectoronic acid, alectosarmentin, alpha-collatolic acid, squamatic acid, mannitol, arabitol, usnic and physocid acids.
*A. ochroleuca-* diffractaic, thamnolic, barbatic, alectoronic, chloroatranorin, and (-) usnic acid.

Recent studies indicate that a new anti-microbial dibenzo-furanoid lactol called alectosarmentin has been isolated from Witch's Hair. The compound exhibits activity against *Staphylococcus aureus*, and *Mycobacterium smegmatis*.

Usnic and physocid acids in this lichen were found effective against these two bacteria as well as *Candida albicans*.

Studies by Gollapudi et al, at the University of Kansas showed four anti-microbial compounds, including usnic acid, physodic acid, 8'-0-ethyl-beta-alectoronic acid, and alectosarmentin, the newly discovered dibenzofuranoid lactol. *J Nat Prod* 1994 57:7.

Witch's hair shows significant inhibition of human lung cancer cells. Yang Y et al, *PLoS One* 2016 11(1).

It contains a yellow dye, and at one time was used by distillers to make alcohol.

Previous studies have indicated the presence of mannitol and arabitol, active anti-tumour polysaccharides.

Green Witch's Hair contains (-)-usnic acid. It was compared with (+)usnic acid from *Cladonia arbuscula* against breast cancer cell line T-47D and pancreatic cancer cell line Capan-2; and found equally effective inhibitors of DNA synthesis. Einarsdottir E et al, *Planta Medica* 2010 76(10): 969-74.

Green Witch's Hair (*A. ochroleuca*) shows strong activity against *S. aureus*. Stoll et al, *Experientia* 1947 3.

The closely related Gray Witch's Hair (*A. nigricans*), lacks usnic acid, but does contain alectorialic acid.

An extract was found to exhibit notable inhibition of ODC activity induced by 12-0-tetradecanoylphorbol-13-acetate in cultured mouse epidermal 308 cells.

The IC50 value was only 2.6 ug/ml. Work by Ingolfsdottir et al, *Pharm Bio* 38:4 found this lichen active against leukemia cell lines and to exhibit quinone reductase activity.

**BLACK TREE LICHEN**
**EDIBLE HORSEHAIR**
(***Bryoria fremontii*** [Tuck] Brodo & D. Hawksw.)
(***Alectoria fremontii*** Tuck.)
**HORSE HAIR LICHEN**
(***B. trichodes*** [Michx.] Brodo & D. Hawksw.)

Black Tree Lichen, known as **WILA**, was mixed with mud by the Interior Salish to chink log cabins. Others made a fibre that could be made into clothing such as vests, ponchos, shoes and leggings.

It was twisted together with strands of Wolf Willow bark or other fibers to give it strength.

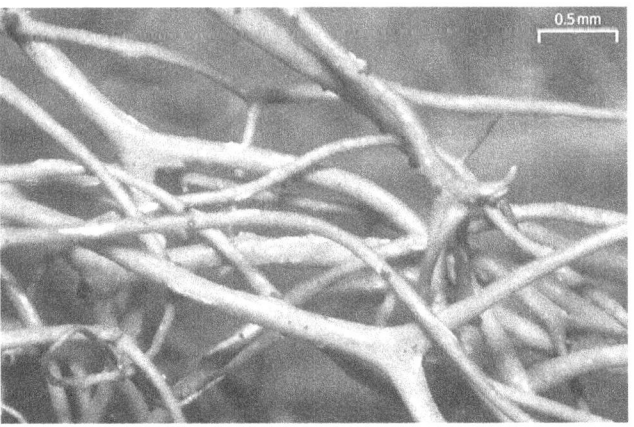

BRYORIA FREMONTII CLOSE UP
(Courtesy of Jason Hollinger)

Northern flying squirrels build their cozy nests from it.

The lichen used by native tribes for food. Some aboriginals say it tastes like candy, if properly prepared; while others maintain it is strictly a survival food. In the Okanagan, young natives would bring back lichen from various areas to their grandmother to taste. If sweet, the family would claim the area where it was growing.

It can be collected at any time of year, and the flavour is definitely influenced by the tree it grows on.

The Northern Okanagan preferred that growing on Ponderosa or Lodge pole Pine; whereas the Southern Okanagan preferred the Douglas fir or Western Larch. Probably whatever was in your area, I imagine.

Long poles were utilized to pull the lichen from branches or youngsters would climb into the trees to throw it down. In a good site, five or six trees would yield sufficient harvest for one family for the year!

The fresh lichen is light and bulky and was soaked in water; then cooked in a steam pit, created by putting hot rocks at the bottom and covering with green leaves and masses of lichens. It was left for the night, removed after cooling in the morning, and cut into jelly like loaves. It can be eaten then or stored for several years, and soaked before eating.

It compacts when cooked; a 20-centimeter thick layer reduces to 4 cm after steaming. It is rather bland, so it was often cooked with layers of nodding onions, mixed with Saskatoon berries, or dipped in berry juice after cooking. The Okanagan would also cook it the False Solomon Seal rhizomes, while others would sweeten it with Douglas fir sugar.

The Carrier mixed it with flour and baked it like fruitcake and before flour with grease.

The Okanagan also used another method for cooking Black Tree Lichen. They would roast it until dry and crumbly, then boil it until molasses like. Further south, the Coeur D'Alêne also ate the lichen they call **SKOLA'PKEN**.

The Nlaka'pamux still prepare it to this day in modern ovens, and serve it as a form of taffy, called **WE'IA** with the texture and flavour of licorice.

The lichen is incredibly rich in iron containing 8.3 mg per 100 grams.

The dried cakes were used for long journeys. Pregnant women did not eat this, as they believed it would make their babies dark. The Okanagan Colville mixed the dry lichen with grease and rubbed it on the navel of newborns to prevent infection. They also gave a mixture of Saskatoon berry juice and syrup of *B. fremontii* to babies after weaning.

Natives of the northern Boreal forest heat the various horsehair lichens into a powder for burns. Further south, the Nez Perce used it for treating diarrhea and ingestion.

Some black spruce forests of northern Saskatchewan produce over 500 kilograms of horsehair lichen per hectare.

It contains some vulpinic acid, atranorin, thamnolic and alectorialic acid.

Horsehair Lichen (*B. trichodes*) is found isolated in central Saskatchewan, but common in eastern North America. The related subspecies *americana* is found in British Columbia and in parts of southern Alaska. It was gathered and piled on a sick person in steam baths to help hold in heat, and used to staunch bleeding wounds. The lichen was also gathered and burned into a black powder for wood paint, as was Shiny Horsehair Lichen (*B. glabra*).

Horsehair Lichen contains fumar-protocetraric acid and atranorin.

One related lichen, Inedible Horsehair (*B. tortuosa*), which looks somewhat like Black Tree, contains high concentrations of the poisonous vulpinic acid and is a potential toxin. This is mainly a coastal species and not present east of the Rockies.

Another species, *B. capillaris*, found on spruce and fir trees of the Rocky Mountain foothills, was traditionally burned into a black powder for paint as above.

Imazalil is a common fungicide used in agricultural and clinical settings, with very serious toxic effects. A water extract of this lichen may help protect human lymphocytes from genetic damage. Turkez H et al, *Toxicol Ind Health* 2014 30(1): 33-9.

The related B. *fremontii* was eaten as food, spun into fiber for clothing, and dye color. Natives of Oregon called it **WA KAMWA**. They dried, powdered and added it to soups. It is said to taste like acorns.

Bryoria species extracts inhibit proliferation of CD8[+] T cells. The extract is non-toxic in spleen cells and suppresses the growth of splenocytes induced by anti-CD3. It significantly suppressed the IL-2 associated with T cell growth and IFN-gamma as the CD8[+] T cell marker; as well as CD86 expression in DCs. This suggests an anti-immuno-suppressing agent that may be useful for organ transplants. Hwang YH et al, *J Microbiol Biotech* 2017 April 3.

Bryoria species contain five mycotoxins: sterigmatocystin, mycophenolic acid, citrinin, emodin and alternariol. Burkin AA et al, *Izv Akad Nauk Ser Bio* 2015 4:361-7.

## SPIRITUAL PROPERTIES

The coyote is the trickster and transformer of all things in their present state. The Black Tree Lichen was originally derived from Coyote's Hair braid which became tangled on a tree branch he was climbing.

He cut himself loose and fell to the ground, without his braid. Looking up he said" You shall not be wasted, my valuable hair. After this, you shall be gathered by the people. The old women will make you into food".

It was changed into lichen and has been used as food ever since.     **MOURNING DOVE 1933**

**ALPINE CORAL LICHEN**
(*Stereocaulon alpinum* Laurer & Funck)
**EASTER LICHEN**
(*S. paschale* [L.] Hoffm.)
**VARIEGATED FOAM LICHEN**
(*S. vesuvianum* [Sm.] Ach.)

Stereocaulon is from the Greek **STEREOS**, meaning hard or firm; and **KAULOS**, meaning stem; referring to the firm brittle texture when dry.

Easter Lichen, and other flat lichens, was used by the Barrens-Keewatin Inuit as a filler in caribou skins to make rafts for crossing rivers and streams. It was used in parts of Europe as an ash-green dye for wool.

*Stereocaulon alpinum* is a rose-white, grayish lichen common to sub-alpine forest floors. It is often confused with the closely related *S. tomentosum*, which is silvery grey.

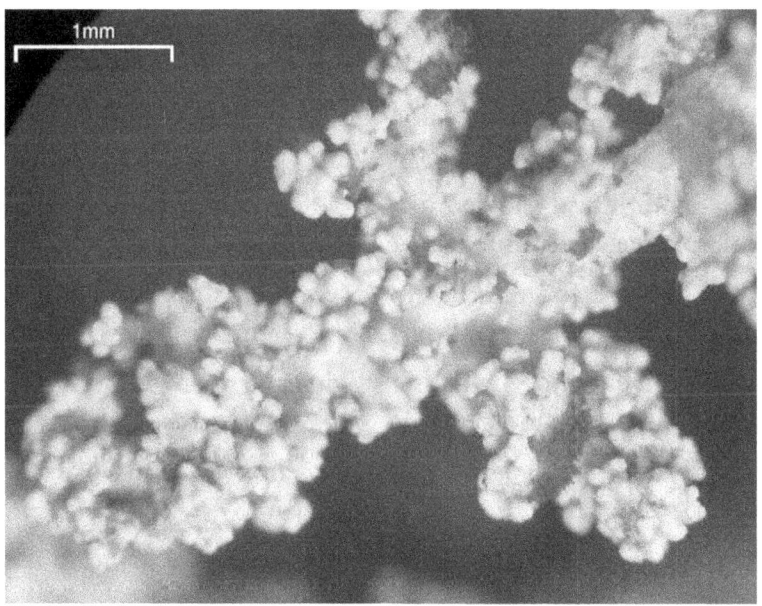

EASTER LICHEN - CLOSE UP
(Courtesy of Jason Hollinger)

Variegated Foam Lichen is a northern species ranging from Alaska to Newfoundland.

# MEDICINAL

**CONSTITUENTS-** *S. alpinum-* methyl beta-orsellinate, lobaric acid, atranorin, 9-cis-octadecenamide, lobastin, lobarstin. *S. paschale-* dextro mannose, dextro galactose, atranorin, lobaric acid, dibenzofurans.

Several studies indicate that the active ingredient of *S. alpinum* (methyl beta-orsellinate) is a superior preserving agent to commonly used methyl and propyl p-hydroxybenzoates. It is anti-fungal and shows signs of gram-positive and negative bactericidal activity.

Early work by Ingolfsdottir et al, *Antimicrobial Agents & Chemotherapy* 1985 28:2 found chloroform and acetone extracts active against *Staphylococcus aureus*, petroleum and acetate extracts active against *Bacillus subtilis*, chloroform extracts active against *E. coli*, and acetone extracts active against *Pseudomonas aeruginosa*. Petroleum, chloroform and acetone extracts all inhibited the fungi *Candida albicans*.

Lobaric acid isolated from this lichen has shown, *in-vitro*, inhibitory effects on arachidonate 5-lipoxygenase, similar to the flavone baicalein, found in Scullcap. Bucar et al, *Phytomed* 2004 11:7-8.

Studies conducted in Iceland, the mecca of polar lichens, by Ogmundsdottir et al of the *Icelandic Cancer Society Laboratory* showed some exciting results in the January 1998 issue of *Journal of Pharm Pharmacology*.

On cultured, human cells, three malignant cell lines from breast carcinomas and erythro-leukemia (K-562) were tested. At concentrations of 20 mcg/mLitre significant cancer cell death was detected.

In contrast, the proliferation and survival of normal skin fibroblasts and DNA synthesis was not affected.

These results open up the opportunity for future studies of protolichesterinic acid, with regards to anti-tumour and anti-inflammatory properties.

Atranorin and lobaric acids, isolated from the lichen, show activity against *Mycobacterium aurum*, a non-pathogenic organism with sensitivity similar to the *Tuberculinum mycobacterium*. Ingolfsdottir K et al, *Eur J Pharm Sci* 1998 6(2): 141-4.

Atranorin, from Stereocaulon species inhibits hepatitis C virus entry. Vu TH et al, *PLoS One* 2015 10:3.

Work by Ingolfsdottir et al, *Phytomedicine* 1997 4:4 shows the presence of an alkamide, called 9-cis-octadecenamide. This compound showed moderate inhibitory activity against cyclooxygenase from sheep seminal vesicle microsomes with an IC50 of 64.3 uM, indicating anti-inflammatory properties.

Recent work found lobastin (pseudodepsidone) maybe an important regulator of inflammation in the atherosclerotic lesion and a possible treatment of atherosclerosis. Lee K et al, *Arch Pharm Res* 2016 39(1): 83-93.

Lobarstin enhances chemosensitivity in human glioblastoma T98G cells, and may be useful when cancer cells are resistant to temozolomide. Kim S et al, *Anticancer Res* 2013 33(12): 5445-51.

The related Rock Foam Lichen (*S. saxatile*), Grand Foam (*S. grande*) and Easter Lichen (*S. paschale*) contain lobaric acid, while Woolly Foam Lichen (*S. tomentosum*) contains stictic acid.

Easter Lichen is used in Traditional Chinese Medicine.

Early work by Burkholder et al, *Bull Torrey Botany Club* 1945 72:2 showed activity against *Staphylococcus aureus, Bacillus subtilis, B. mycoides* and *Sarcina lutea*.

Isolated ascomatic acid dibenzofuran derivatives show activity against the oral pathogens *Porphyromonas gingivalis* and *Streptococcus mutans*. Carpentier C et al, *J Nat Prod* 2017 80(1): 210-14.

Snow Foam Lichen (*S. rivulorum*) usually contains lobaric acid, with some areas containing perlatolic and anzaic acid, and others only atranorin.

The related Variegated Foam Lichen (*S. vesuvianum*) is found on newly exposed rock in the Rocky Mountains as well as throughout the northern territories. It contains stictic and norstictic acids.

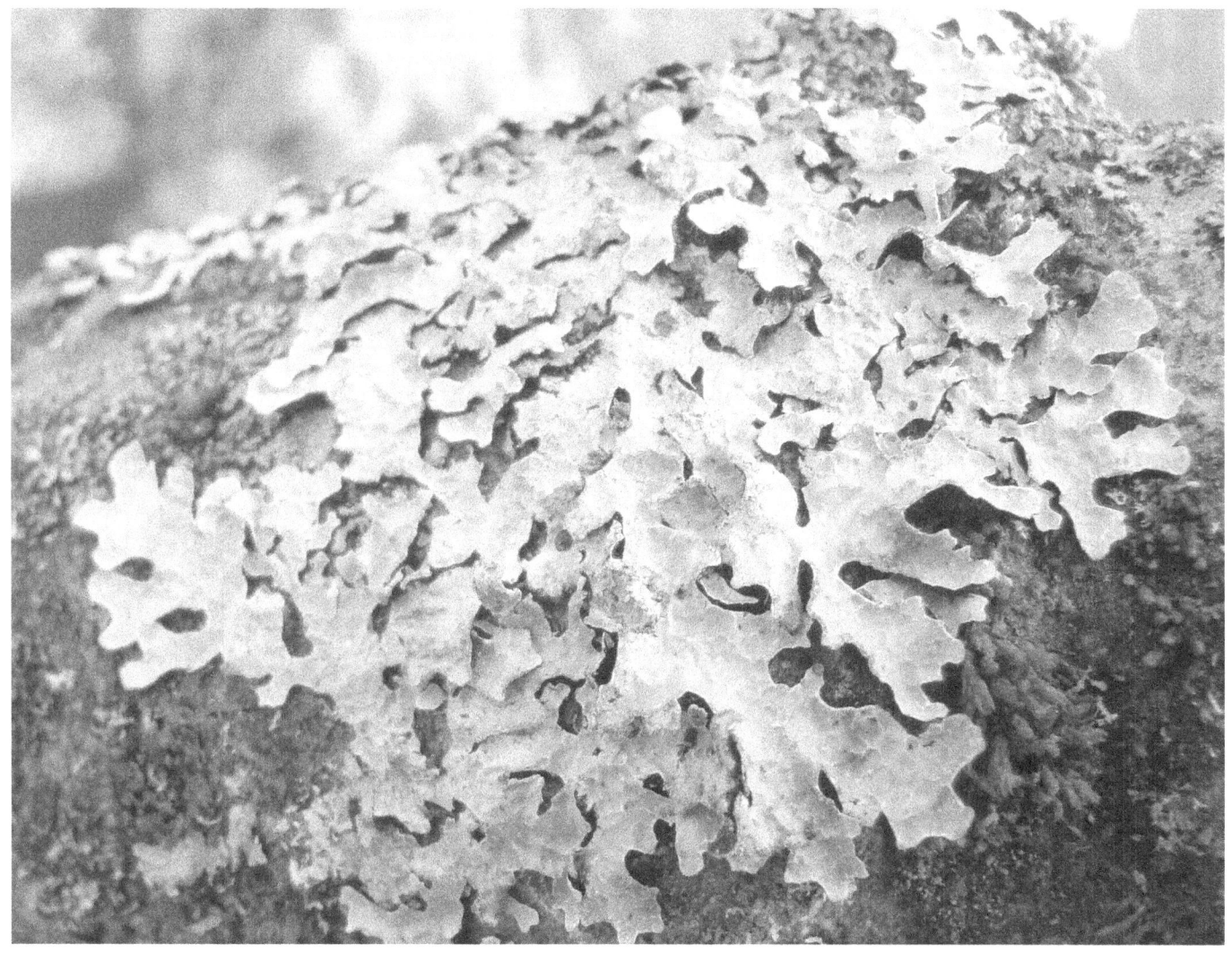

ROCK SHIELD

Petroleum extracts show activity against *Pseudomonas aeruginosa*, and water extracts against *Candida albicans*. This work by Ingolfsdottir et al, *Antimicrobial Agents & Chemotherapy* 1985 28:2 also found chloroform extracts active against *Staphylococcus aureus* and *Bacillus subtilis*.

## LICHEN ESSENCE

Variegated Foam Lichen essence is like the lichen, the first plant to grow on cooled lava. It gives us the power to begin over again. It strengthens our resolve to move forward even in small steps.  **KORTE PHI**

**ROCK SHIELD**
**SALTED SHIELD**
**CROTTLE**
(***Parmelia saxatilis*** [L.] Ach.)
**SMOKY CROTTLE**
(***P. omphalodes*** [L.] Ach)

*Parmelia* was divided into a number of different genera starting in 1974. Research conducted before that year referring to *Parmelia ssp.* can be extremely confusing.

Saxatilis is from the Latin **SAXUM** meaning a rock.

*Parmelia saxatilis* is found abundantly on acidic rocks and outcroppings in boreal forests. It increases in size by an average of 3.4 mm per year.

This lichen may be of significance in the treated of tuberculosis from a natural source.

Various *Parmelia* species have been used traditionally in both India and China for medicinal purpose. In TCM, *P. saxatilis* is known as **SHIH HUA**.

This lichen accumulates the rare mineral beryllium.

In Sweden, country people call this Dye Lichen, or Stone Moss. It is collected from rocks easily after a rain with a table knife. It yields various shades of brown, depended on the quantity used.

In Scotland, it is used to dye wool for Harris Tweed, and does not require a mordant. The scent of Harris Tweed is that of the lichen itself, even more pronounced when wet. In 1850, a factory in Glasgow covered 17 acres and processed 254 tonnes of lichen annually. Human urine was used for ammonia, and required collection of over 13,000 litres daily.

The dried lichen was sprinkled in stockings in parts of the Highlands to prevent foot inflammation and pain from long journeys. In parts of Ireland it was applied to bad sores under the chin, as well as burns and cuts. During the 15th century, the lichen was known in parts of Europe as Muscus cranii humanii, when found growing on a human skull. This was much prized for treating epilepsy and sold for its weight in gold.

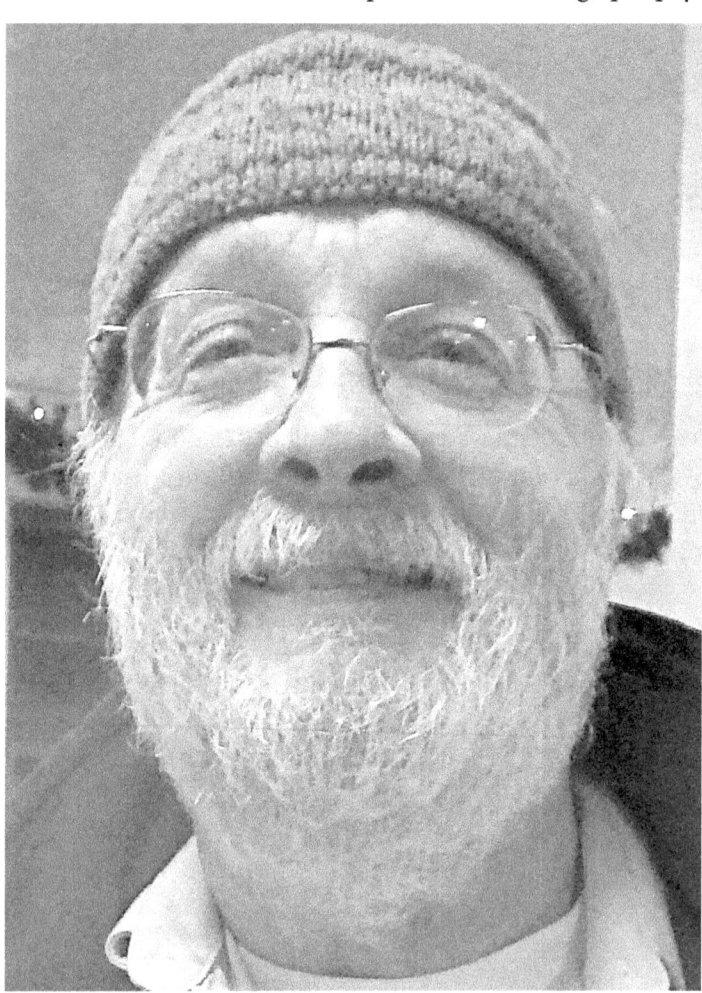

AUTHOR WITH LICHEN DYED CAP

The lichen was used for well-dressing, a tradition from the early 19th century in England. Ritual plant and fungi materials were used to create miniature scenes up to ten feet long, and during the summer festival were leaned up against wells for several weeks.

The Nishinam of California call it **WA'-HAT-TAK**. It was infused as a tea for colic.

Smoky Crottle (*P. omphalodes*) more often found in the northern territories, was also used traditionally for dying the deep red browns and rusty oranges prized by weavers.

The brown shades produced are known as Crottle, and the red shades, Corkir. Studies have shown that the dye is produced by a reaction between the free amino groups of the wool with aldehyde groups on the lichen acids. There is no correlation between the colour of the lichen and the colour obtained on boiling with wool.

Lichen substances such as gyrophoric, evernic and lecanoric acid, as well as erythrin convert to a purple compound in the presence of oxygen and ammonia. August picking yields the richest dye material.

Concentric Ring Lichen (*Arctoparmelia centrifuga*) has been used traditionally in the north as a red brown dye for wool.

## MEDICINAL

Smoky Crottle contains salazinic acid, sometimes accompanied by lobaric acid.

Rock Shield contains both altranoric acid (0.5%) and salazinic acid (3.1%) a compound with myco-bacterial activity. In studies conducted by Ingolfsdottir et al in Iceland, the latter compound showed MIC values of 125 mcg per milliliter. *Eur J Pharm Sci* 1998 6(2): 141-4.

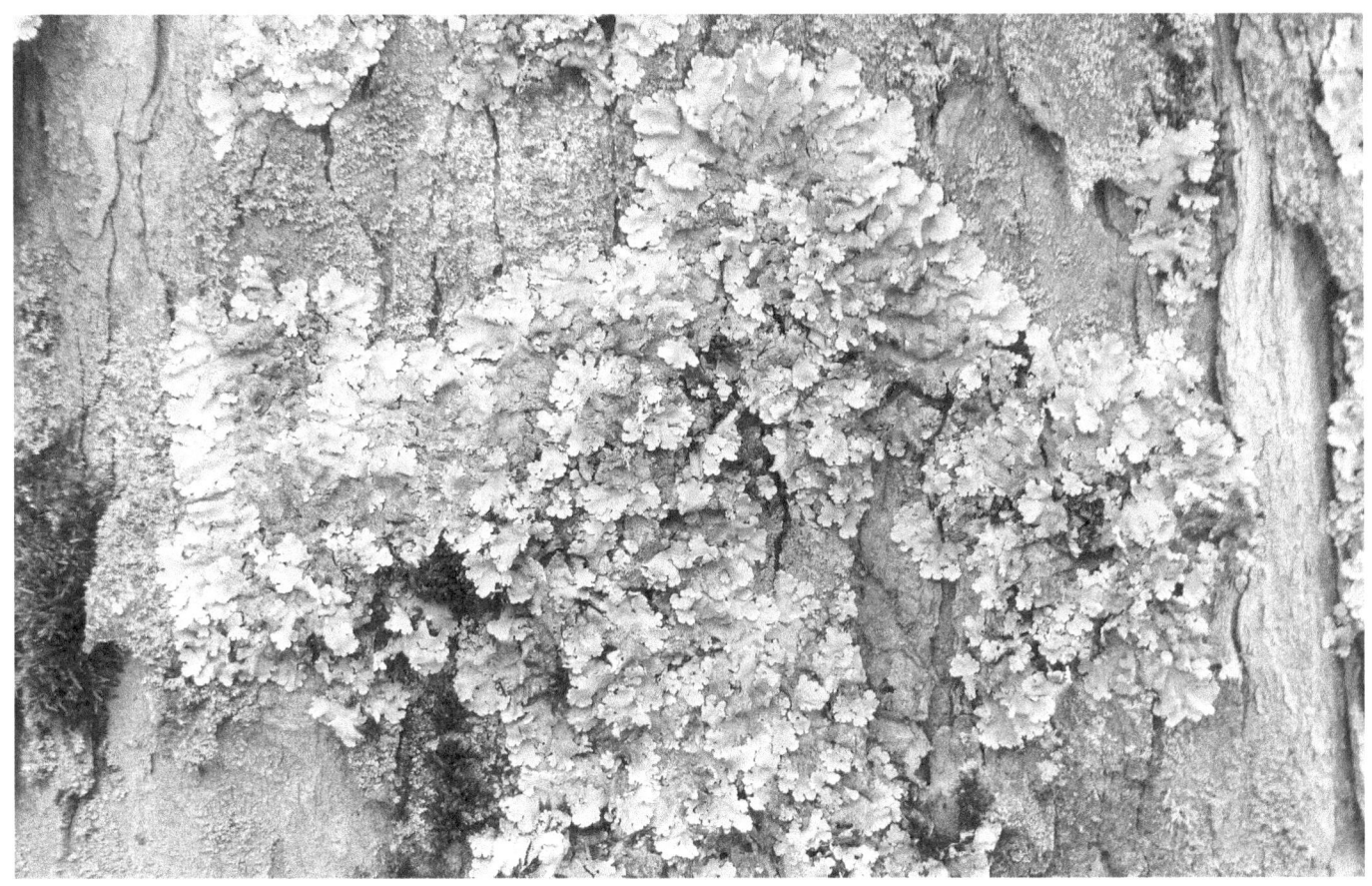

WAXPAPER LICHEN

## WAXPAPER LICHEN
## HAMMERED SHIELD LICHEN
### (*Parmelia sulcata* Taylor)

Sulcata is derived from the Latin **SULCUS**, meaning a furrow or groove.

Also known as Powdered Shield Lichen, this is a common branch lichen on dead spruce branches throughout the north. The Rufus hummingbirds use it to decorate and hide their nests.

The lichen was rubbed on the gums of teething babies to help make them less restless and sleep. The lichen acids, including salazinic and lobaric, are antiseptic.

In Italy, various species of *Parmelia* are used as a cholagogue.

Because it contains salizinic acid, it can be used for dyeing wool.

*Parmelia entotheiochria* contains secalonic acid A, related to the ergochromes from ergot.

The related *P. andina*, which contains lecanoric acid, is used in pipe-smoking mixtures in the southern Sahara.

Alpine Camouflage Lichen, previously known as *Parmelia stygia*, but now moved to the *Melanelia* genus, is found in the western mountains and throughout the former Northwest Territories.

Spotted Camouflage Lichen (*M. olivacea*) has been used previously to produce a brown dye in Great Britain.

The genus contains lecanoric, fumarprotocetraric, stictic and perlatolic acids, as well as echinocarpic and galbinic acids.

Thioredoxin reductase (TrxR) protects cells from oxidative stress. But over-expression has been found in many aggressive tumors. Inhibition of TrxR is a fairly new approach to treating cancer. Both lecanoric acid and vulpinic acid show very strong inhibition of TrxR, much better than chemotherapy drugs. Ozgencli I et al, *Anticancer Agents Med Chem* 2016 May 3.

Type 2 diabetes and obesity are a growing problem. Selective inhibition of PTP1B may be helpful. Lecanoric acid, gyrophoric acid and methyl orsellinate exhibit significant inhibition in a non-competitive manner. Seo C et al, *J Enzyme Inhib Med Chem* 2009 24(5): 1133-7.

Perlatolic acid shows neurotrophic activity in neurite studies, and inhibits acetylcholinesterase associated with Alzheimer's disease and other brain cell function. Reddy RG et al, *Phytomedicine* 2016 23(12): 1527-34. The compound also increased protein levels of acetyl H3 and H4 in Neuro2A cells.

Atranorin and physodic acid show neurotrophic activity in same study.

Ground Lichen (*P. molliuscula*) is a flat species that grows from Nebraska to South Dakota and west to the Rockies. It causes severe paralysis and death to range cattle and sheep when forage is scarce.

## MEDICINAL

Waxpaper lichen shows activity against *Aeromonas hydrophila, Bacillus cereus, B. subtilis, Listeria monocytogenes, Proteus vulgaris, Yersinia enterocolitica, Staphylococcus aureus, Streptococcus faecalis, Candida albicans, C. glabrata, Aspergillus funigatus, A. niger* and *Penicillium notatum*. Candan et al, *Zeit Naturforschung* 2007 62:7-8; Rankovic et al, *Mikrobiologya* 2007 76:6.

The lichen induces apoptosis in human lung, liver and rat glioma cancer cell lines. Ari F et al, *Cell Prolif* 2014 47(5): 457-64.

It induced caspase-independent apoptosis against human breast cancer cell lines. Ari F et al, *Cytotechnology* 2015 67(3): 531-43.

*Parmelia* species exhibit astringent, resolvent, aperient and diuretic properties.

Ethanol extracts of *Parmelia* species are potentiated by colloidal silver in the treatment of *Staphylococcus aureus*. Momoh et al, *Afr J Pharm Pharmacol* 2:6.

**PLATED ROCK TRIPE**
(***Actinogyra muhlenbergii*** [Ach.] Schol)
(***Gyrophora muhlenbergii*** Ach.)
(***Umbilicaria muhlenbergii*** [Ach.] Tuck)
**FROSTED ROCK TRIPE**
(***U. vellea*** [L.] Hoffm.)
(***G. vellea*** [L.] Ach.)
**AMERICAN ROCK TRIPE**
(***U. americana*** Poelt & T. H. Nash)

Rock Tripe is flat, brown, circular lichen that attaches to rocks with a cord.

The Woods Cree of Saskatchewan call it **ASINIWAKON**, and used it for food by cleaning and breaking small pieces into fish broth to thicken it.

Very hot water was poured over the pieces and after cooking for 5-10 minutes the pieces softened and the broth thickened as it cooled. It was considered good nourishment for those who were sick, because it does not upset the stomach. Tripe lichen, harvested from slain caribou, is added to raw fish eggs as a form of stomach ice cream. Hence the name rock tripe, in reference to the stomach of cows, eaten as delicacy in dim sum, and other dishes.

The Chipewyan also used this "rock dirt", or **TTHE TSI** as a food source. The flakes were cleaned off and boiled in soup, giving a sour, mushroom flavour. The soup helps to fatten up sled dogs.

The Chipewyan burned it to ash, and then boiled it to make syrup for tapeworms.

Usually the lichen is added to boiling water that is discarded first to remove some of the more irritating and bitter acids. Wood ashes are sometimes added to the water to neutralize the acidity; even baking soda will make rock tripe more digestible.

The lichen contains gyrophoric acid.

One species *Umbilicaria esculenta*, or "rock tripe" is considered a delicacy in Japan. It is sold as a delicacy, under the name Iwatake, and taken as part of a special tea ceremony or natural food in mountain inns. There is some confusion as to the exact identity of the lichen, with *Dermatocarpon miniatum*, sometimes identified as the same lichen. It is either boiled until tender, and then seasoned with rice vinegar or sesame paste; eaten as a vegetable in soybean soup; or deep fried as a tempura. It has the earthy, unami-taste of mushrooms.

In Japan, a sulfate isolate from rock tripe showed an inhibitory effect on the replication of HIV-1 in vitro. The compound (GE-3-S) appears to work in a manner similar to dextran sulphate and heparin, preventing attachment of HIV to the surface of T4 cells. This partially acetylated pustulan sulphate is only one of four polysaccharide that show weak animal toxicity, with GE-3-S showing no acute toxicity in mice at very high doses. *Chem Pharm Bull* 1989 37:9.

The lichen is active against gram-positive bacteria. A substance similar to pustulan, an acylated B-1-6 glucan, has shown anti-tumour activity against sarcoma 180.

Iwatake (*Umbilicaria esculenta* or *Gyrophora esculenta*) known as "stone mushroom" is collected in the mountains of Japan, and exported to China as a luxury item. Properly prepared, it resembles tripe. As food, the bitter constituents were neutralized by soda ash from fires to lessen stomach irritation. The blacker the lichen the less content of usnic acid, that causes irritation. Work by Moo Sung Kim et al, *J Ethnopharm* 105:3 found the lichen possesses anti-thrombotic properties due to anti-platelet activity. The same author has identified the ability to reduce melanin in human melanoma cells and inhibit tyrosinase glycosylation. *J Microbiol* 2007 45:6.

Petaled Rock Tripe (*U. polyphylla*), mainly found in the far north, but also on the west coast; and Fringed Rock Tripe (*U. cylindrica*), mainly northern, have been studied for their *in vitro* anti-oxidant, anti-microbial and anti-cancer activity. Kosanic M et al, *J Food Sci* 2012 77(1): T20-5. The former lichen showed largest free radical scavenging activity, similar to standard synthetic antioxidants. It was also the most active anti-microbial, while both showed activity against human melanoma and human colon carcinoma cell lines.

Netted Rock Tripe (*U. proboscidea*) is also widespread from Alaska to New England and across the north. It contains fourteen compounds including acylated umbilicaxanthosides. Rezanka T & VM Dembitsky, *J Chromatogr A* 2003 995(1-2): 109-18.

Plated Rock Tripe (*U. muehlenbergii*) can be transformed by *Agrobacterium tumefaciens*. This makes it the only known genetically tractable lichen found to date. A draft genome assembly for the lichen, shows a size of 34,812,353 bp and a GC content of 47.12%, consisting of seven scaffolds. Park SY et al, *Genome Announc* 2014 2(2).

Umbilicaria lichens contain mycotoxins, with the highest content being alternariole.

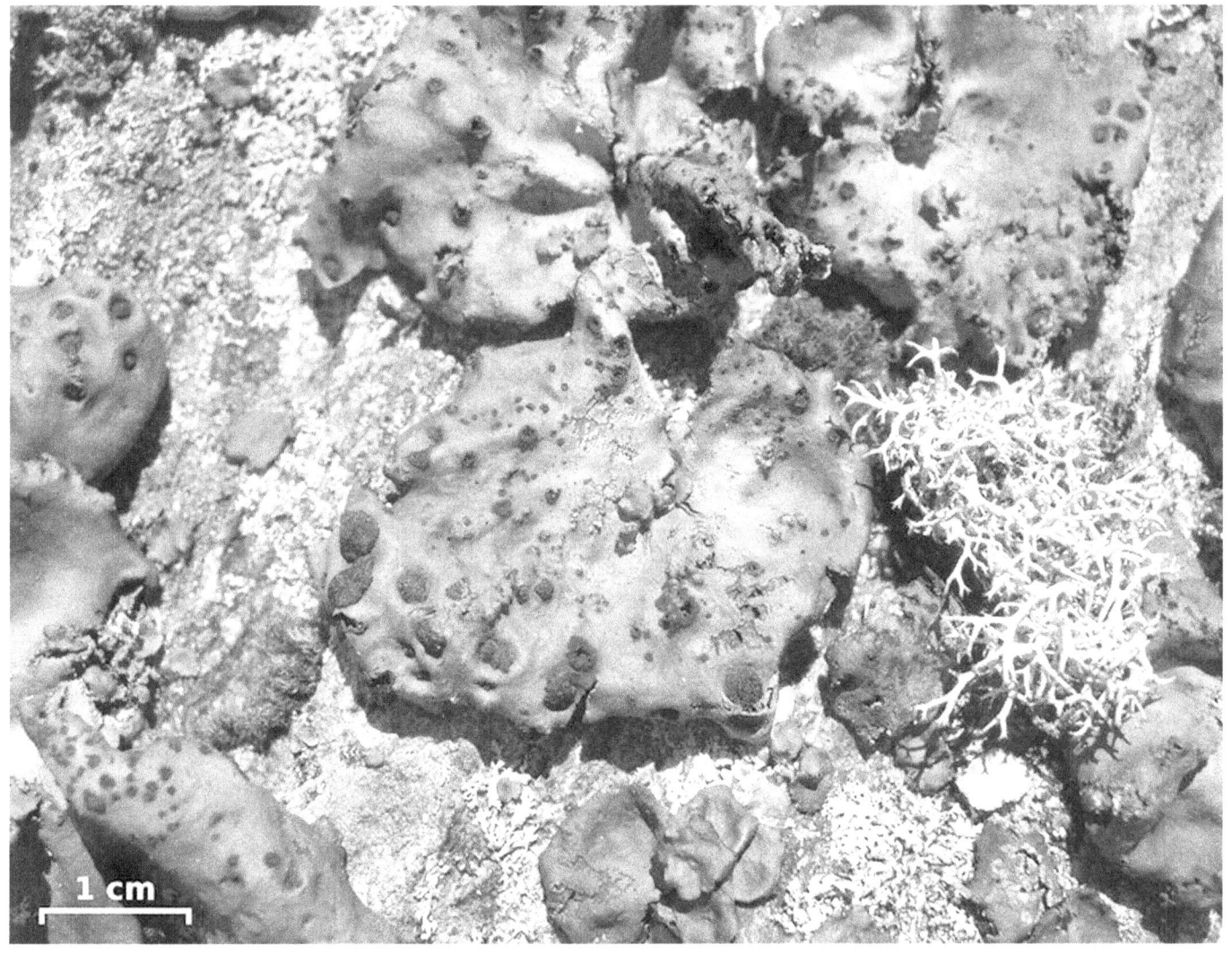

UMBILICARIA MUEHLENBERGII (Courtesy of Jason Hollinger)

In Scotland, rock tripe was used to make **CORKIR**, a brilliant red dye to colour tartans. When treated with urine, it yielded purple.

The Inuit know Rock Tripe as **QUAJAUTIT**, a word associated with slippery underfoot. They absorb blood for cleaning a wound and ripe boils. A spoonful of the boiled lichen is considered good for any illness, but the lichen is not eaten. The tripe was used to absorb oil from the dried skins of baby seals on Baffin Island.

Decoctions can be used as a gargle for soothing canker sores and bleeding gums.

Leather Lichen, or Stippleback Lichen (*D. miniatum*) is found on limestone rock. It is used as a source of ash green dye for wool in some parts of Europe.

The lichens *U. vellea* and *U. americana* have recently been separated into two distinct species. The former was used in Sweden to dye wool a violet color. It contains gyrophoric acid.

The latter lichen is found in a sweeping arc from Lake Winnipeg to Great Slave Lake in the territories.

Work by Swanson and Fahselt found that UV-A increased, and UV-B decreased their content of secondary compounds.

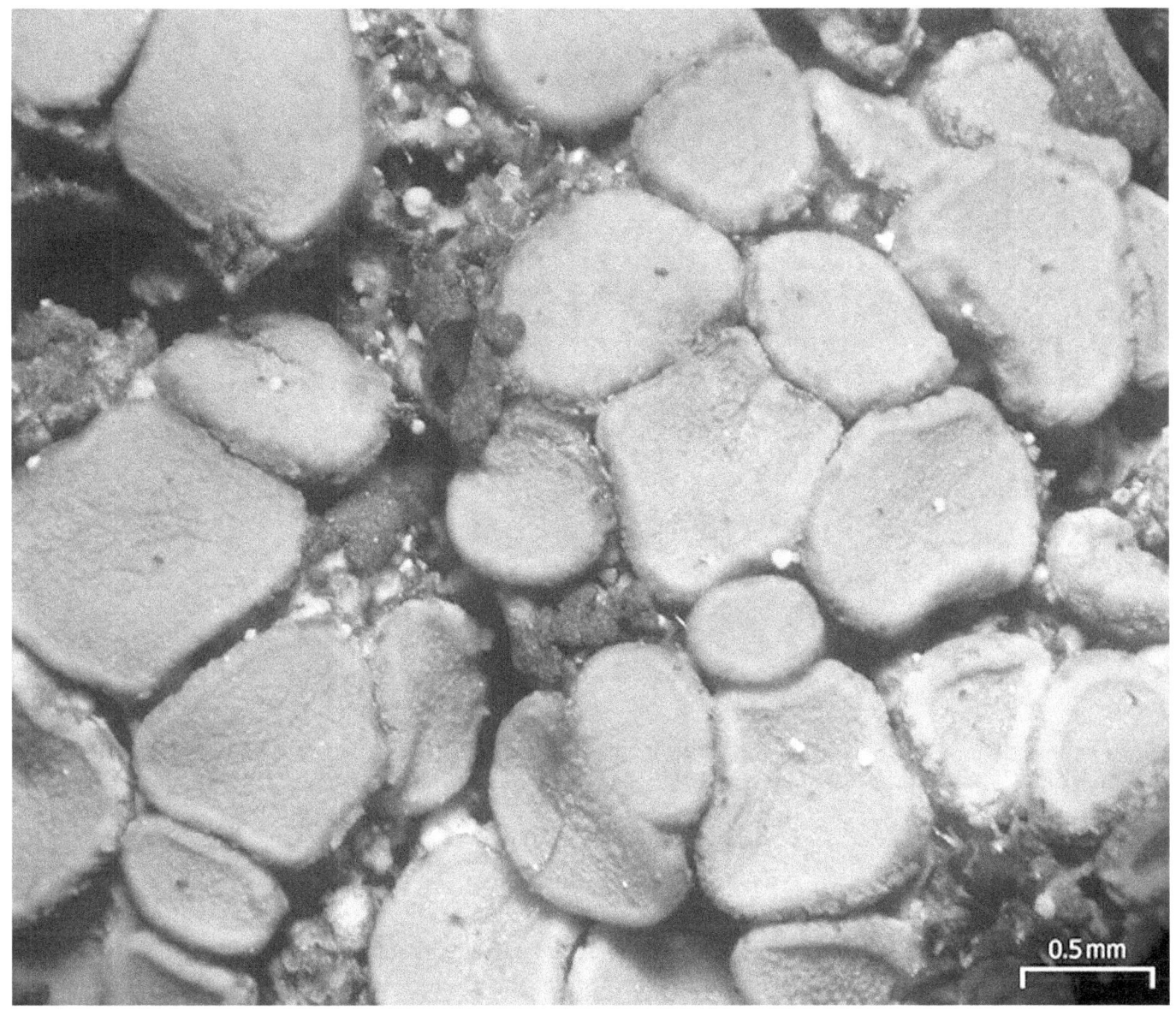

CALOPLACA CERINA (Courtesy of Jason Hollinger)

## FIREDOT LICHENS
## (*Caloplaca spp.*)

Various *Caloplaca* species grow on arctic alpine soil, and others on the bark of aspen poplar trees. They appear as orangey, rusty dots on the bark, or on granite rocks and sidewalks.

A fungus occurring in the genus has been found to produce physcion. This is identical to the monomethyl ester of emodine.

Work by Manojlovic et al, *Pharm Bio* 43:8 on various *Caloplaca* species suggest both anti-microbial and anti-fungal activity. They contain anthraquinones.

Gray Rimmed Firedot Lichen (*C. cerina*) contains parietin, found by same author to possess anti-fungal activity. *Fitoterapia* 2005 76:2.

The related *C. regalis* shows immune modulating effects. Choi HS et al, *Mar Biotechnol* (NY) 2009 11(1): 90-8.

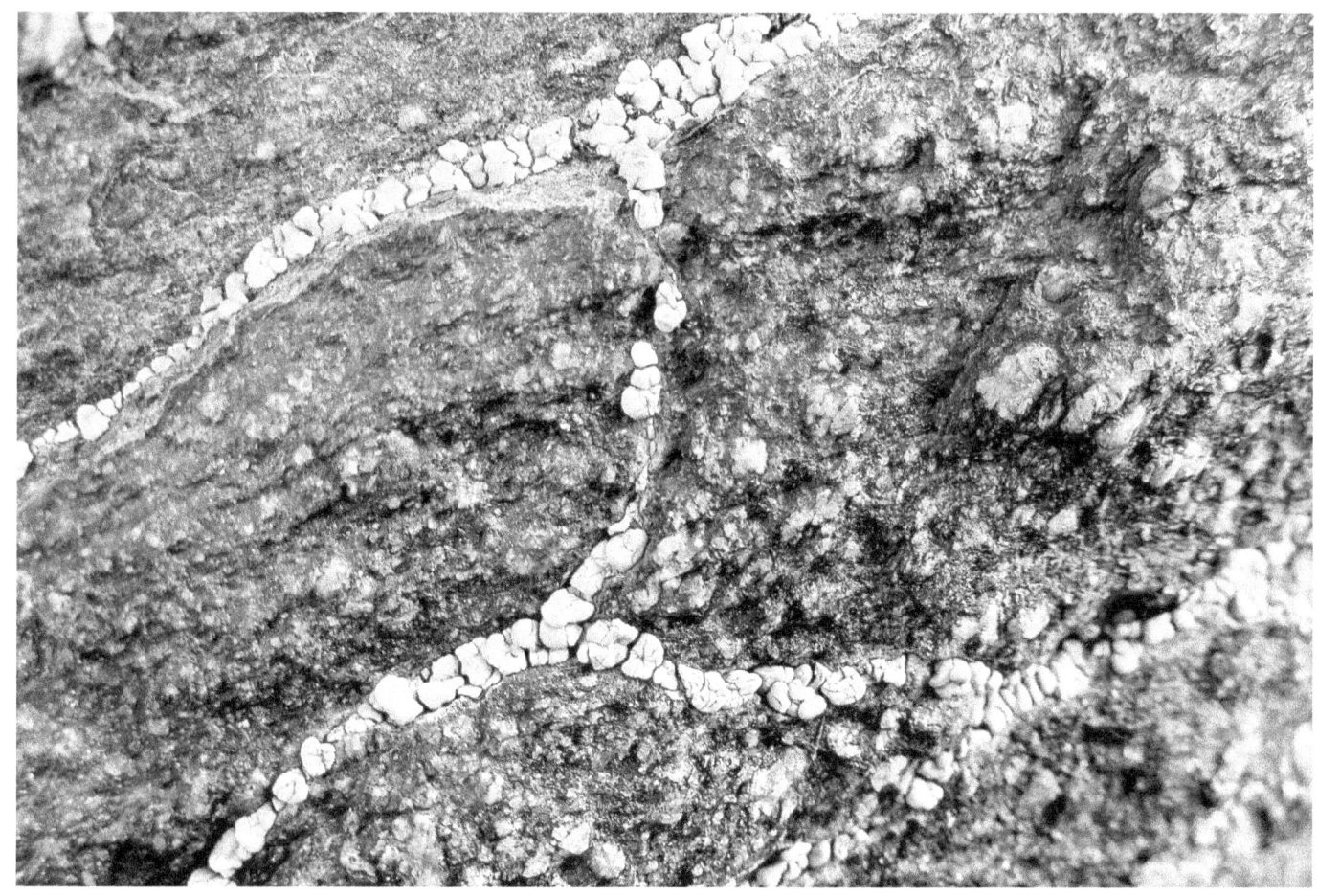

COMMON GOLDSPECK

## LICHEN ESSENCE

Sulphur Firedot Lichen (*C. flavescens*) leaf lichen essence acts as an energy support for the skin. It helps us change or redefine our contact with the outside world. For people who are too "thin-skinned in their relationships.

**KORTE PHI**

**COMMON GOLDSPECK**
(***Candelariella vitellina*** [Hoffm.] Mull. Arg.)

The fungus from this lichen, an egg yolk colored species, with scattered and flattened growth on acid and calcareous rocks, and tree bark, contains stictaurin.

They all contain calycin, a yellow pigment, formerly used in Sweden for dyes.

**ROCK ORANGE LICHEN**
**ELEGANT SUNBURST LICHEN**
(***Xanthoria elegans*** [Link] Th. Fr.)
**TUMBLEWEED SHIELD LICHEN**
(***X. chlorochroa*** [Tuck] Hale)
**MARITIME SUNBURST LICHEN**
**WALL LICHEN**
(***X. parientina*** [L.] Th. Fr.)
(***Teloschistes parientinus***)

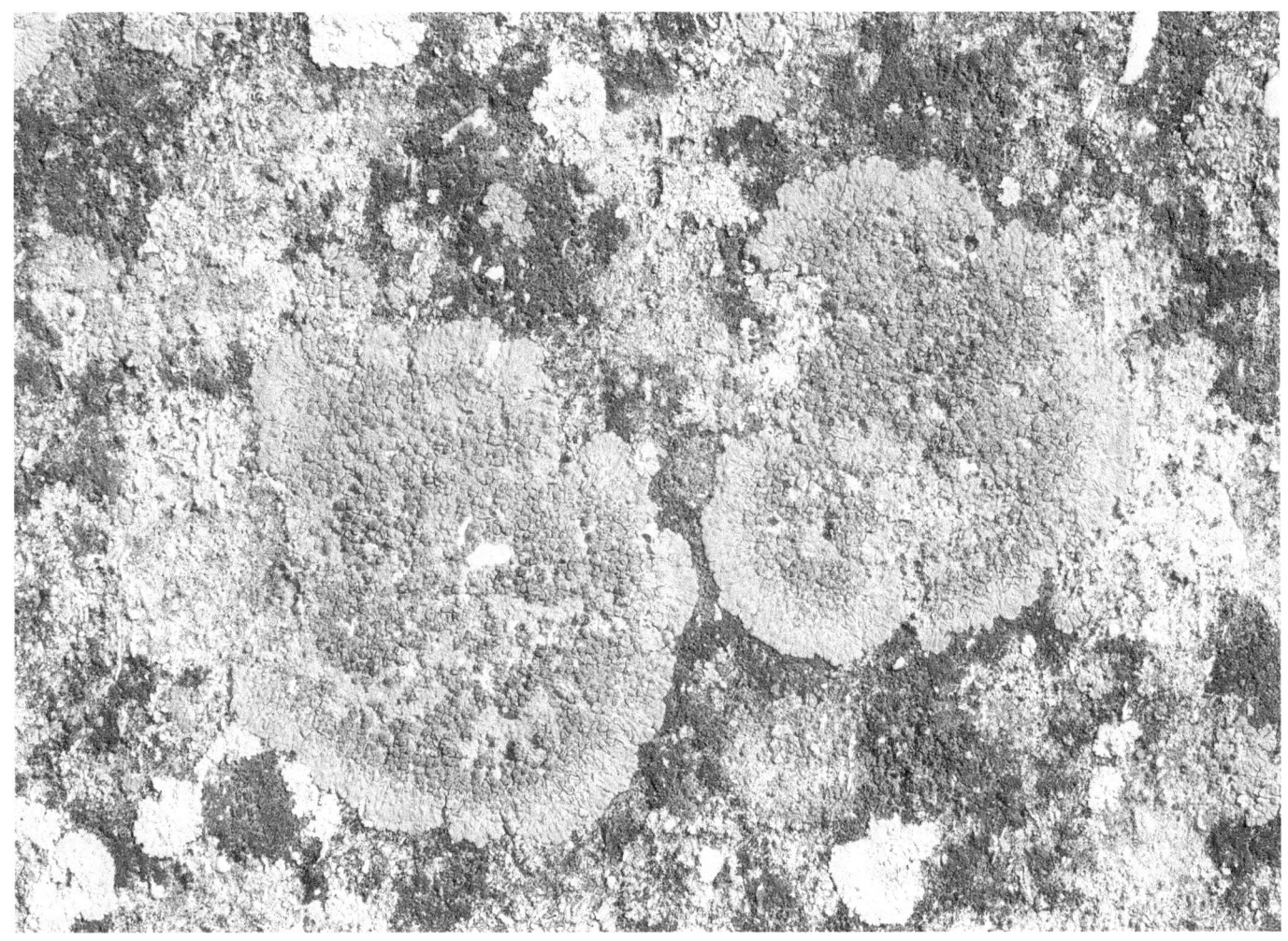

*XANTHORIA PARIETINA*

These rock lichens, are easy to notice, with their flat, fan shape and bright orange colour contrasting against a limestone type rock. Occasionally they may be found on old wood or bones, but they seem to prefer the carbonic environment.

In fact, this lichen is sought by Inuit hunters to locate the burrows of animals such as the hoary marmot. The nitrogen from bird or mammal waste encourages its growth.

Various natives used the pigment for face paint.

The Rock Orange Lichen was found growing on the graves of crewmembers of Franklin's last expedition. The lichens are slow growers, and after more than 100 years only grew 4.4 cm. in diameter. But the lichen is hardy. It has been found on Himalayan mountain rocks at 7000 metres.

The related Wall Lichen (*X. parietina*) was thought, due to its orange colour, of use for jaundice, based on the doctrine of signatures. This is one of many cases, which does not run true. It is sometimes called Maritime Sunburst Lichen. It is bright yellow in sunny regions, and grey in the shade, suggesting a protective mechanism from UV radiation.

The lichen is used as part of hair powder in India. In England, it is known as Gold Moss or Gold Lichen to be more accurate.

Its bright yellow color led to the plant signature of treating jaundice in 15th century Europe, and to its use as a yellow dye for woolens.

Tumbleweed Shield Lichen is prepared as a warm brown dye by Navajo weavers. It contains salazinic and norstictic acid.

The related Hooded Sunburst Lichen (*X. fallax*), commonly found on elm and poplar, contains fallacinal.

Shrubby Sunburst Lichen (*X. candelaria*) is called the Candle Lichen in Sweden and used to color animal fat to make candles. Other shield lichens would work just as well.

Work by Ingolfsdottir et al, *Pharm Bio* 2000 38:4 found Rock Orange Lichen showed significant induction of quinone reductase against hepatoma cells. The concentration to double activity was determined to be only 4.8 µg/ml. This is significant, because many plant constituents with cytotoxic activity are also harmful to healthy cells. Work by Gerhauser et al, *Z Planz und Boden Kunde* 1997 160 found significant induction of QR activity in an assay using cultured Hepa 1c1c7 hepatoma cells.

Xanthoric acid, besides possessing cytoxicity, is anti-convulsive, anti-bacterial and anti-fungal. Activity against *Bacillus subtilis*, *E. coli* and *S. aureus* has been found in work by Karagoz et al, *J Med Plant Res* 2009 3:12. All *Xanthoria* species contain various anthraquinone pigments such as parietin, and xanthroin.

## MEDICINAL

Rock Orange Lichen (*X. elegans*) water extracts may help prevent DNA damage and oxidative stress of mitomycin C in human lymphocytes. Turkez H et al, *Cytotechnology* 2012 64(6): 679-86.

Wall Lichen is decocted in wine in Spain to treat menstrual problems, and simply decocted for kidney disorders, toothache, and as part of a cough syrup. Throughout Spain it is known as Flor de Piedra (stone flower) or Rompiedra (stonebreaker).

It contains bromoperoxidase and significant amounts of beryllium and vanadium as well as parietinic and atranoric acid. Parietin pigment levels are strongly influenced by UVB radiation. It shows activity against *S. aureus*, and is anti-viral. Karagoza et al, *Biologica* 2005 60.

## LICHEN ESSENCE

*Xanthoria parietina* essence facilitates an awakening, bringing wisdom and understanding. It can help to relieve fears, nervousness and confusion. It is for those who walk around in circles. It helps balance the solar plexus, CNS, liver, skin, lungs and nerves. **SILVERCORD**

**FRAGILE SPHAEROPHORUS**
**FRAGILE CORAL LICHEN**
(*Sphaerophorus fragilis* [L.] Pers)
**ALPINE SPHAEROPHORUS**
**CORAL LICHEN**
(*S. globosus var. gracilis* [Huds.] Vain)
(*S. globosus var. globosus*)

Fragile Sphaerophorus is an Arctic species that grows in dense cushions and has very fragile branches. Alpine Sphaerophorus has two variations, one var. *gracilis* that grows on coniferous forest west of the continental divide, and var. *globosus*, a rare type that grows on the ground or in rock crevices.

They both contain hypothamnolic acid, with Coral lichen sometimes containing squamatic acid.

Both lichens exhibit significant inhibition against the estrogen precursor, sulfatase. When tested at 40 ug/ml, the former showed inhibition of 95%, and the latter 90%.

Alpine Sphaerophorus exhibits inhibition against aromatase, another estrogen precursor. While only at 74%, the combined inhibition of both precursors makes this a potentially exciting prospect for the future.

## HOODED BONE
## HOODED TUBE LICHEN
## MONK'S HOOD LICHEN
## PUFFED LICHEN
### (*Hypogymnia physodes* [L.] Nyl.)
### (*Parmelia physodes* [L.] Ach.)
## POWDER HEADED TUBE LICHEN
### (*H. tubulosa* [Schaer] Hav.)

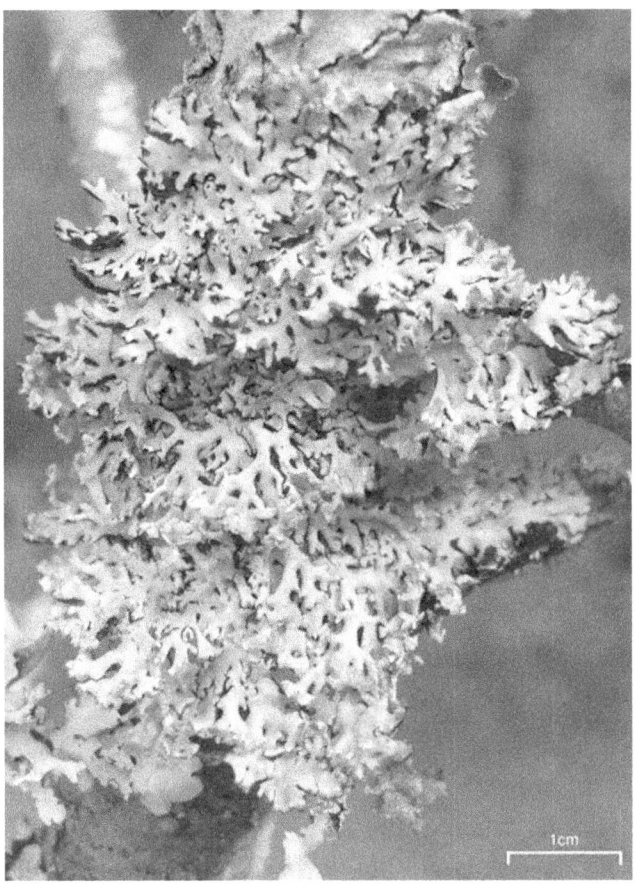

HYPOGYMNIA PHYSODES
(Courtesy of Jason Hollinger)

This pale grey green lichen, Hooded Bone, is commonly found on coniferous and birch trees in the boreal forest. Research shows it is more tolerant of pollution from sulphur dioxide than most macro-lichens, but is still used as an indicator of pollution.

It has been used for both food and medicine. The Potawatomi used it in soup, and as a treatment for constipation. In 15th century Europe, it was combined with *Evernia prunastri*, and *Evernia furfuracea*, in creating the mixture Lichen Quercinus Virides.

In Sweden and Scotland, the lichen is used to yield a brown dye for wool.

Many of the compounds in Hooded Bone lichen are also found in the associated trees.

One study detected physodalic, 3-hydroxyphysodic, physodic acids as well as atranorin in the bark of spruce branches abundantly colonized by lichen. The benefit or harm to the host trees is not fully understood.

## MEDICINAL

**CONSTITUENTS-** *H. physodes-* atranorin, physodic acid, orcinol, as well as beta- orcinol depsidones including protocetraric and physodalic acids, 3-hydroxyphysodic acid, 2'-O-methylphysodic acids, and chloroatranorin; as well as conphysodalic acid, 4-O-methylphysodic acid and alpha-alectoronic acid.
*H. tubulosa-* 3-hydroxyphysodic acid.

Work by Vainshtein et al, reported in the Russian journal, *Mikologiya-i-Fitopatologiya* 1992 26:6 studied the effect of water extracts of the lichen. They found it to inhibit many of the common wood destroying fungi such as *Heterobasidon annosum, Laxitextum bicolor, Schizophyllum commune, Stereum hirsutum,* and *S. rugosum.*

This work could lead to some innovative inoculants or anti-fungal treatments for woodlot management.

Physodic acid, at 6-12 mcg/ml inhibits *Mycobacterium tuberculosis.*

Early work by Burkholder et al, *Bulletin Torrey Botanical Club* 1945 72:2 found the lichen active against *Staphylococcus aureus, S. albus, Bacillus subtilis,* and *Sarcina lutea.*

Hooded Bone lichen extracts and physodic acid are cytotoxic to breast cancer cell lines, MDA-MB-231, MCF-7 and T-47D. Studzinska-Sroka E et al, *Pharm Biol* 2016 54(11): 2480-5.

Powder-Headed Tube Lichen contains 3-hydroxyphysodic acid.

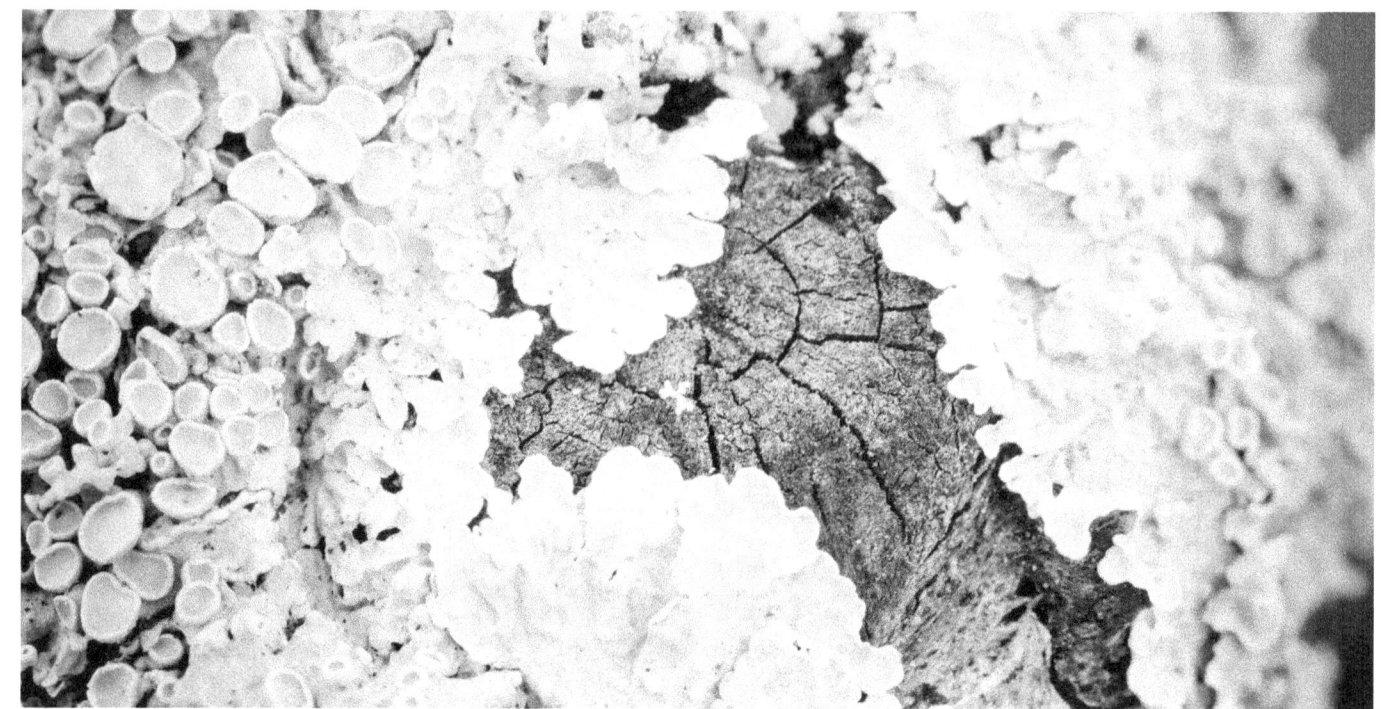

LECANORA MURALIS

Work by Yilam et al, *Zeit Naturforsch* 2005 60:1-2 found this compound active against *Aeromonas hydrophila*, *Bacillus cereus*, *B. subtilis*, *E. coli*, *Klebsiella pneumoniae*, *Listeria monocytogenes*, *Proteus vulgaris*, *Salmonella typhimurium*, *Staphylococcus aureus*, *Streptococcus faecalis*, and *Candida albicans*.

Varnished Tube Lichen (*H. austerodes*) contains oxyphysodic acid, physodic acid, and sometimes 3-hydroxyphysodic acid, in addition to above constituents.

Gyrophoric acid and stenosporic acid from this genus show anti-microbial potential. Candan et al, *Zeit fur Naturforsch* 2006 61:5-6

Hooded Bone appears to be able to bio-remediate arsenic, both by arsenite excretion and methylation of the toxic mineral. Mrak et al, *Environ Pollut* 2007 July 17.

**SMOKY RIM LICHEN**
(***Lecanora cenisia*** Ach.)
**GRANITE SPECK RIM LICHEN**
(***L. polytropa*** [Hoffm.] Rebenh.)
**WHITE RIM LICHEN**
(***L. sordida*** [Pers.] Th. Fr.)
(***L. rupicola*** [L.] Zanblr.)

Smoky Rim Lichen is found commonly throughout North America, and contains atranorin and fatty acids, especially roccellic acid. It sometimes contains gangaleoidin.

The related *L. californica* contains norgangaleoidin and a fatty acid known as nephrosteranic acid.

Granite Speck Rim Lichen (*L. polytropa*) found in the Canadian Shield contains usnic acid, zeorin and fatty acids. It is found worldwide including at the 24,000 feet level on the south side of Makalu.

White Rim Lichen (*Lecanora rupicola*) contains atranoric acid, rocellic acid, and thiophanic acid; as well as sordidone, eugenetin and eugenitol, mycobionts not found in the thallus.

## TRADITIONAL USE

The related *L. esculenta* grows on cliffs of the Middle East, and is believed to be the manna that fed the Hebrew people fleeing from Egypt, as told in the Bible.

Moses told everyone to gather it up because "this is the bread which the Lord hath given you to eat"…tasting "like wafers made with honey". High desert winds sometimes scatter it, even to this day, falling on Bedouin settlements like rain.

It does have a naturally sweet flavour, and edible, hence the species name. Locals call it the "fat of the Earth", and it is sometimes flavored with anise and honey into Panakarpian, a type of bread popular in Alexandria.

Three parts lichen and one part meal are made into a bread called **SCHIRSAD**, and can today be bought in the bazaars of Tehran to encourage breast milk production.

In 1829, during the war between Persia and Russia, a Caspian town was covered with lichen, which literally fell from heaven. This was made into bread and helped stave off starvation.

## MEDICINAL

The related *L. sordida* contains roccellic acid. Work by Barry and McNally in *Nature* 1945 156 found the isolated acid had low activity against *Mycobacterium phlei* and *M. tuberculosis,* but its monoesters and mono amides inhibit growth at very high dilutions. Some of these compounds inhibited *M. phlei, M. smegmatis* and *M. rabinowitz* at 1:20,000 to 1:40,000, and bovine type of *M. tuberculosis* at 1:200,000 to 1:400,000.

Activity against *S. aureus* and *C. diphtheriae* was found.

The related *L. muralis* shows activity against *Bacillus subtilis.* Karagoz et al, *J Med Plant Res* 2009 3:12.

**GREEN LIGHT**
**ARCTIC KIDNEY LICHEN**
(*Nephroma arcticum*)
**POWDERY KIDNEY LICHEN**
(*N. parile*)
**MUSTARD KIDNEY LICHEN**
(*N. laevigatum*)

**CONSTITUENTS-** *N. arcticum-* emodin, 7-chloro-emodin, 1-O-methyl-emodin, 7,7' dichlorohypericin, 2, 2', 7, 7'-tetrachlorohypericin, usnic acids, phenarctin. *N. laevigatum-* various anthroquinones, nephromin, nephrin, usnic acid, fatty acids, hydroxyglutamicol (mycosporine).

Green light lichen is found in the extreme north following the Canadian Shield, and on the extreme tops of the Rocky Mountains. The Yup'ik of Alaska call it **KUSSKOAK**. The lichen is collected and stored until winter and then boiled with fish eggs. A hot water infusion was given to people with weakened constitutions.

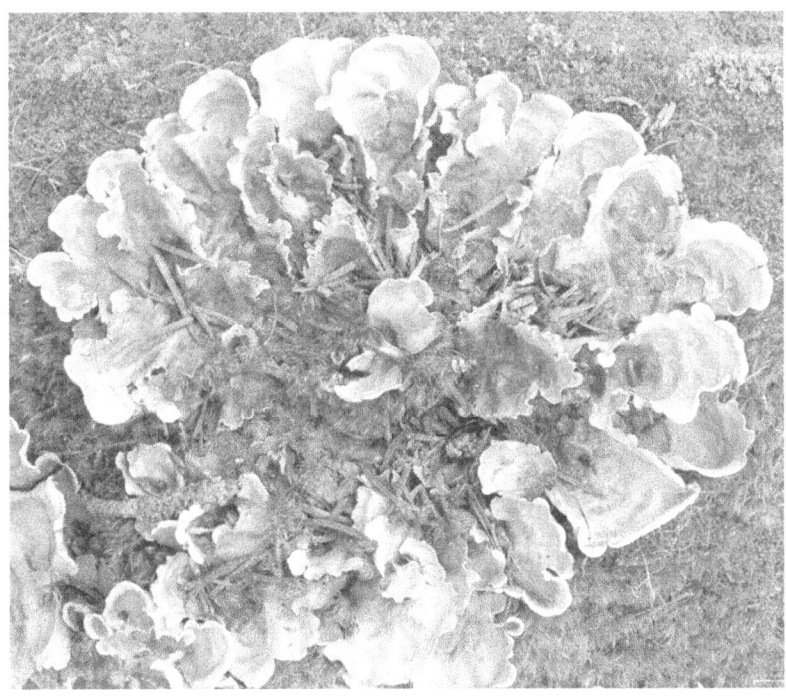

NEPHROMA ARCTICUM
(Courtesy of Jason Hollinger)

It contains emodin and 7-choro-emodin, compounds which possess activity against herpes simplex virus at low concentrations.

Peter Cohen wrote his PhD thesis at UBC in 1995 on this lichen and *Hetereodermia obscurata*. He identified hypericin compounds in both that possess anti-viral activity. It also contains usnic acid, zeorin and phenarctin.

The lichen contains eight mycotoxins, with mycophenolic acid in high quantities, compared to other lichens. Burkin AA & GP Kononenko, *Izv Akad Nauk Ser Biol* 2015 6: 573-80.

Powdery Kidney Lichen is found in the sub-alpine regions and mountains.

Natives of Alaska cooked also cooked this lichen with crushed fish eggs, or alone as an infused tonic after a lengthy illness. The lichen was picked in summer and then stored until needed.

Powdery Kidney Lichen has been used in Scotland as a blue dye for wool. It may contain zeorin. It shows mild activity against *Staphylococcus aureus*. Work by Rankovic et al, *Central Eur J Biology* 2010 April 1 found it weak against various bacteria and fungi tested.

Mustard Kidney Lichen (*N. laevigatum*), found on the west coast, contains usnic acid and nephrin.

**STIPPLEBACK LICHEN**
(***Dermatocarpon moulinsii***)
**LEATHER LICHEN**
(***D. miniatum***)

This fairly common lichen is found on gravel. When wet, the upper part turns green, and becomes translucent. It can be soaked in water and then chewed slowly as a food source. When boiled for about 15 minutes with a little salt, it has a flavour reminiscent of mushroom. It is a good addition to help thicken and flavour rock soup.

Leather Lichen has been used as an ash-green dye for wool in Europe.

Crude extracts inhibit the growth of *Staphylococcus aureus*. *Dermatocarpon miniatum* contains a powerful anti-oxidant identified in work by Aslan et al, *Pharm Bio* 43:8.

**TUMBLEWEED SHIELD LICHEN**
(***Xanthoparmelia chlorochroa*** Tuck.)
**PEPPERED ROCK SHIELD LICHEN**
(***X. conspersa***)

**CONSTITUENTS**- *X. chlorochroa*- usnic, salazinic, constictic and norstictic acids.

Tumbleweed Shield Lichen is common to the Great Western Basin and down through the mid west. The common name is due to its detaching from rock and tumbling around with the wind.

It is an indicator of good antelope grazing territory. Up to 126 kg/ha communities have been found in parts of Montana. The lichen is toxic to domestic sheep, cattle and elk, resulting in red urine, ataxia and muscle weakness.

The entire plant, called Ground Lichen by the Navajo, was boiled for a red, brown, or orange dye for leather, baskets and wool.

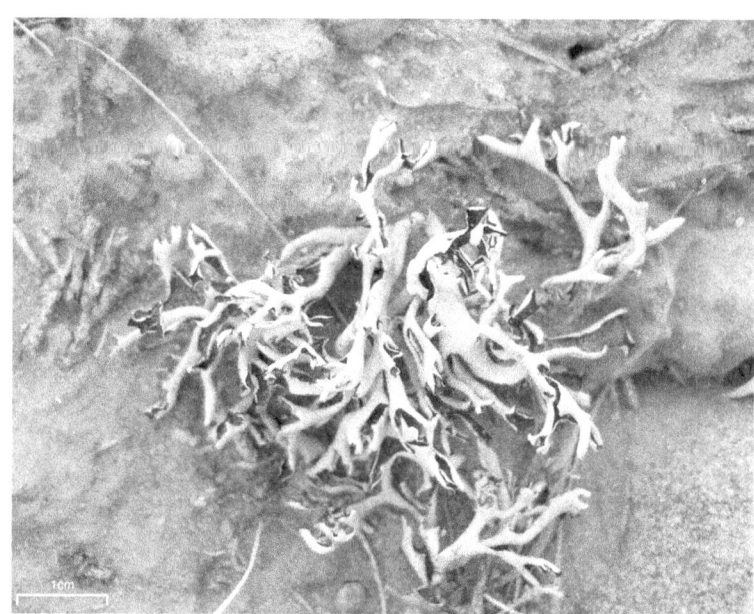

XANTHOPARMELIA CHLOROCHROA
(Courtesy of Jason Hollinger)

They used it medicinally to treat impetigo, possibly due to its content of salazinic and norstitic acid. It contains 2% usnic acid, compared to 1.5% in *Usnea barbata*.

Norstictic acid inhibits triple-negative breast cancers, due to C-Met inhibition. Ebrahim HY et al, *Phytotherapy Research* 2016 30(4): 557-66.

The lichen extracts are cytotoxic to Burkitt's lymphoma (Raji) cells, due to upregulation of p53, decreased proliferation, and apoptosis. Shrestha G et al, *Phytotherapy Research* 2015 29(1): 100-7.

Peppered Rock Shield Lichen is present in eastern and western North America.

It has been used in England for dye, producing a red-brown colour for wool.

The lichen is used in southeastern Africa for medicine, both internally and applied as a powder to treat snakebites and venereal disease, especially syphilis.

It contains a sticitic acid complex including cryptostictic acid, and variable amounts of norstitic acid. A crude extract inhibits *Bacillus subtilis*.

Work by Stoll et al, *Experientia* 1947 3 showed weak activity against *S. aureus*.

The related *X. taractica* is common throughout the boreal forest, on exposed rock associated with gravel and slides. The lichen is a hyper-accumulator of zinc, and may be a prospecting tool for mining companies.

The related *X. scabrosa* has been found to induce smooth muscle relaxation, that promotes arterial dilation and increased blood flow. It is a main ingredient in a novel sexual stamina formula, a sort of natural Viagra approach to arousal.

Various species of this genus may contain phosphodiesterase type 5 inhibitors. Not only is blood flow to genital area increased, in both men and women, but it may also be helpful in pulmonary hypertension.

The related *X. pokornyi* contain vulpinic and gyrophoric acids, that photo-protect human skin cells from UVB. Varol M et al, *Phytother Research* 2016 30(1): 9-15.

Salazinic, usnic and stictic acid from Xanthoparmelia species exhibit protection of U373 MG human astrocytome cell lines, suggesting anti-oxidative effect for neurodegenerative disorders such as Alzheimer's disease and Parkinson's disease. dePaz GA et al, *J Pharm Biomed Anal* 2010 53(2): 165-71.

Acetone and ethyl acetate extracts of *Xanthoparmelia mexicana* inhibit gram positive bacteria. Yeash EA et al, *J Sci Food Agric* 2017 April 2.

## CURLED SNOW LICHEN
### (*Flavocetraria cucullata*)
## CRINKLED SNOW LICHEN
### (*F. nivalis*)

**CONSTITUENTS-** *F. cucullata*- usnic acid, salazinic acid, squamatic acid, baeomycesic acid, d-protolichesterinic acid and lichesterinic acid.
*F. nivalis*- thallus- 4-8% usnic acid (highest in late autumn), divaricatic acid.

Other interesting lichens include the Snow Lichens, such as Curled (*Flavocetraria cucullata*) and Crinkled (*F. nivalis*).

The former, previously classified as *Cetraria cucullata*, has been used in northern Canada as a condiment for fish or duck soup. The Yup'ik call it **NINGUUJUG** meaning, "would like to be stretched", perhaps in reference to its filling nature on the stomach.

Curled Snow Lichen has been used as a food, and was used by Russia during the Second World War to produce glucose molasses, yielding 71% by dry weight.

It produces a violet dye with addition of ammonia. It contains usnic and protolichesterinic acids.

Lichen extracts were the most potent cytotoxic against several cancer cells lines, of seventeen species tested by Nguyen TT et al. It was more potent than usnic acid alone, reducing levels of epithelial-mesenchymal transition markers and inducing apoptosis. *PLoS One* 2014 9(10). Normal cells were unharmed at lower doses, but still decreased cancer cell motility, and inhibited both *in vitro* and *in vivo* tumorigenic potential.

Crinkled Snow lichen is widespread at elevated mountain zones.

Near the Peru/Bolivia border, Crinkled Snow lichen is known as Beard of the Rock. The lichen is infused in hot water as a cardio-pulmonary tonic for heart attack and altitude sickness. It is weakly active against *Staphylococcus aureus*. According to the *Pharmacopoeia Universalis* of 1846, the medicinal uses are similar to Iceland Moss.

Its content of (+)-usnic acid has been studied and found to inhibit non-small cell lung cancer cell motility. When combined with cetuximab, the inhibition was even higher, suggesting (+)-usnic acid has potential for inhibition of metastasis. Yang Y et al, *PLoS One* 2016 11(1).

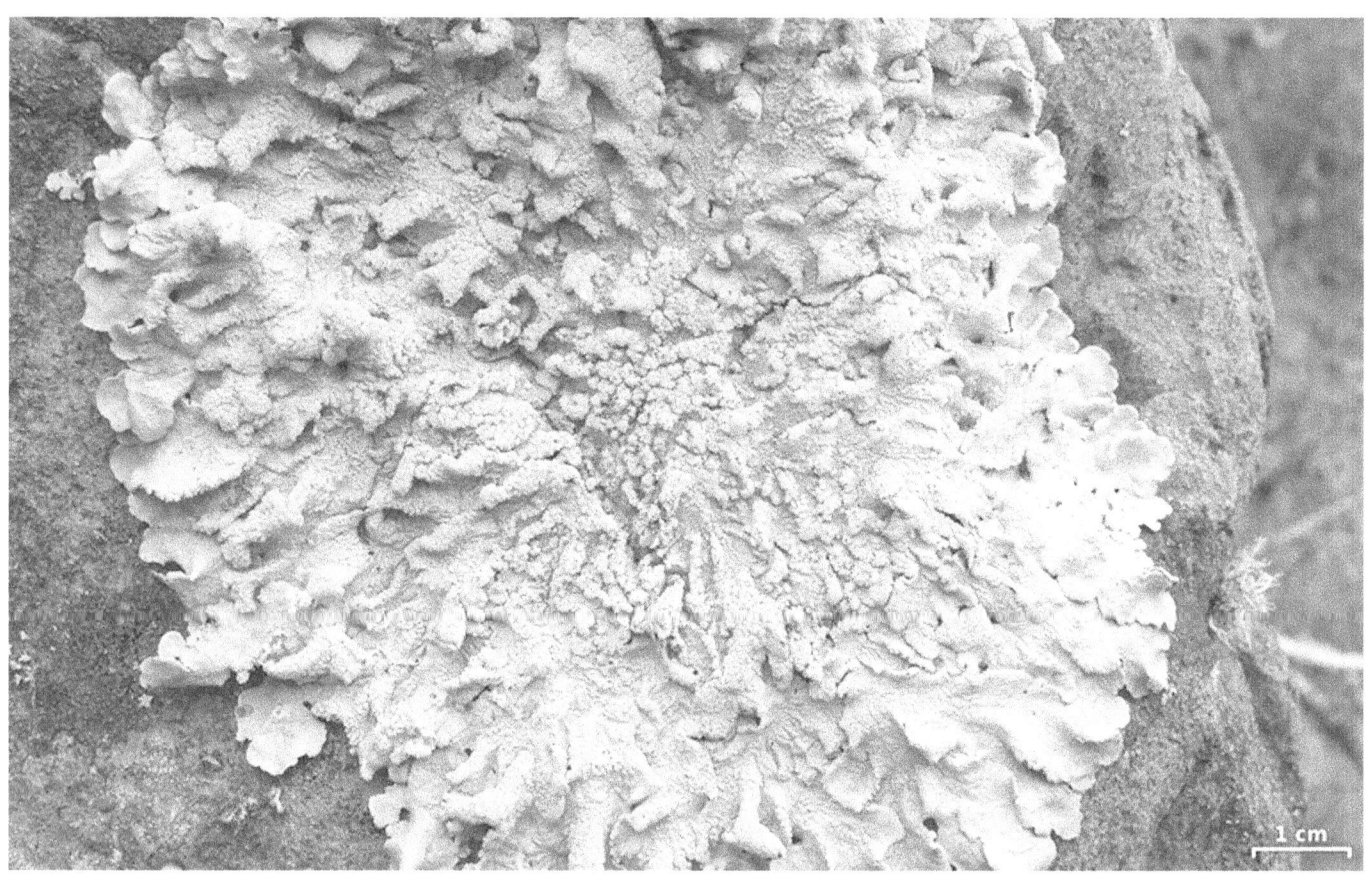

FLAVOPARMELIA CAPERATA (Courtesy of Jason Hollinger)

**COMMON GREEN SHIELD LICHEN**
(***Flavoparmelia caperata*** [L.] Hale)
**ROCK GREEN SHIELD LICHEN**
(***F. baltimorensis*** [Gyelnik & Fóriss] Hale)
(***Pseudoparmelia baltimorensis***)

Common Green Shield Lichen (*Flavoparmelia caperata*) is throughout northeastern Canada and United States, as well as the southwest.

It has been used as an orange-brown to yellow dye on the Isle of Man, and a dried powder was applied to burns by the Tarahumara of Mexico.

It contains usnic, protocetraric and caperatic acids as well as atranorin.

Ethanol extracts were found activity against the virulent strain of *M. tuberculosis* H$_{37}$Rv. Gupta et al, *Pharm Bio* 2007 45:3.

Early work by Burkholder et al, *Proced Nat Acad Sci USA* 1944 30:9 found activity against *Staphylococcus aureus, Diplococcus pneumoniae, Streptococcus hemolyticus, S. viridans, Bacillus subtilis, B. mycoides* and *Sarcina lutea.*

Lichen extracts induce apoptosis in HCT-116 (colon) cancer cell lines. Mitrovic T et al, *Int J Mol Sci* 2011 12(8): 5428-48.

Rock Green Shield Lichen is common in eastern North America, usually found on sun-exposed rocks.

An alpha(1-3)glucan containing fraction appears to influence the dentate gyrus (part of hippocampus), associated with a high rate of neurogenesis and influence on formation of new memories, and the modulation of stress and depression. Edagawa Y et al, *Neurosci Research* 2005 53(4): 363-8.

Powder-edged Speckled Greenshield (*Flavopunctelia soredica*) is found on bark in open woods. It contains usnic and lecanoric acid.

The Navaho of New Mexico use it to produce a flesh colored dye.

Green Starburst Lichen (*Parmeliopsis ambigua*) is widespread, and contains divaricatic acid.

## DOTTED RAMALINA
## (*Ramalina farinacea*)

There are a number of interesting *Ramalina* species. Worldwide there are approximately 250 species, and about 118 with published papers on any activity.

Only 13 species have been studied to any degree, and only 18% of the 153 identified compounds have undergone clinical study.

Dotted Ramalina, or The Dotted Line (*R. farinacea*) has been used traditionally as a light brown dye for wool, and has a history of use in cosmetics and perfumes throughout Europe.

The lichen contains ramalinolic acid, sekikaic acid, arabitol, mannitol, and d-usnic acid.

Work by Tay et al, *Z Naturforsch* 59 found (+)-usnic acid from this lichen active against *Bacillus subtilis, Listeria monocytogenes, Proteus vulgaris, Staphylococcus aureus, Streptococcus faecalis, Yersinia enterocolitica, Candida albicans* and *C. glabrata.*

Work by Karagoz et al, *J Med Plant Res* 2009 3:12 found methanol lichen extracts active against *B. subtilis, S. aureus, S. epidermidis* and *E. coli.*

In fact, fractions from this lichen were more active against *S. aureus* isolates than tetracycline or ampicillin. Esimone CO et al, *Phytotherapy Res* 2002 16(5): 494-6.

Norstictic acid showed activity against all the above except *Y. enterocolitica* as well as *Aeromonas hydriphila*, and protocetraric acid showed activity against the yeasts.

Ethyl acetate fractions have shown the ability to inhibit lentiviral and adenoviral as well as HIV-1. Esimone CO et al, *Chemotherapy* 2009 55(2): 119-26.

Work by Esimone CO et al, *Int J Exp Clin Chemotherapy* 2009 55:2 tested fractions of dotted ramalina against herpes simplex virus type 1, and the respiratory syncytial virus. Both were potently inhibited (IC$_{50}$ + 6.09 and 3.65 mcg/ml, respectively). It also inhibited HIV-1 reverse transcriptase with an IC$_{50}$ of only 0.022 mcg/ml.

Sekikaic acid shows potent inhibition against respiratory syncytial virus, and interferes with viral replication at the post-entry step. In fact, it is over 1.3 fold more active than ribavirin at four-hour post-infection stage. Lai D et al, *Plant Medica* 2013 79(15): 1440-6.

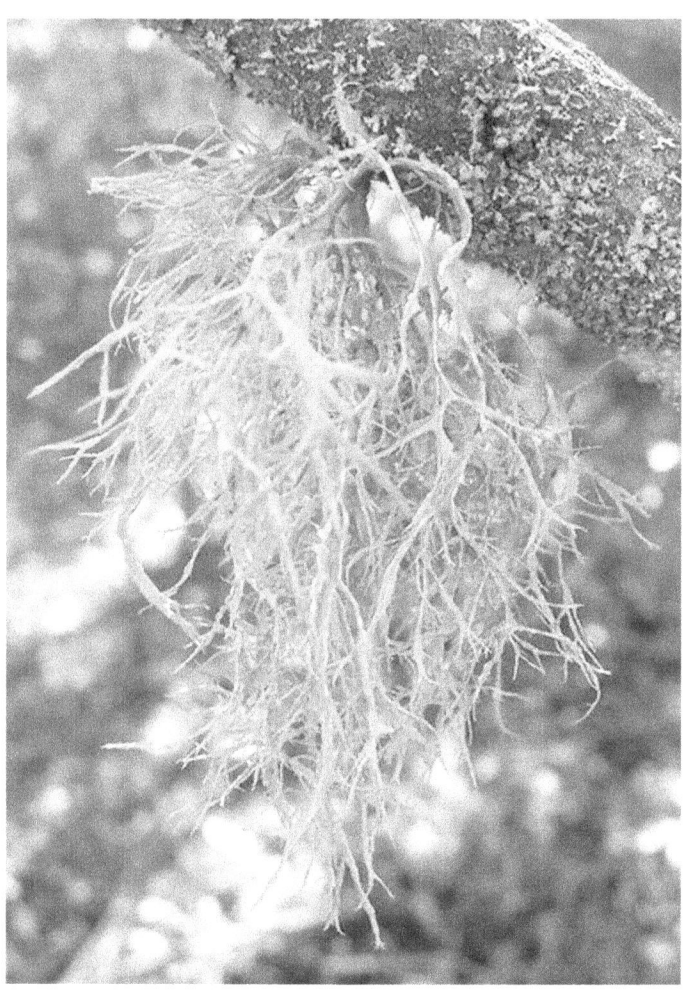

RAMALINA FARINACEA
(Courtesy of Jason Hollinger)

Rock Ramalina (*R. intermedia*) which resembles the Dotted species in some respects, contains sekikaic acid.

Palmetto Lichen (*R. celastri*) is confined to southern Texas. It contains parietin that shows anti-viral activity against arenaviruses Junin and Tacaribe. Fazio AT et al, *Zeit fur Naturforsch C* 2007 62:7-8. The former is associated with hemorrhagic fever.

An alpha glucan from this species is cytotoxic against HeLa cancer cell lines, suggesting biological response modification. Stuelp-Campelo PM et al, *Int Immunopharmacol* 2002 2(5): 691-8.

The related *R. bourgeana* is used in Europe to dissolve kidney stones.

The Manchurian drug **SHIH HUA**, which translates as stone-flower, and known to the Japanese as **SEKI KA** consists of a mixture of Ramalina species.

Dusty, or Chalky, Ramalina (*R. pollinaria*) is common. It has a long history of use in the preparation of cosmetics and perfumes. It contains usnic, obtusatic, evernic, and sekikaic acid.

Infections caused by *Pseudomonas aeruginosa* are common in cystic fibrosis. Evernic acid, found in various lichens, including Ramalina and Usnea species, inhibits the quorum sensing systems of the bacteria, leaving it vulnerable to adjunct therapies. Gokalsin B & Sesal NC, *World J Microbiol Biotechnol* 2016 32(9): 150.

Polysaccharides derived from this lichen are 1,3 and 1,4 linked beta D glucans. Sulphated derivatives of these glucans show cytotoxicity against HeLa cell lines, and induced cell death via apoptosis. Leão AM et al, *J Submicrosc Cytol Pathol* 1997 29(4): 503-9.

Ramalin, isolated from *R. terebrata*, mitigates Th2 immune response and production of inflammation in mast cells and keratinocytes, suggesting benefit in atopic dermatitis. Park HJ et al, *Phytother Res* 2016 30(12): 1978-87. Ramalin induces apoptosis in breast cancer cell lines, MCF-7 and MDA-MB-231. Lee E et al, *Phytother Res* 2016 30(3): 426-38.

It may also have therapeutic benefit in modulating inflammation within atherosclerosis. Park B et al, *Biosci Biotechnol Biochem* 2015 79(4): 539-52.

Stereocalpin A appears to exert a protective effect by modulating inflammation with the atherosclerotic lesion. Byeon HE et al, *Int Immunopharmacol* 2012 12(2): 315-25. A patent was given for this compound in Korea. KR 20,130,043,995.

*Ramalina fraxinea* and *R. fastigiata* have been studied for constituents, that include usnic acid, protocetraric acid, evernic acid, obtusatic aicd, sekikaic acid and atranorin. Significant activity was noted against HeLa, A549 (lung) and LS174 (colon) cancer cell lines. Ristic S et al, *Curr Pharm Biotechnol* 2016 17(7): 651-8.

Frayed Ramalina (*R. roesleri*) is found in widely isolated parts of North America. It contains atranorin, protolichesterinic acid, usnic acid, 2-hydroxy-4-methoxy-6-propyl benzoic acid, homosekikaic acid, sekikaic acid, benzoic acid.

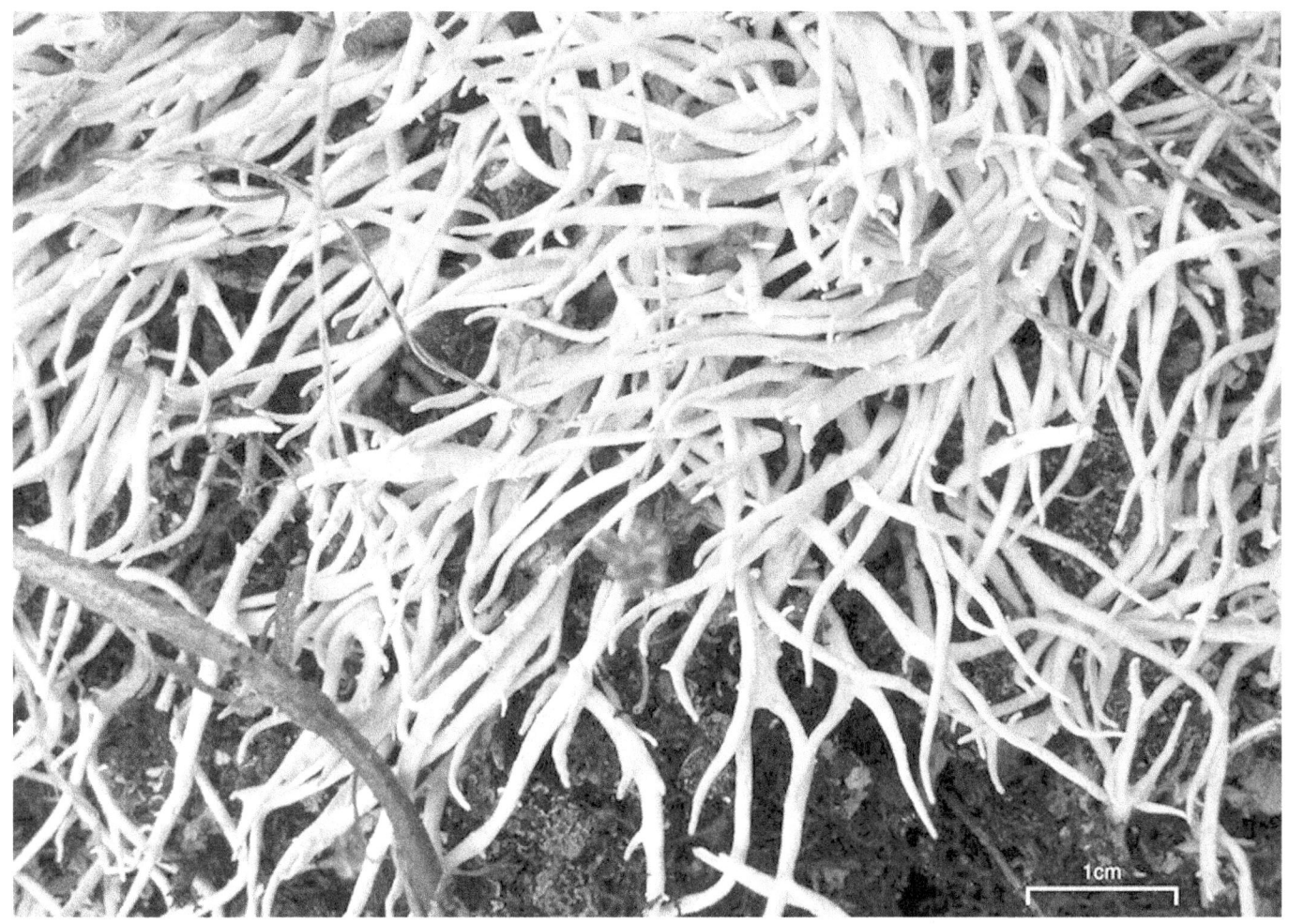

WHITEWORM LICHEN (Courtesy of Jason Hollinger)

Extracts show high activity against *Staplylococcus aureus* and *Streptococcus mutans*. Sisodia R et al, *Nat Prod Res* 2013 27(23): 2235-9.

Lace Lichen (*R. menziesii*) contains usnic acid, identified as active against *Mycobacterium tuberculosis* in 1883. Zopf W. *Liebigs Ann* 1905 340:276-309.

A great review of the chemistry and activity of Ramalina species has been written by Moreira AS et al, *Molecules* 2015 20(5): 8952-87.

*Lobothallia alphoplaca* lichen, also known as *Aspicilia alphoplaca*, is found from southern Canadian prairies, and down through the mid-West to Arizona and New Mexico. It prefers granite and sandstone rocks.

Acetone extracts inhibit the growth of breast cancer MCF-7 cancer cells lines, at the G2 phase. Yeash EA et al, *J Sci Food Agric* 2017 April 2.

**WHITEWORM LICHEN**
(*Thamnolia vermicularis*)

**CONSTITUENTS-** baeomycesic acid, hypthamnolic acid, 3'-methylevenic acid, squamatic acid, methyl 3'methyl lecanorate, barbatinic acid, atranorin, beta-orcinol-type depsides, thamolan, beta glucans, evernic acid, beta-resorcylic acid, ethyl orsellinate, vermicularin, heteroglycans.

Whiteworm Lichen (*Thamnolia vermicularis var. subuliformis*) is frequently found on tundra and arctic alpine areas. Birds like the Golden Plover use the lichen for nesting material. It is used in Nepal for its antiseptic properties, and in China as a medicated tea. Wang et al, *The Lichenologist* 2001 104:3.

It contains baeomycesic acid, a beta-orcinol depside, which shows weak inhibition of platelet type 12 (S) lipoxygenase. Ingolfsdottir et al, *Phytomed* 1997 4. The activity was comparable to the flavone baicalein. Bucar F et al, *Phytomedicine* 2004 11(7-8):602-6.

There are two distinct strains, one containing thamnolic acid and another with squamatic and baeomycesic acid, the former found more coastal, and the latter in the Rocky Mountains. The lichen is strongly anti-oxidant, albeit not as strong as BHA nor quercitin.

Work by Omarsdottir S et al, *J Phytomed* 13:9-10 and *Phytomedicine* 2007 14(2-3): 179-84 identified thamnolan as an immunomodulating polysaccharide.

Earlier work identified a lentinan-type 1,3 beta-D-glucan, also found in shiitake mushrooms. It proved to be strongly active in anti-complement testing. Olafsdottir ES et al, *Phytomedicine* 2003 10(4): 318-24.

Various lichen polysaccharides show immune modeling effects on dendritic cells, including thamnolan and related heteroglycans. Omarsdottir S et al, *Int Immunopharmacol* 2006 6(11): 1642-50.

Stoll et al, *Experientia* 1947 3 found strong activity against *S. aureus*. Early work by Ingolfsdottir et al, *Antimicrobial Agents and Chemotherapy* 1985 28:2 found petroleum extracts active against *S. aureus, B. subtilis, E. coli* and *Candida albicans*.

Thamnolia depside A have been found to inhibit prostate cancer cell production. Guo J et al, *Planta Medica* 2011 77:18 2042-6.

An ethanol extract has been found to improve learning in APP/PSI mice and markedly reduce the number of senile plaques in the hippocampus and cortex. This suggests possible benefit in the treatment of Alzheimer's disease. Li C et al, *Acta Pharmacol Sin* 2017 38(1): 9-28.

Blue Grey Rosette Lichen, or Powderback Lichen (*Physcia caesia*) contains atranoric acid, haematommic acid, and zeorin. Star Rosette Lichen (*P. stellaris*) contains atranorin.

As mentioned above, Physcia species were previously combined with pine resins to produce a yellow staining paint.

The distinct shiny bluish grey appearance of this genus is due to a thin layer of calcium oxalate crystals that deflect light and help lichens survive extreme conditions.

Physica species have been found to inhibit *Staphylococcus aureus* and *Bacillus subtilis*.

Gold Eye Lichen (*Teloschistes chrysophthalmus*) contains usnic acid that shows activity against the arenaviruses Junin and Tacaribe. Fazio et al, *Zeit fur Naturforschung* 2007 62:7-8.

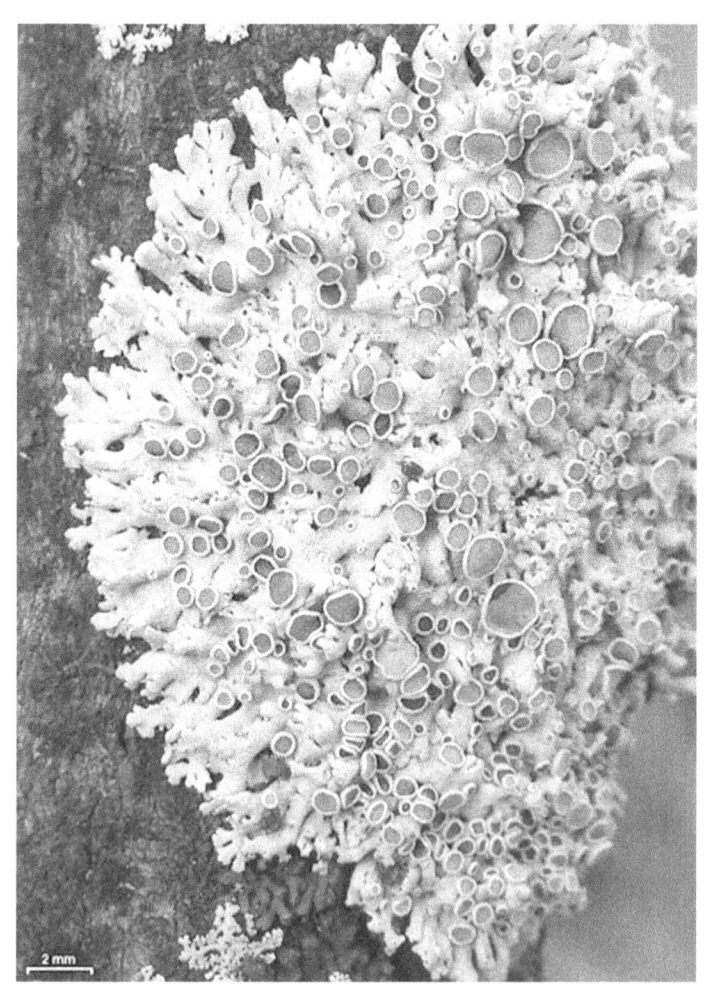

PHYSCIA STELLARIS
(Courtesy of Jason Hollinger)

Powdered Orange Bush Lichen (*T. flavicans*) contains parietin, an efficient photo-screening pigment with promising application in anti-bacterial therapy. Comini LR et al, *Photochem Photobiol Sci* 2017 16(2): 201-10.

The lichen and parietin extracts possess anti-edema and anti-inflammatory activity, but were not effective on sub-chronic inflammation. Pereira EC et al, *Pharmacognosy Research* 2010 2(4): 205-10.

This lichen is increasingly rare on east coast, but still found occasionally on Pacific Ocean trees. It contains pullulans, also found in the fungi Yellow Witch's butter (*Tremella mesenterica*).

Powdered Loop Lichen (*Hypotrachyna revolta*) is a gray-green species found on trees, rocks and ground. It is not widely found. It contains hypotrachynic, deoxystictic, 8'-methylconstictic, 8'-methylstictic, 8'-methylmenegazziaic, stictic, 8'-ethylstictic and gyrophoric acids, as well as atronorin, and cryptostichinolide.

Bitter Wart Lichen (*Pertusaria amara*) is found on the west coast and eastern seaboard of North America. It contains arabitol, mannitol, and emulsin, as well as picrolichenic acid.

It is extremely bitter, as the name suggests, is the basis for its medicinal use in treating high fever. The decocted medicine was said to be a quinine replacement.

The related *P. communis* (*P. pertusa*) was said more useful for men than women. The genus contains a variety of depsides, depsidones and xanthones.

Eight lichens, including Varied Rag Lichen or *Platismatia glauca,* found on lodgepole pine and white spruce, were studied for cytotoxic activity. Bezivin et al, *Phytomedicine* 2003 10:6-7. All demonstrated activity on human cancer cell lines.

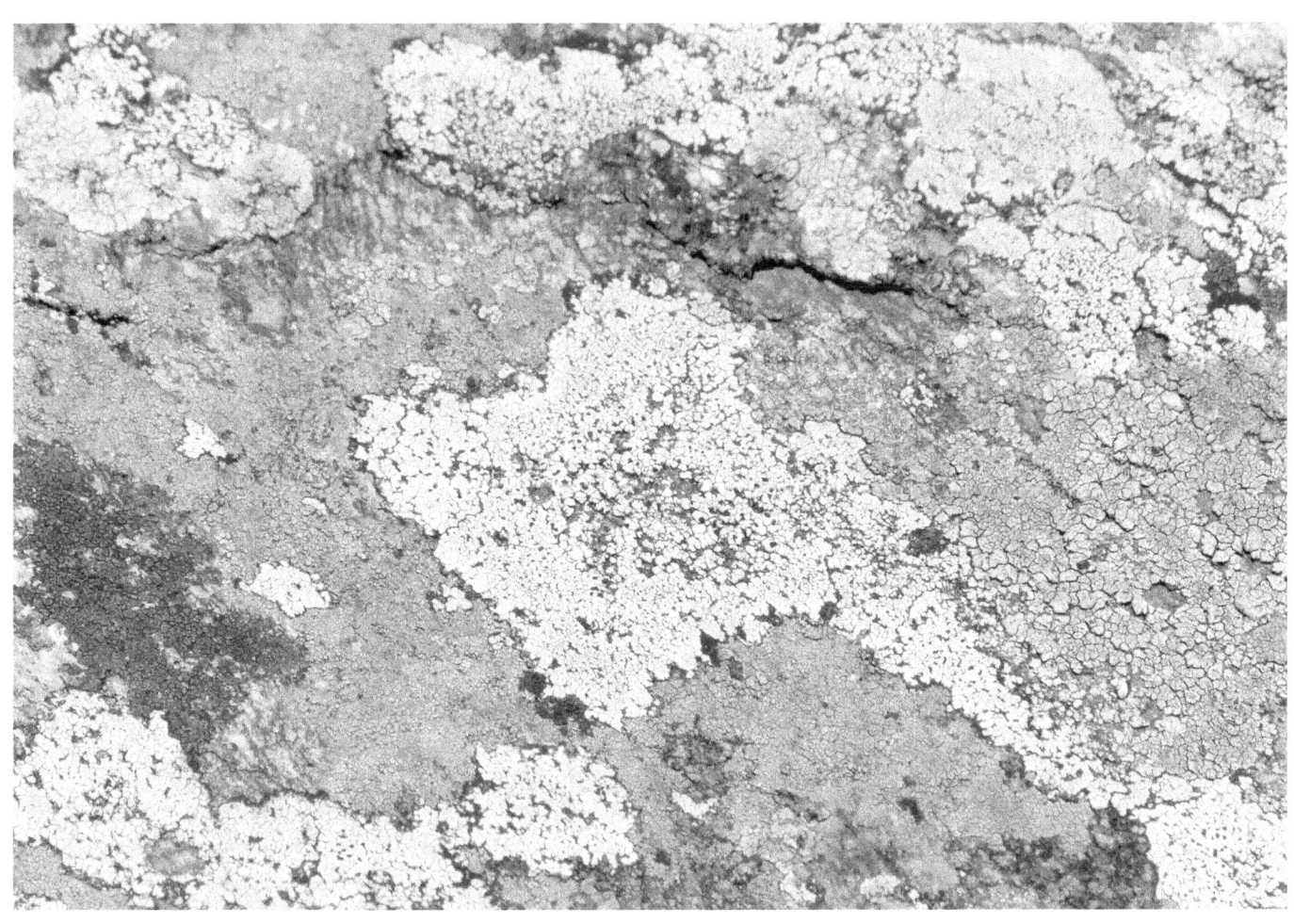

RHIZOCARPON GEOGRAPHICUM

*Platismatia glauca* contains proto-lichesterinic acid, caperatic acid, atraric acid, atranorin and chloroatranorin. The lichen is strongly anti-oxidant and active against all eleven bacterial species and nine fungal species tested. Anti-biofilm activity against *S. aureus* and *Proteus mirabilis* was noted. Mitrovic T et al, *EXCLI J* 2014 13:938-53.

Elders of Haida refer to the lichen as Red Cedar Goat Wool or Light Clouds.

Yellow Map Lichen (*Rhizocarpon geographicum*) is a popular lichen used in Scandinavia for producing a brown dye for woolens.

It contains the pigment rhizocarpic acid, as well as parellic, psoromic and rhizonic acid, and tetronic acid derivatives.

Rhizocarpic acid and various depsidones found in various lichens are active against methicillin resistant strains of *Staphylococcus aureus*. Work by Kokubun et al, *Planta Med* 73:2 found hybocarpine the most active compound.

Fine Rock Wool (*Pseudephebe pubescens*) derives its common name for its appearance of black steel wool. The Haisla of British Columbia used it to make a black wood paint.

Candle Flame, or Lemon Lichen (*Candelaria concolor*) contains callopismic acid, also known as ethylpulvic acid; stictaurin or dipulvic acid, barbatic acid, and dipulvic dilactone; as well as tetronic acid derivatives, vulpinic acid, calycin and 5-chloroatranorin.

The Dust Lichen (*Lepraria latebranum*) contains lepraric acid, and fuciformic acid, while Fluffy Dust Lichen (*L. lobificans*) contains atranorin, stictic and constictic acids as well as zeorin. *Siphula ceratites* contains siphyulin.

Orange Chocolate Chip Lichen (*Solorinia crocea*) contains solorinic and norsolorinic acid, as well methyl gyrophorate and gyrophoric acid. Solorinic acid is an anthraquinone.

It was used for coloring woolens in Scotland at one time.

As the name suggests, it is unmistakable with its bright orange medulla and red born apothecia. Common throughout the mountains, it contains at least two lacasses. Lisov et al, *FEMS Microbio Lett* 2007 275:1.

Crater Lichen (*Diploschistes scruposus*) has a zinc content up to 9.34% of its dry weight, showing unusual ability to absorb ions from the soil.

It makes a red-brown dye after treatment with urine, or ammonia. It contains atranorin, lecanoric and diploschistesic acid.

Blood Spot Lichen (*Haematomma lapponicum*) and other species of this genus contain porphyrillic acid, which shows antibiotic activity, as well as divaricatic and usnic acids. The related *H. coccineum* contains 20% usnic acid dry weight, a phenomenal amount.

The poetic Pepper Spore Lichen, *Rinodina oreina* (*Dimelaena oreina*) contains gyrophoric and fumarprotocetraric acids.

Brown Cobblestone Lichen (*Acarospora fuscata*) is widely found on granite rocks throughout the continent, from Alaska to Texas. It contains stictic, norstitic, gyrophoric, usnic and atranorin acids. Gyrophoric acid was found most effective radical scavenger and most active anti-microbial. Kosanic M et al, *EXCLI J* 2014 13: 1226-38.

The related *A. socialis* ethanol extract shows significant anti-oxidant activity. Yeash EA et al, *J Sci Food* Agric 2017 April 2.

*Evernia prunastri*, mentioned below, contains evernic acid. This compound shows activity against mycobacterium at rates similar to usnic acid. It was used traditionally to leaven bread, and as a hop substitute for beer.

It shows moderate activity against *S. aureus* in work by Stoll et al, *Zeit fur Naturforsch*.

Flaccid Jelly Lichen (*Collema flaccidum*), found on the east coast, has been found to possess antitumor activity. Renzanka et al, *Nat Prod Res* 2006 20:10. Two colleflaccinosides A & B were identified, the former more active.

The related Finger Jelly Lichen (*C. cristatum*) is somewhat rare, but I have seen it in Nova Scotia, Colorado and British Columbia. A mycosporine derived from this species prevented UV-B induced erythema when applied to the skin prior to irradiation. Torres A et al, *Eur J Biochem* 2004 271(4): 780-4.

Powdered Loop Lichen (*Hypotrachyna revoluta*) found in small, scattered areas of North America, contains beta-orcinol metabolites hypotrachynic acid, deoxystictic acid, cryptostictinolide, and 8'-methyl-constictic acid. Papadopoulou P et al, *Molecules* 2007 12:5.

Anxiaic acid, a depside from the genus, is a topoisomerase poison inhibitor and shows potential as a source of new anti-bacterial and anti-cancer compounds. Studies by Cheng B et al, *PLoS One* 2013 8(4) found anziaic acid inhibits both *E. coli* and *Yersinia pestis*.

*Parmotrema* species containing atranonin and chloroatranonin exhibit COX 1 and 2 inhibition, suggesting anti-inflammatory activity. Bugni et al, *Fitoterapia* 80:5.

Powder edged Ruffle Lichen (*P. stuppeum*) is found in the Appalachians and west coast of California. It contains methyl orsenillate, orsenillic acid, atranorin and lecanoric acid that show moderate antioxidant activity. Jayapraksha & Rao, *Zeit fur Naturforsh* 2000 55:11-12.

Unwhiskered Ruffle Lichen (*P. austrosinense*) is found in Texas and adjacent states. It contains (3R)-5-hydroxymellein, which is a potent anti-oxidant and recovered skin damage caused by UVB radiation and inhibited melanin synthesis. This suggests development of skin protectant products. Zhao L et al, *Molecules* 2016 22(1).

It also contains lecanoric acid, which stimulates high growth of *Lactobacillus casei*, an important probiotic bacteria. Galkwad S et al, *J Food Sci Technol* 2014 51(10): 2624-31.

Palm Ruffle Lichen (*P. tinctorum*) is common to the southeastern United States. It contains atranorin and lecanoric acid. Oxaspirol B was isolated from *Lecythophora* sp. FL 1375, an endolichenic fungus isolated from Palm Ruffle Lichen. It shows moderate p97 ATPase inhibition. Wijeratne EM et al, *J Nat Prod* 2016 79(2): 340-52.

N-butyl orsellinate, modified from orsellinates obtained from this lichen, was more active against B16-F10 melanoma cells than cisplatin. Ethyl orsellinate was active against HEp-2 larynx carcinoma. Bogo D et al, *Z Naturforsch* C 2010 65(1-2): 43-8.

Lecanoric acid exhibits anti-oxidant activity. Lopes TI et al, *Chem Pharm Bull* (Tokyo) 2008 56(11): 1551-4.

This lichen shows significant anti-oxidant activity and inhibitory potential against carbohydrate digestive enzymes, and significant anti-glycation potential, including inhibition of aldose reductase. Its development into a functional food/nutraceutical is possible. Raj PS et al, *Nat Prod Res* 2014 28(18): 1480-4.

Cracked Ruffle Lichen (*P. dilatatum*) is found along the southeastern Atlantic coastline. A study including this species, examined atranorin, lichexanthone, (+) usnic, diffractaic, divaricatic, perlatolic, psoromic, protocetraric and norstictic acids, from various lichens.

All showed activity against various melanoma cells line. Protocetraric acid was highly selective against UACC-62 cells, followed by norstitic, perlatolic, psoromic and divaricatic acids; while norstictic and divaricatic acids were more selective against B16-F10 cells. Brandao LF et al, *Chem Pharm Bull* (Tokyo) 2013 61(2): 176-83.

*Parmotrema reticulatum* (*Rimelia reticulata*), another Cracked Ruffle Lichen, has been found to have moderate activity against virulent strain of *Mycobacterium tuberculosis* strains $H_{37}Rv$ and Ra. Gupta et al, *Pharm Bio* 2007 45:3.

Various flavonoids and usnic acid possess anti-bacterial activity and anti-inflammatory effect in work by Jain AP et al, *Indian J Pharm Sci* 2016 78(1): 94-102.

An 70% alcohol extract induced apoptosis in MCF-7 breast cancer cell lines. Ghate NB et al, *PLoS One* 2013 8(12). No cytotoxicity was found against lung (A549) carcinoma and normal lung (WI-38) fibroblast.

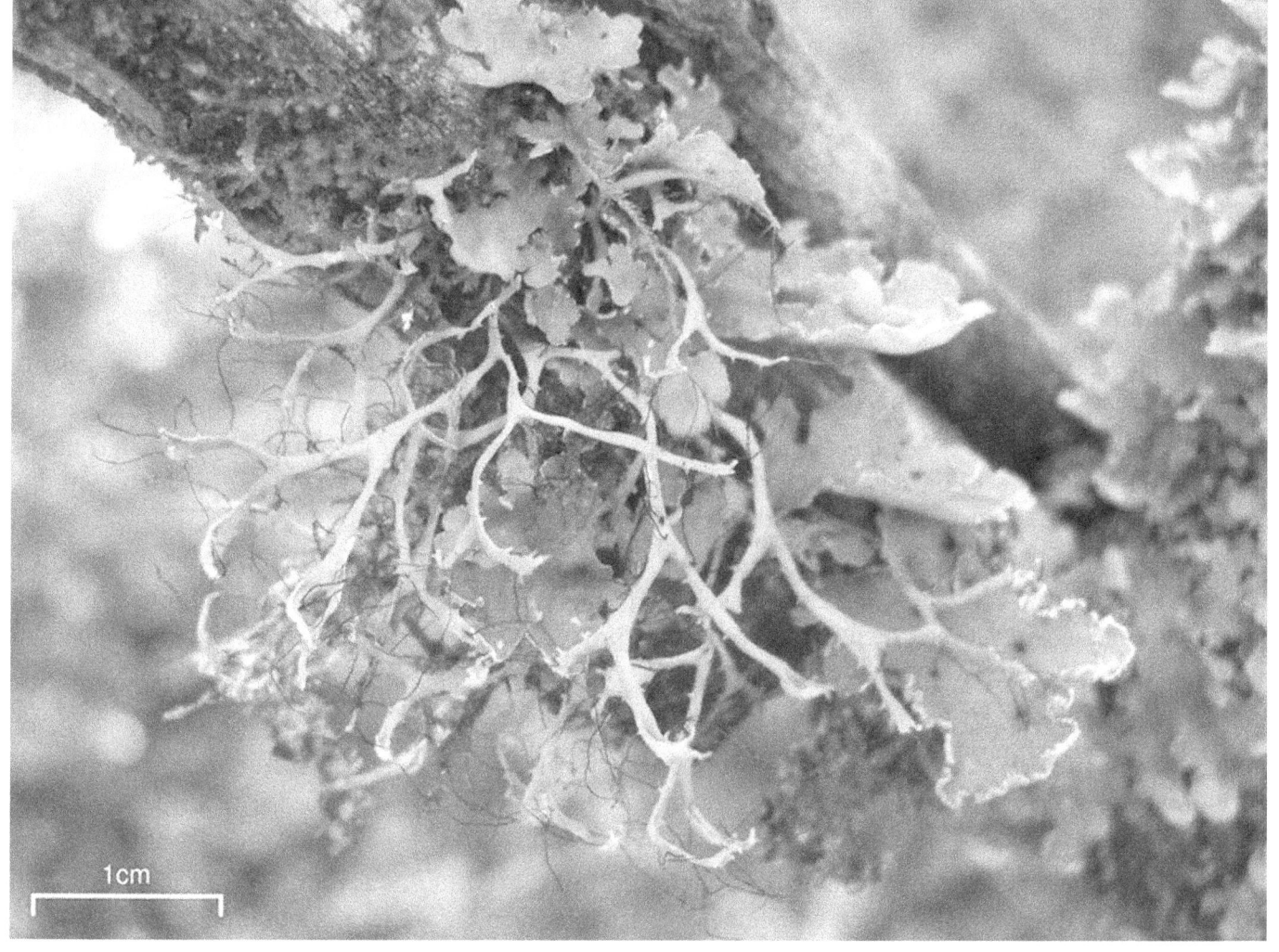

HETERODERMIA LEUCOMELA (Courtesy of Jason Hollinger)

Perforated Ruffle Lichen (*Parmotrema performatum*) is found mainly in southeastern United States. It is used in India for food and medicine under the name Chharila. It is used for a wide variety of conditions including dyspepsia, spermatorrhea, amenorrhea, kidney stones, enlarged spleen, bronchitis, hemorrhoids, sore throat and pain in general. It is mentioned in various Indian materia medicas, under both *P. performatum* and *P. chinense*.

The smoke is used to relieve headaches. It is powdered and used as snuff or applied to bleeding wounds. Chharila is widely adulterated with other lichens. It contains atranorin and norstictic acid.

Atranorin, from Parmotrema species, inhibits COX-1, suggesting anti-inflammatory activity. Bugni TS et al, *Fitoterapia* 2009 80(5): 270-3.

Green Rock Posy (*Rhizoplaca melanophthalma*) is widespread from the northernmost points of Canada down to New Mexico. It shows activity against both *Bacillus subtilis* and *S. aureus* bacteria.

Psoromic acid may be useful for the treatment of glioblastoma multiforme, based on preliminary studies by Emsen B et al, *Pharm Biol* 2016 54(9): 1748-62.

Psoromic acid, also found in Usnea species, exhibits competitive type of HMGR inhibition and mixed type of ACE inhibition, suggesting cardiovascular protecting properties. Behera BC et al, *Pharm Biol* 2012 50(8): 968-79.

Rab geranylgeranyl transferase inhibitors may be potential agents for treatment of cancers and osteoporosis. Psoromic is a potent inhibitor. Deraeve C et al, *J Am Chem Soc* 2012 134(17): 7384-91.

Elegant Centipede or Elegant Fringe Lichen (*Heterodermia leucomela* [L.] Poelt) is found in New England, the Appalachians, Florida, and along the west coast of North America.

Work by Gupta et al, *Pharm Bio* 2007 45:3 found ethanol extract quite active against the virulent strain of tuberculosis $H_{37}Rv$. More work should follow. It contains a number of interesting compounds of which hydroxy-4-methoxybenzoic acid that shows mosquito larvicidal activity is most interesting. Kathirgamanathar et al, *Pharm Bio* 2006 44:3

Orange Tinted Fringe Lichen (*H. obscurata* [Nyl.] Trevisan) was studied by Peter Cohen for a PhD thesis at UBC in 1995. It contains a number of interesting compounds, including blastenin, zeorin, atranorin, 7-chloro-emodin, emodin, flavoobscurin A-B, 7,7'-dichlorohypericin, and 5,7-dichloroemodin. The latter compound has anti-viral activities that respond in the presence of light. Emodin and 7-chloro-emodin both show activity against the herpes simplex virus at 2 mcg/ml.

Glucomannan extracts from this species, shows analgesic and anti-inflammatory properties. Pereira et al, *Phytochemistry* 2010 719(17-18): 2132-9.

Recent work suggests the glucomannan exhibits significant relief in both acute and chronic pain. Cordova MM et al, *Carbohydr Polym* 2013 92(2): 2058-64.

The lichen is found from Nova Scotia to the Great Lakes down to Florida and over to Texas.

Cupped Fringe Lichen (*H. diademata*) is confined to southern Arizona and New Mexico. In Nepal, it is known as **DHUNGO KU SETO JHAU**. The lichen is mixed with leaves of *Ageratina adenophora* and made into a poultice for cuts and wounds, and protect against infection. It contains atranorin and zeorin.

Lobed Button Lichen (*Diploicia canescens*) is rare and confined to the islands off of southern California. It contains various secalonic acids, diphenyl ether and other compounds. Cytotoxicity is found against B16 murine melanoma and HaCaT human keratinocyte cell lines. Millot M et al, *J Nat Prod* 2009 72(12): 2177-80.

Common Toadskin Lichen (*Lasallia pustulata*) is a common lichen from Europe, that has been reported in North America, but may well be *L. papulosa*.

The lichen possesses strong anti-oxidant, anti-microbial activity against five different species of bacteria and fungi; as well as inhibition of FemX (human melanoma) and LS174 (human colon carcinoma) cell lines. Kosanic M et al, *Cytotechnology* 2016 68(4): 999-1008.

Powdery Axil-Bristle Lichen (*M. aurulenta*) syn. *Parmelina aurulenta*, is confined to the eastern half of North America. It contains 16-O-acetyl-leucotylic acid which exhibits anti-proliferative activity against HL human leukemia cell lines. The activity is greater than leucotylic acid, also found in this lichen and the structurally related anti-tumor compound betulinic acid. Tokiwano T et al, *Biosci Biotechnol Biochem* 2009 73(11): 2525-7.

Various Ochrolechia species from the Arctic have been studied for anti-bacterial and anti-oxidant activity, and show positive results. Kim MK et al, *Pol J Microbiol* 2014 63(3):317-22.

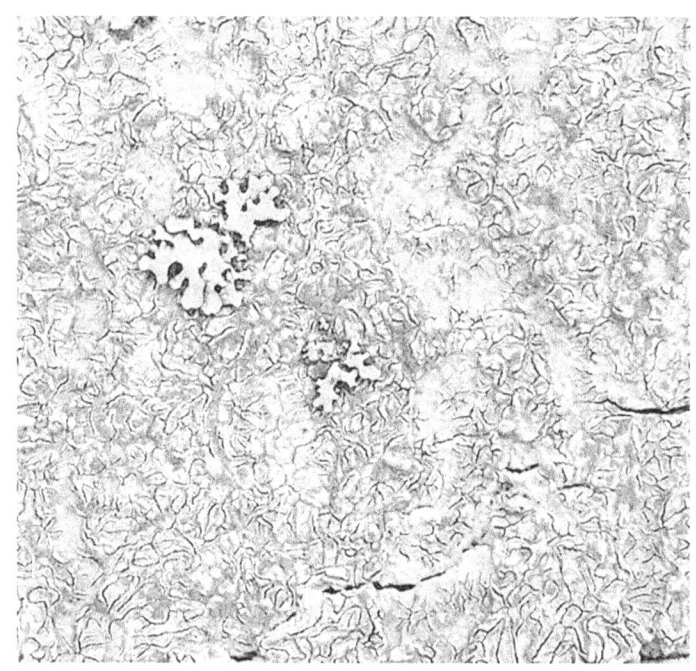

*GRAPHIS SCRIPTA*
(Courtesy of Jason Hollinger)

179

Common Script Lichen (*Graphis scripta*) appears scribbled on birch and other hardwoods, mainly in eastern North America, but occasionally on the west coast. It has been found to contain anti-oxidant ability and inhibit tyrosinase and xanthine oxidase. Higuchi et al, *Planta Med* 1993 59; Yamamoto et al, *Bryologist* 1993 96.

Work by Behera et al, *Current Science* 2004 87:1 looked at the tyrosinase and xanthine oxidase activity of various *Graphis* species in India. Tyrosinase plays a role in melanin production and may play a role in some human cataracts. Xanthine oxidase is found in those individuals suffering gout due to excess uric acid and observed in patients with hepatitis, and brain tumors. More study is needed on our local species.

Abraded Camouflage Lichen (*Melanelia subaurifera*) and Shiny Camouflage Lichen (*M. fuligonsa*) are both found in southwestern Alberta. The former is widespread from Alaska to California at higher elevations and east to Newfoundland, down to South Carolina.

Shiny Camouflage is more spotty, but still found in British Columbia and down the west coast, isolated in Colorado mountains, as well as eastern Canada.

They contain usnic acid, lecanoric acid, gyrophoric acid, atranorin, anziaic acid and 2'-O-methyl anziac acid. The latter showed the highest anti-microbial activity.

Abraded Camouflage lichen exhibited high cytotoxic activity against a variety of cancer cell lines. Ristic S et al, *J Food Sci Technol* 2016 53(6): 2804-16.

Blood Comma Lichen (*Arthonia cinnabarina*) is common in Florida, sometimes found in the Appalachians, and northern California. It contains bostrycoidin, 8-O-methylbostrycoidin, arthoniafurnes A and B (isofuranonapthoquinone derivatives). Yamamoto Y et al, *Phytochemistry* 2002 60(7): 741-5.

Alpine Blood Spot (*Ophioparma ventosa*) grows on non-calcareous rocks in the high Arctic. The fruiting bodies contain quinonoid naphthopyranonones such as ophioparmin, 4-methoxyhaemoventosins and 4-hydroxyhaemoventosin; as well as anhydrofusarubin lactone, miriquidic acid and haemoventosin. Moderate, to strong, anti-oxidant activity was exhibited by various compounds. The pigment haemoventosin exhibited significant cytotoxicity towards nine cancer cell lines. Le Pogam P et al, *J Nat Prod* 2016 79(4): 1005-11.

The Speckle Belly Lichens (*Pseudocyphellaria* species) look very similar to Sticta and Lobaria species. They are generally found in old growth forests

*Pseudocyphellaria coriacea* extracts show significant inhibition of human lung cancer cells. The compound physciosporin works through a variety of novel mechanisms to halt migration and invasion of cancer cell motility. Yang Y et al, *PLoS One* 2015 10(9): e0137889.

Cracked Ruffle Lichen (*Rimelia reticulata*) syn. *Parmotrema reticulatum*, is commonly found in the southeastern United States and north, into New England.

In the western Sahel of Africa, the lichen is known as Yari, and grows on ebony trees. It is contains moderate levels of good quality protein and 14.7 mg/g of calcium and 1.4 mg/g of iron.

Warty Script Lichen (*Sarcographa tricosa*) is confined to southern Florida. Three eremophilane-type sesquiterpenes have been isolated, in addition to six eremophilanes and ergosterol peroxide. These are 3-epi-petasol, dihydropetasol and sarcographol.

Blister Lichen (*Toninia candida*) contains norstictic acid, which possesses significant antioxidant activity. Rankovic B et al, *Int J Mol Sci* 2012 13(11): 14707-22.

Wrinkle Lichens (*Tuckermannopsis* species) are also taxonomically known as synonyms of Cetraria species.

*T. ciliaris* has been studied for potential as an anti-cancer agent. The viability of normal lymphocytes was not affected by extracts that show cytotoxicity against Burkitt's lymphoma (Raji) cells. Protolichesterinic acids were main compounds identified. Shrestha G et al, *Phytotherapy Research* 2015 29(1): 100-7.

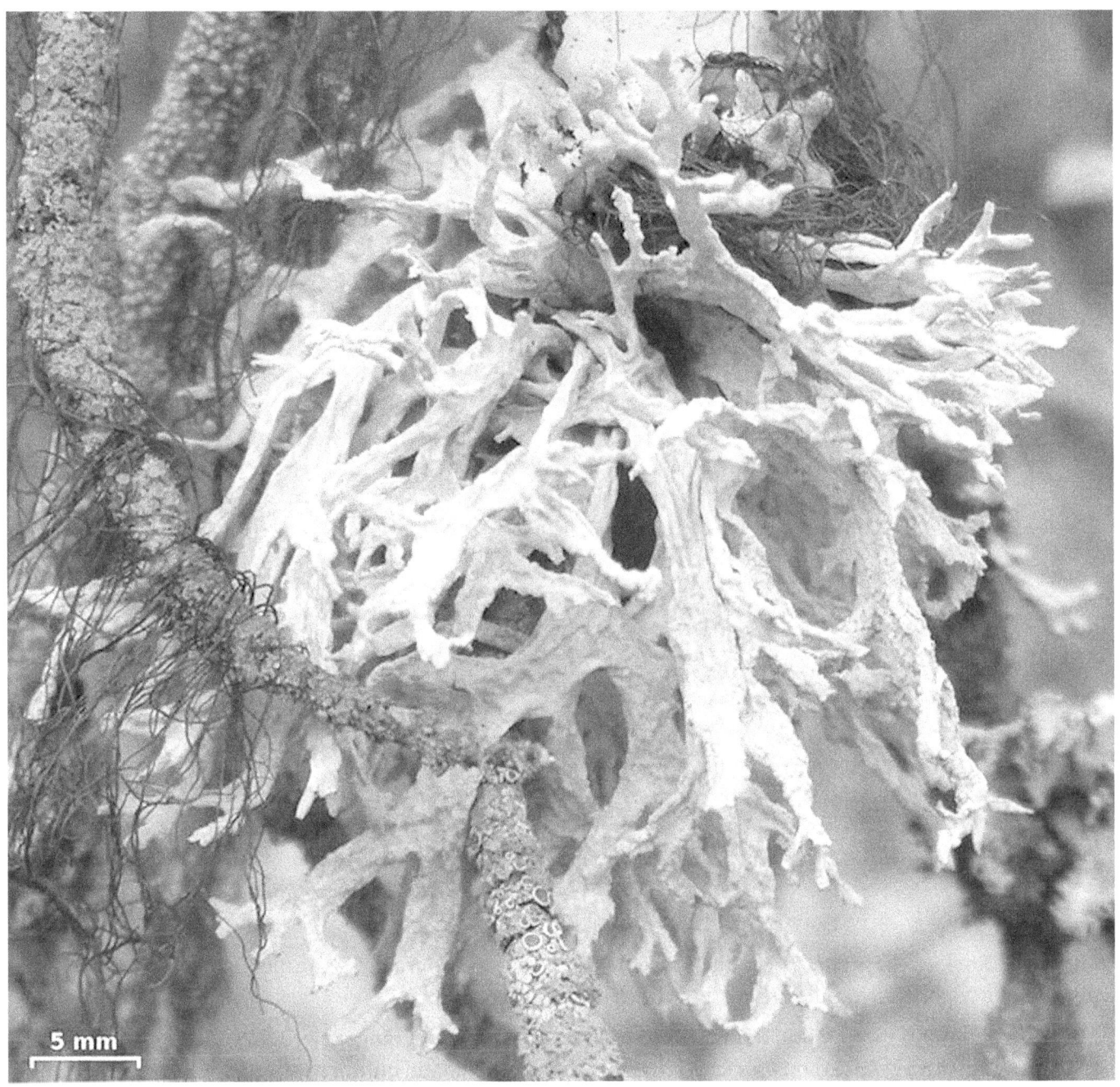

5 mm

EVERNIA PRUNASTRI (Courtesy of Jason Hollinger)

## ESSENTIAL OILS

All lichens will give up a certain percentage of essential oils. Certain varieties like the oak moss lichen (*Evernia prunastri* [L.] Ach.) have been used in Europe for centuries by the perfume industry as fixatives and bass notes. It was shipped from Cyprus and Greece to Egypt for packing embalmed mummies.

From the northern boreal muskegs, spruce moss or Boreal Oak moss Lichen (*E. mesomorpha* Nyl.) grows on the branches and bark of black spruce, larch, and birch. The Chipewyan call it **K'TSA"JU**, or birch lichen. They would use a cooled decoction of the lichen from birch trees as treating snow-blindness.

Solvent extractions of spruce moss have been used since the 16th century for perfume.

181

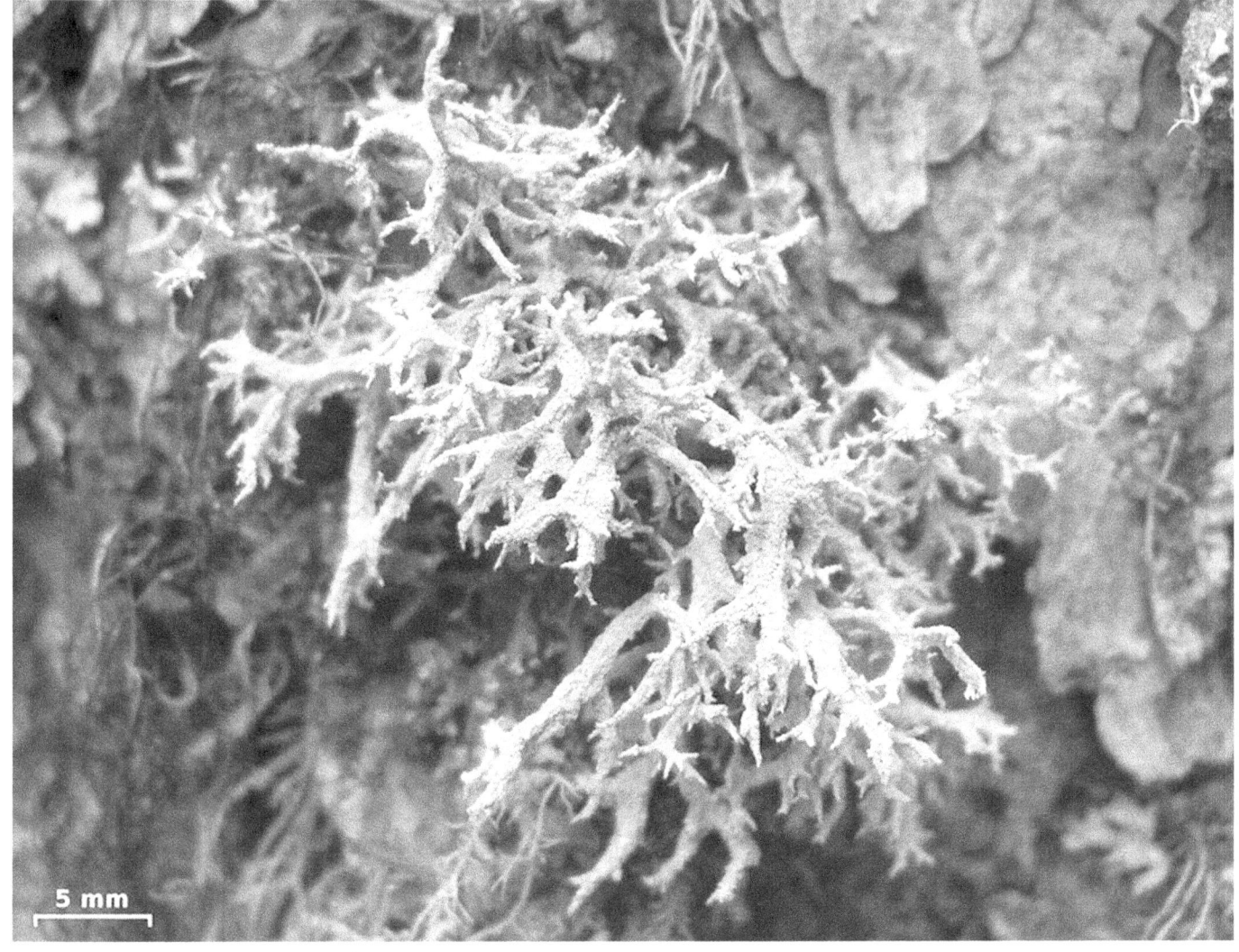

EVERNIA MESOMORPHA (Courtesy of Jason Hollinger)

West of the Rockies, *E. prunastri* is quite prominent, and a good source of perfume fixatives as well as usnic acid, and heteropolysaccharides. I have also found it in Nova Scotia.

About nine thousand tons are still today, shipped from Macedonia to France to produce Oak moss absolute. It is often mixed with *Pseudoevernia furfuracea*, which is more aromatic but inferior as a perfume fixative. This lichen is not found in North America.

Oak moss is used today in aromatherapy for its grounding nature, and to create a sense of security and personal prosperity. It helps one work with nature spirits and prevents slipping of secrets.

Oak moss Lichen has been used in Egypt as a bread additive, and by the Turks to make a type of jelly.

Dr. Schweinfurth, traveling through the Nile Valley in 1864 found a scrap of *Evernia furfuracea* in a vase of the 18th Dynasty (1700 BC). It does not grow in that country so was procured through trade.

Over the centuries, certain lichens have been dried and powdered for the white powdered wigs of aristocrats and to repel lice. Lichen extracts are also found in soups and deodorants, due in part to their anti-bacterial activity, which in turn, helps reduce underarm odour.

It has been used to dye wool a violet color when treated with urine or ammonia. It is slow growing, only about two millimeters a year, so do not over-harvest.

Various *Ramalina* and *Parmelia* species are useful for the production of absolutes by alcohol and aldehyde free petroleum ethers. Punctured Gristle (*R. dilacerata*) and Dusty, or Chalky Gristle (*R. pollinaria*) is commonly found near my home.

Iceland moss has been distilled and yields 0.051% of a brownish oil from which unidentified crystals separate upon standing. It contains cetrarine, a phenol-ketone.

Lungwort (*Lobaria pulmonaria*) makes a fine perfume by alcohol extraction.

Dilute Lichen absolutes can be rubbed into the forehead and over sinus area for pain relief.

Some lichens such as *Sticta fulgininosa* have an oceanic or fishy smell, not appreciated by all, but prized by perfumers and aromatherapists.

Considering the vast expanses of raw material available, there are great possibilities for creating viable business opportunities.

They all possess the ability to retain scent, and are used extensively in potpourri for this purpose.

## PERSONALITY TRAITS

Lichens are an amazing partnership between fungi and algae, the one providing support and structure, the other nutrients and sustenance.

Lichens can live several hundred years on trees and in harsh habitats such as wind ravaged mountain rocks. They even adapt happily to life on graveyard tombstones. They draw nutrients from dew and rainfall, and store the food in their bodies for very long periods, releasing nourishment gradually as needed. The lichen can thus sustain itself almost indefinitely in a tough environment.

What provisions do you need to sustain you tomorrow? A certain amount of food, money, clothing and household goods are only a start. What about the sustenance that comes from family, friendships, and sound values? It's never too soon to stock your storehouse with these treasures that nourish over a lifetime.

**GINA MOHAMMED**

Many people are familiar with litmus papers, those little pH indicator strips that turn either red or blue when dipped in acid or alkali. Litmus papers are imbued with special dyes derived from several species of lichen. In modern times, the *litmus test* has been used in a philosophical sense as well. We may say something is a litmus test of success, or love, or commitment, meaning that it is a discriminating test that will produce a definitive answer.

I wonder how many of us would be willing to subject our priorities to a litmus test. What if we chose peace of mind as our litmus, and held it against each of the priorities, large and small, that we hold at this very moment. Take a few moments to run the test, and see what doesn't pass. Perhaps these are burdens we shouldn't be carrying.

**GINA MOHAMMED**

In certain districts of Scotland, as Aberdeenshire, almost every farm or cotter had its tank or barrel (litpig) of putrid urine (graith) wherein the mistress of the household macerated from lichens (crotals or crottles) to prepare dyes for homespun stockings, nightcaps or other garments. The usual practice was to boil the lichen and woolen clothes together in water or in the urine treated lichen mass until the desired colour, usually brown, was obtained.

This took several hours, or less on the addition of acetic acid, producing fast dyes without the benefit of a mordant or fixing agent. The colour was intensified, by adding salt or saltpeter. This method was prevalent in Iceland as well as Scotland for those homespuns best known to the trade as Harris Tweed.

**G. A. LLANO 1951**

## SPIRITUAL PROPERTIES

I have always felt lichens spoke to the essence of unconditional love. They consist of two unrelated living entities, a fungus and an algae, dependent on each other for nourishment, protection and habitat...Their biological systems become so intermingled that they act as a single living entity we call a lichen. When speaking botanically this is pure symbiosis, in human terms could it not be unconditional love?                    **K. KEANE**

Usnea's keyword is clairvoyance. Usnea gives one trust in their higher consciousness. Usnea supports all the extrasensory perceptions and heightens any kind of clairvoyance.                    **MULDERS**

## RECIPES

**TINCTURE**- One to two ml. up to three times daily. The mother tinctures of lungwort, Iceland moss, usnea and ground liverwort are made from the fresh thallus in alcohol. Generally lichen tinctures can be made at 1:5 and 50%. I prefer Usnea tincture of 1:3 at 95%, but hey that's me. Let it soak for up to two months, longer if you can.

Hot alcohol tincture is best but not to be tried by the amateur. A Soxhlet extractor is needed for this precise extraction.

**COLD INFUSION**- Take one teaspoon of the dried shredded lichen to one cup of cold water and let sit overnight. Warm slowly before drinking one ounce every hour as needed.

**DECOCTION**- In order to remove the bitter principles in lichens, a quick boil, and discarding of first water can be followed by a standard decoction. When the demulcent and antiseptic properties are needed this is a good idea. Bitter decoctions are better in cases of stomach deficiency, vomiting, and night sweats.

**SODIUM USNATE**- 30 mg three times daily/ or 1.5 mg/kg/day. Take one week off every twelve and continue.

**DYES**- Various constituents of lichens decompose to produce orcin, that in the presence of ammonia and oxygen produce orecein, and a purple colour.

**CAUTION**- All lichens have the tendency to mold. If not handled properly, this can create bronchial or dermal irritation, allergies. Usnea tincture is contraindicated during pregnancy. Iceland moss may aggravate gastric or duodenal ulcers, and is contraindicated in cases of excessive catarrh or mucous congestion.

Usnea is a cold medicine and overuse for colds, flu and infections can damage spleen Qi.

Aromatic lichen acids are UV-absorbing substances and several are evidently able to photosensitive human skin. Atranorin is the most frequently involved.

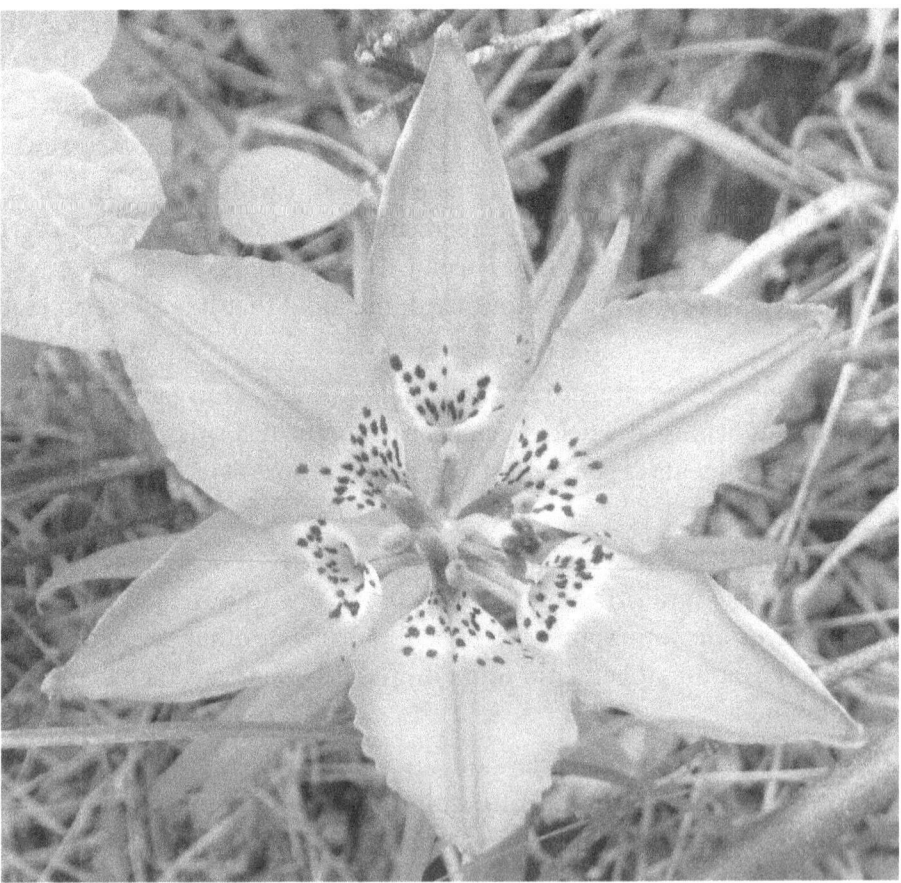
WESTERN WOOD LILY

184

WESTERN WOOD LILY
ORANGE RED LILY
PRAIRIE LILY
ROCKY MOUNTAIN LILY
(*Lilium andinum*) not accepted
(*L. philadelphicum* L.)
(*L. philadelphicum var. andinum* [Nutt.] Ler-Gawl)
not accepted
EASTERN WOOD LILY
(*L. philadelphicum var. philadelphicum*) not accepted
(*L. philadelphicum* L. )
TIGER LILY
COLUMBIA LILY
(*L. columbianum* Leichtlin ex Duch) not accepted
(*L. canadense var. parviflorum* Hook.)
TIGER LILY
(*L. tigrinum* Ker-Gawl.) not accepted
(*L. lancifolium* Thunb.)
WILD TIGER LILY
AMERICAN TIGER LILY
SWAMP LILY
(*L. superbum* L.)
(*L. canadense subsp. superbum* [L.] Baker) not accepted
CAROLINA LILY
(*L. carolinianum* Michx., non Bosc ex Lam)
not accepted
(*L. michauxii* Poir.)
TURK'S CAP LILY
(*L. martagon* L.)

TAIWAN LILY
(*L. formosanum* A. Wallace)
MADONNA LILY
WHITE LILY
(*L. candidum* L.)
EASTER LILY
(*L. longiflorum* Thunb.)
BROWN'S LILY
(*L. brownii var. colchesteri* Wilson)
MEADOW LILY
CANADA LILY
(*L. canadense* L.)
TAWNY DAY LILY
(*Hemerocallis flava* [L.] L.) not accepted
(*H. lilioasphodelus* L.)
CITRON NIGHT LILY
(*H. citrina* Baroni)
CORAL LILY
(*L. pumilum* D.C.)
STAR GAZER LILY
(*L. speciosum* x *L. nobilissimum*)
SPANISH LILY
(*L. pyrenaicum* Gouan.)
BLACKBERRY LILY
LEOPARD FLOWER
(*Belamcanda chinensis* [L.] DC)
DAVID'S LILY
(*L. davidii* Duch. Ex Elwes)
PARTS USED- bulbs, seeds, flowers

Fair white lilies, having birth
In their native genial earth —
These in scent and queenly grace,
Match thy maiden's form and face.

HOWITT

This time she came upon a large flower bed, with a border of daisies, and a willow tree growing in the middle. "Oh, Tiger-lily!" said Alice, addressing herself to one that was waving gracefully about in the wind, "I wish you could talk!"
"We can talk," said the Tiger Lily, "when there's anybody worth talking to."     **ALICE IN WONDERLAND**

Pale as the duskiest lily's leaf or head,
Smooth-skinned and dark, with bare throat made to bite,
To wan for blushing and too warm for white.

**ALGERNON C. SWINBURNE**

Lilium is from the Greek **LEIRION**, meaning white, or possibly from the Celtic **LI**, or Persian **LALEK.** Both stem back to the Egyptian **HRR**, meaning lily.

Philadelphicum is so named because a plant collector of Linnaeus lived in that city. Andicum means "of the Andes", and to be honest, I have never seen them there. Hemerocallis is from the Greek **HEMERA**, meaning Day, and **KALLOS**, meaning beauty. It comes from the Emerokallis of the 1st century Greek physician Dioscorides.

Superbum means, superb.

Candidum means pure or white, referring to the flowers, which according to legend sprang from a drop of milk that fell from the lips of the baby Hercules as he fed at Hera's breast, after drugging her to sleep. The initial mother's milk flowed into the universe and created the Milky Way.

When Aphrodite saw the pure white lily she became jealous and made an enormous, obscene stamen, the "donkey's penis" grow of the middle. The plant guardian of chaste marriage became a symbol of the amorous adulteress, but reverted back in Catholic Middle Ages as a symbol of the Immaculate Conception, and the Virgin Mary.

Roman candidates wore shining white togas. In Spanish folklore, eating lily petals restored humans cursed to take the shape of beasts.

Turk's Cap refers to the turban worn by Sultan Muhanned I of Turkey. Pumilum means small, and *brownii* is named after either Dr. Robert Brown, an English botanist, or F. E. Brown, a nurseryman from Slough, England. Michauxii is named in honor of Andre Michaux, a French botanist who compiled North America's first flora. He received the recognition posthumously in 1813 from another French botanist, Jean Louis Marie Poiret.

The Lily has six petals, and at their base are an outer whorl of three and inner whorl of three. Because the showy parts are all alike, they have been given the name tepals. Within the tepals, you will find a circle of six long filaments, each bearing an anther. There are three sticky stigmas, six stamens in series of two, and three locules.

The Hebrew word for lily, **SHUSHAN**, may derive from **SHESH**, the root word of six.

Britomartis, the goddess of Crete, whose name means "sweet virgin", had lily as her emblem. In Spenser's *Faerie Queen*, she becomes Britomart, the female knight personifying chastity and purity.

The Greeks attached the lily to Hera and the Romans to her equivalent Juno.

The bright orange Western Wood Lily is a pleasant sight of summer on the prairies, and is often called Prairie Lily.

Wood Lily was chosen the provincial flower of Saskatchewan in 1941, and survives very dry conditions.

The Eastern Wood lily is found in southeastern Manitoba, and has all its leaves in whorls, as opposed to only the uppermost. They are used the same. In fact, taxonomists believe they are small species.

Know as the Red Spotted Flame lily, or dwarf lily of Acadic, the plant found a following in Europe. Linnaeus assigned philadelphicum to the species, due to his lack of geographic acumen. Acadia is a former French colony, founded in Nova Scotia, hundreds of miles north. The halved root was favored as a love charm by various indigenous tribes.

Tiger Lily is more common to the montane and foothills, and up into sub alpine zones from Alberta to New Mexico. It grows up to five feet hall and can have as many as thirty blossoms to a plant, although five is more common.

Both Wood Lilies have been used traditionally for good, the fresh or dried tubers, the size of a large rice grain, having a bitter, peppery flavour. The flower and seeds were also consumed.

Natives of the boreal forest used the root decoctions of Wood Lily for stomach troubles, coughs, including tuberculosis and fevers.

Externally the tiny roots were poulticed and applied to swellings, sores, and wounds on the skin.

The root tea was given to expel the afterbirth of new mothers.

The Cree call it **WAPAYOOMINUSK**, meaning Rice Plant or the shorter **WAKICAN**.

The root is part of a compound medicine for heart trouble; or a dried tuber is placed in a tooth cavity to relive the pain of toothaches.

The root can be decocted to relieve appendicitis.

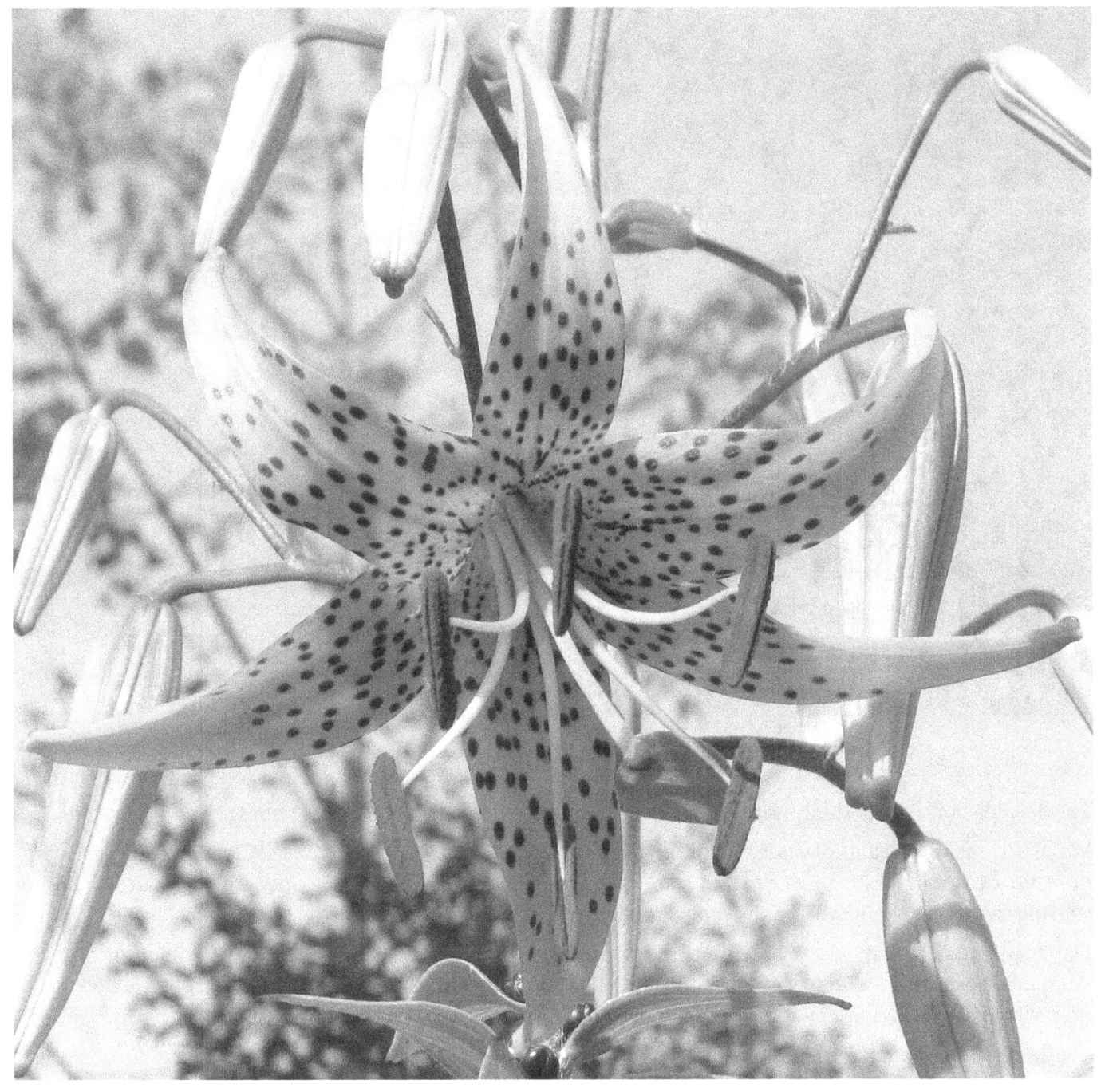

AMERICAN TIGER LILY (*L. SUPERBUM*)

Both the Blackfoot of southern Alberta, and the Dakota put a poultice of the flowers on "small, brown poisonous spider" bites. The Lakota name for Western Wood Lily is **MNAHCA' HCA**, meaning " very smelly flower".

The flower is quite edible; but is was mainly the bulb that was eaten fresh or added to soups.

They called it "Bee's Tooth", because it breaks into small rice grain sized pieces when rubbed.

The Esquimaux of British Columiba call it Mouse Root, due to the fact that field mice feed upon the root. It is also a favourite of porcupines, who dig it from sandy soil.

Further east, the Ojibwa used **MISKODE-PIN** bulbs for wounds and dog bites. The neighboring Algonquin boiled the root for stomach problems, and the Malecite for cough, fever and consumption.

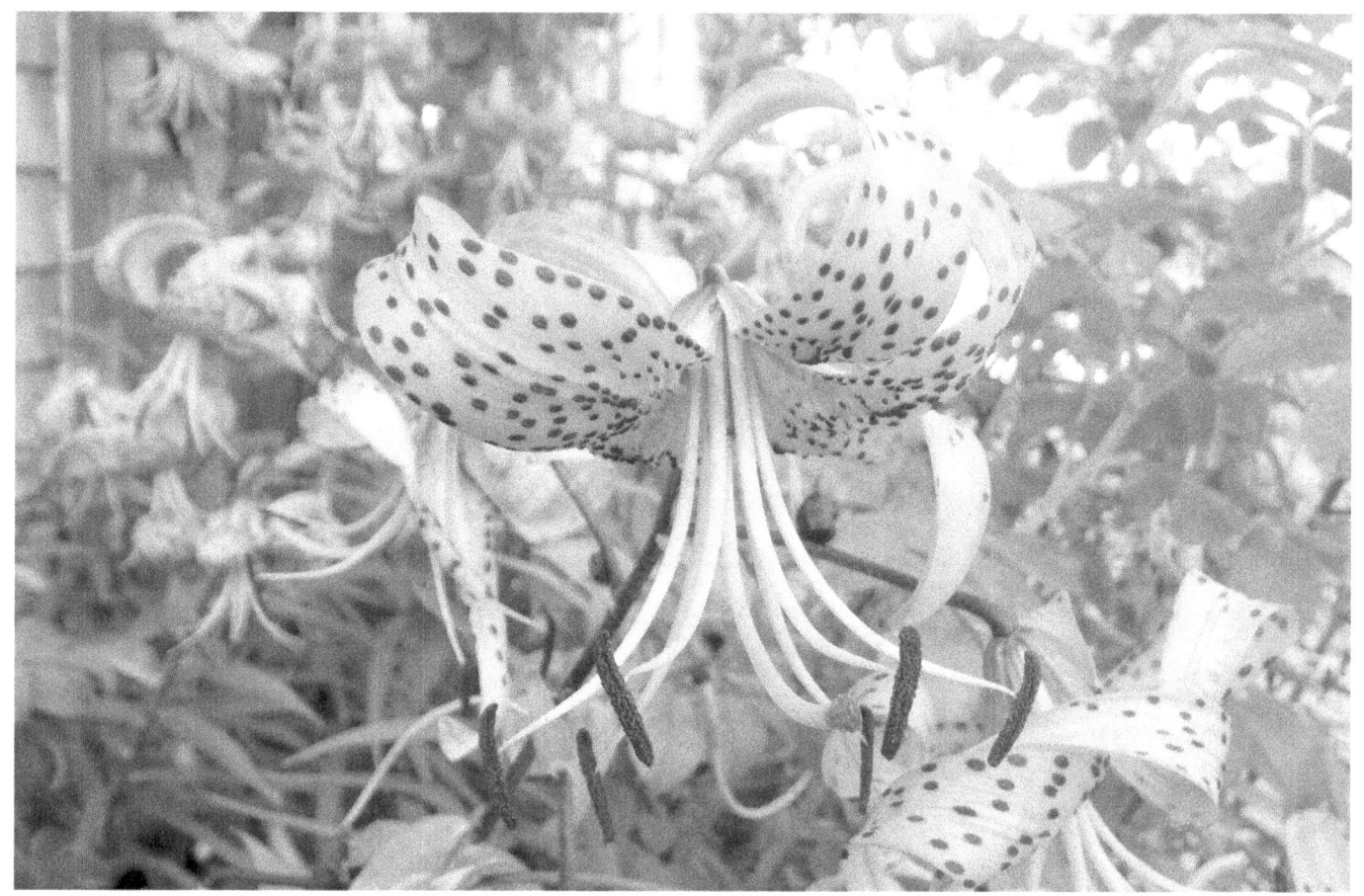

COLUMBIAN TIGER LILY

The halved roots of Wood Lily were considered powerful love medicine by some tribes.

Wood Lily makes a beautiful garden addition, but due to the relative scarcity in the wild, and its protected status in some areas, it is best cultivated from seed. The first year plant will produce only one leaf, but will bloom starting in the second. Mature bulbs can be transplanted and later divided.

Dr. Ieuan Evans, a plant specialist with Alberta Agriculture, found a small site just west of Edmonton that had 40 prairie lilies with 8 different colors and shapes. Tissue cultures of yellow and pink varieties are now being propagated at D'n A Gardens at Elnora, Alberta. You can view them at www.dnagardens.com.

Tiger Lily (*L. columbianum*), is more common to British Columbia and south, but was known to the Cree, and called **YOSKIHTEPAKWA**. Both plants were used in a similar manner.

Various tribes ate the bulbs from blooming time until late fall, usually by steaming. The taste is said to be similar to bitter roasted chestnut flesh.

The flavor is better after flower, but then it is more difficult to find.

Tiger Lily (*L. lancifolium*) is a native of China and Japan, commonly cultivated in prairie gardens. It is hardy to the zone, and does very well. In Japan, it is an important ingredient in the traditional "namono" eaten to celebrate the New Year. Starch is extracted from the bulbs and used to make steamed mochi cakes. They must be parboiled to remove bitter flavour.

The bulbs appear like gray flattened garlic cloves. In Japan, it is known as Devil Lily or **ONI-YURI**. This lily has been cultivated, over two millennium, for food and medicine.

The bulbs were mentioned in the *Divine Husbandman's Materia Medica*, dating from the 1ˢᵗ century AD; and used to moisten the lungs, stop dry coughs, and calm the spirit.

They arrived in North America around 1800 and are triploids and sterile, probably due to longtime cultivation.

Grieve mentions Tiger Lily for menopausal complaints associated with uterine prolapse.

The orange red coloring of the flowers, called capsanthin, has been used as a dye for foodstuffs. The flowers have no fragrance.

The introduced Tiger Lily was featured in Lewis Carroll's *Through the Looking-glass*, written in 1872, the sequel to *Alice's Adventures in Wonderland*.

Meadow Lily, or Spotted Martagon (*L. canadense*) is an eastern species used by the Malecite for irregular menstruation. The Algonquin used the root for stomach disorders, and the Chippewa used root decoctions of **WINABOJO'BIKWUK**, or Winabojo's Arrow, externally to treat snakebites. It was selected by Andre le Notre to be in gardens he designed for King Louis XIV of France. There are two distinct forms, one with golden-yellow petals, and the other, orange-red flowers. John Parkinson, the royal apothecary herbalist, grew the lily in his garden. The secret to growing it is yet undiscovered, as in one yard it will flourish, and in the neighboring soil do well for a few years and then fade. Can we pronounce mycorrhizal?

Brown's Lily (*L. brownii* var. *colchesteri*) is used in Traditional Chinese Medicine.

It was probably introduced about 1600 AD from Korea to Fukuoka, and today almost all the collections in Japan and Korea are hybrids of this lily and Taiwan lily (below).

Recent studies suggest *L. brownii* is closely related to both Taiwan lily and *L. longiflorum*. Nishikawa Y et al, *Breeding Science* 2001 51:36-46. The flowers of *L. brownii* are pure white, while the hybrid funnel is pale yellow on opening and a cream color, fading to white within a day. The former are nearly odorless, and the hybrid flowers are very fragrant. In other words, it is a taxonomic mess.

It is called **BAI HE**, in Mandarin, or **BAAK HAP**, in Cantonese, with the bulb most commonly used. Other names include **PA FAN HUA**, white-petal flower, or **PAI HUA PAI HO** meaning white flower lily.

Sometimes the root, **BAI HE GEN** or **BAAK HAP GAN** is preferred to the bulb in relieving apprehension or anxiety, as well as dysuria and edema. Traditionally, drinking Lily flower tea or eating the petals was said to help one overcome worry and sorrow, making it easier to get over unpleasant or unfortunate experiences.

The petals contain capsanthin, and capsorubin, both orange red colouring.

Wild Tiger Lily (*L. superbum*) is hardy to zone 3 and looks a lot like tiger lily. It is indigenous to North America, extending in Canada to the Rockies. It is a popular garden flower.

Thoreau mentions the bulbs eaten by indigenous people, who sometimes used them to thicken gruel and soups. The bulbs are "somewhat like raw green corn on the ear."

Also known as Virginia Swamp lily, it reached Britain by mid-17ᵗʰ century.

Taiwan Lily (*L. formosanum*) is also hardy to our extreme climate. The seed is often substituted for Birthwort fruit (*Aristolochia contorta* or *A. debilis*) in Taiwan herb markets.

They require a strongly acid soil, and even so, are prone to viral infection. The flowers possess a scent reminiscent of Easter lily.

Tawny Day Lily is a very common and prized plant in prairie gardens. There are nearly 30,000 named varieties of Day Lily (*Hemerocallis*).

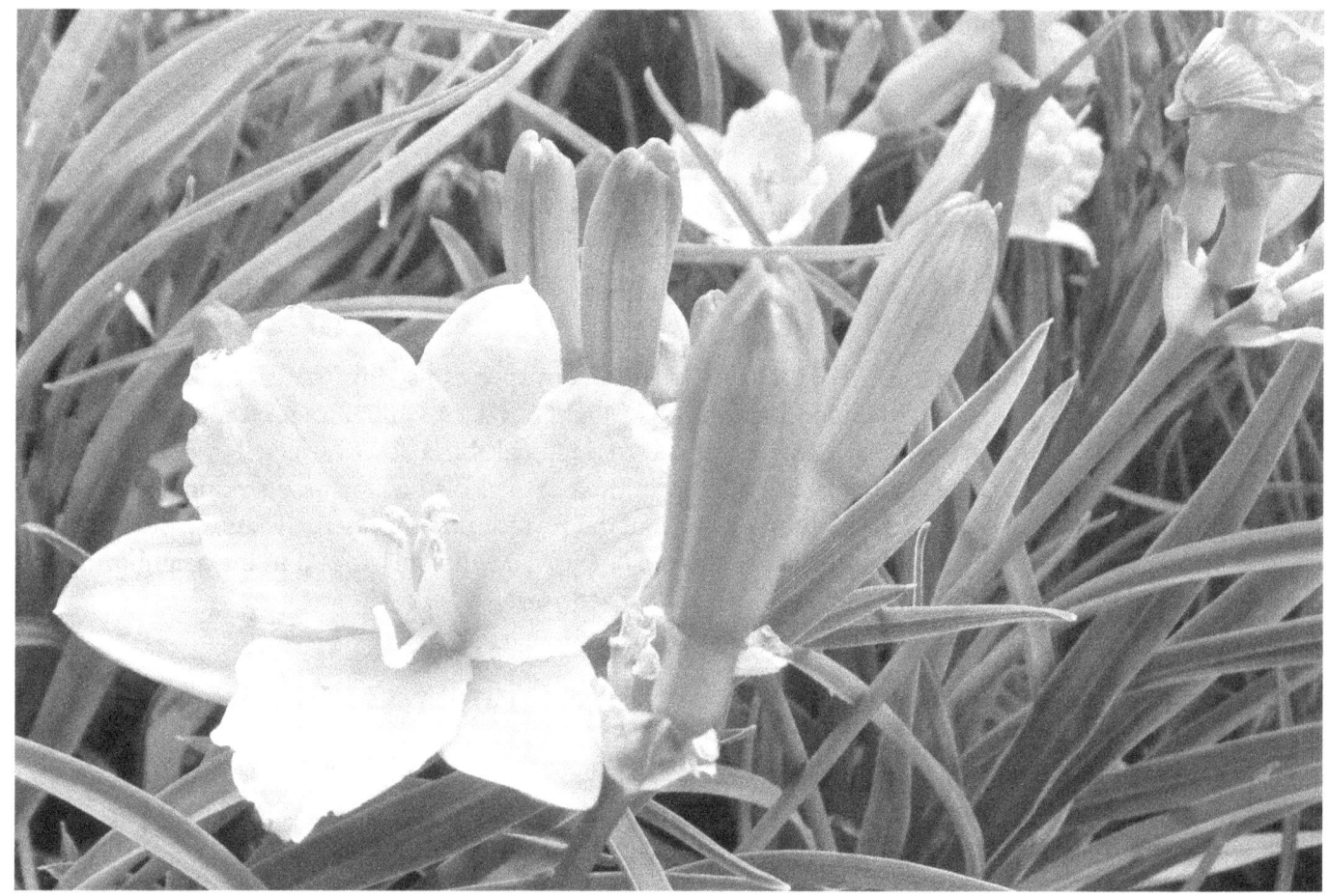

DAY LILY

In fact, it has somewhat naturalized to eastern North America; the famous botanist Thomas Nuttall observed it near Philadelphia in 1812. They became known as Outhouse Lily, due to the popularity of planting them around outhouse foundations.

Tawny Day Lily symbolizes coquetry, and related to birth date of July 15th.

In Chinese literature, the Day lily is first mentioned in songs attributed to Confucius in 500 BC. A treatise called *An Introduction to the Day Lily* by Chi Han was published in 304 AD; in which he suggests using the flower as a vegetable.

The flowers open at midnight, and last about twenty-four hours, hence the name.

The flavour of the cooked young shoots is like creamed onions. The juice of the root was used at one time to antidote arsenic.

The buds can also be steamed, and served with herb butter or pickled.

The dried or fresh unopened flower buds are sold as a vegetable in China and called **JIN-ZHEN-CAI**. They have a mucilaginous, sweet taste. In stores they are called Golden Needles or Gum Jum. In Japan, it is called **YABU KANZO**.

The flower and buds parts are also known as **WANG YOU CAO**, meaning "forget-one's sadness plant."

The mature bud, the day before opening, tastes like a cross between green beans and eggplant; the open flower much milder.

The seedpods can be steamed as a vegetable, or stir-fried. You can also pickle them in vinegar.

The tubers are sweet, resembling faba beans with a background of sweet corn.

Do not eat the stringy root, which is toxic, but only the small yellowish tubers. You can even rob them, like you would for new potatoes. Simply dig around the roots, snip off the tubers, and put the root back in the ground. At one time these were used as a sweetener in Japan.

Duke mentions that people who suffer from gout and have taken colchicine, and become sensitized, may suffer diarrhea following root ingestion. He believes it is due to colchicine or a very similar alkaloid in the roots; and if he had no other medicine, would ingest the roots. I think I would stick with dandelion root and cherry juice.

They can be cooked, or eaten raw like radishes, or Jerusalem Artichokes.

The day lily flower can be dipped in plain fritter batter and deep-fried. Serve hot with white sugar sprinkled over!

The flowers taste like lettuce/green beans, after removing the white base of each petal.

When the flower expands the can be fried or added to soups as an aromatic thickener. Those who have eaten hot and sour soups in Chinese restaurants have consumed day lily flower petals. New York City imports more than two tons of the dried petals each year alone.

They can be dried or preserved in salt, and need to be soaked in water before use. The flowers can be cooked with duck, my favourite, or pan fried with pork and onions, wrapped in pancakes, or in stir-fries. Soak the dried flowers or buds overnight, cutting off only the hard end.

The fresh buds can be dusted with flour, dipped in a batter and deep-fried, or blanched and frozen for up to 8 months.

The young shoots, considered potentially hallucinogenic in large doses, are used in Chinese folk medicine (see below).

Cats have shown nephrotoxicity after feeding on *H. fulva*. Hadley et al, *Vet Hum Toxicol* 2003 45:1.

Citron Night Lily (*H. citrina*) looks indentical save the flower color. Day lily opens in the morning and is pollinated by butterflies, whereas Night lily opens at night and is pollinated by hawkmoths.

Madonna Lily is not supposed to be hardy to the prairies, and yet, there it is in some Edmonton gardens. Probably only possible in protected areas, but a beautiful Lily up to six feet tall, with shiny white flowers. It was the official emblem of Quebec from 1963 until very recently. The Lily will not flower until at least its third year.

The first mention of the bulb and flowers dates back to 3000 BC. It was depicted on Cretan vases and frescoes on walls near Knossos in 1500 BC. The lily paintings of Thera confirm the Minoan's love of lilies, along with the prized saffron crocus.

It adorned the capitals of columns in various ancient civilizations, including Assyrians.

To the Greeks, it was the flower of flowers.

It was a favorite of the ancient Greeks and Romans, being originally a Mediterranean flower. In the early days of Christianity, it was dedicated to the Madonna, to symbolize purity, chastity and virginity. To the Greeks, it was the flower of Hera, who represented marriage and childbirth. The Egyptians and Greeks used lily flowers in their perfumes, or ointments. Dioscorides describes the manufacture of perfumes in great detail. He suggested the lily is warming and softening, and effective for inflammation of the vulva, as well as scaly scalp, varicose veins, dandruff and fever marks on the skin. The leaves were useful for burns, snakebite, and indolent ulcers.

Pliny mentions the use of petals and stamens for unguents and oils.

In Crete, the flower was sacred to the "sweet virgin" Britomartis, who later became Dictynna, the "mother of the nets", She was saved by the nets of a fisherman when she tried to escape King Minos, who pursued her for the symbolic nine months.

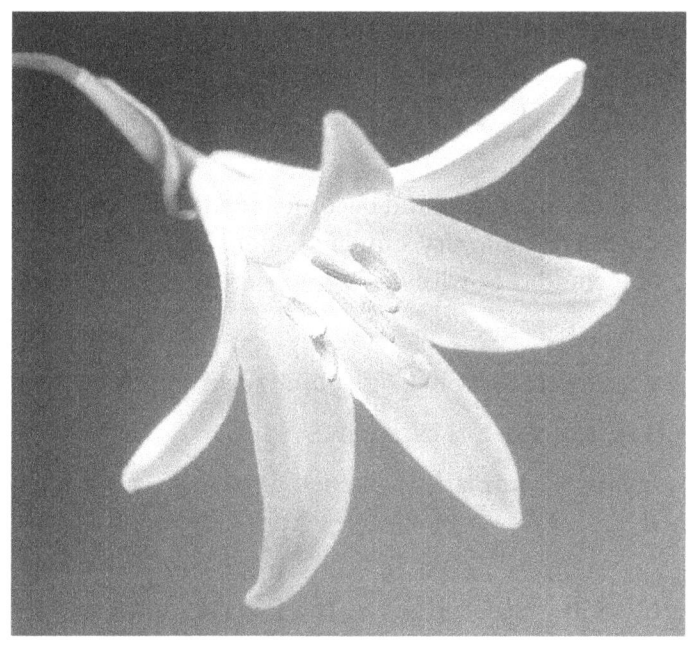

**MADONNA LILY**

In one Roman legend, Jupiter ordered Somnus, the God of Slumber, to concoct a sleeping potion disguised as nectar. While Juno slept, he placed his son Hercules at Hera's breast so that he could drink the celestial milk and become immortal.

As he withdrew Hercules from the breast, some of the milk spilt and formed the Milky Way. Some dropped back to earth and became the Madonna lily. Another name is Juno's Rose.

Aphrodite was so jealous of its whiteness that she gave the flower an enormous pistil, which some have likened to a donkey's phallus.

Des Esseintes, the anti-hero of Joris-Karl Huysman's 19th century novel, Against Nature, spied a row of white lilies, and his lips curled up with a smile, as he remembered the writings of Nicander of Colophon, who, "likened the pistil of a lily to the testicles of an ass."

Mary is often depicted holding lilies in older, church paintings. Lilies were shown to bloom on Joseph's staff, symbolizing his own virginity. Immaculate deception.

Madonna lily was one of the oldest perfume crops of the Mediterranean area.

The Romans made **LIRIUM**, a popular perfume from the flowers. They also macerated the root steeped in wine to apply to leprous sores and scurfy skin. The petals in vinegar were a plaster for wounds, and the powdered seed in ale used for erysipelas.

Pliny suggested it as cure for foot complaints and skin problems.

The early Christian church tried to ban the flower from its rituals. Wearing floral crowns was considered a pagan practice.

The Roman Catholic Church formally adopted the lily in the 5th century as a representation of the Virgin Mary. It was firmly linked with the mother of Jesus in Spain in 1043, after the bulbs were introduced, by the Moors.

In 1618, this was formalized, with a papal edict that "the introduction of the white lily into pictures of the Immaculate Conception."

During Victorian times, the yellow stamens were removed from lilies to "remain ever virgin".

Vermeulen notes. "Nothing can be so perfect as to be flawless. That might have crossed Satan's mind when viewing the Madonna lily. Perceiving that a flower so sublime and immaculate could not pass for real, Satan fitted it out with sexual organs of a size impossible to overlook."

The Benedictine monks in Switzerland grew the lily in their monastery in 812 AD. An early Benedictine monk, Venerable Bede, wrote this poetic description of Madonna and Mary:

"The white petals signifying her bodily purity, the golden anthers the glowing light of her soul."

Hildegard de Bingen recommended the juice of Madonna lily bulb for persons who cannot digest their food.

In medieval times, the bulbs and flowers were boiled and applied "to dissolve and ripen hard tumours, inflammations and swellings-to break boils- and cleanse foul and rotten ulcers."

Gerard, the English herbalist wrote, "the root of Garden lily stamped with honey, gleweth together sinews that be cut asunder, it bringeth the hairs again upon the places that have been burned or scalded, if it be mingled

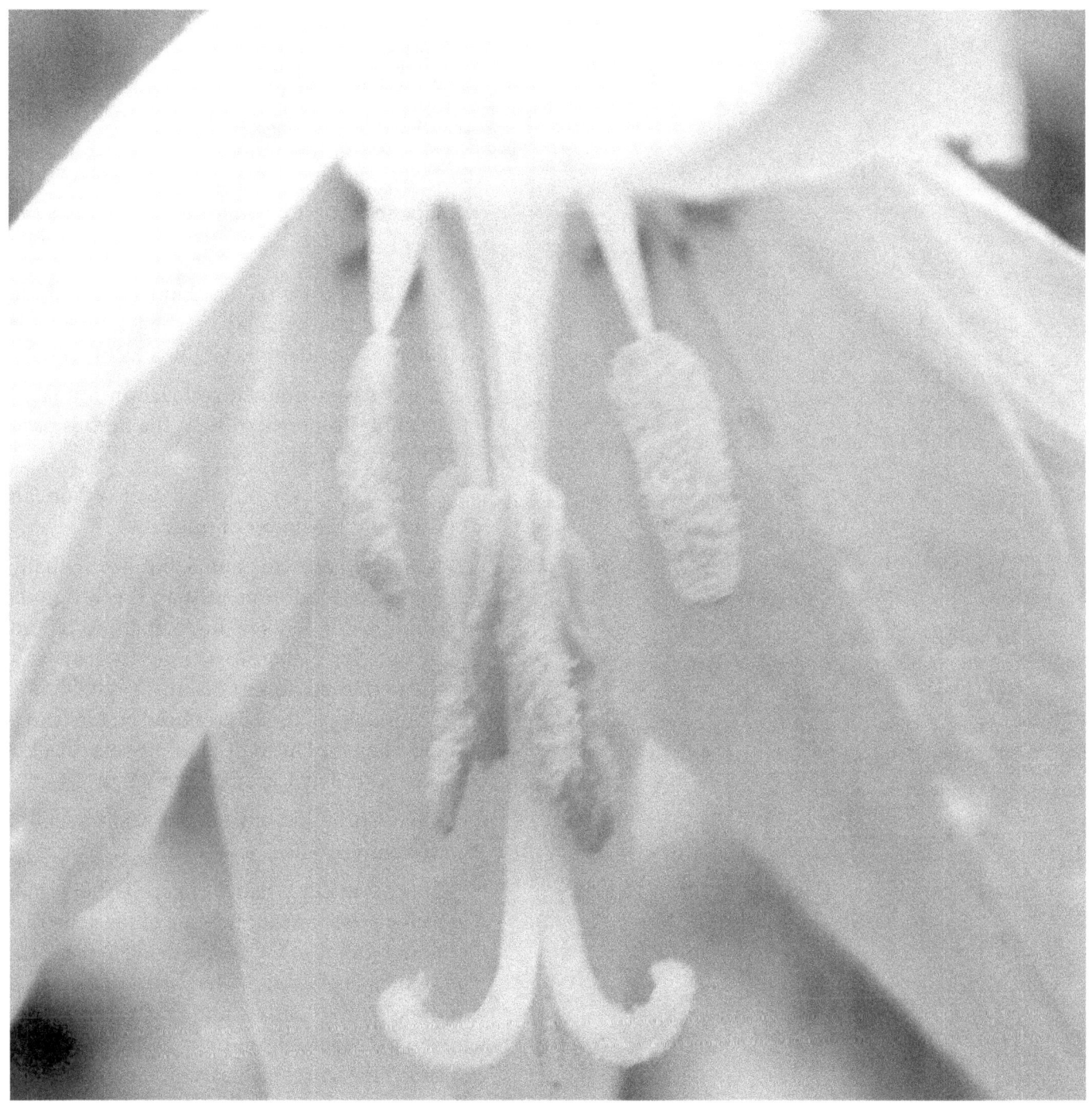

EASTER LILY

with oil or grease. The root of the white lily, stamped and strained with wine and given drink for two or three days together, expelleth the poison of the pestilence." He recommended the distilled lily water for easy and speedy childbirth and expelling the afterbirth.

Culpepper wrote, "the juice of it being tempered with barley meal baked, is an excellent cure for dropsy." This idea was probably borrowed by William Godorus, surgeon to Elizabeth I, who baked the plant juice into cakes for treating this affliction.

Culpepper continued, "the rot roasted and mixed with a little Hog's grease, makes a gallant poultice to ripen and break plague sores.

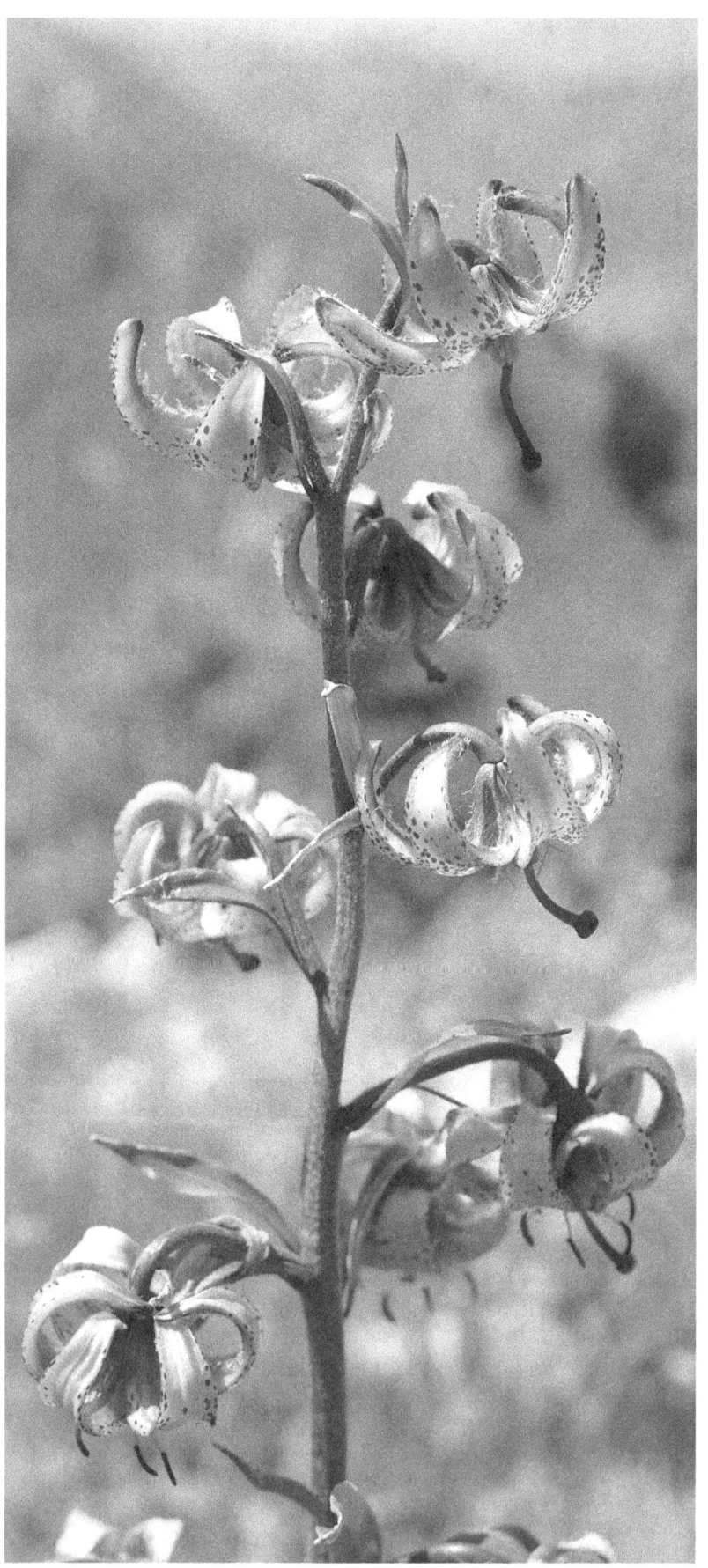

TURK'S CAP LILY

The ointment is excellently good for swellings and will cure burnings and scaldings without a scar and trimly deck a blank space with hair."

Early German settlers brought them to the New World. The root was used as an emollient to bring boils and abscesses to a head. The Japanese roast or boil the bulbs, and serve them with a white sauce.

Originally from the Liu-kiu Islands, off the coast of southern Japan, the Easter Lily is know as Blunderbuss Lily, or **TEPPO-YURI**.

It loves well-drained soil rich in lime and calcium. In northern Italy, the herb is used for herpes zoster.

Easter Lily is the official flower of Vatican City; and the flower of funerals.

It is only hardy to zone 6, but has virtually replaced Madonna Lily as the religious symbol, due to its being forced into bloom in time for Easter. It is easier to grow and the perfumed flowers last many days. Some 12 million plants are produced annually in a region on the Oregon/California border called the Easter Lily Capital of the World.

It has a beautiful scent that is reminiscent of hyacinth and lily.

Turk's Cap Lily is native of Europe, but grows well on the prairies. It is one of the principal flower motifs of the people living in the Tatra highlands of Poland. They use it in their folk dress as well as arts and crafts, the flower being a beautiful soft pink-purple with dark spots. The flower scent is rank and unpleasant. Turk's Cap has been a cultivated plant since the 15th century.

The Kamschatka Lily root is the source of food called savanne, which was made into bread by natives of that region of Russia. They boil them like other lilies.

Collecting the roots is easy. They simply wait for field mice to do the collecting and then rob their hoards.

It has been used traditionally as a cooling tonic and healing root.

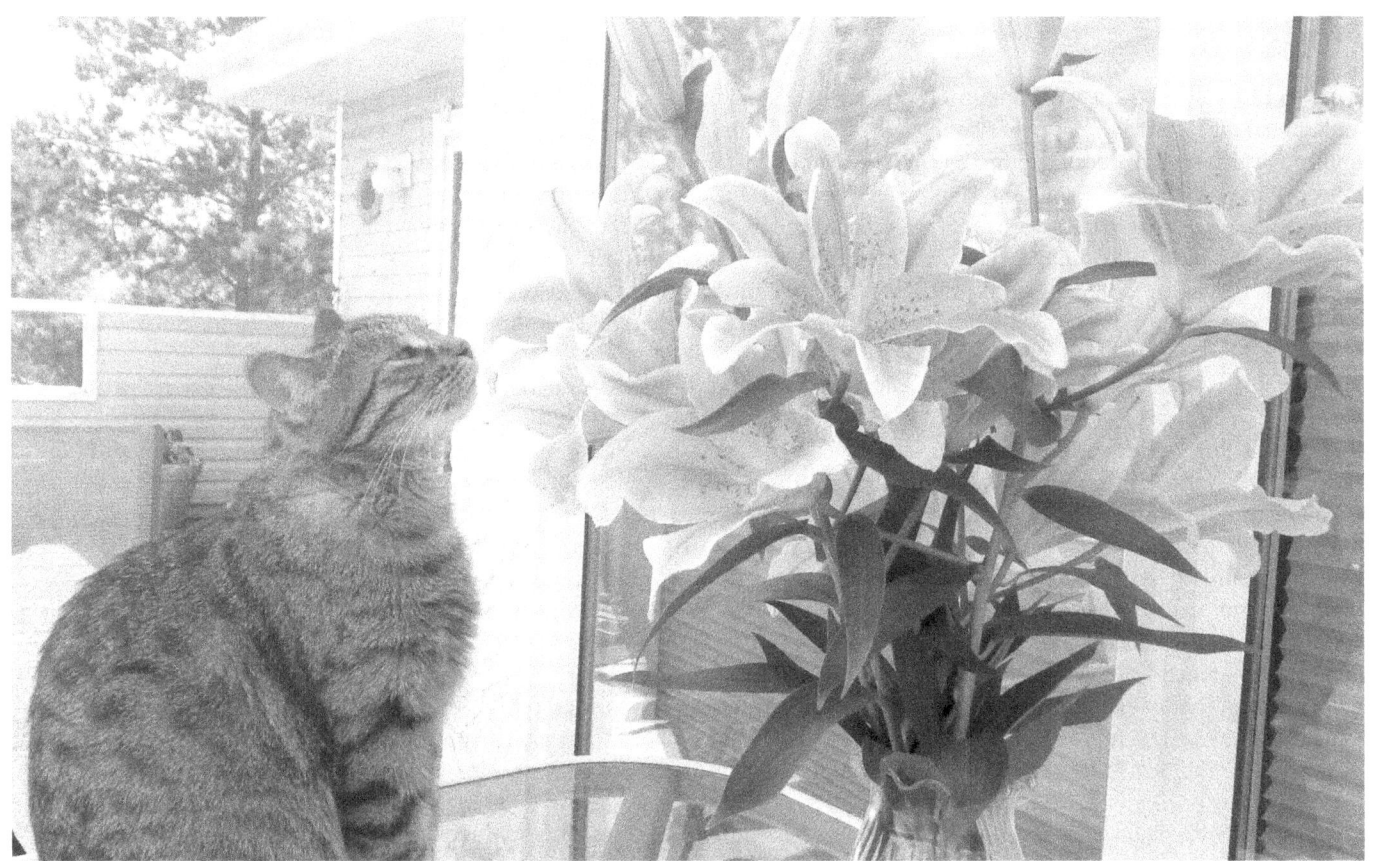

CERES AND STARGAZER LILY ON OUR FRONT DECK

My wife and I both love Stargazer Lily, both the beautiful appearance, and especially the narcotic, sweet floral scent. We chose the flowers for our wedding, which makes them all the more special.

It is hardy on the prairies to -34° C, and well worth trying to obtain a perfumed scent from the flowers as either an essential oil (doubtful), or as an absolute.

The Spanish Lily (*L. pyrenaicum*) has long been in cultivation, and is hardy to zone 3. Alcohol macerates of the bulbs have been used traditionally as anti-inflammatory agents.

Coral Lily has been used for over two thousand years in both TCM and Kampo medicine. The bulb is harvested in the fall, after the aerial parts have been killed by frost. The flowers are rose purple on the outside, and pure white inside. The fresh bulbs are eaten raw or lightly cooked.

Blackberry Lily is planted from rhizomes in zones 3-4, and will display yellow-orange flowers with red dots that only last one day, with new blossoms that go on for weeks. The round seed capsules split open and reveal the black seeds that give the plant its name.

In Nepal, the lily root is juiced as an expectorant, hepatic and carminative. About one half teaspoon of the juice is taken to abort 2-3 month pregnancies. Its medicinal use was first recorded in *Shennong Bencao Jing*, as a monograph in 300 A.D.

David's Lily, also know in TCM as Lan Zhou lily is a choice edible.

The town of Neepawa, Manitoba has set a world record of the most lilies per capita in the world. A World Lily Festival is held in mid July, with around 780,000 blossoms.

Oregon is considered the Lily State.

**CAUTION**- several lily species are nephrotoxic to cats.

# MEDICINAL

**CONSTITUENTS-** Day lily bulb/root- asparagin, chyrsophanol, various alkaloids including colchinin, friedelin, hemerocallin, and obtusifolin; methyl rhein, trehalase 1,8-dihydroxy-3-methoxy-anthragnium, beta sitosterol, rhein, hydroxy-chrysophanol, quinines, various glycosides including sweroside, laganin, picraquassioside C, puerarin, HN saponin, and 3'methoxypuerarin.

flower- 23.4% protein (63% solubility), and a relative feed value of 299. The flowers are rich in potassium, iron (88 ppm), zinc (66ppm) manganese (40), and boron (16), carotenoids, polyphenols, caffeoylquinic derivatives, flavones, a tryptophan derivative, adenosine, guanosine, fluvanine lactams, anthocyanins and anthraquinones.

fresh flower-stelladerol, longitubanine, various glycosides, rutin, gallic acid, (+)-catechin

leaf- 20.6% protein ( 26.4% solubility), extremely rich in iron (203 ppm) and boron (49 ppm), choline, pinnatanine, roseoside, phlomuroside, lariciresinol, adenosine, and various flavonoids.

*H. lancifolium*- scaleleaf- regalosides A & C, methyl-a-D-mannopyranoside, methyl-ca-D-glucopranoside, daucosterol, adenoside, berberine.

*H. citrina* bulb/root- hesperidin, rutin, chrysophanol, 2-methoxy-obtusifolin, rhein, aloe-emodin, hemerocallone, hemerocallin.

*L. philadelphicum*- 3-rutinoside, phytomelin, ilixathin, rutin, eldrin.

*L. candidum*-bulb- mucilage, boron, calcium sulphate, iron chloride, potassium chloride, potassium sulphate, sodium and magnesium salts; soluble polysaccharides such as glucomannans, starch, gamma-methylene glutamic acid, tuliposide, two spirostanol saponins, two pyroline derivatives, jatropham and its glucoside; etioline (steroidal alkaloid), kaempferol, methylsuccinic acid

aerial parts- linaline, lilanine, lilyn

flower- isorhamnetin rutinoside.

*L. longiflorum* flowers- kaempferol, kaempferol glycosides, quercitin glycosides, regaloside, a chalcone and fatty acid.

*L. pumilum*- alkaloids, starch, glucose, manna, iliosterin, colchiceine, anthocyanion, vitamin C.

flower- carotenoids consisting of beta carotene, capsanthin, capsorubin; and waxes, n-nonakosane, n-heptakosane, and n-pentakosane

*L. martagon* bulb- phenylpropanoid ester of pyrroline derivative, two steroidal saponins; soluble polysaccharides, starch, gamma-methylene glutamic acid, jatropham, and tuliposide.

aerial- lilidine

*L. brownii* var. *colchesteri*- bulb- beta sitosterol, daucosterol, colchicine, n-butyl-beta-D-fructopyranoside, lilin (an arginine and glutamate rich protein), various steroidal saponins, brownioside, deacylbrownioside, tigogenin, beta-1-solamargine, and diosgenin; steroidal alkaloids including solamargine.

*L. speciosum x L. nobilissimum* "Star Gazer"- bulbs- steroidal saponins.

*L. pyrenaicum* bulbs- 1-0-p-Coumaroylglycerol, (2S)-1-0-p-coumaroy 3-0-bea-D-glucopyranosyl-glycerol, and D-glucose

*B. chinensis* rhizome- iridin ( irigenin 7-glucoside), apocynin, testosterone 5-alpha reductase, tectoridin, tectorigenin., shikanin, belamcandin (C24H24O12), mangiferin, resveratrol, iriflophenone, belalloside A-B, belamphenone, 58 flavonoids, 17 terpenoids including 12 iridal type triterpenes including iridobelamal A, isoiridogermanal, 28-deacetylbelamcandal, anhydrobelachinal; four pentacyclic triterpenoids, ursolic acid, betulin, betulonic acid and betulone, as well as pentacylci triterpenoids, cycloartanol.

Seeds- 9 quinones including belamcandones A-D, belamcand aquinone A-B, ardisianone A and belamcandols A-B.

*L. davidii*- flowers/pollen- testosterone, beta sitosterol, stigmasterol, emodin.

Day Lily flower is an effective analgesic, anti-spasmodic and fever-reducing herb. The remedy is often given for pain relief during labor; to treat depression, and promote digestion.

The flower buds are also used, to promote urination, eliminate wetness heat, and remove oppression and hotness from the chest. The buds are decocted for blood astringent urine, jaundice, piles, bloody stools, sleeplessness, and lung problems.

The root is more commonly used and called **XUAN CAO GEN**, in Mandarin; and **SAN CHOU** in Cantonese.

This part is considered a bitter, cool, calming and decongestant herb, and used primarily as a liver decongestant in hepatitis, and jaundice.

In Fukien province in China, the fresh root is used to treat arthritis. The roots can also be boiled with sugar (6:1 ratio) and taken for treating mumps, or combined with Wood Ear mushroom for rectal prolapse, or blood in the stool or urine.

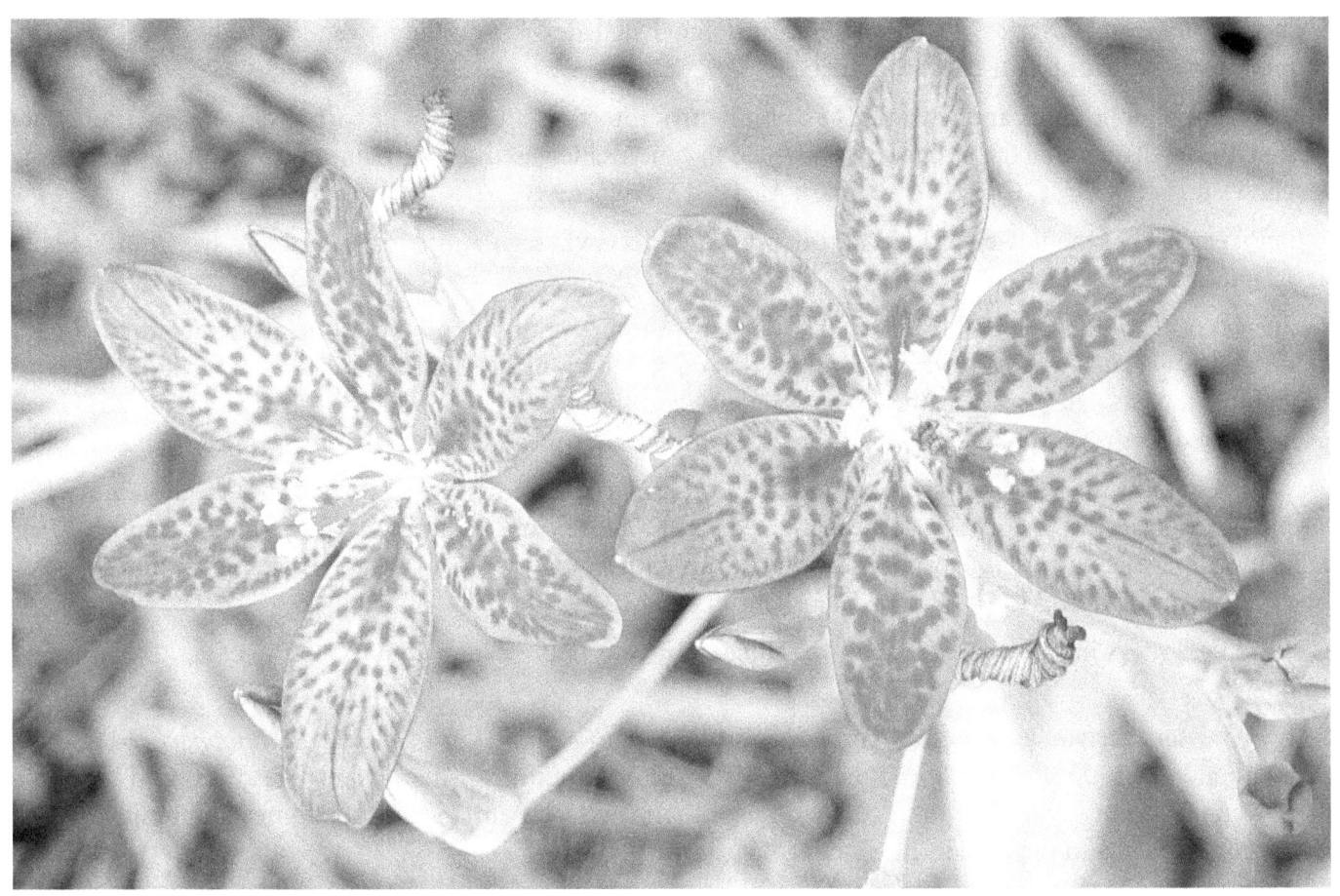

BLACKBERRY LILY

It helps clear infection from the urinary tract, as well as helping pass sand, gravel and stones. To this end it is a resolving diuretic, when the kidneys are not functioning optimally.

Mastitis, parotitis and cervical lymphadenitis are likewise resolved using the decoction or tincture internally, and applying a poultice to the breast for mastitis, breast abscess or tumours.

It is used for nosebleeds, and for blood from the lungs, urine or stool, including dry constipation.

The shoots are sweet and cool and used to promote urination, eliminate wetness and heat, remove oppression and hot feelings in the chest, alleviate digestive problems, and used for jaundice or bloody urine.

The leaves of *H. fulva* show activity against gram positive and negative bacteria, as well as *Candida albicans*. Zhang Y et al, *Life Sci* 2004 75:6 identified novel compounds in day lily leaves with strong anti-oxidant properties.

Interesting studies on the ability of the freeze-dried flowers to induce significant sleep, were conducted by Vezu et al in Japan in 1998. In laboratory studies, the extracts did not change the daylight sleeping time of lab animals. The Day Lily flower is known in Traditional Chinese Medicine as **XUAN CAO HUA**.

The flower is considered analgesic, anti-spasmodic and anti-pyretic. It is sometimes used, for pain relief during labor, and are rich in organic iron.

Other work by Hsieh et al, *Journal of Ethnopharmacology* 1996 52:2 showed that water extracts decrease the concentration of norepinephrine in the cortex of the brain, and a concentration of dopamine and serotonin in the brain stem.

Cichewicz and Nair, *J Agric Food Chem* 2002 50 isolated stelladerol from the flowers. This glycoside has been found to possess strong anti-oxidant activity.

The flower phenolic acids and flavonoids exhibit neuroprotection. Phenolics in corticosterone and glutamate treated PC12 cells elevated dopamine levels, whereas flavonoids increased acetylcholine and 5-hydroxy-tryptamine levels. Tian H et al, *BMC Complement Altern Med* 2017 17(1): 69.

Ethanol extracts of the flowers exhibit anti-depressant effects via regulation of serotonergic system. Lin SH et al, *J Tradit Complement Med* 2013 3(1): 53-61.

Cichewicz et al, *Life Sci* 2004 74(14): 1791-9, isolated root compounds that inhibit proliferation of human breast, colon and lung cancer cells. The research found that co-incubation of the anthraquinones with vitamins C and E potentiated cytotoxic effects against colon cancer cells. Other research found day lily extracts induced G1 cell cycle arrest of various human colon carcinoma cell lines. Kaneshiro T et al, *Asian Pac J Cancer Prev* 2005 6(3).

Day Lily contains a novel lipolysis promoter that can sensitize response of adipocytes to catecholamine and amplify the intracellular signaling pathway related to PKA or in some manner modifies the other mechanism regulating lipase activity. This may improve adipose mobility in obesity, or sub-cutaneous adiposity and suppress body fat accumulation. Mori et al, *Exp Biol Med* 2009 234:12.

Citron Lily flowers in the form of ethanol extract exhibit anti-depressant activity. Gu, Lan et al, *J Ethnopharm* 139:3 780-7.

Anti-depressant activity was found in cortisone-induced rat models by Li Tao Yi et al, *J Ethnopharm* 144:2 328-334. Other work by Xu P et al, J Ethnopharm 2016 194:819-26 found anti-depressant-like effects and cognitive improvement in unpredictable, mild stressed rats. Ethanol extracts enhance monoamines and brain-derived neurotrophic factor in depression-like models.

Flavonoids from Citron Lily inhibit liver injury by decreasing oxidative stress. Shen N et al, *Yao Xue Xue Bao* 2015 50(5): 547-51.

Extracts attenuate the upregulation of proinflammatory cytokines. Liu XL et al, *J Ethnopharm* 2014 153(2): 484-90. Hesperidin, a flavonoid, also found in citrus peels, is believed responsible, in part, for the reduction of pro-inflammatory cytokines. Carballo-Villalobos AI et al, *Inflammopharmacology* 2017 24(2): 265-9.

Hesperidin may be useful for preventing diabetic osteoporosis. Shehata AS et al, *Exp Toxicol Pathol* 2017 Jan 26. Pubmed listed over 1600 studies on this one flavonoid.

Dried bulb tinctures increased serotonin and dopamine levels in the central nervous system. Du B et al, *BMC Complement Altern Med* 2014 14: 326.

Chrysophanol, aloe-emodin and rhein are all present in rhubarb root as well. The former compounds induces apoptosis of choriocarcinoma, and minimizes side effects of conventional treatments. Lim W et al, *J Cell Physiol* 2017 232(2): 331-9.

It exhibits neuroprotection against inflammation in middle artery occlusion in mice, suggesting benefit in ischemia/reperfusion. Zhao Y et al, *Neurosci Lett* 2016 630: 16-22.

**CAUTION**- Do not take the root on continuous basis due to cumulative toxicity. Urinary incontinence, dilated pupils, diarrhea, and difficulty breathing are signs to observe. Do not use the fresh flowers, only dried.

Modern science indicates that the root of *H. citrina* is anti-bacterial and kills blood flukes, and used clinically for the latter and tuberculosis.

Colchicine and rhein have been shown in laboratory studies to reduce tumors. Colchicine is the active ingredient of Autumn Crocus, a well-known reliever of gout.

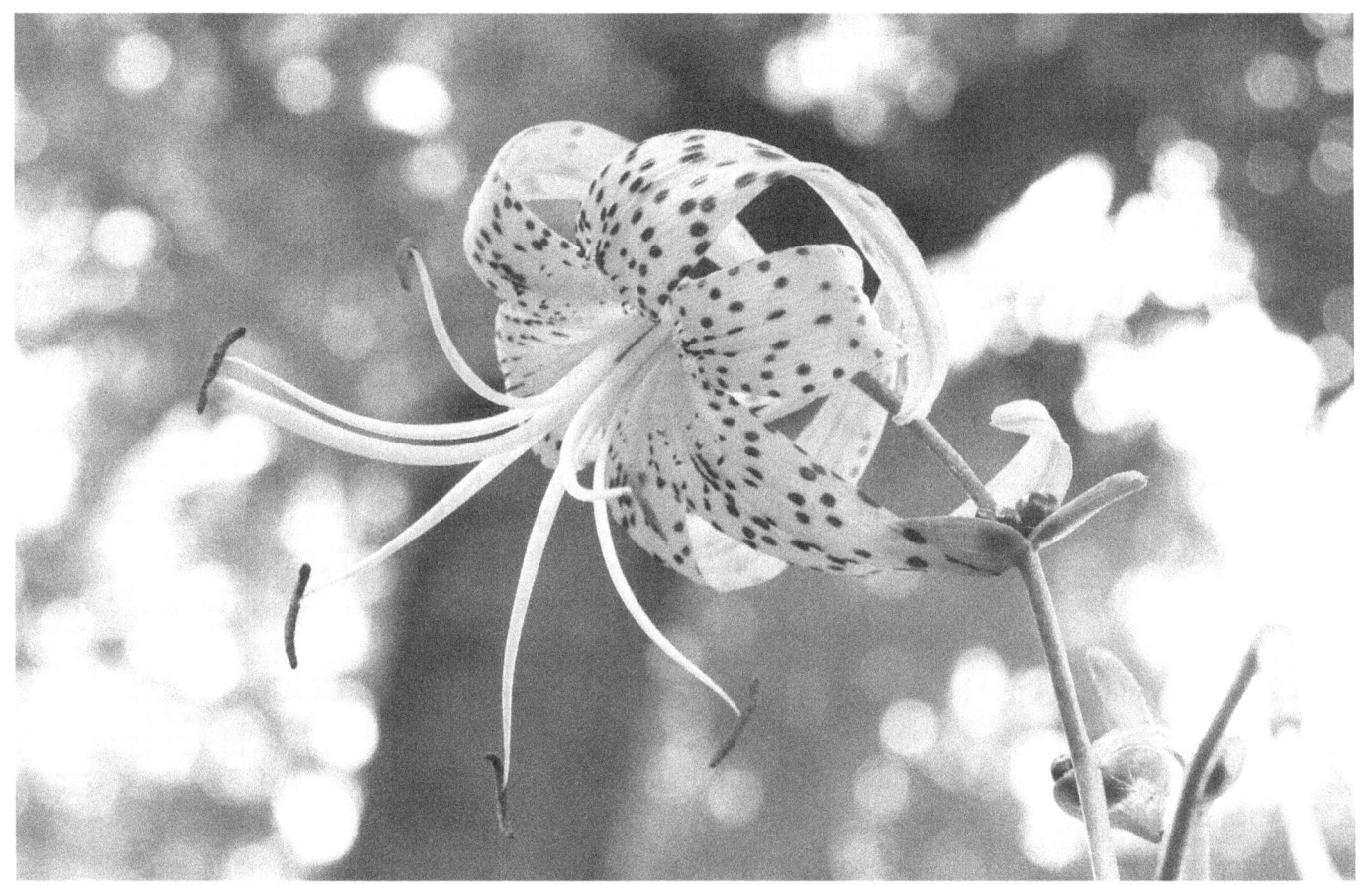

TIGER LILY (*LILIUM LANCIFOLIUM*)

Tiger Lily (*L. lancifolium*) tinctures of the leaves, stalks and flowers are still prescribed in the treatment of various women's complaints such as morning sickness in pregnancy, or the pain of uterine prolapse and ovarian neuralgia.

Consider using one tsp of tincture for depression with anxiety, muttering under the breath, weeping and fear of being alone associated with menstrual or menopausal problems. The leaves contain polysaccharides with anti-oxidant activity.

Polysaccharides from the bulbs possess hypoglycemic effect on streptozotocin-induced diabetic mice, and significantly decreased kidney weight, but not liver nor pancreas. Zhang T et al, *Int J Biol Macromol* 2014 65:436-40.

Another mouse study found root extracts reduce lung inflammation and airspace enlargement in cigarette smoke-exposed models. The authors suggest its therapeutic possibilities for pulmonary inflammation and emphysema. Lee E et al, *J Ethnopharm* 2013 149(1): 148-56.

The root/bulb anti-inflammatory effects were studied, and found due to downregulation of iNOS and COX-2. Kwon OK et al, *J Ethnopharm* 2010 130(1): 28-34.

Madonna Lily bulbs, or corms are demulcent, astringent, resolvent and vulnerary. When the scales of the corm are made into an ointment, it helps remove corns and hard growths, takes away pain and inflammation caused by scalds and burns, without leaving a scar.

It is also effective in contracted and painful tendons, or tendonitis.

Creams and ointment lighten periocular hyper-pigmentation. Alsaad SM & M. Mikhail, *J Drugs Dermatol* 2013 12(2): 154-7.

Infusions are an excellent remedy for inflammation of the stomach, intestines, kidney and bladder; as well as gynecological conditions such as severe period pains.

Madonna or White Lily corm is useful in leucorrhea and prolapsed uterus, the decoction taken internally and used as a douche; combining well with Life root (*Senecio aureus*).

Dr. George Winterburn, speaking of his clinical observations, noted. "From these imperfect observations I am inclined to give it a place in neuralgia of the uterus."

He used *Lilium candidum* 2x. He noted, "besides its use in such cases, *Lilium candidum* has a defined value in ascites and in inflammations of the middle ear."

When boiled in milk it is an excellent poultice for ulcers, tumours and skin inflammation.

When available, the fresh root has been found useful in treating dropsy.

For local application as a poultice to swollen glands, tumours, hard lumps and unresolved skin ulcers use a thick paste from the fresh or cooked bulb. Alopecia is sometimes restored to hair growth with daily use of the bulb ointment.

Extracts of the bulb have been found to stimulate phagocytosis in laboratory studies by Delaveau et al, *Planta Medica* 1980 40.

In fact, the bulb contains a number of carcinogenic and inhibitory compounds. Vachalkova A et al, *Neoplasma* 2000 47(5): 313-8.

Alcohol extracts induce p53-mediated apoptosis on human breast cancer cell line MCF-7. Tokgun O et al, *J Med Food* 2012 15(11): 1000-5.

Vachalkova et al, *Neoplasma* 2000 47:5 have identified several compounds with tumor inhibition, including spirostanol saponins at more than 70% inhibition, and jatropham glucoside at nearly 50%.

Etioline, a steroidal alkaloid, exhibits strong activity against liver damage. Lin CN et al, *Planta Medica* 1989 55(1): 48-50. The compound exhibits significant cytotoxicity against human PLC/PRF/5 cells, in vitro. Gan KH et al, *J Nat Prod* 1993 56(1): 15-21. This is a marker for Alexander cell line that produces hepatitis B antigen.

Both bulbs and flowers show anti-yeast activity, the former much more active. Mucaji et al, *Ceska Slov Farm* 2002 51(6): 297-300.

Etioline, also found in various Solanum species, exhibits high cytotoxicity against the cervical cancer cell line, Hela. El-Sayed MA et al, *Z Naturforsch C* 2009 64(9-10): 644-9.

In Italy, the bulbs are fried in olive oil as an anti-viral to heal shingles (*Herpes zoster*). Pieroni A et al, *J Ethnopharm* 2000 70 235-273.

Leaf extracts strongly inhibit herpes simplex virus-1, in vitro. Yarmolinsky L et al, *N Biotechnol* 2009 26(6): 307-13.

The leaf shows activity against herpes simplex virus 1. Yarmolinsky et al, *N Biotech* 2009 August 21.

The bulbs contain kaempferol and jatropham. Both compounds were shown to possess a potential to modulate and decrease the cytotoxic and genotoxic/clastogenic effect of the antibiotic, zeocin. Jovtchev G et al, *Environ Toxicol* 2016 31(6): 751-64.

The flowers give up their fragrance to low heated oil and this too may be used for local skin inflammations, pains of the womb or otitis.

Turk's Cap (*L. martagon*) bulb powder is used as a diuretic and in the treatment of dysmenorrhea, and prolapsed uterus.

It has been used medicinally, according to Duke, for cancer, gas, scleroma and water retention. Externally, the bulb is poulticed and applied to skin ulcers. Note that the bulb constituents are very similar to Madonna Lily above.

Easter lily flower tincture may be useful in a variety of female reproductive issues, ranging from cysts of the ovaries, breasts and skin. It appears to be well suited to androgenic excess, according to Matthew Wood, associated with infertility, frustration, intense sexual desire, acne and polycystic ovarian syndrome.

Mucus in fallopian tubes may prevent fertility and conception, as the egg is unable to descend and implant.

The flowers contain kaempferol, which shows 94% inhibition of COX-1, and 37% inhibition of COX-2. Francis JA et al, *Life Sci* 2004 76(6): 671-83.

Studies have found the steroidal glycosides, and furostanol saponins, in bulbs play a role in the wound healing process. This is due to promotion of dermal fibroblast migration. Esposito D et al, *J Ethnopharm* 2013 148(2): 433-40.

In Traditional Chinese Medicine, it is used to treat coughs, haemoptysis, insomnia and fidgetiness in the latter stages of febrile disease.

It is anti-asthmatic, anti-tussive, expectorant and sedative.

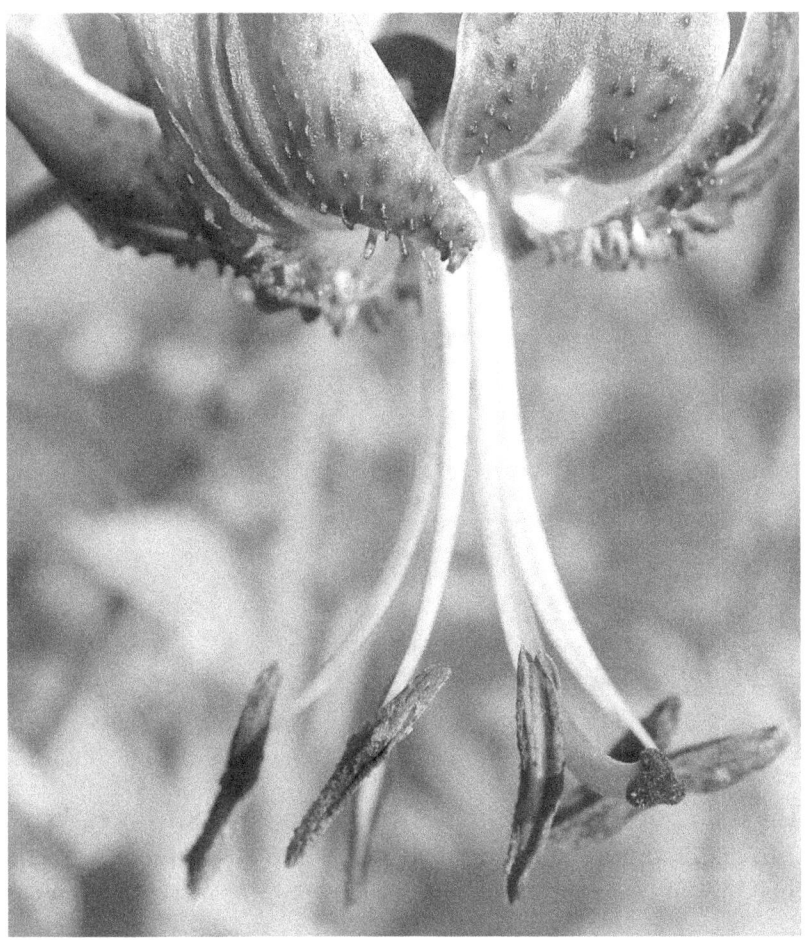

TURK'S CAP

Tinctures of the bulb improve liver and pancreas response in diet-induced mice. Tang W et al, *J Agric Food Chem* 2015 63(44): 9722-8.

Brown's Lily (*L. brownii var. colchesteri*) bulbs are used in TCM for their sweet, cool, moist, and slightly bitter and oily properties. The dried bulb, known as **BAI HE**, meaning "hundred meetings", or **PAI HO**, is considered restorative and calming to the respiratory system. Japanese Kampo medicine knows it as **HYAKUGO** or **BYAKUGO**, meaning "hundred meetings", and Korean practitioners call it **PACK HAP**.

It is decocted or used in tincture form for hot, dry coughs associated with bronchitis, laryngitis, TB, hemoptysis, sore throats, allergic asthma and spasmodic coughing.

It is used in low-grade fevers, hot spells or heat exhaustion.

As a neurocardiac sedative, it helps soothe unrest, irritability, heart palpitations, insomnia, anxiety, apprehension, neurosis, headaches and visual disturbances.

Tinctures (50%) of the bulb inhibit MAO-B, suggestive of use in treating neurodegenerative conditions. Lin RD et al, *Phytomedicine* 2003 10(8): 650-6.

The flower tea, or simply eating the petals helps overcome anxiety, worry and sorrow, helping one get over unpleasant situations.

Bulb tea, it is used to encourage more breast milk when needed. In new mothers the relaxation and sedative action is much appreciated, a very good combination for both mother and child.

When honey mix-fried, the energy is more neutral, and useful for coughs associated with lung damage and bleeding, as well as night sweats, and dry sore throats.

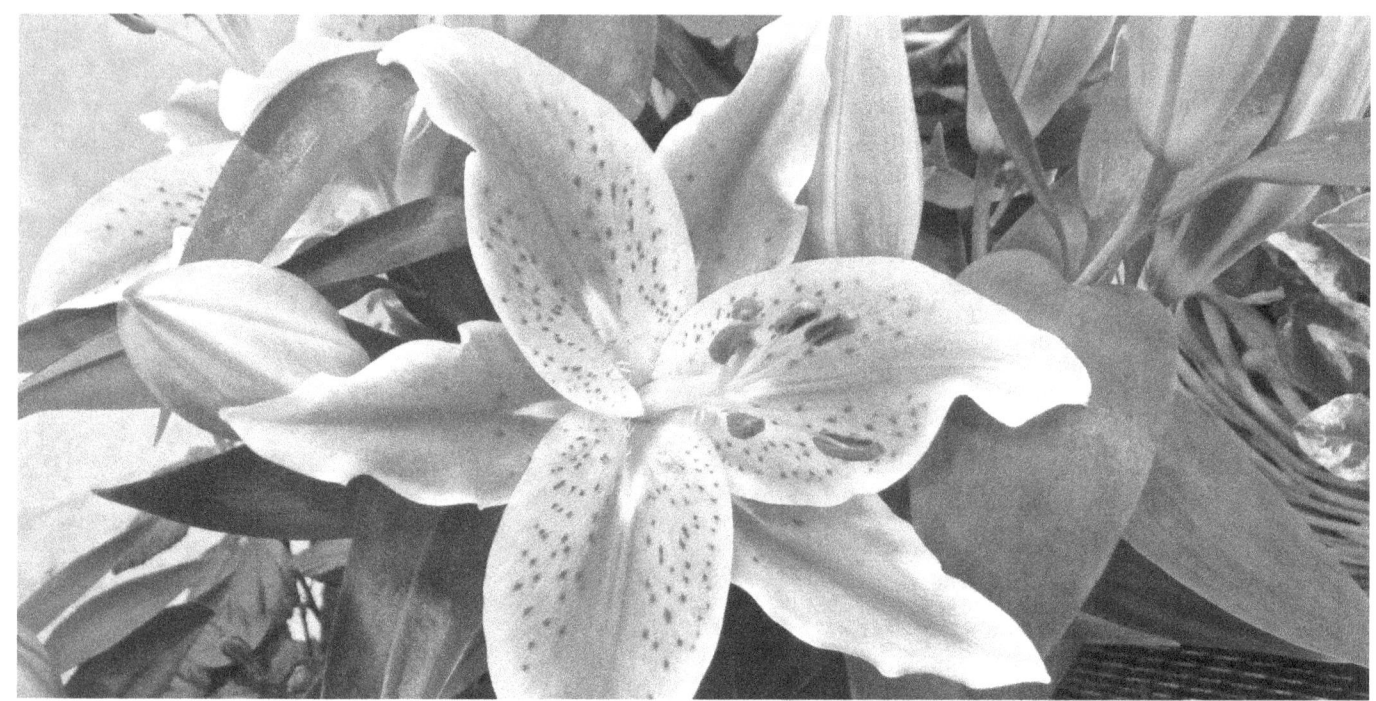

STAR GAZER LILY

The bulb powder can be used topically to dust skin sores. When made into a cream, by stirring the powder into distilled water and gradually heating to 60 degrees C, it is then applied when cooled to post surgical nasal bleeding. It begins to dissolve after three hours and disappears after 14 hours. *Chinese J of ENT* 1954 1:20.

A new weight loss formula, containing barley and *L. brownii* has been developed for commercial sales. Laboratory testing indicates efficacy in reduction of adipose tissue.

Studies have shown the bulb to contain anti-histamines. It combines well with Job's Tears seed to treat dry coughs, thick mucous and lung abscess.

Mimaki et al, *Biological and Pharmaceutical Bulletin* 1995 18:3 showed compounds from the bulbs active against human cervical cancer cells, human malignant tumor cells, pancreatic cancer, osteosarcoma, human gastric cancer, pheochromocytoma and HeLa cells.

Lilin, is a recently identified protein with strong anti-fungal and mitogenic activity; as well as inhibition of HIV-1 reverse transcriptase. It is similar to a polypeptide from *Luffa cylindrica* seed. Wang H et al, *Life Sci* 2002 70(9): 1075-84.

**CAUTION**- Do not use in cold windy conditions with phlegm, or in spleen deficiency with diarrhea.

Lily flower is known by the Chinese as the plant for forgetting care and sorrow. They believe eating or drinking a tea of the flower helps one to forget unpleasant memories and sadness. It is high in iron and helps build the blood. It is often prescribed for fright-induced palpitations, insomnia and dreaminess.

The Star Gazer lily bulb contains steroidal saponins with anti-tumor activity. Work by Nakamura et al, published in *Phytochemistry* 1994 36(2): 463-7 found a methyl ester showed potent inhibitory activity on 12-0-tetradecanoylphorbol-13-acetate (TPA)-stimulated 32P incorporation into phospholipids of HeLa cells.

Blackberry Lily rhizomes are used in Traditional Chinese Medicine. The plant is called **SHE KAN,** or **SHE GAN** due to the long stem, which looks like a launching rod. It is know as arrow shaft or shooting dryness. It is also known as **JIAO JIAN CAO.**

The root is bitter and cold, and affects mainly the lung and liver meridians.

It is used for dispelling heat, soothing swollen or sore throats, expelling phlegm and relieving coughs, and painful chest conditions. If excessive yellow phlegm, combine with balloon flower root or licorice root.

The root reduces the pain and swelling of lesions, removes toxins and dispels blood stagnancy. Various studies suggest both anti-inflammatory and anti-oxidant properties.

In laboratory studies, ethanol extracts of the root lower blood pressure of rabbits, while increasing, at the same time, the amplitude, or strength of the pulse.

The root also possesses anti-fungal properties, useful in a variety of skin conditions. A decoction of the root is also used as a gargle for treating halitosis, and abscessed tonsils.

In one clinical trial, 87 patients with galacturia treated with decoction showed an 85% rate of effectiveness. In another, 104 patients showed over 90% relief. Zhong *Yi Zz Zhi* 1986 11:66.

The rhizomes contain tectorigenin and tectoridin that exhibit anti-angiogenesis activity and reduction of sarcoma 180 cancer cell lines. Jung SH et al, *Planta Medica* 2013 69:617-22.

The herb suggests estrogenic receptor activity, at least, *in vitro*. Zhang et al, *J Ethnopharm* 98 295-300. Tectorigenin may be a clinically useful estrogen receptor modulator. Seidlova-Wuttke D et al, *Phytomedicine* 2004 11: 392-403.

Tectorigenin and irigenin regulate prostate cancer cells by inhibiting proliferation through cell cycle regulation. Morrissey C et al, *Journal Urol* 2004 172: 2426-33.

Work by Thelen P et al, found isoflavones disrupt steroid receptor signaling in hormone sensitive cancers, and may be useful to prevent, or treat human prostate cancer. *Carcinogenesis* 2005 26: 1360-7.

Tectorigenin inhibits aldose reductase, and significantly inhibited sorbitol accumulation in the eye lens, sciatic nerves and red blood cells of diabetic rats. Jung SH et al, *Arch Pharmacal Res* 2004 27: 184-8.

Isoflorentin may be useful for the treatment of Parkinson's disease. Chen YM et al, *Anti-Corros Methods Mater* 2015 5(1): 238-42.

The above ground herb is sometimes substituted for Knotweed (*Polygonum aviculare*) in TCM, and known as **PIEN HSU** or **PIEN CHU**.

Do not use during pregnancy. A good review is Zhang L et al, *J Ethnopharm* 2016 186: 1-13.

David's Lily, or Lan Zhou lily contains testosterone as well as beta sitosterol, and stigmasterol. Beta sitosterol is a gonadotrophic compound that stimulates the ovaries and testes, increasing and optimizing steroid hormone production. In human men, it is both androgenic and anti-estrogenic.

It contains emodin, found in Rhubarb and Rumex species, and possesses anti-cancer activity.

The bulbs are used for coughs and colds, as well as lung and breast cancer. It is often used interchangeably with Brown's Lily.

## HOMEOPATHY

Tiger Lily (*L. tigrinum*) is indicated in complaints associated with prolapse of the uterus during menopause; various bearing down sensations and left sided ovaritis. Hot tempered, violent, cursing and swearing.

There may be burning and heat in the palms of the hands and soles of feet.

There are accompanying nervous cardio-circulatory complaints, and a lot of irritable emotional discord or upset.

It is worthy of trial in the nausea and vomiting of pregnancy when nothing else has worked.

Exaggeration of one's importance, fault finding, envious, averse to or aggravated by consolation. Feel better by being busy.

Sleep is un-refreshed, with disagreeable dreams. There may be great heat and lassitude in the afternoon, with throbbing throughout the body. Better from fresh air.

**DOSE**- The middle and higher potencies have done best (30-200th). The curative action is sometimes slow in developing itself. The mother tincture is made from the whole fresh plant in flower.

Provings collated by Payne on nine provers with tincture, 1x, 3x, 5c, and 300th dilution in 1867-9; proving by Dunham on six females at tincture, 3x, 30x in 1869; Payne with five provers with crude drug or 1x in 1886, and then collation of six male provers with crude drug in 1888. Kenyon contributed clinical effect on 48 year old patient from 30th dilution three times daily for four days.

*Lilium superbum* is for mental exhaustion, headache, dullness of the eye, epistaxis, paleness and sickly expression of countenance; bitter taste in mouth; burning of the mouth and esophagus' increased appetite; spleen discomfort; constipation; oppression of chest; acceleration of the pulses; weakness of the extremities; languor, debility, prostration and restlessness.

**DOSE**- Turk' Cap Lily tincture was prepared from the fresh bulb and proved by Dr. E Reading at unknown attenuations. See Allen.

### MATERIA POETICA

*Lilium tigrinum*

She came into the office
Impatient, in a stew
Snapping at the office staff
Complaining about you
She said you didn't treat her
The way she felt you should
I do declare her furious
No one could make things good
*Her head was feeling crazy*
*Wild, with strange ideas*
And sexually excited
With much religious fear
She certainly keeps busy
With iron on the fire
All this fruitless stuff she does
To suppress her hot desire
Lilium Tigrinum
Despairs to walk in sin
She is angry and hysterical
And you can never win
Nothing will ever please her
Except perhaps some meat
She has two conflicting sides
That cause her endless grief
Tiger Lily does not smile
It's not a joyful state
When sex and religion intertwine
Despair is oft their fate.

**SYLVIA CHATROUX MD**

## ESSENTIAL OILS

Although no essential oils are produced, the Madonna Lily (*L. candidum*), yields an absolute that is sometimes produced in Bermuda and available on a limited basis.

The ancient Greeks made a perfume from the Madonna Lily, called **SUSINON**.

The absolute is a dark orange to yellow colour. The odour is delicately floral with a pronounced oily, waxy top note. Its balsamic sweet body is reminiscent of narcissus and boronia; with an undertone that is sweet like figs or plums. The odour is tenacious and would mix well with other exotics in perfumes. One high quality perfume, Zinnia, uses the true product. It is estimated that less than 2 kilograms of the product is produced.

Head space analysis has identified phenylethyl alcohol 24% as the major constituent, as well as linalool 15%, heptadecane 8% alpha heptadecane 5.5%, phenylacetaldehyde 4.2%, methyl palmitate 3.5% and palmitic acid 2.5%.

Kappus of Germany use *L. candidum* extract in soap; useful for those prone to acne.

Stargazer Lily would certainly make an interesting absolute, and is hardy to the prairie zones.

## PETAL OIL

The oil of white lily is prepared thus. Take a half-pound of good quality olive oil and a quarter pound of fresh flower petals. Put this together in a glass vessel and set it in the sun for 14 days.

Used warm, this oil brings sores quickly to a head, eases swellings and is very good for oozing scale on the scalp. The petals that sink to the bottom of the oil are of special use for all manner of livid sores, or burns from fires, boiling water and oil, and so forth. They ease the pain promptly, draw out the burn, and heal the injury. These petals are also good for plague blisters. The oil of white lily should not be ignored in clysters, particularly in cases of hard, inflamed constipation, colic of the bowels and diarrhea. **SAUER**

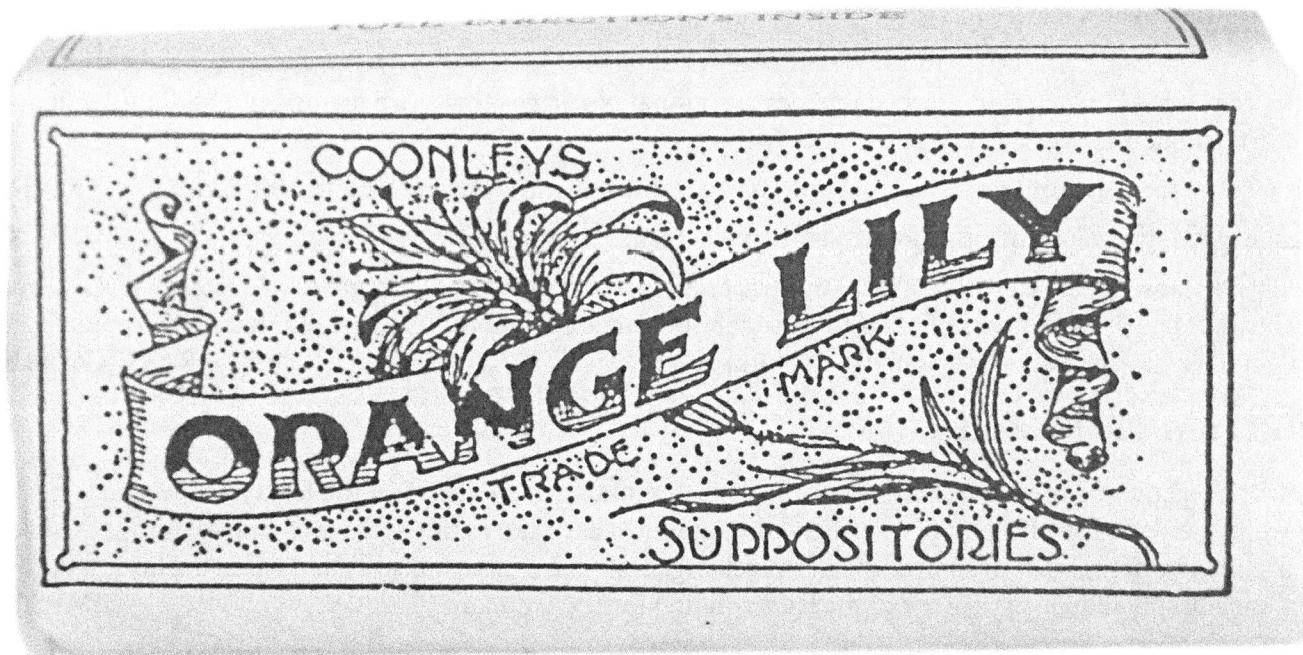

ORANGE LILY SUPPOSITORIES

## HYDROSOL

The distilled water takes away all manner of freckles and burns on the face that are caused by the sun. Dip a little piece of cloth in it and lay it over the sunburn sores where they are tender. Also, for the mouth and throat, gargle it in the throat, and rinse the mouth with it. It will hinder putrefaction and inflammation. Internally, Lily water strengthens the head, restores speech and is good for coughs, congestion of the lungs, and pulmonary consumption.                                                                                                      **SAUER**

Brunschwig, in the Book of Distillation, notes that the petal distillation of Madonna Lily yield a water that is good for reducing redness of eyes, cleansing and clearing face, clearing heat about heart and liver. It is taken internally by women whose womb has fallen (prolapsed uterus), or during labour to ease delivery. It was also combined with rose water for women with diseases of the reproductive system, pain about navel, provoking menses or expelling a dead fetus. It may be mixed with honey for impetigo. It was also suggested to women inclined to lechery.

## FLOWER ESSENCES

Day Lily essence is a practical remedy, especially the yellow variety, which helps us to make decisions and commitments and stick to them. It will help you realize just how precious days and moments are. When you take the essence, you may find yourself first taking care of mundane matters. Old baggage wastes energy and prevents us from becoming all we were meant to be.                                                      **JADE MOUNTAIN**

Easter lily flower essence is for those who have feelings that sex is impure or unclean, or those who suffer inner conflict over sexuality. The flower essence will help one get in touch with the inner purity of soul, especially the ability to integrate sexuality and spirituality.                                            **FLOWER ESSENCE SOCIETY**

Stargazer Lily opens the pathway in the heart between the creative impulse, centered in the second chakra, and the sixth chakra (or third eye) through which creative vision moves out into the world. This essence doesn't increase creativity, but helps ease the bottleneck in the heart chakra caused by fear or lack of confidence.                                                                                                      **OLIVE**

Stargazer lily creates clarity of vision. It helps one to feel more secure in one's inner knowing and wisdom.                                                                                                      **ILMINSTER**

Turk's Cap Lily (*L. martagon*) essence releases emotional blockages that were formed in childhood when we couldn't defend ourselves against abuse or bullying.

This essence frees us from uncertainty about our own abilities and restores our self-confidence.          **KORTE**

Orange Day Lily essence helps re-found self-respect, resulting from bullying.                    **MIRIANA**

Daylily is the essence of self worth. It helps one trust our inner knowledge and improves self-esteem. It is symbolic of rebirth. It helps us see how futile it is to worry about things beyond our control and that being centered and living in the present is the way to change the future.                                            **RAVENWORKS**

## SPIRITUAL PROPERTIES

There is a legend in Korea which tells how a hermit found a tiger, wounded in the leg by an arrow. He healed the wound and the tiger became his constant companion. Years later, as the tiger was dying of old age, he asked his friend to keep his body near him. The hermit changed the beast into a tiger lily and when the hermit himself died, the lily spread to every corner of the land, looking for the old man.                                            **SIMPSON**

If we look at the petals of the...Easter Lily we will see that the union of opposites is portrayed in the structure of the plant itself. The petals are a beautiful, luminous, milky white, embodying the ideal of purity. At the same time the sexual parts of the flower protrude beyond the ends of the petals in an obvious and unabashed fashion.

The male parts, the anthers, are coated with an abundant, heavy golden pollen. The female part, the stigma, drips with a white exudate. (It) represents a picture of what would normally be considered opposites: purity and sexuality. Yet it is able to unite these under one vegetable roof.

The contention and reconciliation of opposites corresponds to the healing qualities embodied in the plant. In the mental/emotional state we will usually see evidence of the contention of idealism with the need to fulfill personal desire. The female patient will often suffer from a "nun/whore complex". She may be sexually indiscriminant, feel unclean, or that her partner makes her unclean. On the other hand, she may entertain a puritanical restraint which cuts her off from a healthy relationship.

In men, there is a tendency to idealize women or the opposite....any excessive idealism tend to create the Lily state of mind.                                                                                            **WOOD**

The fire of the (Easter) Lily is noticeable and cannot be overlooked. The sticky substance that oozes from the stamen has an intoxicating perfume. The luminous petals and the milk white pearl relate to the feminine divine and the fertilizing power of the moon. The flower is a vessel of Divine Love in which the sexual fires of passion and the waters of emotion join in perfect harmony.                                                **RUDGINSKY**

Tiger Lily is associated with the vitality and the headstrong competitive nature of Aries, ruled by Mars; which gives us the ability to act and assert ourselves based on our personal desires.

In times when there is much to do, we try to avoid hasty and rash decisions. In times when the best action is no action, we can try to not force things to happen. The tiger teaches the importance of taking one step at a time to meet the demands of each moment and each situation. Each movement relates to the whole and is key to the desired goal.                                                                                           **RUDGINSKY**

Blackberry Lily flower is related to attachment for the divine. It wraps itself around the Divine and find all its support in Him so as to be sure never to leave Him.                                        **THE MOTHER**

A fundamental expression of individuality is sexuality and reproduction…This family's biology perpetuates conventional uniformity in its tendency to asexual reproduction, which produces homogeneous progeny. Its activity is fruitless, in that no fruit is produced for reproduction. This is in contrast to sexual reproduction, which creates individuals and unique offspring. It is fitting that these flowers signify chastity, virginity, and Immaculate Conception. The family members have been used and associated with both fruitfulness and fruitlessness such as sterility, fertility, brides, blessed unions, conception and successful pregnancy, menses, fecundity and as aphrodisiacs…It is necessary to be sexual to have an earthly presence. A completely celibate population, pure and celestially perfect as it may be, will soon be relinquishing their earth-bound existence for good…Those in this family are convinced it is not possible to be pure and sexual at the same time…Knowledge, including sexual awakening, is the path to a full, fruitful human life of contraindications, temptations, growth and individual expression. Reconciling this dilemma is the essence of Liliales.                                      **VERMEULEN**

## PERSONALITY TRAITS

White Lily is a time-honored remedy for the female genital tract. Its general tendency is to clean and purify the tract. Its relative, Tiger Lily, is used as a cramp remedy. The latter, being red, robust and vibratory in appearance, has a stronger influence on uterine contractions than the former. The traits overlap, however and Easter Lily will sometimes cure (or cause) cramps, while Tiger Lily will remove cysts. The proper prescription depends on the constitution of the patient: Tiger Lily is better suited to those who are vibrant and rowdy, Easter Lily to those who personify purity.                                                                            **WOOD**

"Oh, Tiger lily", said Alice to one which was waving gracefully about in the wind, "I *wish* you could talk"…"we can talk", said the Tiger lily. "When there is anybody worth talking to". When Alice has got over her surprise, she asks 'almost in a whisper, "Can all the flowers talk?"

"As well as you can", said the Tiger lily, "and a great deal louder".                            **ALICE IN WONDERLAND**

...That Hercules, who Jupiter had by Alcumena, was put to Juno's breasts whilest she was asleepe; and after the sucking there fell away abundance of milk, and that one part was spilt in the heavens, and the other upon the earth; and that of this sprang the Lilly, and other the circle in the heavens called Lacteus Circulus, or the Milky Way.

**GERARD**

Even though they're a bit on the weedy side, I love Tiger Lilies.

They are remarkably adept at reproducing themselves, using four routes to new plant production. Bulb offshoots (bulblets), bulb scales, seeds, and even aerial bulbils- little black nodules that appear where each leaf meets the stem- are all able to regenerate a brand new Tiger Lily. In fact, it seems that there's very little that could stop these tenacious tigers. Versatility and variety- words that aptly describe Tiger Lilies. They have truly mastered the art of the backup plan. Have you?

**G. MOHAMMED**

Julia Graves differentiates the mental states between Madonna lily and Easter lily. "The former has more sensitivity, bordering on clairvoyance". She has often verified the indications I found long ago, that this is a remedy for feel who feel a great conflict between the sexual and the spiritual, or are too sexual or too spiritual. She further notes that these lilies have a powerful feminizing element, making one more receptive and intuitive, and reducing fear about being vulnerable or feminine.

**WOOD**

Zhang Zhongjing (c. 200 CE) describes the use of lily bulb in Synopsis of Prescriptions of the Golden Chamber. In fact, he named a disease pattern after the plant: "lily bulb syndrome". He writes:

"The patient wants to eat, but is reluctant to swallow food, and is unwilling to speak. Or he prefers to lie in bed, yet cannot lie quietly due to restlessness. He may want to walk about, but soon becomes tired. Now and then he may enjoy eating certain delicacies, but at other times he cannot even tolerate the smell of food. He may feel either cold or hot, but without fever or chill. He also has a bitter taste in his mouth and passes reddish urine. No drugs appear able to cure the syndrome. After taking medicine, acute vomiting and diarrhea may occur. The disease 'haunts' the patient, and though his appearance is normal, he is actually suffering. His pulse is somewhat speedy".

**WOOD**

The lily was the sign of the prostitute in Paris in the 19th century. It is an intensely sexual-looking flower. It's the combination and conflict of sex and religion. Without sex they are too restless to pray. With sex on the brain, they pray for their soul. They need sex before praying to calm them down, but sex is a sin, they are thinking. They enjoy and they need it, and yet it's a sin. Typically it's needed by the religious widow or divorcee who needs sex and finds her attention drawn to men's genitals or vice versa.

They are irritable, hurried, must do several things at once, and they have an excess of frustrated sexual energy. In extreme there is nymphomania and the same in men. They can have what they describe as a wild feeling in head.

**PETER CHAPPELL**

The principle of opposites and the balancing of tension in counterparts are fundamental to life. As the embodiment of ambiguity between opposites, lilies express double meanings and consequently their healing qualities may serve to promote reconciliation of these oppositions. Reconciliation is defined as restoring friendship or union, bringing to agreement or contentment, adjusting, composing and regaining. All this must be done for the split psyche to be in a state of healthy integrations.

**VERMEULEN**

## RECIPES

**DAY LILY ROOT TINCTURE**- 1-3 ml.

**DAY LILY ROOT DECOCTION**- 6-10 grams

**DAY LILY FRESH SHOOTS**- 15-30 gr.

**DAY LILY DRIED FLOWER BUDS**- 15-30 grams

**TIGER LILY TINCTURE-** A tincture of the whole, fresh flowering plant is prepared at a 1:2 at 50%. Use only 5-10 drops as need. Use with moderation.

**TIGER LILY BULB- DECOCTION-** optimal extract of flavonoids is obtained at 1:30 ration of 80% ethanol, with ultrasonic treatment for forty minutes, twice at temperature of 70 degrees Celsius. Up to 99.25% flavonoids are obtained in this manner.

**EASTER LILY FLOWER TINCTURE-** One drop once daily for 10-14 days before period. It is made from the fresh flower in 60% alcohol.

**MADONNA LILY INFUSION-** Boil 24 ounces of water and pour over two ounces of lily bulb finely cut. Steep for 30 minutes. Strain and sweeten with honey.

Take one tbs. or more 3-4 times daily.

**MADONNA OINTMENT-** In a crockpot place two ounces of fresh, finely cut lily bulb and one pint of sweet almond oil at low heat for 24 hours. Strain and while hot combine with four ounces of beeswax. Pour and allow to cool.

**BLACKBERRY LILY ROOT DECOCTION-** 6-9 grams.

**CORAL LILY DECOCTION-** 5-15 grams. This remedy is not meant for those with cold and damp constitution.

**BROWN'S LILY DECOCTION-** 10 to 30 grams

**TINCTURE-** 2-5 ml. Do not use in coughing from wind cold or lung phlegm conditions.

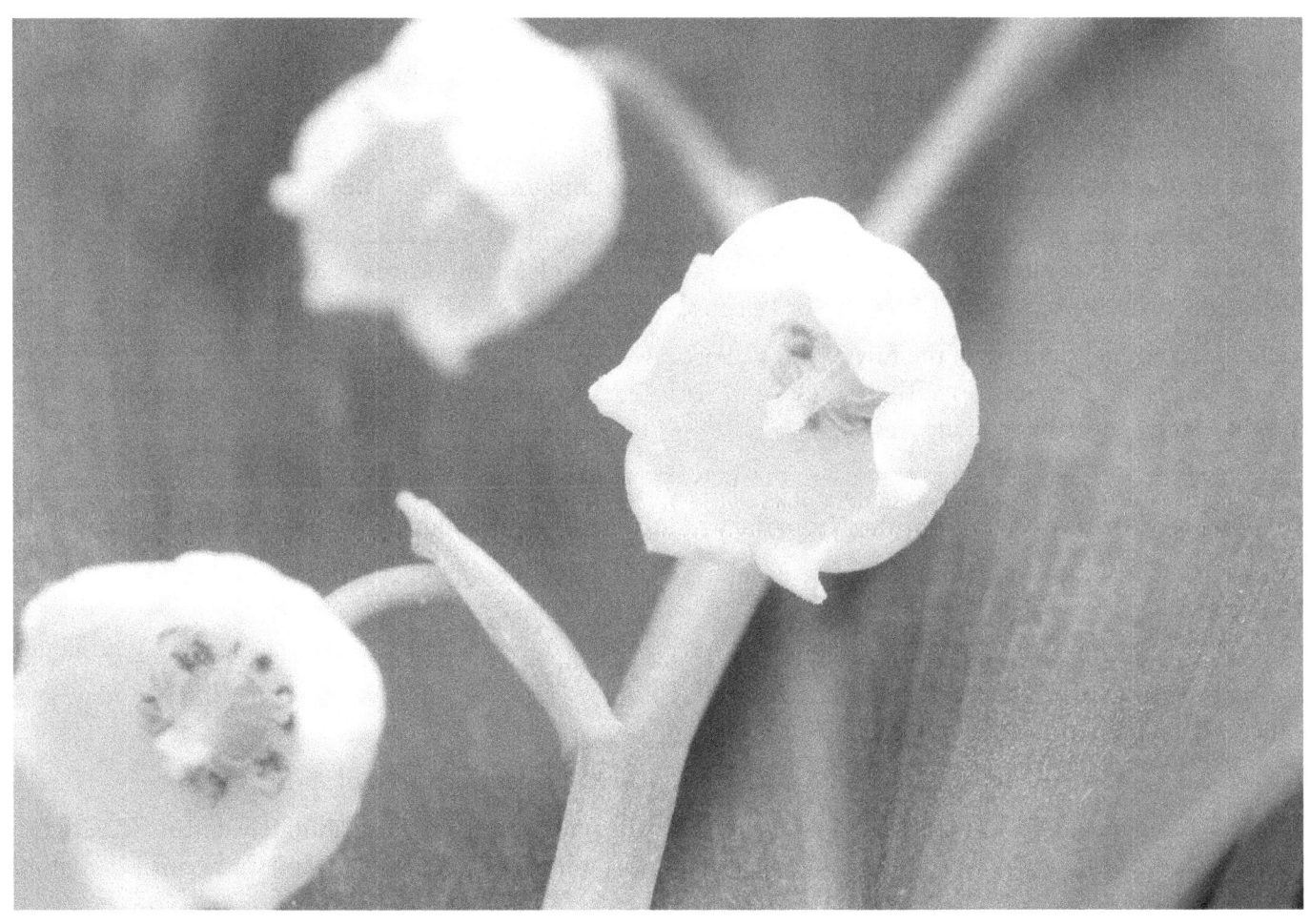

CLOSE UP— LILY OF THE VALLEY FLOWERS

## LILY OF THE VALLEY
(*Convallaria majalis* L.)
**PARTS USED**- roots, leaves, flowers

No flower amid the garden fairer grows
Than the sweet lily of the lowly vale,

The queen of flowers.                                                                                                           **KEATS**

The Naiad-like Lily of the Vale,
Whom youth makes so fair and passion so pale,
That the light of its tremulous bells is seen
Through their pavilions of tender green.                                                             **P. B. SHELLEY**

And stooping Lilies of the Valley,
That love with shades and dews of daily,
And bending droop on slender threads
With broad hood-leaves above their heads like white robed maids in summer hours
beneath umbrellas shunning showers.                                                           **JOHN CLARE**

Convallis is from the classic Latin meaning a valley enclosed on all sides; **VALLUM**, an earthen wall or palisades. Hence **VALLUS**, meaning stake or pale, then onto Old French **VAL** meaning, valley. The plant was originally named *Lillium convallium*.

Majalis suggests the month of May; named after the ancient Italic Earth Goddess **MAIA**, the daughter of Atlas. This, in turn, is from the Latin **MAIOR**, meaning greater.

May is the month of increase, greater and renewed growth, and hence major. May 26 is the birth date of the herb. In the language of flowers, it depicts the return of happiness and unconscious sweetness associated with May.

The plant and fragrance are sometimes called Muguet, also from French meaning valley. The flowers are a customary May Day gift in Paris. It is the national flower of Finland and former Yugoslavia. In old astrology books, the plant is placed under Mercury or Hermes.

Legend has it the fragrance of the Lily of the Valley draws the nightingale from hedge to bush, and leads him to choose his mate in recesses of the glades. Another legend suggests chaste white flowers are a symbol of the Virgin Mary, appearing in many painting.

The flower is considered, by some, as a sign of Christ's second coming.

An older legend relays the plant sprang from the wounds of St. Leonard during his battle with a dragon.

The even, step-like arrangement of the flowers along the stalk inspired medieval monks to name it Ladder to Heaven.

Lily of the Valley flowers are small but sweetly perfumed, and over the centuries came to be associated with spring festivals and Whitsuntide. An old custom in Germany was to gather bunches on Whit Monday, and called May Bloom, or **MAIGLOCKCHEN**.

Earlier, the plant was sacred to Ostara, the Anglo-Saxon and Germanic goddess of spring.

A famous carnival near Rambouillet, France, held in May has carts, and floats all elaborately decorated with the flower spikes. The flowers formed the bridal bouquet at the wedding of Prince William and Catherine Middleton.

At one time, bonfires were lit and flowers thrown into the flames as an offering.

In the 4th century *Herbarium of Apuleius*, it was known as Glovewort, and prized for care of the hands.

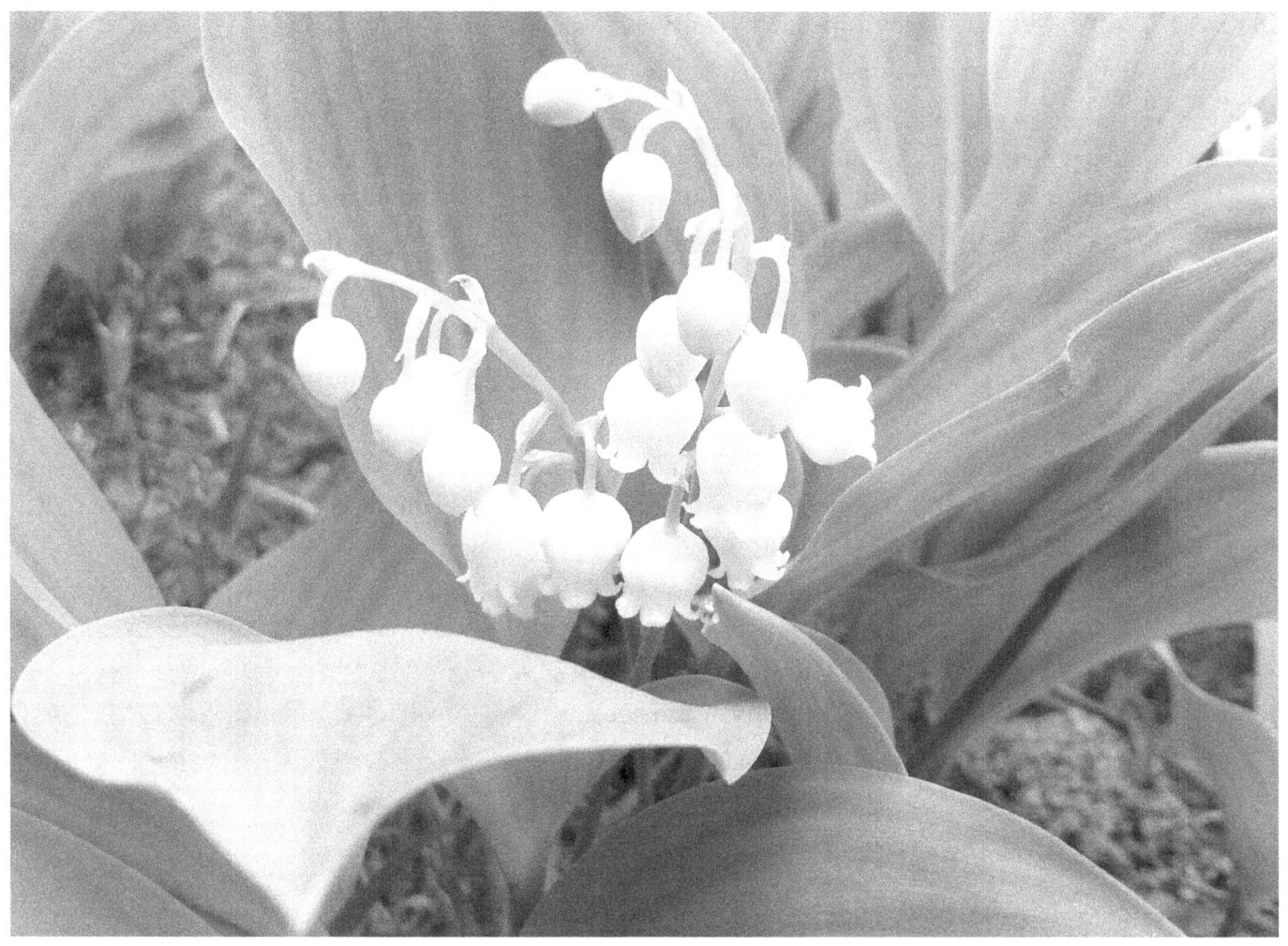

LILY OF THE VALLEY

In the 16<sup>th</sup> century, herbalists recommended infused flowers for gout; the whole plant steeped in wine to strengthen the memory and soothe inflamed eyes.

William Cole (1657) wrote the plant, "recrutes a weak memory".

Culpepper agreed that the distilled water of the flowers in wine, "restores lost speech, helps the palsy, and is excellently good in the apoplexy; comforts the heart and vital spiritual."

Matthiolus observed it strengthened the heart and alleviated spasms and palpitations. Porcher wrote the flowers, "have a delightful odour, resembling that of musk, and when dried and powdered are much employed as a sternutatory, acting sometimes quite violently." The dried, powdered flowers are today still used as snuff.

Russian peasants relied on it for dropsy caused by pulmonary edema and other cardiac insufficiencies.

Early Ukrainian settlers in Alberta ate the fresh flowers or made an infusion of the dried flowers for breathing problems.

Traditionally, the herb was used for weak contractions in labour, epilepsy, conjunctivitis and leprosy, uses no longer having much scientific basis.

For relieving headaches, including migraines, a few flowers dipped in wine, and eaten are said very effective. "An infusion of the flowers constantly taken instead of tea is an excellent remedy for nervous headaches, trembling of the limbs and other similar complaints."

In parts of Germany, a wine is made from flowers and raisins, while the root was traditionally powdered as a snuff.

Golden water, the hydrosol was stored in golden or silver containers.

The whole plant can be utilized for healing farm animals, according to Juliette de Bairacli Levy. She considered the flowers most potent for helping quiet heart disorders, and the mild narcotic properties for nerves, hysteria and epilepsy. The leaves cool skin inflammation; the seeds reduce fevers and kill round and thread worms.

The roots are mildly aperient and soothing to the intestines.

During Victorian times, the forced flowers were a popular winter decoration, and exported from Germany as Berlin Crowns.

The plant is hardy to zone 2, in protected nooks. Work by Oinonen, *Acta For Fenn* 1969 97 estimates plants can live more than 670 years.

Un-developed plant growth can be sped up by use of anaesthetics such as chloroform. Simply wet a cotton swab with a few drops and let the winter buds absorb vapors for a few hours. Plant the bulbs and you'll be amazed at how much sooner they develop leaves and flowers.

This is interesting as during the First World War, it was used to treat soldiers who had suffered from the effects of mustard gas, due to a strengthening of the nervous system. Leaf infusions were traditionally used in Wiltshire, England as a nerve tonic, to strengthen the memory and restore speech after stroke.

It was the floral emblem of the former Yugoslavia, and became the national flower of Finland in 1967.

Lily of the Valley (*C. majalis var keiskei*) is cited by taxonomists as a sub-species or variety. In China and Japan, it is known as *C. keiskei*.

## MEDICINAL

**CONSTITUENTS**- whole plant- convallarin desglucocheirotoxin, convallosaponins, convallogenin B, thymidine, rhodexin A, rhodexoside, sarmentosigenin A, tholloside, bipindogenin, convallatoxin (40-45% of total alkaloids) locundioside, nearly 40 cardenolide glycosides, associated with nine different aglycones (23 in aerial parts) have been isolated so far; as well as 8 flavonoids, saponins, essential oils, asparagine, convallarinic and chelidonic acid, malic acid, citric acid, caffeic acid, carotene, sugars.
flower- 0.1-0.4% cardiac glycosides (cardenolides), isorhamnetin (quercitin), convallamarin (glucoside). The main glycoside is convallatoxin, which converts to strophanthidin and (-)-rhamnose.
seeds- 0.5% cardiac glycosides (highest content of cardenolides in plant.
leaves- 0.2-0.4% cardiac glycosides, flavonoid glycosides, vitamin C, silver, trace of progesterone (57 mcg/100 grams) in fresh leaf.
leaves, flowers and seed- lokundjoside, saponins.
root- canarigenin-3-0-alpha-rhamno-pyranosyl (cardenolide); saponin convallamaroside, convallasaponins A-D.

Lily of the Valley is most useful for treating cardiac arrhythmia due to mitral stenosis and coronary diseases, such as pericarditis.

It vasodilates, and opens capillary circulation, making it invaluable in chronic nervous depression, memory loss, and peripheral artery deficiency.

Strokes, concussions, paralysis and cerebro-vascular ischemia may all benefit from doses of this herb. Infusions are useful for restoration of speech after cardiac arrest.

In the case of cardiac asthma, left-ventricular heart failure, and congestive heart failure, the diuretic activity of the herb is excellent. It lowers the elevated left ventricle diastolic pressure, and pathologically raised venous blood pressure. It is worth noting that vitamin E supplementation is contra-indicated in left ventricular disorders.

The herb slows the ventricular rate in atrial fibrillation or flutter, and acts only on the heart muscle, and not the vagus nerve, like digitalis.

Work by Hoffmann and Bigger, in Goodman and Gilman's *The Pharmacological Basis of Therapeutics*, 8th Edition 1990, suggest both mechanical and electrical modification of the vascular system. The cardiac glycosides exert a number of effects on neural tissue and thus indirectly influence the heart and modify vascular resistance and capacitance.

Chronic nervous depression and catatonic states may respond to Lily of the Valley leaf and flower.

Pulmonary edema and severe heart failure in the elderly can be greatly relieved. This is without the toxicity of digitalis, or foxglove, and acting more rapidly.

When I had a clinical practice, I had the opportunity to observe the potency of this herb.

One evening, my colleague received a call of distress at our clinic, from a client whose father was in hospital, with uncontrollable pulmonary edema. He begged for help, and so the two of us took a small 10ml vial of lily of the valley tincture to the hospital. It was about 8 pm, just before the end of visiting hours. Two drops, every ten minutes were given for the next four hours. By morning, there was significant improvement and he turned the corner of concern. The medical staff knew none of this, and accounted for it as a "miracle".

Nausea and vomiting may present itself in some patients, but this is generally mild and rare. It combines well with hawthorn for treating arteriosclerosis and gout; and with dandelion leaf for dropsy (left-sided heart failure).

The principal cardenolide glycoside is convallatoxin, but the plant contains many minor cardenolides.

Convallatoxin is poorly absorbed as a pure product, but according to Weiss, other compounds aid in its absorption.

Convallatoxin may be useful for treating triple negative breast cancers, derived largely from African Americans. The antiproliferative effects are via a variety pathways. Kaushik V et al, *Cell Death Discov* 2017 3:17009.

The compound possess potent anti-cancer effect on non-small cell lung cancer (A549) cells, via non-classical inhibition of Na,K-ATPase. Schneider NF et al, *Mol Cell Biochem* 2017 428(1-2): 23-39. Additional research suggests the tumor suppressor p53 is important in the action of the compound. Kaushik V et al, *J Cell Physiol* 2016 Sept 23.

Cytomegalovirus is a pathogenic virus that attacks immune compromised patients. The present anti-virals have significant adverse side effect on blood and kidneys. Convallatoxin inhibits primary isolates of the virus, including those resistant to ganciclovir, at doses low enough for healthy cells to tolerate. Cohen T et al, *J Virol* 2016 90(23): 10715-27.

It also appears to by cytotoxic to colon cancer cells. Feith J et al, *J Nat Prod* 2009 72(11): 1969-74.

Strophanthidin, as a degraded constituent, has been found in animal studies to increase contractility of right ventricle, increase diastolic relaxation of both ventricles and increase pressure of the pulmonary artery. Frantsuzova et al, *Farmakol Toksikol* 1985 48:4.

Like linden flowers and hawthorn, the herb softens accumulated deposits in the arteries, and blood, as well as joints and muscles. It possesses anti-tumour activity, including those of a cancerous nature, by promoting drainage processes in metabolic organs.

For arterial hypertension combine it with gentian root, while for excitation combine with motherwort. In general, I combine it with hawthorn for a wide variety of cardiovascular concerns, usually at 1:10 ratio.

Lily of the Valley relieves urinary tract infections, and when kidney and bladder stones are present. Leaf infusion, taken cold, when the flower is in bloom, is a good diuretic.

Convallamaroside possesses anti-fungal and antibiotic activity. Work by Tschesche, *Pharmacognosy and Phytochemistry*, 1971 suggests these effects are not therapeutically useful, since it forms a complex in the body with cholesterol.

Convallamaroside is a steroidal saponin that shows significant inhibitory effect on angiogenesis. This prevents new blood vessel growth from kidney tumor and sarcoma cancer cells. Nartowska et al, *Acta Pol Pharm* 2004 61(4): 279-82.

Study by Sauter and Wolfensberger found the berry contains cytotoxic activity, as well as preventing replication of the avian influenza virus. However, the berry is toxic, and not used in herbal medicine.

The compound chelidonic acid may help regulate depression associated with inflammation. Jeong HJ et al, *Exp Biol Med* (Maywood) 2016 241(14): 1559-67. This acid is also found in the rhizomes of *Chelidonium majus*, a member of the poppy family.

All other parts of the plant can be used. The flowers are picked in full bloom in May or June, the leaves in June-August, and the rhizomes, if desired in the fall after the tops have died down. Late harvests in July and August give higher yield (0.5%) of glycosides.

Cardenolide glycosides from the root show cytotoxic activity to human sub-mandibular gland carcinoma. Higano T et al, *Chem Pharm Bull* (Tokyo) 2007 55(2): 337-9.

The pulp of berries contains traces of cardenolides but the seeds contain about 0.45% of water-soluble glycosides, mainly cardenolides.

An interesting ouabain compound (cardenolide) has been identified in the adrenals and brains of humans. Discovered by Nakanishi et al in 1996, this cardiotonic factor appears to be involved in renal function, and in the pathogenesis of hypertension. It is a natural hormone that stimulates the parasympathetic nervous system and inhibits the sympathetic.

It is a traditional arrow poison found in the roots, seeds, leaves and stems of *Acokanthera schimperi* and *Strophanthus gratus*, native to east Africa.

Rhodexin A has been found to be more cytotoxic than ouabain against K562 cancer cell lines. It is also a cardiotonic. Masuda T et al, *Biosci Biotechnol Biochem* 2003 67(6): 1401-4.

The cardiac glycosides are only 10% absorbed and 50% eliminated in 24 hours.

An extract of *C. majalis* var. *keiskei* may be useful for treating salivary gland cancer. It targets myeloid cell leukemia-1 and induces apoptosis. Lee HE et al, *Head Neck* 2016 38(suppl 1): E761-70.

A recent U.S. publication found in 2639 cases of lily of the valley ingestion, that although 6.1% of patients suffered symptom side-effects, only three had severe symptoms, and none died. Krenzelok et al, 1996.

See Frohne & Pfander, *Poisonous Plants* volume 2 for more information.

## HOMEOPATHY

Lily of the Valley increases the energy of heart's action, and renders it more regular. It is of use when the ventricles are over-distended and dilation begins, and when there is an absence of compensatory hypertrophy, and when venous stasis is marked.

The patient may be irritable, with a dull headache and intellect, and some degree of depression. The headache moves from the vertex to the temples.

The nose and lips are raw and sore, with a distortion of vision of an imaginary gray spot three inches square. When reading, all letters look the same, and there is a heaviness of the upper eyelids, with a dull right eye pain and a pulsating pain in the left ear with pain.

There is grating of teeth and a copper taste in the mouth upon waking. The tongue may feel scalded or sore, with a thick, heavy, dirty coating.

The back of the throat may feel raw upon inspiring.

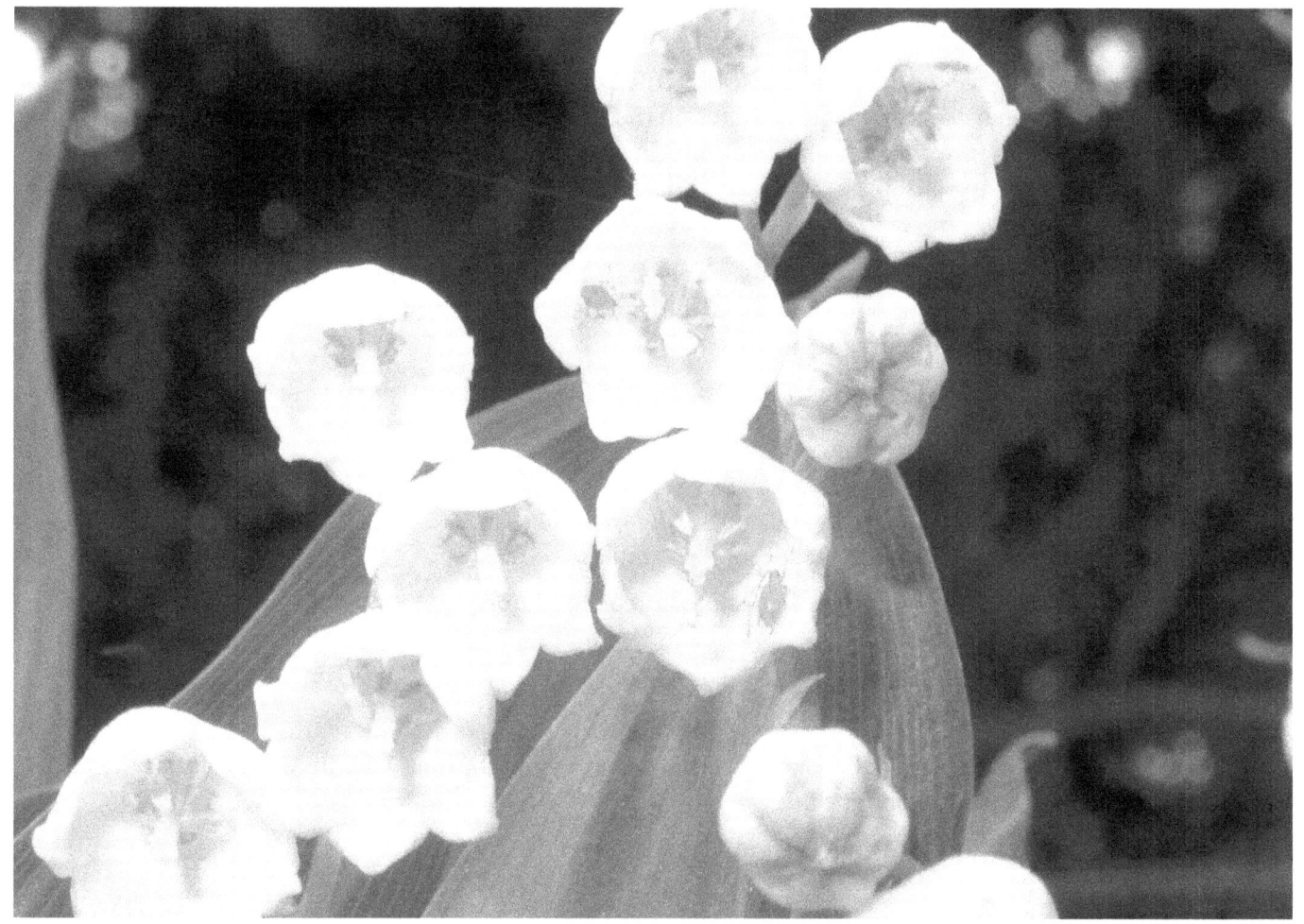

LILY OF THE VALLEY

Clothing feels tight, with movement in the abdomen like the fist of a child. The digestive tract involves fatty-tasting eructations, nausea after meals with mucous vomiting, and a dull colic like pain in umbilical region.

The bladder feels distended, with frequent, scanty, offensive, cow-like odor upon urination.

The female may suffer great soreness of the uterine region, with sympathetic heart palpitations. There may be pain of the sacro-iliac with sciatic pain running down the legs.

Pulmonary congestion and dyspnea while walking, may be accompanied by a feeling as if the heart is beating throughout the chest. Sensation as if the heart ceased beating, then starting very suddenly. Tobacco heart, especially when due to cigarettes, with angina pectoris, and rapid, irregular pulse also present.

Back and extremities are painful, with trembling hands and aching in wrist and ankles. The patient is chilly down the spine, followed by fever, and little sweat.

One distinct symptom is the presence of tiny nodules on the front of the thigh, like insect bites, that itch strongly.

The patient feels better in open air, and worse in a warm room, feeling sleepy and restless during sleep.

A split or dissociation from one's own feelings, helps make one invulnerable to dangerous situations. Indifference takes the place of unpleasant feelings like fear, pain, grief and pain.

**DOSE**- Third attenuation. In cases of heart involvement use 1-15 drops of the mother tincture. This is prepared from the whole fresh plant in flower. Proving by Lane and self experimentation in 1883-4, and Sutherland in 883 with tincture. A dream proving by Santos & Konig of 20 females and 8 males at 30c was done in 1994.

## FLOWER OIL

The fresh flowers may be picked and sun infused in cold pressed canola oil. If the summer temperatures are below normal, you may have to use a gentle simmer on the stove, or in crock pot. The scent is extremely subtle, and after two days of sun infusion, you must squeeze them out and replace with new flowers. Repeat 6 to 10 times, until desired scent appears, or until you run out of patience.

## ESSENTIAL OIL

In early days, Lily of the Valley fragrance could only be captured by sun infusion of the flowers in olive or sweet almond oil. This is known as enfleurage.

In modern perfumery, the flowers are extracted by volatile solvents, into a concrete or absolute. No essential oil is distilled.

It is usually mixed with synthetic hydroxy citronellal up to 50%, and the resulting product sold as Muguet.

This in turn provides perfumers with the most exquisite fragrance used in some 14% of all modern perfumes of any quality. Opium, Roma and Florissa are some examples.

When diluted in ethanol, the oil was 94.6% effective in repelling mosquitoes in field tests in Sweden. Thorsell et al, *Phytomed* 1998 5.

The leaves of Lily of the Valley have been distilled and yield 0.058% green-brown oil with a pleasant odor. It is, however, nothing like the fresh flower scent.

The oil melts at 40.5° C and begins to boil at 120° C. After expressing the liquid, white shiny crystals melt at 61° C and composition $C_{20}H_4O_5$ is obtained.

It is composed of 49.5% hydroxy-citronellal and 10.8% citronellol.

## HYDROSOL

The distilled water of lilies of the valley, taken in one or two spoonful doses, will strengthen a weak head and heart, promote difficult delivery, withstand the falling evil, apoplexy, and dizziness, and restore lost speech. Those small children who are plagued by fits, colic and worms should be given a tablespoonful from time to time.

During this distillation, the first waters to condense are trifling and normally thrown away, but the spirit that follows is especially valued. If it is rectified again, the inherent volatile salts will go off and collect on the sides of the glass. After this comes a very smooth, fine spirit that, as well as the salts, can be stored away for future use. Administer the spirit in 15-20 drop doses each time.                                    **SAUER**

The distilled flower water is used as an astringent and skin-whitening agent, known as **AQUA AUREA**, or Golden Water. It was considered worthy of preservation in vessels of gold or silver.

The water can be taken internally to reduce fluid retention caused by heart problems, and is given as a tonic in China.

Culpepper recommended the flower water for inflammation of the eyes. "Water of the flowers of the Lilies of the valley, strengthens the brain and all the senses."

Brunschwig recommended a water of the flowers only for bee and wasp stings, trembling of the hands, flecks in the eye, trouble in labor, epilepsy, stitches of the heart, heat of liver, comforting mind and brain, excessive menstruation, loss of milk in breasts, and swollen penis and testicles.

The water doth strengthen the Memorie and comforteth the Harte.                                    **DODOENS**

The flours of the Valley Lillie distilled…the water doth strengthen the memory that is weakened and diminished; it helpeth also the inflammations of the eies, being dropped there into.                                    **GERARD**

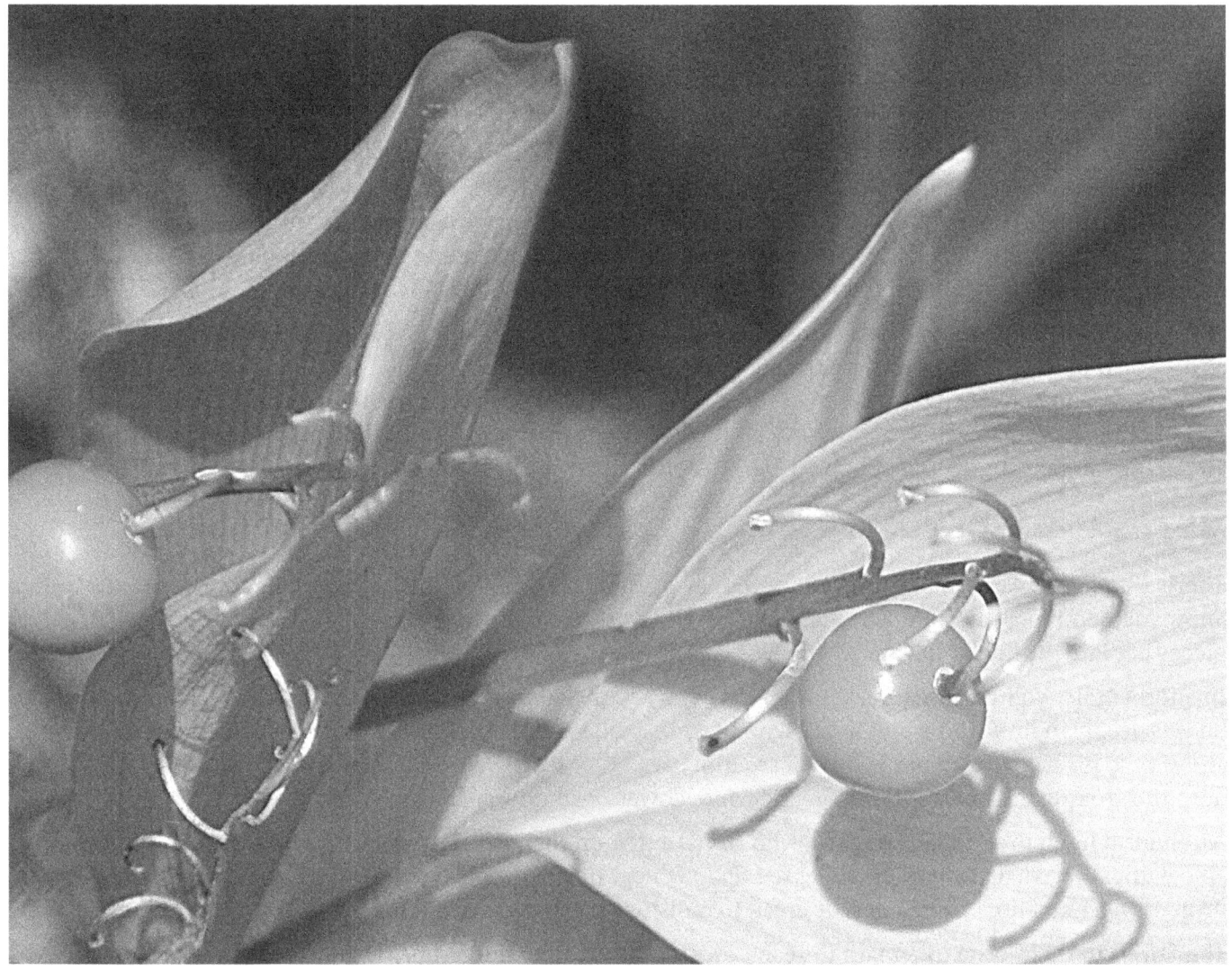

RIPE BERRY

## FLOWER ESSENCES

Lily of the Valley essence brings us back to that state of child-like innocence and wisdom where we only know how to respond with loving behaviour. It puts us in touch with that place within ourselves that existed before our lives were complicated by "shoulds" and all the other layers of conditioning we learned in order to survive and get love and approval.

Lily of the Valley is an emotional tonic which helps us see "through the eyes of a child". People who live their lives bound by convention and seeking social approval can benefit. **PACIFIC**

Lily of the Valley essence helps one begin to express their emotions. **CHOMING**

Lily of the Valley essence helps bring joy and lightness and prevents self-deception and unattainable goals. **MIRIANA**

This is the essence for yearning, for those who desire things that are unattainable. Perhaps they are in love with someone and those feelings are not returned.

Lily of the Valley helps to create "the empty cup" so that what we truly need can find the space within us and enter it. **BAILEY**

## PERSONALITY TRAITS

A herbal remedy such as Lily of the Valley leaves contains several cardio-active glycosides that are released sequentially in the body, the result is a lengthening of the cardiac response and the avoidance of an abrupt and undesirable peak in plasma concentration.

Certain non-cardioactive glycosides also present increase almost 500 times the water solubility of convallatoxin and convallatoxol. Other glycosides act synergistically by occupying protein-binding sites and thereby effecting a high plasma concentration of active glycosides with correspondingly increased bioavail-ability. The combination occurring in the leaf has many therapeutic advantages over the isolated glycosides...   **F. FLETCHER HYDE**

About the lily of the valley there is an atmosphere of innocence and purity, the bell-like flowers hang almost shyly down in their white dresses. Striking is the contrast with the tiger lily which flaunts its spotted orange dress and exhibits its sexual parts for all the world to see. When we turn to the drug pictures we find that the action of the lily of the valley is primarily on the heart or rather vascular system and secondarily on the pelvic and genital organs. In the tiger lily the reverse is certainly true.   **TWENTYMAN**

## MYTHS AND LEGENDS

There are many Russian fairy tales about the lily of the valley. In one tale, a young woman called the White Snow Maiden ran away from her wicked stepmother. As she ran, the necklace she wore fell apart. The fallen pieces became the lily of the valley.

In another tale, Volhva, the Water Queen, was in love with Sadko, a handsome musician. When found out that he was deeply in love with a young girl who lived in a village near the river, she left the water to hear him play and sing to his beloved. When Volhva heard him play, bitter tears welled up in her beautiful blue eyes. They fell onto the ground and became the aromatic white flowers we know as lilies of the valley.   **ZEVIN**

An English myth involves St. Leonard, who slayed a dragon that was troubling the whole countryside. After an epic battle, the exhausted knight collapsed and lay near death. The fairies used tiny buckets and brought one drop of water at a time from a nearby creek to moisture his lips and after much work revive the hero.

The fairies in their haste to remain unseen quickly disappeared, but left behind their tiny buckets on stems of grass. These became the flowers of Lily of the Valley.

Ancient myths depicting patriarchal saints destroying dragons represents the move from matriarchal societies to male dominated ones.

## RECIPES

**INFUSION-** 2-7 grams twice daily. The aerial parts are collected as the flowers begin to open and are dried, or tinctured.

**TINCTURE-** 5-20 drops twice daily. Use a 1:5 tincture at 60% alcohol of the recently dried root. Both leaves and roots can be used, but wait until after flowering. If fresh, use 1:2 ratio. For 1:8 tincture use 1.2 ml 3 times daily. A flower tincture is made 1:8, with dosage of 5-15 drops in water three times in 24 hours.

**STANDARDIZED EXTRACT-** 600 mg (0.2-0.3 % glycosides).

**POWDER-** One gram of lily of the valley equals 120 digitalis units in potency. Toxicity occurs more rapidly, but is non-cumulative. Maximum allowable dosage in Britain is 150 mg, with a daily maximum of 450 mg.

**CAUTION-** Overdoses can cause diuresis and purging. Use emetics, or activated charcoal, atropine if necessary, and watch potassium imbalance and treat serum insulin if needed. Take for ten days, and then ten days off. Avoid in Yin deficient conditions or where fatty heart degeneration is already present.

Do not use simultaneously, according to Commission E, with quinidine, calcium salts, saluretics, laxatives or glucocorticoids. Do not combine with gotu kola!

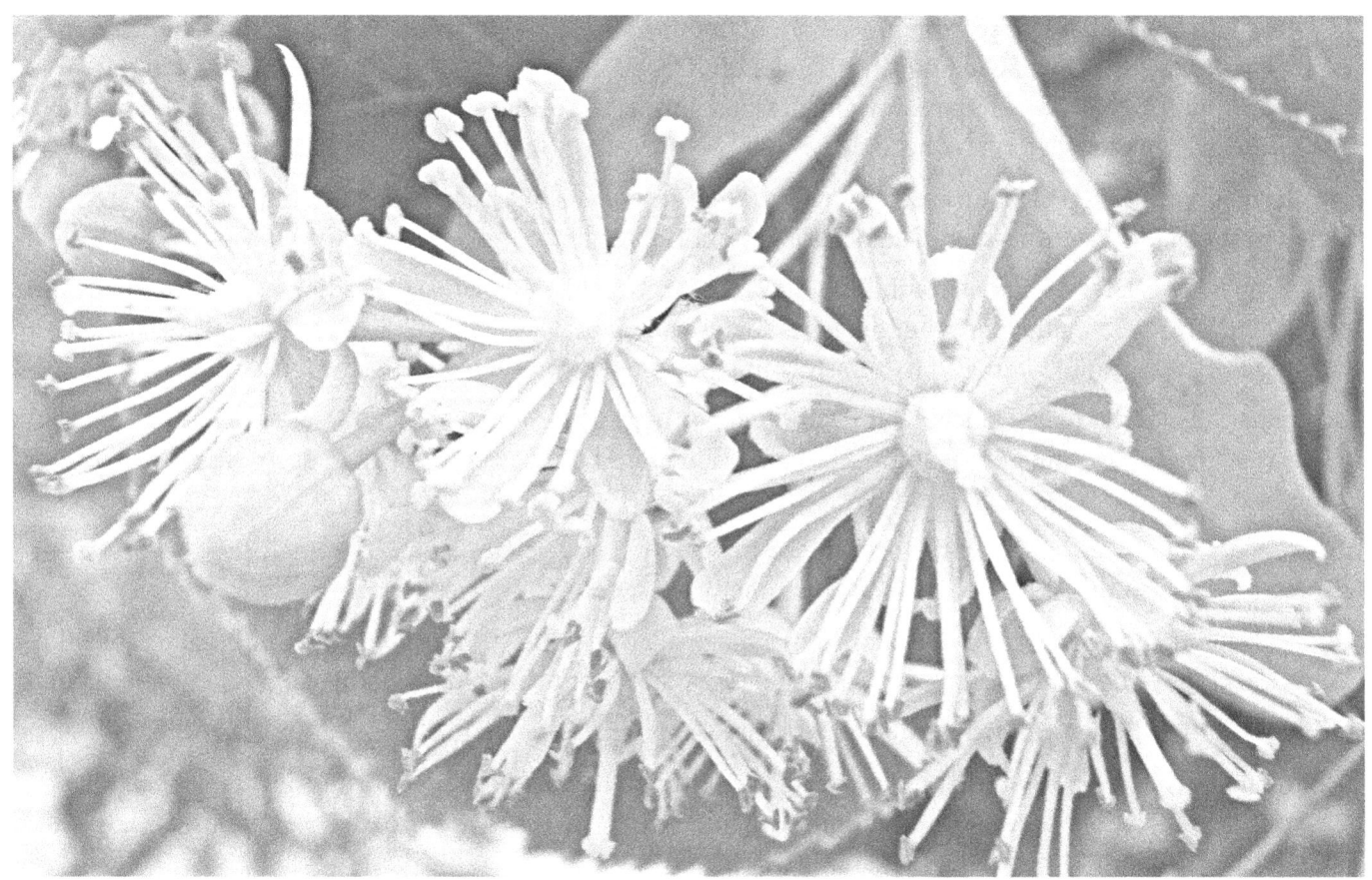

LINDEN FLOWERS

**LITTLE LEAF LINDEN**
**LIMEFLOWER**
**LIME TREE**
(***Tilia cordata*** Mill.)
(***T. parviflora*** Ehrh.) not accepted
**BASSWOOD**
(***T. americana*** L.)
**DROPMORE LINDEN**
(***T. X flavescens*** A. Braun ex Döll)
**MONGOLIAN LINDEN**
(***T. mongolica*** Maxim.)

**SILVER LINDEN**
**SILVER LIME**
(***T. tomentosa*** Moench.)
**MANCHURIAN LINDEN**
(***T. mandshurica*** Rupr. & Maxim)
**BROAD LEAVED LINDEN**
(***T. platyphyllos*** Scop.)
(***T. grandifolia*** Ehrh.) not accepted
(***T. rubra*** DC.) not accepted
**PARTS USED**- leaves, flowers, sapwood

If thou lookest on the lime-leaf, Thou a heart's form will discover.
Therefore are the lindens every chosen seat of each fond lover.                    **HEINRICH HEINE**

The linden in the fervours of July, hums with a louder concert.                    **W C BRYANT**

Now, tell me thy name, good fellow, said he, under the leaves of Lyne.                    **SHAKESPEARE**

Tilia is from Greek **TILLEIN**, "to pluck or extract fibre". Other authors suggest it is an alteration of **TELIA**, in turn from **TELUM**, a dart, in reference to use of wood. And yet, other authors suggest it derives from **PTILON** meaning feather, in reference to the floral leaf appearance.

Basswood is from bast, the fibre from inner-bark of linden, later applied to other fibre like hemp or flax. Linden was originally an adjective of Old English or Norse **LIND** tree. The root **LI**, from the Indo-European root means flax thread, with **LENTUS** coming to mean "flexible". Linné, the father of taxonomy, was Swedish and **LINN**, meant linden. Lyne may later have become lyme.

The German verb **LINDERN** means, "to soothe". Cordata means heart-shaped, referring to leaf. Lime tree is related to the plants usefulness as an antacid or systemic alkalizer of the body system. Maybe.

According to Greek legend, the nymph Philyra was raped by Saturn, disguised as a horse. She eventually gave birth to the famed Centaur, Chiron. Philyra was so devastated that she begged the gods not to leave her among mortals. The gods granted her wish by transforming her into the mother spirit of the linden tree.

Linden has been a shade tree since the time of the Egyptians. It was a holy tree in Greece, sacred to Venus due to heart-shaped leaves, and Germans and Slavs, who attributed the power to ward off destruction by lightning. Linden is female, as Oak is male in the Teutonic tradition.

The trees are long-lived, in part due to an interesting stem production. As one stem matures, the next begins to form below it, so that it can replace the older one when it dies.

Siegfried, a famed mythical hero, was dipped in a magical river by his mother to make him invulnerable. But a linden leaf clung to his heart, leaving one vulnerable spot that later proved his undoing. Sound familiar, Achilles?

In many cultures, linden was believed to absorb disease by simply being touched.

In Lithuania, for example, women made sacrifices to linden as part of religious rites. It was believed bark of linden, if carried, would prevent intoxication, while the leaves and flowers were used in love spells. In Poland, the inner bark was said to be able to tie up the devil.

In Sweden, many surnames such as Lindemann, Tiliander and Linné derive from the guardian tree.

Pliny noted in ancient Rome that bast fibre, known as **LIBER**, was used to make paper, and hence the origin of words such as library.

In Russia, the corky outer bark forms a sole, and strips of the plaited bast were used to form the top of a shoe. This footwear was short-lived and so were the lime flower forests.

Linden oil is a personal favourite fragrance of my wife Laurie. Whenever the various trees boom in July, we make a point of visiting and sniffing the fragrant emissions.

In Germany, the flowers were never brought into the house due to their ability to induce erotic dreams.

The tree was associated with Freya, the guardian of life and goddess of fortune, love and truth. It was believed the tree would un-earth the truth, so town meeting were held under the trees in central squares. Over 850 place names can be traced back to linden.

Honey produced from the blossoms is regarded as one of the most delicately flavored in the world.

Little Leaf Linden is the national emblem of Slovakia, Slovenia and the Czech Republic.

Both American Basswood and Little Leaf Linden are hardy to the prairies, the former to zone three and the small import from Europe, to zone two.

Dropmore Linden is a hardy hybrid of the two, resistant to the linden mite, and well adapted to dry prairies.

Mongolian Linden is a much shorter tree, only getting to five metres, about half the average of others. Silver Linden is not quite as hardy (zone 4) in our region. It is native to Turkey and Eastern Europe, with fragrant flowers that are somewhat intoxicating to bees. Manchurian and broad-leaved linden have been grown successfully at Morden Research Station.

All Linden flowers have exquisite perfume. American Basswood scent is similar to grape flowers, while *T. cordata* and *T. tomentosa* are more honey-like, and *T. platyphyllos* flowers are sweet like watermelon with a touch of clove and fringe tree flower.

Green Sunday, or the Feast of the Pentecost, held in the Russian Orthodox Church, is decorated with linden blossoms to symbolize new life in the Spirit.

It is said that eleven different varieties are grown in Russia, with an estimated 27 million acres of linden tree plantations (Zevin, 1997).

The bark was removed in spring and soaked in water until soft by various Native peoples. The tough outer bark then easily separates from the desired inner bark, separated into mainly one-inch strips, and coiled for future use.

Sometimes the bark was boiled with wood ash and peeled off the soft fibrous inner bark and cut into lengths. This was used to make belts, fishing nets, snowshoe webbing; and when cut thinner, as thread to sew robes, moccasins, pouches, birch bark containers, fishing line and even sutures for severe skin cuts.

False facemasks were carved by the Iroquois on the living tree, and when finished cut off to hollow out the back.

Wide strips were cut by Chippewa to weave mats and tie large and small packets. The width of fibre determined the strength, but also the softness; and it was often re-boiled after separation to add additional toughness.

Pehr Kalm, traveling through Quebec in 1749 wrote, "I could have sworn it was a fine hemp cord."

The inner bark of American Basswood was infused by the Cherokee for dysentery, or mixed with cornmeal as a poultice for boils.

They used the inside bark and twigs in pregnancy to relieve heartburn, morning sickness, weak stomach and bowels.

A jelly was made from the bark and used for cough of tuberculosis.

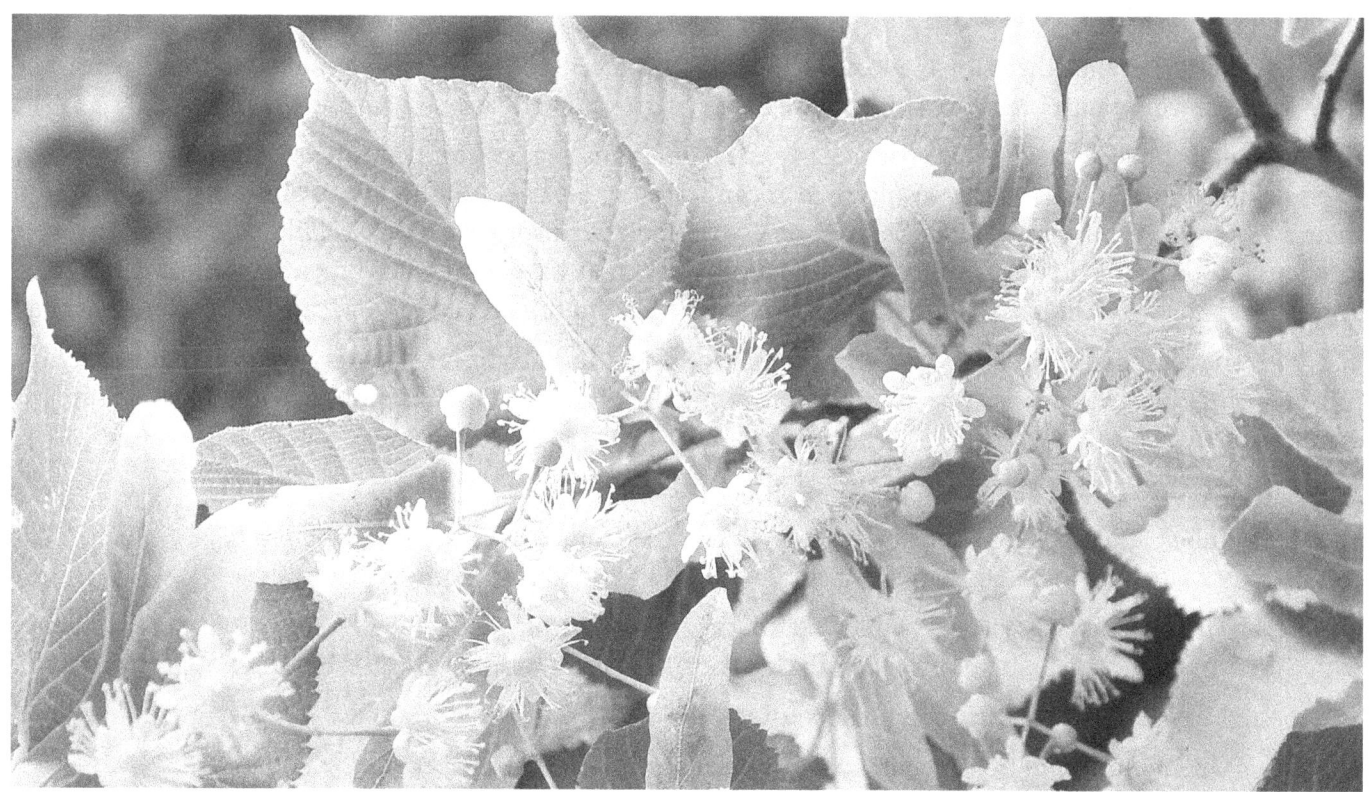

LINDEN FLOWERS, LEAVES AND BRACTS

The Fox tribe used inner bark poultices for drawing boils, while a twig decoction was reserved for lung trouble.

The Iroquois infused the bark to increase urination, and the shoots for those feeling worn out. The bark was part of a compound decoction for internal hemorrhage, and part of a leaf poultice for broken bones and swollen areas.

The Mi'kmaq used the roots as treatment for worms, while the bark was used for suppurating wounds. The Onondaga decocted the bark to promote urination.

The Mohawk drank the flower tea to induce sweating and relieve spasms, and the twigs, when combined with staghorn sumac bark, were considered a tonic tea during pregnancy.

Linden has been used for timber, and the fibrous inner bark or bast has been used for baskets, ropes, and mats. The Swedes used the fibre as a source of thread for fishing nets, while the Polish used inner bark to make rough shoes called **CHODAKI**, baskets and hats.

Archeological digs have un-earthed woven basswood necklaces, strung with copper beads from before the time of Christ.

The wood is prized for carving, being close-grained, white and very smooth. Over three centuries ago, Grinling Gibbons used it for many of his exquisitely detailed carvings; and because linden wood is never worm-eaten, well-preserved today. Good luck charms are often carved from the wood.

The wood carvings found along Gaspe Peninsula are often made of basswood.

The keys and sounding boards of musical instruments are often made from linden wood; as well as yardsticks and Venetian blinds. During the Second World War, the Mosquito fighter planes were crafted from this hardwood.

The wood is burned without oxygen to produce medicinal grade charcoal, useful for dyspepsia and other digestive complaints.

The twigs can be placed in a burning fireplace, and later removed, powdered and put into empty gelatin or vegetable capsules in an emergency.

A sticky black substance that drops onto parked cars is produced not by the tree, but a aphid that lives on the tree. This honeydew sugar can cover one square metre of ground with as much as one kilogram of syrup.

As mentioned above, honeybees are particularly attracted to the sugary sap. This sap quickly ferments, so they often drink an alcoholic cocktail, resulting in meandering paths back to the hive. Collisions with trees and their own hives are common. Guard bees are on the outlook for disorderly bees, and like night club bouncers forcibly eject drunks from the premises. Persistent offenders may have their limbs bitten off, resulting in a most unpleasant hangover. Linden flowers of *T. tomentosa* have a hypnotic constituent that causes drowsiness in bees.

The tree can be tapped, for a sweet, sugary juice in the spring. In Europe, an electuary from linden was highly prized during the middle ages, especially when combined with linden blossom honey. The fermented sap was drunk as wine.

A mucilaginous sap from inner bark is very useful for healing skin burns.

The seeds, or berries can be collected and powdered, and used for treating diarrhea; or put into a pepper grinder and used as a salt substitute. The fruit, commonly called "monkey-nuts" contains rich oils.

The French chemist Missa discovered in the 1700s that grinding the fruit, with linden flowers, produced a substance with the scent of chocolate. It was even commercialized in Prussia for a short time, but did not preserve well.

The roasted fruit can be used as a coffee substitute.

The leaves when young and translucent, added to salads, or cooked to thicken soups and stews.

The leaves are simmered down to half the water, becoming quite mucilaginous when cooled, and used for chapped skin, cuts, sores, burns and other minor problems.

Linden extracts are used in hair products such as Freeman Botanicals Hair Rescue and Intensive Conditioner.

During the Second World War, the older, tough leaves were dried, pulverized and powdered to make a nutritious "green flour" to supplement bread and cakes. The leaves contain inverted sugars, easily used by diabetics. Elsewhere, the leaves can be dried like hay, and used for winter feed for livestock.

In France, and elsewhere, afternoon tea is served under scented linden trees helping calm hyperactive children, and creating a quiet, peaceful moment of time. Linden leaf tea is a good choice for those with poor protein digestion, due to lack of tannins.

It was linden flower tea into which Proust dipped his madeleine, evoking the nostalgia of his childhood and inspiring the masterwork *A LA RECHERCHE DU TEMPS PERDU*. I haven't taken the time to read it. My loss, no doubt.

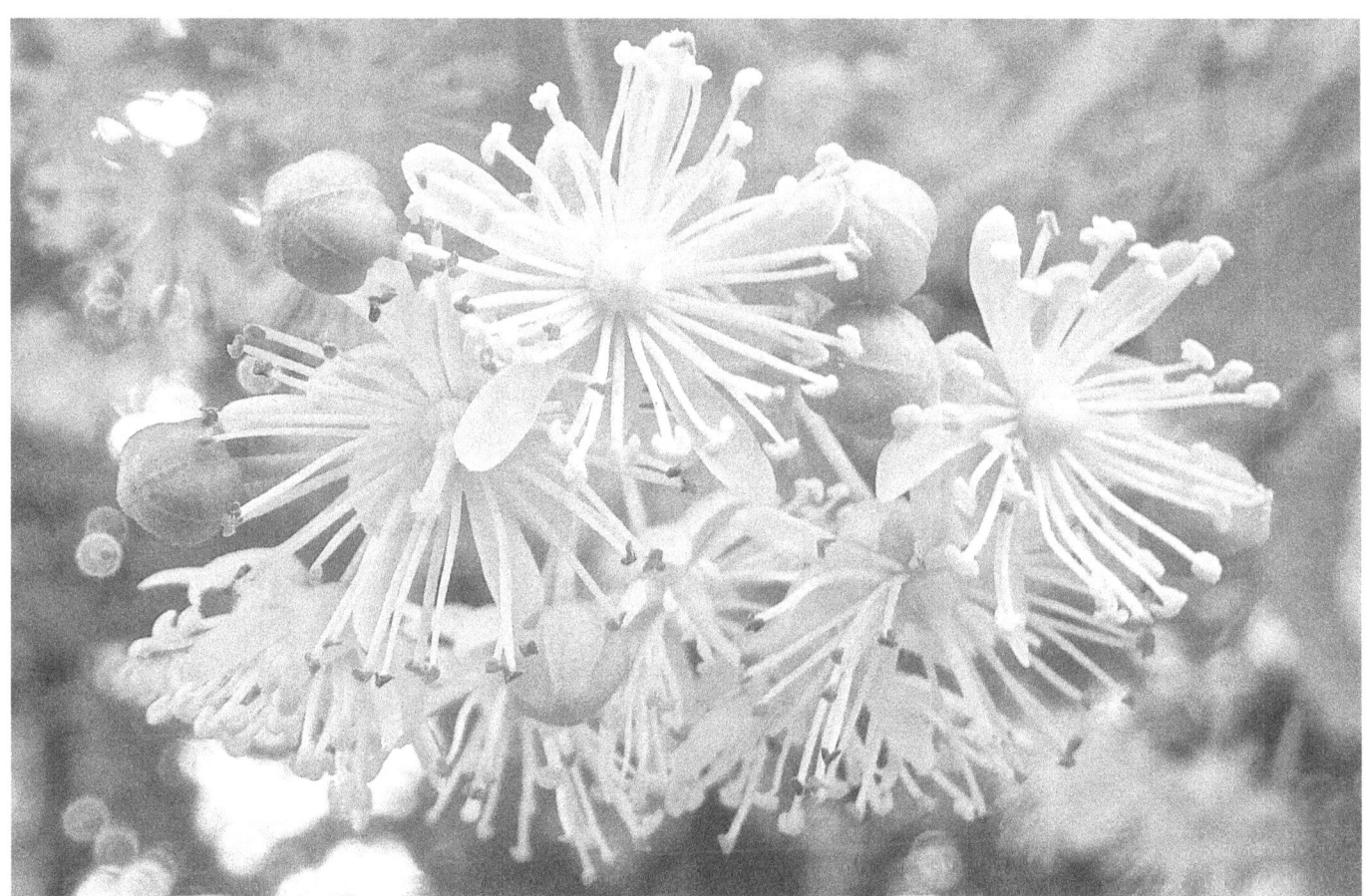

YOUNG LINDEN BLOSSOMS

# MEDICINAL

**CONSTITUENTS-** *T. cordata* flowers- organic acids p-coumaric, caffeic and chlorogenic; tiliacin; proanthocyanidins, tannins and especially flavonoids (1%), mainly quercitrin, isoquercitrin, tiliroside, hyperoside, hesperidin, rhamnosyl-7-kaempferol, etc; essential oil (see below); and mucilage composed of D-galactose, L-arabinose, L-rhamnose, and uronic, malic, acetic and tartaric acids. Also contains the amino acids phenylalanine, alanine, cysteine, and cystine. Fresh flowers contain 40 mg/100 g of vit C, carotene, scopoletin (coumarin) and benzodiazepine-like compounds.
sapwood- phenolic acids, tannins, fraxoside, esculoside, cichorioside, amino acids, 1.5-7% polyphenols.
leaves- 16.5% protein (11.9% soluble), relatively high calcium (2.79%), iron (198 ppm), and boron (52 ppm).
fruit- squalene
*T. tomentosa* leaves- flavonoids: quercitroside, kaempferine, astragaline, quercitol 3, glucose 7 rhamnoside, tiliroside quercitroside, soquarcitro-cide; scyllitol; coumarin derivatives, tillroside amino acids including aspartic acid, proline and indol-3-acetic acid.
*T. platyphyllos*- protocatechuic acid, (-)-epicatechin and caffeic acids.

223

Linden flowers and bracts are gathered and used in herbal teas for their sedative and relaxing quality, and cooling and drying nature.

The stalks of dried linden flowers are used in France for Tilleul tea.

The flowers have been used traditionally in France, and elsewhere for the symptomatic treatment of neurotic states, especially minor sleep disturbances, nervous vomiting and heart palpitations. This may be due to the binding of GABA receptors, similar to valerian.

Just walking or sitting under the trees can be soothing to nervous people.

The flowers are poulticed or infused for treating itchy skin, or other dermatological irritations. Cold infusions, gently-warmed and added to baths, are said useful for hysteria, and overly-excited nervous states.

As a febrifuge, linden is especially good for cooling the entire system, in cases of excessive heat, or acute fever states. Linden flower is better than Catnip for this purpose. Peter Holmes puts it best "The remedy excels for heavy-set, tense-muscled people with acute upper or lower respiratory infections manifesting heat and lack of sweat."

Matthew Wood says the tongue calling for linden flower is usually red, sometimes flame-shaped, and usually somewhat moist.

In Germany, the flowers are specific for children with influenza. They are anti-catarrhal and used in various respiratory infections. Recent research in India indicates linden extracts are effective against various virus cultures.

Isoquercitrin, and tiliroside are some of the flavonoids responsible for its diaphoretic effect. The former compound inhibits lens aldose reductase (prevents cataracts), and is active against *Pseudomonas maltophilia* bacteria.

Tiliroside shows liver protective activity. Matsuda et al, *Bioorg Med Chem* 2002 10:3.

It also exhibits neuroprotective effects in human neuroblastoma SH-SY5Y cells, *in vitro*. Yuan Z et al, *Chem Biodivers* 2017 Mar 11.

Tiliroside inhibits neuro-inflammation in neuro-degenerative disorders. Velagupudi R et al, *Biochim Biophys Acta* 2014 1840(12): 3311-9.

Tiliroside is also present in rose hip seeds. It inhibited lipid accumulation in induced obese mice models, probably related to reduction in expression of peroxisome proliferator-activated receptor gamma.

A 12 week double-blind, randomized, placebo-controlled trial of 32 subjects given either rosehip seed extract (with tiliroside) or placebo. All measures of abdominal visceral fat was lower in herbal group. Nagatomo A et al, *Diabetes Metab Syndro Obes* 2015 8:147-56.

A study, by two pediatricians at Chicago University, involved 55 children with flu symptoms, treated with bed rest, linden blossom tea and at most one or two aspirin. Thirty-seven other children, in addition to above, were given sulfa drugs, and another 67 antibiotics only. The authors were surprised children taking linden tea and bed rest not only recovered quicker, but had the fewest complications. Children given antibiotics needed longer to overcome the condition, with more complications.

The flowers and leaves are used to treat disorders associated with Earth, Wood and Fire Yang. To use traditional Chinese terms, by draining the Fire of the Heart, it is useful for treating insomnia, anxiety, anguish, neurosis, hysteria, epilepsy, vertigo, migraines and apoplexy.

Matthew Wood explains its use this way. " It is suited to symptoms of kidney heat and irritation, including increased blood volume, essential hypertension, orthostatic hypertension, moist, warm skin, congestion of the kidneys, scanty, dark urine and edema. It is cooling enough to work on herpes."

The flowers and bracts are useful for Wind Heat in lungs, with cough, chronic bronchitis and yellow phlegm.

Taken hot, the flower or leaf infusion will often stop head or respiratory infections from fully manifesting. This is External Wind Heat.

Steam containing linden flower extracts has been shown superior to steam alone in alleviated un-complicated colds.

Linden, or Lime Flowers, as they are sometimes called, remove excess uric acid from the system, and slowly dissolve cholesterol from the arterial walls.

In the treatment of hypertension, for example, the slow steady influence of linden flower can be helpful on several levels. Linden balances the central nervous system, calms the nerves and scrubs the buildup of plague and/or calcification of arteries. Add to this a stimulation of sluggish renal function and elimination, and you have a good hypertensive tonic. The vaso-dilating action reduces constrictor tone in the peripheral blood vessels.

Linden flowers are effective in conditions of abnormally high blood viscosity and hyper-coagulation. Tiliroside induces anti-hypertensive activity through an L-type $Ca^{2+}$ influence on smooth muscle. Grazielle C. Silva et al, *Planta Medica* 79:2 1003-8.

Extracts show anti-thrombin activity. Goun EA et al, *J Ethnopharm* 2002 81 337-342.

There appears to be a synergistic effect between the saponins and flavonoids on the blood vessels. It shares a similar saponin with horse chestnut, and thus is useful in varicose veins, phlebitis, migraine and arteritis.

Tinctures or cool infusions are best for conditions of hypertension and neuro-cardiac concern over the long term. It is similar to, and work well with chrysanthemum flower.

Slanc et al, *Phytother Res* 2008 Dec 23 found linden leaf (*L. platyphyllos*) possesses lipase inhibition. Experimental work supports it reputation as an anti-spasmodic and relaxant, and demonstrated estrogenic effect.

Like bupleurum root, it relieves headaches and blood pressure associated with Liver Yang. Water extracts of *T. cordata* flowers have been found, in vitro, to stimulate lymphocyte proliferation. Anesini et al, *Fitoterapia* 1999 70:4.

They found the same effect from two different agonists of peripheral benzodiazepine receptors, leading to speculation that *Tilia* extracts bind to these sites.

Work by Arcos et al, *Phytother Res* 20:1 found flowers of *T. cordata* exhibit anti-proliferative activity against tumor cells.

Scopoletin (coumarin) derived from the flowers of *T. cordata* show anti-proliferative activity on BW 5147 lymphoma cancer cells. Barreiro Arcos ML, *Phytotherapy Research* 2006 20(1): 34-40.

The flowers are one of our few stomachic herbs with very low levels of tannin. This, of course, favors digestion, as tannins, even in ordinary tea, inhibit true protein digestion.

The leaves create some astringency useful in diarrhea, or bleeding from the nose and mouth, due to protocatechic leaf tannins. The leaves are mildly diuretic.

The flowers combine well with hawthorn for high blood pressure, with hops for nervous tension and anxiety, and with elder flowers for colds and flu.

Think of linden flowers for hyper-adrenal conditions, combining well with burdock root.

Various French physicians do not consider the flowers of American basswood to be useful medicinally. They suggest the flowers are hexamerous, not pentamerous, like *T. cordata*, and do not contain adequate concentration or proportions of the active principle.

I don't know if this is geocentric or scientific in basis, as both have pronounced odiferous properties. There appears bias with some authors suggesting the flowers of American Basswood can cause nausea. This has not been my experience, however.

In fact, linden flowers with higher tannin levels and low mucilage content as found in *T. cordata and T. platyphyllos* are more flavorful teas.

Schmidgall et al, *Planta Medica* 2000 66:1 found polysaccharides from *T. cordata* show moderate bio-adhesion to isolated epithelial tissue.

Tiliroside appears to interact, at least *in vitro*, with CYP3A4, CYP2C9 and CYP2C8 pathways, suggesting influence on possible herb/drug interactions, or absorption of drugs with the herb. Sun, DX et al, *Phytother Res* 2010 24:11.

The sapwood decreases bile flow in humans. This is useful in the treatment of biliary dyskinesia, or when dandelion root is contra-indicated. Work by Debray showed this was due to inhibition of T.G.P transaminase.

At the same time it is a uric acid dissolver and hepato-biliary drainage remedy.

It combines well with horse chestnut, fleabane, meadowsweet and goldenrod for the treatment of cellulite.

Laboratory studies in early 1960s have found sapwood to be anti-spasmodic, serotonin antagonist, diuretic and hypotensive agent. It is a coronary dilator, acting to ease tension in the whole cardiovascular system.

Sapwood tea, decocted from the dried strips of wood, is useful for epigastric bloating, and impairment of digestion.

It can be useful in certain types of migraine associated with coronary syndromes, such as angina and maintenance treatment, after infarction.

The decocted bastwood can be used in relief of rheumatism.

The wood charcoal, made from dry linden twigs or bark, is used internally for intestinal disorders, including hyperacidity, gallbladder and liver complaints and cases of poisoning. Externally, the charcoal has been used for skin ulcers.

Coumarin anti-coagulant content in *T. tomentosa* decreases from the stalk toward the leaf. When compared with amino acids and particularly flavonoids, the quantity of active ingredients is higher in buds.

Bud extracts mimic GABA and benzodiazepine agonists, by targeting hippocampal GABAergic synapses. They also inhibit network excitability by increasing the strength of inhibitory synaptic outputs. Allio A et al, *J Ethnopharm* 2015 172: 288-96.

Flowers of *T. tomentosa* exhibited anxiolytic activity in a mouse study by Viola H et al, *J Ethnopharm* 1994 44(1): 47-53.

The flowers, bracts and developing seeds of *T. americana* show activity against *Staphylococcus aureus*. Borchardt et al, *J Med Plants Res* 2008 2:5.

Both hexane and water extracts of *T. americana* flowers possess neuroprotective effects against neuronal damage induced by ischemia. Angeles-Lopez GE et al, *Neurochem Res* 2013 38(8): 1632-40.

The bark shows activity against methicillin-sensitive *Staphyloccus aureus*, and *Mycobacterium phlei*. Omar et al, *J Ethnopharm* 2000 73 161-70.

Squalene is an intermediary in cholesterol synthesis, found in shark liver oil and some plants such as olive and linden. Squalene is anti-bacterial, anti-tumour and immune stimulating.

## HOMEOPATHY

Lime Tree/Linden is indicated for uterine prolapse, passive hemorrhages and urinary incontinence. It is of value in muscular weakness of the eyes; neuralgia that is first right sided and then left; and a dimness of vision as if a veil is over the eye.

The patient may find difficulty using binoculars, for example.

The female may suffer intense soreness of the uterus with bearing down pain, and sweating with no relief. Profuse slimy leucorrhea is produced while walking. The external genitalia are sore and red; while the skin suffers intense itching and burning, made worse by scratching. Eruptions of small, red, itching pimples may occur.

Sweating is profuse and warm soon after falling asleep, with the sweating increasing as rheumatic pain increases.

The patient feels worse in the afternoon and evening, or in a warm room or bed. Symptoms are better from cold, and motion. Feeling separated from family, laughing and joking about death, injury and suffering-black humor.

Strong desire to smoke, vertigo with tendency to fall backwards or to right. Deep cracks in skin of heels. Dreams of fire, flood, military, shooting, black water and yellow colours.

**DOSE**- Mother tincture to 6th potency. The mother tincture is prepared from the fresh flowers of the Tilia species, particularly *T. cordata* and *T. platyphyllos* in Europe. On the prairies, use *T. cordata* or *T. americana*.

The first proving with *T. cordata* was by Robert Bannan with 31 provers at 30c in 1995.

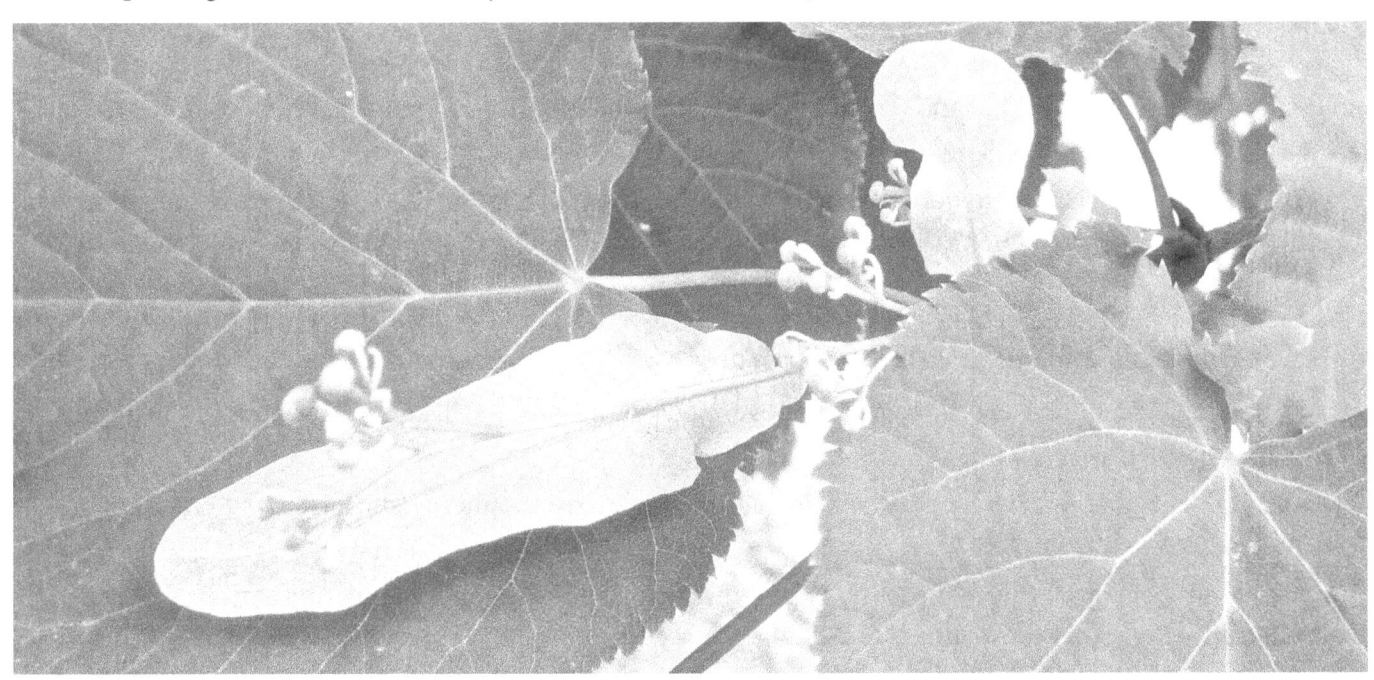

LINDEN BRACTS AND FLOWERS GOING TO SEED

# GEMMOTHERAPY

The buds of Silver Leaf Linden (*T. tomentosa*) are rich in farnesol, a terpene with neuro-regulating sedative properties.

Experiments in laboratory animals confirm that it clearly holds sleep-inducing capacities.

It is not a hypnotic, but a sleep-inducer without toxicity, and non-habit forming. It is particularly recommended for treating the nervous system of fragile persons, such as children, pregnant women and the elderly.

Not only is Tilia sedative, but it anxiolytic. In too high a dose, it has the reverse effect and will prevent sleep.

It works well with *Pinus montana* 1D for neuralgia and other nerve related pains. However, do not combine gemmotherapy drops, but alternate from the individual bottles.

**DOSE**- Bud macerate 1D, 50-100 drops at bedtime or after the evening meal. For children, 25 drops, depending upon age, both with water.

# ESSENTIAL OIL

**CONSTITUENTS-** bracts- rich in phenylacetyaldehyde and other aldehydes.
flowers- dominated by monoterpenoid hydrocarbons, tricosane, isocyclocitral, notrienol.
Both contain oxygenated mono- and ses-quiterpenes such as linalool, geraniol, farnesol, camphor, carvone, and cineole; aromatic alcohols like phenyl-ethanol, benzylic alcohol, phenols, and aliphatic compounds.

Linden blossom oil is strongly affected by urban pollution. In one study the content of oxygenated compounds reduced from an average of 47-55%, to 20-27% in dirty city environments.

The oil is used in nervous tension, insomnia, and anti-depressant. It combines well with rose, and some citrus notes, as well as jasmine and frankincense.

Work by Buchbauer et al, *Arch Pharm* 1992 325 April, found linden species oil sedative to mice upon inhalation. It is a personal favorite of my wife, Laurie.

# HYDROSOL

Linden hydrosol is slightly floral and heady, like yeasty-beer in odor. It has a pH of 4.3-4.6, is slightly unstable, but good for at least one year.

The distilled water of linden blossoms, taken in spoonful doses, is highly praised for treating the falling evil, convulsions, dizziness, and other cold distempers of the head. It is also good for colic, and will benefit injured bowels following bloody flux. If someone has been struck by convulsions, administer often a spoonful of linden blossom, lily of the valley and black cherry water mixed together. When young children are afflicted with the fits, give them often a tablespoon dose of one part peony water and one part linden blossom water.

Linden blossom water is used by women, to remove spots on the face. It will also heal blisters in the throat and a scurvied mouth.

If young children develop a large, bloated belly (cardiology), they should be administered a tablespoonful of linden blossom water from time to time.                                                    **SAUER**

A hydrolat may be prepared from the leaves. Viaud says this distilled water is stimulating and a vasodilator, low doses calming and higher doses more stimulating.

Jeanne Rose suggests the hydrolat in a spray for shingle pain, as it is very soothing. She finds it calming, relaxing and sedative, helping to relieve anxiety and depression.

Susan Catty finds it useful in headaches, including migraine, and nervous exhaustion. It may be put to good use in dry eczema, itchy skin eruptions, or puffy skin.

A hydrolat prepared from the wood is used for arthritis, gout, and rheumatoid arthritis, according to work by Viaud.

A water from the blossoms is good for falling sickness, pain in gut, trembling heart, sunburn, clearing sight, cold uterus or womb, causing to speak and for much milk.                                **BRUNSCHWIG**

# SEED OIL

The seeds of American Basswood yield oil that solidifies at -10° C. It has a specific gravity of 0.938, a saponification value of 178.1, and an iodine value of 111.

Linden seed oil has been used for consumption, in days past, as well as oil lamps.

# FLOWER ESSENCES

Linden (*T. platyphylla*) flower essence is for helping develop receptivity to human love. It strengthens the relationship between mother and child. It eases communication and exchanges with respect and cordiality. It helps bring out qualities of protection, nourishing warmth, softness and calmness.                    **DEVA**

Basswood or Linden flower essence will help make you more outgoing. It will also help people to notice you instead of having to always be the one to stick out your hand first. Linden will help you to lighten up at a party and if you want to let go and be romantic, it will help you do so. Linden essence is excellent for cultivating love for humanity and in overcoming prejudices.                    **JADE MTN**

Linden essence is for people who feel alienated and never welcome anywhere. It is symbolized, by Hestia, the Goddess of Hearth and Temple.                    **HORUS**

Limeflower (*T. platyphylla*) flower essence helps us open our hearts to the light and loving of our universal being. From this awareness we experience our inter-relatedness on earth and create harmonious relationships in our lives.

It is indicated when individuals are too introspective or focused on self; or there is over identification with lower self/personality.

Limeflower essence supports us in overcoming feelings of separation from our spiritual self or others, and can empower and encourage us to work for peace and spiritual harmony on earth.                    **FINDHORN**

Linden (*T. x europea*) leaf essence is a great pick-me-up after a period of stress or illness. It can also be taken continuously to deal with ongoing stress.                    **FALLING LEAF**

Linden (*T. cordata*) leaf essence releases the pattern of "male chauvinism"- being authoritarian, domineering, controlling, or insensitive in intimate relationships with females.                    **FALLING LEAF**

Lime essence helps to decrease an oversensitive cross energy, allowing the body to focus on a spiritual endeavor. It is useful for when you want to shift levels of consciousness without disorientation, helping to lessen past behavior programming, erase doubts and fears, and calm the anxiety related to the practical use of your psychic and healing potential.                    **OLIVE**

# PERSONALITY TRAITS

When Zeus and Hermes visited Phygria in human form they were refused hospitality ...until they came to the cottage of Philemon and his wife Baucis, who entertained them kindly. Zeus gave them practical thanks by taking them to the top of a high hill where they survived while a flood devastated the lowlands. There was a temple of Zeus on this crest, and he made them it guardians. The only wish the old couple had was that they should die at the same moment, and this was granted to them by Zeus.

As they died he changed them into trees- Philemon into an oak, and Baucis into a linden, the emblem of conjugal love.                    **POWELL**

On a cold winter day the tall Mississauga chief, Niniboju was tramping the shores of a frozen lake. He stopped suddenly and inspected a large basswood tree that stood on the shore. He peeled off a strip of the bark and with it tied two stones to his heels. Then he tried leaping on the ice and laughed at the tinkling sounds that the stones made as they hit the ice. Attracted by the tinkling sounds, a little fish came up through a hole in the ice.

Quickly Niniboju caught the fish in his hands and ate it. Then he danced vigorously and the sounds of the stones grew louder. Soon more fish came up through holes in the ice and Niniboju caught them all.

He tore the basswood strip down the centre and strung the fish as he caught them. By night he had a long string of fish which he carried back to camp. All the Indians had a good laugh and helped to eat the fish. Niniboju praised the basswood tree and called it Niniboju's helper. Other Indians tried dancing on the ice, but they caught no fish.

**GUILLET**

Confident with who they are from an early age, Lindens will be determined to follow the path they set for themselves, carrying on regardless of any opposition to their plans. These are open and up-front people, helpful when the mood takes them. They are a very interesting personality as they can change and wear many guises.

Lindens are perfectly happy to reside in the shadow of their partner or family, nurturing their growth and encouraging their ambitions…Due to lack of ambition, Lindens are often found in jobs that do not suit their temperament.

In negative mode, Lindens are possessive of their partner or children, always reminding everyone of what could go wrong. They become the worriers.

**WORWOOD**

The southern American basswood likes its taste of flesh. *Tilia tomentosa* sneaks a hypnotic potion into its floral nectaries because it is hungry for nitrogen. The pollinating bees take a hit. They slowly die in the cool shade, their bodies supplying just enough nitrogen for the trees to make maternal protein for another season of sex.

**BERESFORD-KROEGER**

## MYTHS AND LEGENDS

Old words for dragon—the German **LINDEWURM**; the Old English **LINDWORM**—and the name of the tree have a common root, the Indo-European **LENTOS** (flexible). In all cultures the dragon is a personification of the Earth's life force, which flows along the dragon or ley lines. A person encountering a place of intense Earth or dragon energy is charged both physically and spiritually.

**HAGENDER**

## RECIPES

**TINCTURE**- 2-4 ml as needed. The tincture is made with fresh flowers and/or bracts at 1:3 in 35% alcohol. I personally prefer flowers only, but the fresh bracts are useful.

**INFUSION**- One tsp of dried herb to one pint of boiled water for 15 minutes.

When collecting the flowers, they should be picked early with the whole flower cluster including the bract. They are dried in the shade.

**NIGHT CREAM**- Take 25 grams of beeswax, and blend with 100 ml of cocoa butter in a double boiler. As it is cooling, add 5 drops of linden blossom absolute or its essential oil. Bottle, label and cool. Store in a cool, dark spot.

**CAUTION**- Linden flowers may bind up iron supplements. They should be taken 2 hours apart. Do not use in cases of low blood pressure.

Low concentrations of *T. cordata* water extracts stimulated biofilm formation in *E. coli* BW25113, by up to three times.

**COMMON LIVERWORT**
**LUNG LIVERWORT**
**GREEN TONGUE LIVERWORT**
(***Marchantia polymorpha*** L.)
**GREAT SCENTED LIVERWORT**
**SNAKE LIVERWORT**
(***Conocephalum conicum*** [L.] Lindb.)
**PARTS USED**- aerial

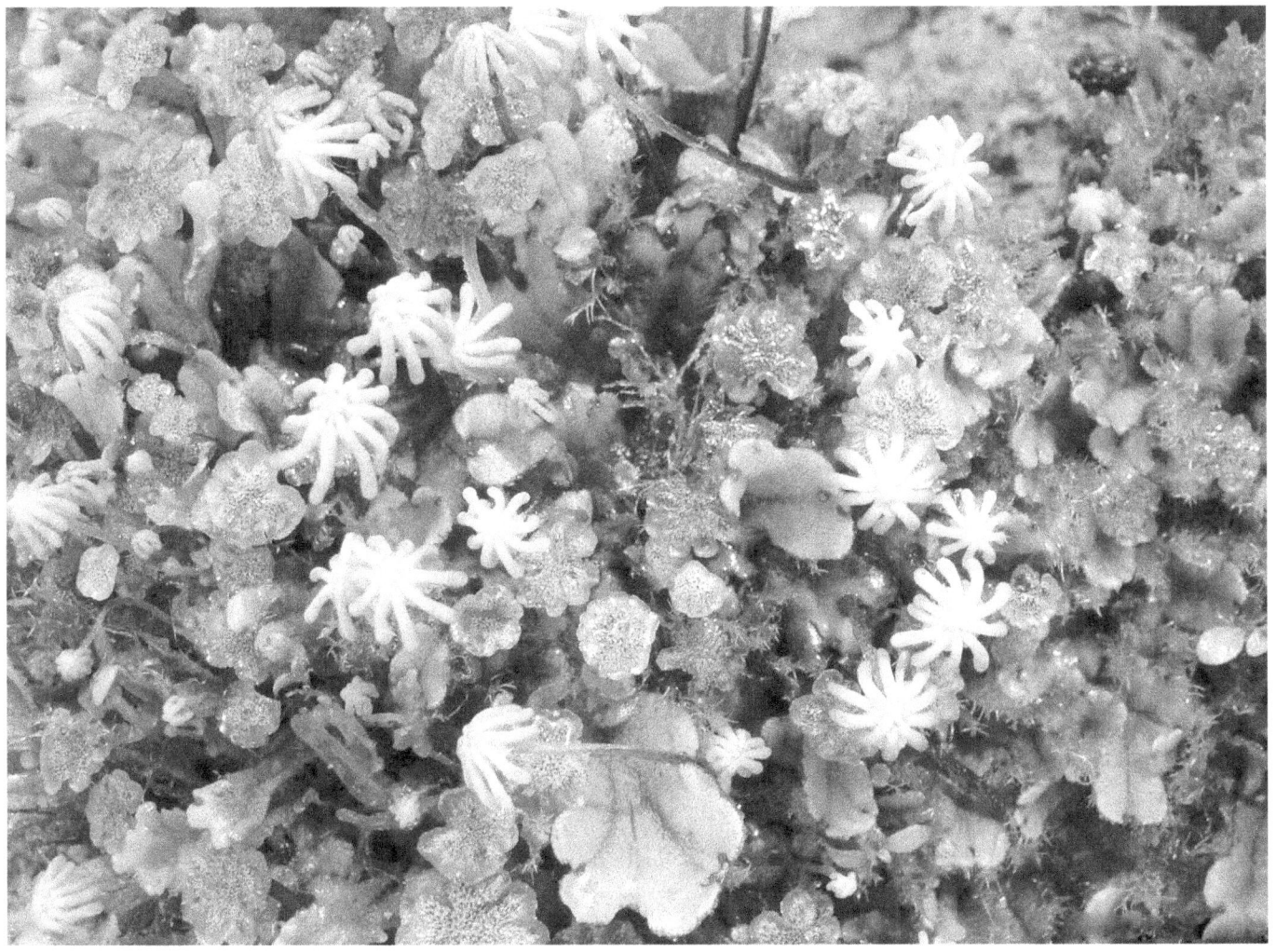

COMMON LIVERWORT (Courtesy of Alfred Cook- Creative Commons)

Concephalum means "small cone head". Polymorpha refers to the fact that there is more than one form or morph.

Liverworts have many features in common with mosses, and therefore are one division of Bryophytes. Mosses and hornworts are the other two classes. However, they are different in ten ways:

1. Most liverworts have complex oil bodies in leaf cells, mosses do not.

2. Most liverworts have fused leaves, mosses do not.

3. Liverworts are either thalloid or leafy, mosses are always leafy.

4. It is very rare for mosses to have the ventral rank of leaves reduced or absent.

5. The seta of liverworts is soft, hyaline and short lived.

6. Liverworts never have a peristome.

7. Liverworts produce spirally twisted, hygroscopic threads called elaters among the spores, mosses do not.

8. Liverworts have much more complex chemistry than mosses.

9. The lateral leaves in liverworts have lobes, mosses do not.

10. Rhizoids are unicellular in liverworts, and multicellular in mosses.

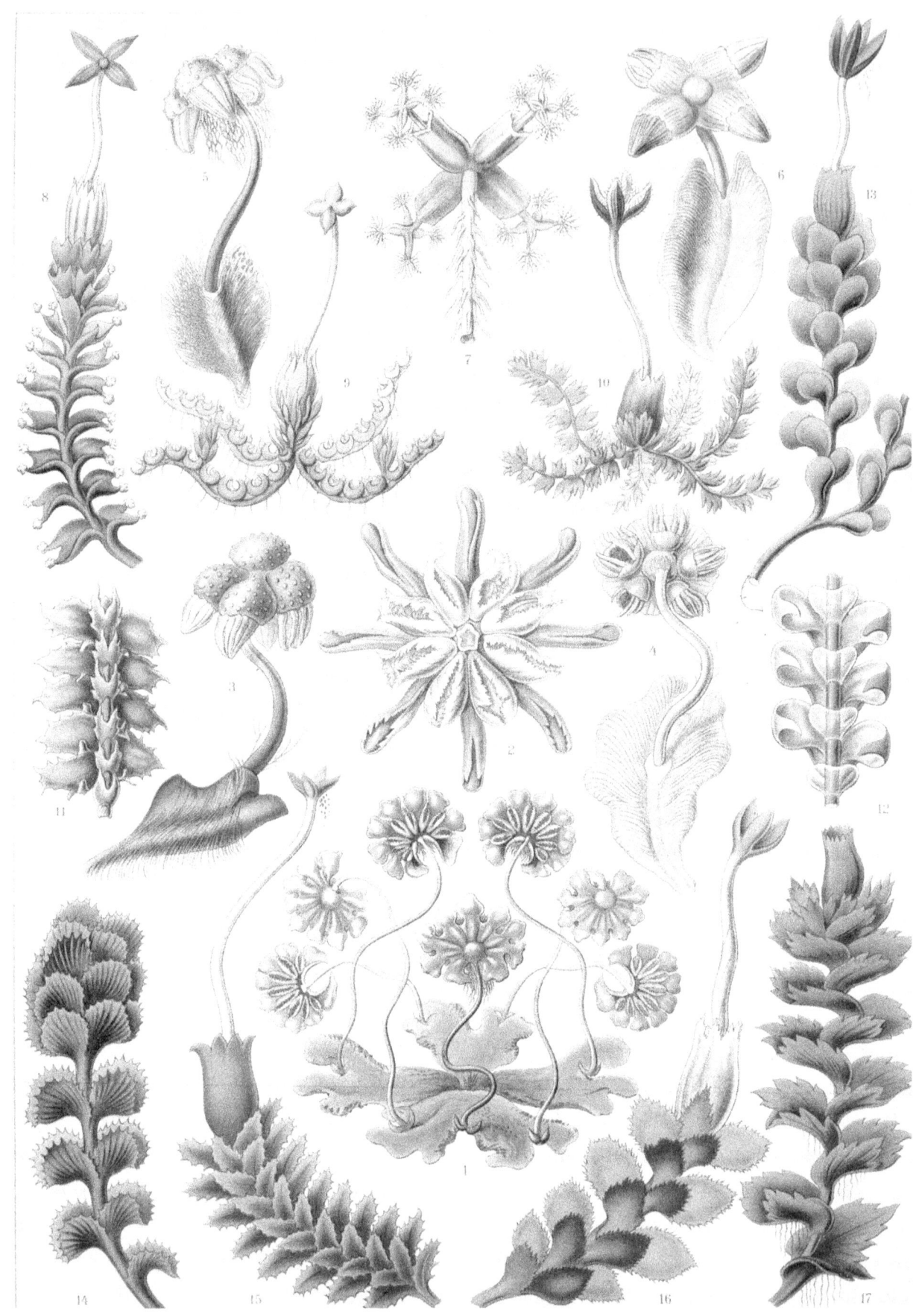

LIVERWORT POSTER

Common or Lung Liverwort is often found as a garden weed, and as a pest in tree nurseries, where it can kill the young seedlings.

*Marchantia polymorpha* is both a good luck charm and love medicine to a number of First Nations people.

It can be chewed, sprinkled on objects, or drunk as a tea, the latter ensuring the consumer will think only of the secret admirer that fixed the tea!

The Iroquois used it as a cure for "caddis fly love medicine." It was made into a tea, drank and then vomited, to rid one of the malady. The Menomini used it for liver complaints.

An older English herbal author commented upon Marchantia, based on its plant signature of liver shaped leaves. "It is a singular good herb for all the diseases of the liver, both to cool and cleanse it, and helps the inflammations in any part, and the yellow jaundice likewise."

It has been used for boils and abscesses, due to the doctrine of signatures as well. The young archegoniophore resembles a boil when it first emerges from the thallus.

Casper Schwenckfeld was a late 16ᵗʰ century, who published *Stirpium et Fossilium Silesiae Catalogus* in Leipzig (1600 AD).

Under the original name *Hepatica fontana,* he wrote:

"It is refrigerant, dessicant, gradually astringent, and it cleans away. Due to a great affinity to a liver, its heats, acute and ternary fevers, which originate from the bile. It stops the blood, and protects against inflammation."

The liverwort has been used ethnopharmacologically in at least ten countries. In Papua New Guinea, Marchantia species are known as **NAGAMI SEVA**. It was traditionally used as part of an herbal mixture to treat someone with pain or fatigue, if a victim of enemy sorcery.

In China, it is called **DI FU PING**, meaning "earth-duckweed".

In the Kumaun region of India, it is known as **PHODI** meaning, "a small boil". In China it is known as Earth Money, or Stone Moss and mixed with oils as an ointment for boils, eczema, cuts, wounds, ringworm, foot sores, and burns. It was used for damp heat in the liver and gall bladder, and to treat pulmonary tuberculosis.

In Columbia, it was used to treat stones in the bladder, and for general liver maladies.

Snake Liverwort is so named for the hexagonal markings that resemble a snakeskin. It has a very pleasant odour when crushed. It is used in different countries, mainly for various skin conditions.

Various First Nations including Haisla and Hanaksiala ground the dry liverwort and mixed it with mountain goat fat for sunburns. It was also used to make a green paint for wood, including totem poles.

The Kwakwaka'wakw call it "tongue on ground", and used it for oral canker sores and rashes. The Kwakiutl also used same term and similar usage. For small children it was put in water and the diluted form was used to wipe a child's mouth.

The Nitinaht used the brophyte for kidney problems, and eye medicine, probably cataracts.

The Haida call it **XUD T'AANGAL**, or Hair Seal's Tongue, while the southern Kwakiutl name is Tongue on the Ground. Native tribes such as the Ditidaht used it as an eye medicine.

According to Nancy Turner, various groups used the liverwort for stoppage of urine. One respondent mentioned the species was eaten by people, with recurrent dreams of sex with the dead. If the treatment did not stop this night-time occurrence, it was believed that the dreamer would soon be joining their ancestors.

In China, it is known as snake moss, or snake earth money, and used to clear heat, relieve toxicity, reduce swellings and pain. It was used for venomous snake bites, carbuncles or gangrene on the back, burns or scalds, knife wounds, broken bones, gallstones, and boils.

In Vietnam, it was called "first land plant", and used for similar purposes.

A number of Bryophytes are used in North America, China, and Europe for curing burns, bruises, and external wounds.

In France it was traditionally used to pass urine, resulting from urinary sand and gravel. In England, its was also used for stones, and a diuretic.

Many bryophytes have fragrant odors, and a hot and bitter or saccharine taste.

Bryophytes such as *Marchantia polymorpha* bio-accumulate lead. Others like *Dicranella heteromalla* accumulate cadmium, copper and zinc and may have application in bryo-remediation.

*Scapania* species can survive pH of 3.9 and hyper-accumulate zinc, lead and cadmium.

# MEDICINAL

**CONSTITUENTS-** The liverworts (about 6,000 species) contain mainly mono-sesqui- and diterpenoids, as well as lipophilic aromatic compounds, oligosaccharides, polysaccharides, sugar alcohols, amino acids, fatty acids, aliphatic compounds, prenylquinones, etc.

In China, 30-40 species of bryophytes are used medicinally. A mixture of the two major liverworts are combined in vegetable oils for bites, boils, burns, cuts, eczema and wounds.

Various liverworts have cytotoxic, anti-fungal, anti-HIV-I, and antimicrobial activity. They possess superoxide anion radical release inhibitory activity, muscle-relaxing activity, and cardiotonic and vasopressin antagonist activity.

Liverworts emit volatile terpenoids or aromatic compounds when crushed. These are responsible for intense sweet-woody, intense turpentine, and sweet, mossy, fungal like, carrot-like or seaweed-like scents (See below).

Common liverwort (*Marchantia polymorpha*) is used in China to treat jaundice, hepatitis, and external therapy to reduce inflammation.

In the Himalayas, it is used for boils and abscesses, and mixed with vegetable oil for boils, cuts, wounds, eczema and burns.

It was used traditionally in France as a diuretic drug. The fresh plant was soaked in white liquor, and then drunk as a medicine. In the Shetland Islands, it is known as Dead Man's Liver, and used to treat asthma. In Berwickshire, England it was traditionally used for colds and consumption, as a diuretic in dropsy, and "a binding at the heart". The similar texture to lungs led to its use in pulmonary tuberculosis.

The gametophyte contains marchantin A-D; chalcone synthase protein, as well as various flavonoids and terpenoids.

Marchantin A tri-methyl ether has been isolated from this interesting liverwort. The molecule possesses both convex and concave surfaces, with a central hole on the concave surface.

A pharmacological study by Taira et al in Japan showed that the skeletal muscle relaxation activity is about 3.5 times less potent than d-tubocurarine. Marchantin is structurally similar to later alkaloid .

Marchantin A has been shown to increase coronary blood flow, and may turn out to be a valuable coronary vasodilator. It inhibits growth of bacteria and fungi in various ways.

Marchantin A inhibits MCF-7 breast cancer cell lines. Huang 2010

Against *Candida albicans,* Plagiochin E induces apoptosis, accumulates reactive oxygen species, induces mitochondrial dysfunction and interferes with cell wall chitin synthesis. Wu et al, *Biochim Biophys Act Gen Subj* 2010 1800 439-447.

It is cytotoxic against P-388, lymphocytic leukemia cells.

Marchantins A, B and D inhibit the biosynthesis of 5-lipoxygenase products, and the release of arachidonic acid in Ca2+ inophore A23I87 stimulated human granulocytes. They also show significant cycloxygenase inhibitory activity. Panossian et al, *Phytomedicine* 1996 2:4.

Marchantins A and D, as well as perrottetin and paleatin shows cytotoxicity gagainst KB cancer cell lines. Marchantin C induces apoptosis in human glioma A172 cancer cells. Shi 2008. Marchantin C and neomarchantins A and B, inhibit P388 cancer cell lines. Scher 2002. Marchantin A, B, D and perrottetin F and paleatin B show anti-HIV activity. Asakawa 2008 (see below).

Various marchantins and plagiochin A inhibit influenza A virus endonuclease activity.

Cathepsin l is correlated with osteoporosis and allergy. Enzyme inhibitors from natural products to develop chemopreventative drugs for these diseases have led to marchantin series.

Riccardin D shows anti-fungal activity against fluconazole-resistant Candida albicans, and appears synergistic with the drug. Guo 2008. Isomarchantin C is the strongest inhibitor against both enzymes cathepsin L and B.

Work conducted by Friederich et al, *Phytochemistry* 1999 52:7 discovered two specific cytochrome P-450 enzymes in *M. polymorpha*.

One compound, perrottetin D, was studied extensively by Schwartner et al in 1996 in Germany. This compound gave proof to the verifiably superior radical scavenging capability of the aroxyl radical derived from the phenolic antioxidant.

Perrottetin E exhibits inhibitory activity fwAor thrombin, which is associated with blood coagulation. A lectin has been isolated from *M. polymorpha*. It is a monomeric protein with M9r0 of 16,134.64 +/- 2.93.

Common liverwort has been found to be an aromatase inhibitor, useful in the prevention and treatment of hormone sensitive cancers, such as breast and prostate. Hegazy et al, *Cell Biochem Biophys* 2012 63:1 85-96. See Stinging Nettle.

It inhibits breast cancer cell line A256 and is synergistic with Aurora-A kinase inhibitor MLN8237. Jensen et al, *Planta Medica* 2012 78:5 448-54.

The endogenous plant hormone idole-3-acetic acid was isolated from this liverwort. It produces alpha tocopherol, vitamin K, plastoquinone, plasto-hydroquinone and alpha tocoquinone. Prelunaric acid and (S)-2-hydroxycuparene are present.

This lectin has been shown by Adam and Becker from Germany, to agglutinate erthrocytes of different mammals and exhibits carbohydrate specificity against complex carbohydrate structures.

Plagiochin E is active against Candida albicans, and a DMSO extract shows activity against *Aspergillus versicolor* and *A. fumigatus*.

DMSO extracts were also active against *A. flavus and Penicillium funiculosum*. Sabovlijevic et al, *Methods Mol Biol* 2009 547 117-28.

Methanol and cholorform extracts inhibit *Tilletia indica, Fusarium oxysporum, Sclerotium rolfsii* and *Rhizoctonia solani*. Gahtori & Chaturvedi, *Arch Phytopath Plant Protect* 2011 44 731-6.

Marchantin O and P have been recently synthesized. It is hoped these drugs will retain the microtubular inhibition and anti-tumor activity of Marchantin C, and have reduced side effects. Speicher et al, *Nat Prod Commun* 2011 6:3.

The reproductive organ, or archegoniophore, contains flavonoids that exhibit ten times stronger activity as anti-oxidant, and acetylcholinesterase inhibitors, than gametophyte.

Lung Liverwort was the first plant completely sequenced for chloroplast DNA.

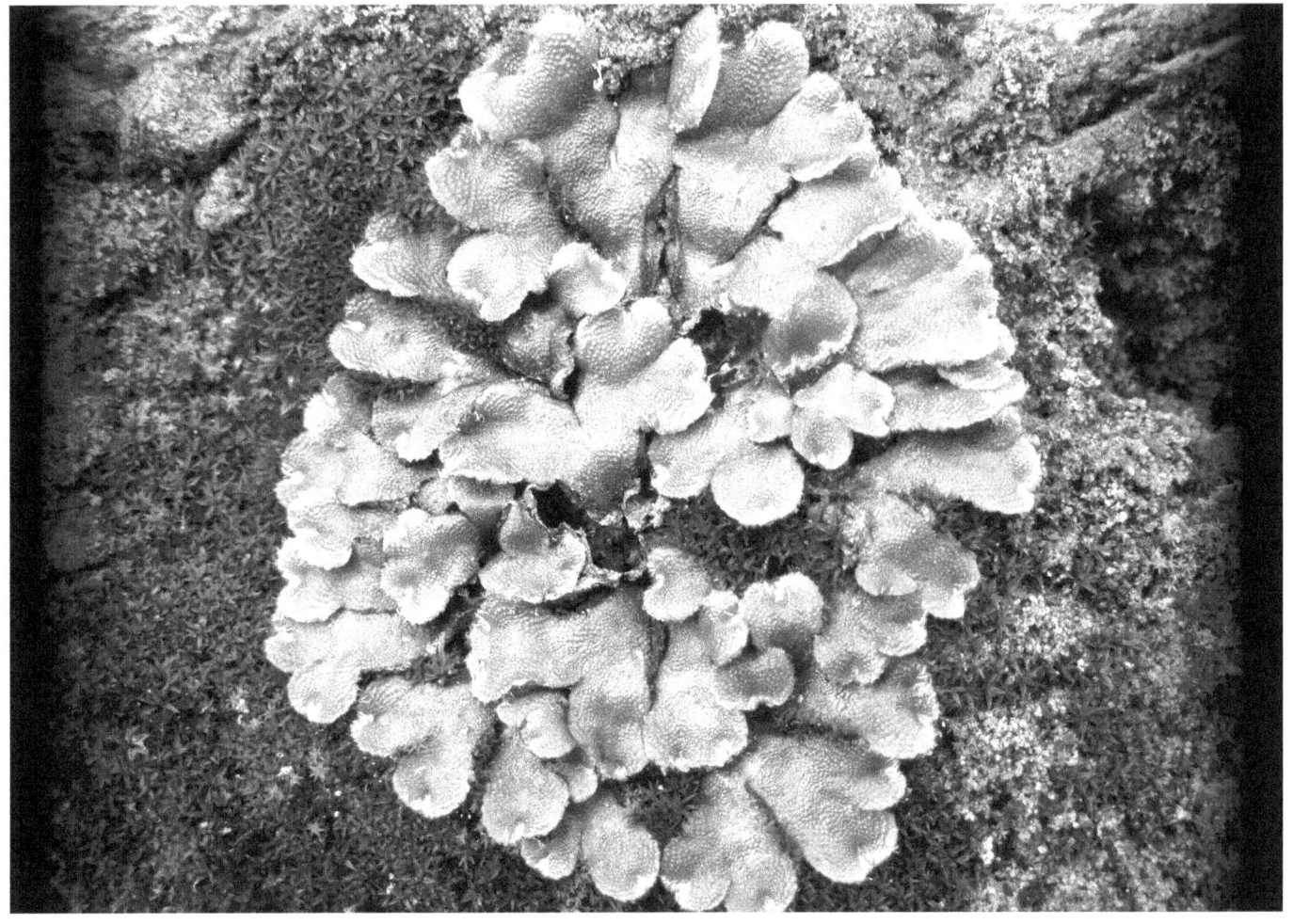

GREAT SCENTED LIVERWORT FOUND IN PALM SPRINGS CANYON

Great Scented Liverwort has a strong mushroom-like smell when crushed. It may be mixed with oils as an ointment for cuts and burns, and inhibits the growth of microorganisms.

It contains tulipinolide and zaluzanin, which are growth inhibitory substances, and require further investigation. It contains trans-methyl cinnamate, as one of the major volatiles. Also, (+)-bornyl acetate is a major monoterpene produced by this liverwort.

Both (-)-Aromadendran-5-ol and (+)-aromadenr-4-en-12-ol have also been isolated from the essential oil.

It has been demonstrated that bornane-type monoterpenes are derived from geranyl diphosphate by the action of bornyl diphosphate synthase in studies by Adam et al, *Phytochemistry* September 1998.

In studies conducted by Allison McCutcheon et al, at the University of British Columbia, great scented liverwort was found to exhibit antiviral activity against bovine herpes virus type 1. *J Ethnopharm* 1995 49:2. Later studies with colleagues, Towers et al, revealed activity against herpes simplex type 1, related to cold sores.

Bicyclogermacrenal inhibits superoxide release from guinea pig peritoneal macrophage. This may be of some importance, since excess superoxide anion radicals cause various angiopathies such as cardiac infarction and arterial sclerosis.

Norpiguisone is a potent anti-microbial. Work by Singh M et al, *Pharm Biol* 2011 49(5): 526-30 found chloroform extracts of liverworts were most active against Gram negative strains of bacteria.

Various guaianolides from *C. conicum* have shown cytotoxic activity against P-388 lymphocytic leukemia.

It is considered antifungal, and has been used traditionally in cases of gallstones.

It can be easily identified from its very pronounced hexagonal markings on the upper leaf surface.

Other liverworts on the prairies have important medicinal properties.

Lunularic acid, found in most liverworts as a minor component has anti-hyaluronidase activity, stronger than that of tranilast, an anti-allergenic agent developed in Japan for oral use. Lunularic acid is an aging hormone found in liverworts, but not mosses, that possesses anti-fungal activity. In fact, liverwort is never attacked by fungi!

*Pellia endivifolia* is a liverwort that is fairly common east and west of the Rockies, and up into Yukon.

The Hesquiat call it **CICIPALKUK** meaning, "resembling fish-scales." The juice was taken or liver was chewed for sore mouth or throat in children. The Nitinaht name was **BAYALSI?**. They used it for pain in the body, taken internally or applied externally.

The whole plant has a unique dried seaweed-like aroma that would be useful in perfumery. It has a persistent pungent taste when the fresh plant is chewed, probably due to sacculatal.

When dried, the liverwort lacks this hot taste.

Extracts have shown cytotoxic activity against P-388 lymphocytic leukemia.

*Radula complanata* is found in the Eastern Rockies, and throughout British Columbia. It contains prenyl bibenzyl, shown in French trials to be a vasopressin antagonist.

These compounds inhibit the growth of *Staphylococcus aureus* at low concentration. Asakawa et al, 1982. The same author found perrottetin E from *R. perrottetti*, cytotoxic against KB cancer cells. Simple bibenzyls from *Radula* species show calmodulin inhibitory activity. The related *R. laxiramea* contains the cannabinoid, perrottetinene.

Many *Plagiochila* species contain plagichiline A, and perrottetin E, both cytotoxic and active against the KB cell.

*P. stephensoniana*, from New Zealand contains a bibenzyl with anti-fungal activity. In India the species *P. appendiculatum* and known as **PATHARSHALI**, was prepared fresh as a paste and applied to burns, boils and blisters, or skin eruptions caused by the sun.

In Peru, the related *P. rupestre*, **MAKI MAKI** meaning, "fist" was used for kidney or rectal problems. It is considered a remedy for fainting by married women. The whole bryophyte is boiled, and used as a tea, or an ingredient in Chicha, or corn beer.

Plagiochilal B and plagiochilide, derived from *P. fruticosa*, accelerate neurite sprouting, but enhancement of chorine acetyl transferase activity in neuronal cells.

*Diplophyllum albicans*, a pacific coast bryophyte, contains diplophyllin, that exhibits cytotoxic activity ED 50 in KB cells of 2.1 micrograms/ml.

*Diplophyllum* species contain ent-eudesmanolide and diplophylline.

*Fissiden* species are used as an anti-bacterial agent for swollen throats and other infectious conditions.

*Porella* species exhibit anti-microbial activity in work by Isoe et al, 1983.

*Frullania, Porella, Lepidozia* and *Phlagiochila* species, as well as *M. polymorpha* contain the tumor inhibiting compounds, tulipinolide and costunolide. In cell cultures, these substances are active against carcinoma of the naso-pharnyx.

*Frullania tamarisci* exhibits antiseptic activity. In China, it is known as pearl ear leaf liverwort, and used to clear an irritated heart, improve blurry vision and red swollen eyes, and reduce heat.

*F. nisqualensis*, found on the west coast, contain costunolide, exhibits inhibition of A549 human non small cell lung carcinoma.

*Frullania* species can cause contact dermatitis, so caution is advised.

*Ptilidium pulcherrimum* methanol extracts show activity against *Aspergillus versicolor, A. ochraceus, A. flavus, A. niger, Tricoderma viride* and *Penicillium funiculosum*. Veljic et al, *Arch Biol Sci* 2009 61.

Various triterpenoids from this bryophyte show inhibition of PC3 human prostate cancer cell lines. Guo 2009

*Porella cordeana* contains drimenin, and aristolone, both moderately toxic to DNA repair deficient mutants of *Saccharomyces cerevisiae*. Harrigan GG et al, J Nat Prod 1993 56(6): 921-5.

It also shows cytotoxicity against both HL-60 and KB cancer cell lines.

Work by Bukvicki D et al, *Molecules* 2012 17(6): 6982-95 found activity against five yeast strains and three bacterial strains including *Salmonella enteritidis, E. coli* and *Listeria monocytogenes*.

Porella species, including *P. cordaeana* and *P. navicularis*, contain polygodial, also found in Bistort species. It is powerful anti-fungal. The former species exhibits anti-inflammatory activity. Tosun A et al, *Pharm Biol* 2013 51(8): 1008-13.

*Diplophyllum albicans*, common on the West Coast contains diplophyllin, a compound that shows significant activity against human epidermoid cancer cells. Ohta et al, 1977.

Diplophyllin is a minor constituent of Elecampane (*Inula helenium*) essential oil.

Extracts show activity against *Coniophora cerebella, Trametes versicolor, Botrytis alli, Fusarium bulbigenum* and *Pyricularia oryzae*. Wolters et al, *Planta Medica* 1962 62 88-96.

*Radula* species have been found to inhibit *Staphylococcus aureus* activity.

A great review of medicinal uses of liverworts can be found in work by Asakawa et al, *Curr Pharm Des* 2008 14:29.

## ESSENTIAL OILS

*Conocephalum conicum*, particularly the male thallus has a pronounced mushroom-like odour. The fragrance of this liverwort is due to a mixture of simple monoterpenoids and the special mushroom components. The constituents are (+)-bornyl acetate, sabinene, trans-methyl cinnamate and 1-octen-3-ol and its acetate. These are similar to flavours in the most prized mushroom of all, in Japan, the matsutake.

There are three distinct chemo-types of this liverwort, exhibiting sabinene, bornyl acetate, or methyl cinnamate as the major component. When stressed, this liverwort shows trans-methyl cinnamate as the major compound.

The sesquiterpene, (-)-(1R, 7S, 1OR)-cadina-3,5-diene) is present, and found only in one other essential oil, Manuka (*Leptospermum scoparium*) from New Zealand. *Phytochemistry* 1997 44:7.

*Marchantia polymorpha* yields an essential oil, containing the sesquiterpenoid, (-)-1(10,11-eremophil-adien-9beta-ol.

Other liverworts worthy of examination include:

*Bazzania* species- sweet balsamic, tree-moss like.

*Frullania* species are mossy and oak moss-like in odor. *F. tamarisci*, in particular, has a remarkable odor reminiscent of hay, costus, violet leaf and seaweed. *Frullania* species are also notable for causing contact dermatitis allergy. *F. boulanderi*, and *F. nisquallensis*, our two local species contain sesquiterpenes with alpha-methylene-gamma-butyrolactones the can cause strong dermatitis.

*Lophozia* species are pleasant with cedar like notes.

*Pellia endivifolia*, usually found east of the Rockies, has a dried, mossy, seaweed-like odor.

*Plagiochila* species have sweet mossy and woody scent; sometimes turpentine-like.

Biocyclohumulenone, isolated from P. sciophila, possesses an aroma reminiscent of patchouli, vetiver, cedar wood, iris, moss and carnations.

*Porella* species will be found to have woody earthy, or malty, earthy odors.

*P. roellii*, in particular, contains very pungent substance.

*Porella cordaeana*, when dry, has a characteristic seaweed-like odor. The volatiles include beta caryophyllene and beta phellandrene.

*Radula* species, especially *R. perrottetii* has a castor-like or animal-like scent.

The *Tritomaria* species is worthy of investigation, as *T. polita* has been investigated in Germany, and contains interesting sesquiterpenoids. Adio et al, *Phytochem* 2003 64:2.

# HYDROSOL

Liverwort water lessens hot dropsy, comforts and strengthens the liver, and for those that too much the work of love or of generation that his liver drys or destroys also.                                    **BRUNSCHWIG**

# LIVERWORT ESSENCE

Lichen (sic) *Marchantia polymorpha* essence is for when we feel alienated from the source of our being; life can be very difficult and unrewarding. Indeed, in extreme circumstances we may feel that there is just no point in going on living.                                    **BAILEY**

Snake Liverwort essence is associated the concept of regeneration, cell division and transmutation.

In the case of regeneration, the essence may help promote increased production of cell growth and strengthen the ability to repair. On the other hand, it may help to slow down the excessive cell growth of cancer cells and skin cells related to psoriasis and related conditions. For the latter, it combines well with Velvet Foot.

The essence is helpful to those who feel vulnerable to parasites. This could involve susceptibility to "energy vampires" in a social, workplace or clinical practice, or individuals who believe their energy is waning due to perceived or real intestinal parasites. It combines well with Lobster mushroom essence.

Another aspect that is helped by Snake Liverwort essence is the impression in pregnancy that the fetus is a parasite. Indeed, the feeding from mother can be interpreted as such, when there is a lack of nurturance or resistance to the new experience. The essence, in this case, may help induce calm and acceptance in both mother and unborn child.

Early *in utero* experiences can influence the developing fetus. Bruce Lipton (2013) writes. "Now we know that the very same chemicals that shape a mother's experiences and behaviors cross the placenta and target the same cells and genes in the fetus that they do in the mother. The consequence is that the developing fetus, bathed in the same blood chemistry as the mother, experiences the same emotions and physiology as the mother.

The fetus, for example, absorbs cortisol and other stress hormones if the mother is chronically anxious. If the child is unwanted for any reason, the fetus is bathed in the chemicals of rejection."

Snake Liverwort essence may reinforce the ability of the body to transmute one element into another. Organic silica, for example, is utilized by the body for the formation of calcium. Organic manganese may be transmuted into organic iron. And so on. For this purpose, add two drops of snake liverwort essence to your herbal preparation at the last minute before ingestion.

For more information, refer to the fascinating work of Dr. Kervran (1972).

Snake Liverwort is associated with the moon sign in Scorpio and the planet Pluto.

# PERSONALITY TRAITS

Step Lightly on Your Liverwort
No exquisite blossom to delight you in the Spring
But a quiet mediocrity this raspy bryophyta brings.
Why is the corrugated interloper so supine,
Puckered green and brown, much maligned?
Lanquishing dejected, unique and bizarre,
This raspy liverwort- sometimes black as tar.
This austere scabrous plant, survivor extraordinaire
Growing for its own sake, requiring no care
On sodden barren ground- requiring only air.
Insects do not relish it, slugs just slip away.
So step lightly on your liverwort. Let it stay.
Every garden needs liverwort to remind the human race
Someday you'll be wrinkled with warts upon your face.

JANET LOGG

**LOMATIUM**
**WILD CELERY**
**INDIAN BALSAM ROOT**
**FERN-LEAVED DESERT PARSLEY**
**CARROT LEAVED BISCUITROOT**
**CHOCOLATE TIPS**
**PURPLE FLOWERED LOMATIUM**
(*Lomatium dissectum* [Nutt.] **var.** *dissectum*
               Mathias & Constance)
(*L. dissectum* [Nutt.] **var.** *multifidum*
               Matthias & Constance)
(*Leptotacnia multifida*) not accepted
(*Leptotania dissectum*) not accepted
**BARE STEM BISCUITROOT**
**INDIAN CELERY**
(*L. nudicaule* [Pursh] J. M. Coult & Rose)
**PRAIRIE PARSLEY**
**NINE-LEAVED DESERT PARSLEY**
**NARROW LVD. DESERT PARSLEY**
**NARROW-FRUITED WESTERN WILD PARSLEY**
(*L. triternatum* [Pursh] J.M Coult. & Rose)
**GREAT BASIN BISCUITROOT**
(*L. simplex* [Nutt. J. F. Macbr.)
**SWALE DESERT PARSLEY**

**SEVALE DESERT PARSLEY**
**WYETH BISCUITROOT**
(*L. ambiguum* [Nutt.] Coult. & Rose)
**LONG FRUITED PARSLEY**
**LARGE FRUITED DESERT PARSLEY**
**INDIAN CARROT**
**INDIAN SWEET POTATO**
(*L. macrocarpum* [Nutt. ex Torr. & A. Gray]
               J. M. Coult & Rose)
(*Cogswellia macrocarpa*) not accepted
(*Peucedanum macrocarpum*) not accepted
**WHITE-FLOWERED PARSLEY**
**NORTH IDAHO BISCUITROOT**
(*L. orientale* J. M. Coult & Rose)
**HAIRY-FRUITED PARSLEY**
**CARROT LEAF DESERT PARSLEY**
(*L. villosum* Raf.) not accepted
(*L. foeniculaceum* [Nutt.] J. M. Coult & Rose)
**BISCUIT ROOT**
(*L. montanum* J.M Coult & Rose) not accepted
(*L. cous* [S. Watson] J. M. Coult & Rose)
(*Peudedanum ambiguum*) not accepted
**PARTS USED**- root, flowers, leaves and seeds.

The Genus name is from the Greek **LOMATION** meaning a little border, referring to the shape of the winged fruit. Macrocarpum is from the Greek **KARPOS** meaning fruit, and **MACRO**, for large.

Lomatium is a perennial member of the parsley family, something obvious when you nibble on the fresh leaf. There are over 70 species in the genus, maybe more. As Stephen Buhner writes, "Trying to pin a taxonomist down is like gluing feathers on a donkey so it can fly."

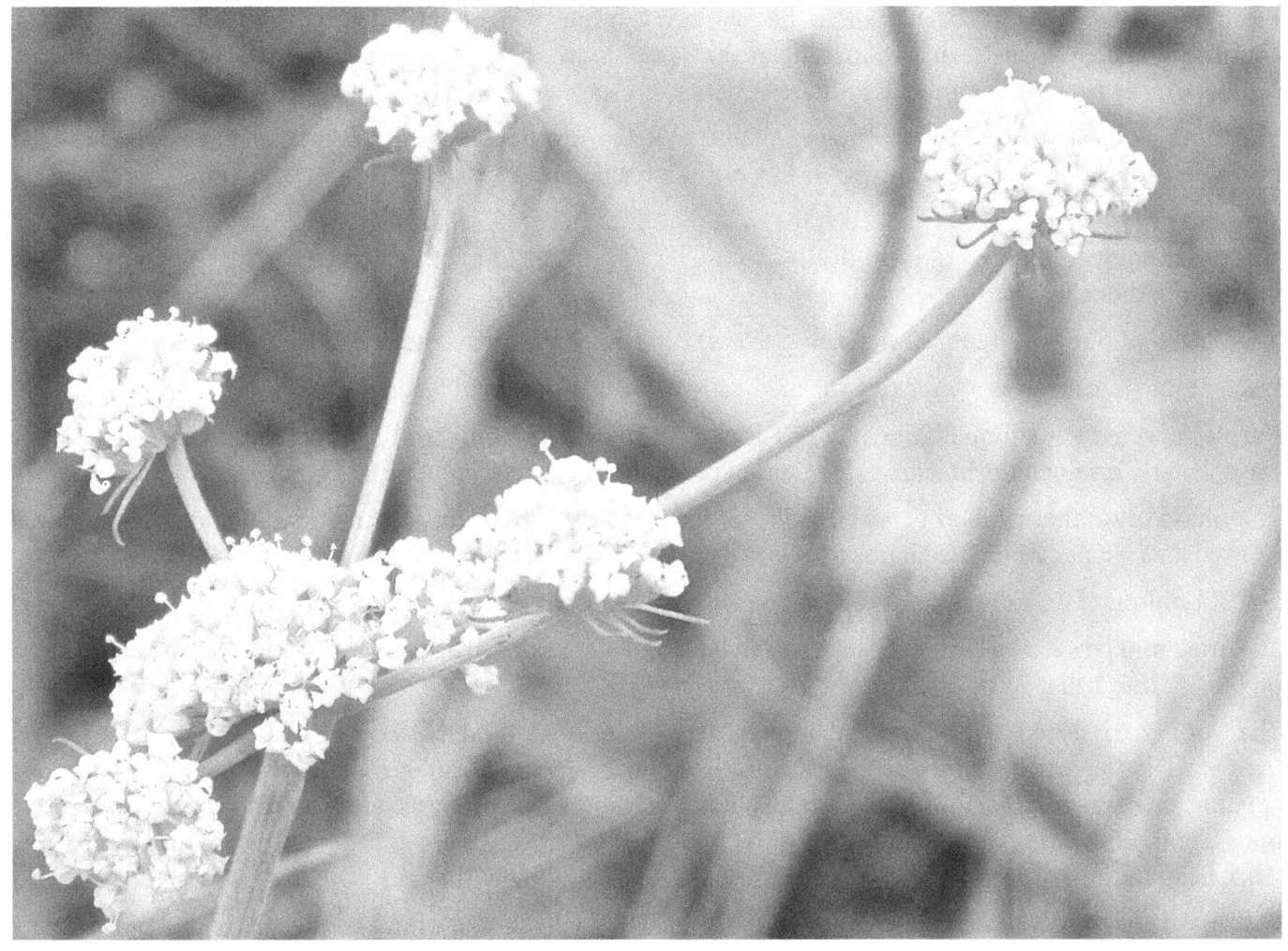

LOMATIUM NUDICAULE

Various native tribes, including the Pawnee, carried lomatium seeds with them to attract love and new friendships.

It is associated with Venus and the water element, even though some species live on steep, rocky hillsides in very dry areas in my region of Alberta.

Many species are rare, and because they take a long time to grow, and cultivation is difficult, be very selective if you are wild crafting. Use species most common to area for medicine, and do not eat them. They are not really that tasty, and why waste valuable medicine.

Some of the species have edible, starchy parsnip-like roots, with many species called biscuit root. *Lomatium dissectum* has a bitter, waxy and oil root that is not that tasty. These roots are best collected in fall after flowering has stopped.

They can be dried, ground into flour and made into biscuits or cakes. The milky sap from the spring roots has skin moisturizing qualities. All lomatium are edible, it is just that some of the roots are tastier than others. Indian Balsam root, or Chocolate Tips, so named for the small, purple flowers, was collected by some tribes, sliced and partially dried, and threaded with a bone needle onto dogbane strings for later use.

The dried roots were soaked in water for two nights and steamed. They are more bitter than other genus members.

The fresh leaves, as mentioned, have a strong parsley taste that spice up salads.

A tea can be made from the leaves, stems and flowers. The seeds can be collected in fall, and eaten roasted or dried.

Fresh *L. dissectum* root has been used, in the past, as a fish stupefacient poured into creeks, and killing fish for about a kilometer downstream. An insecticide for horses to rid them of lice was also made from the root as a solution, or by rubbing the animals with fresh stems and leaves.

The root was also used as a hide-tanning agent, due to its astringency. The fresh roots smell like a cross between parsnips and lemon pledge furniture polish, a distinct resinous oily odor.

An article in *Ecology* 1998 79:7 looked at the multiple consumers of *L. dissectum* over a ten year period. Pocket gophers accounted for 43% of plant deaths, with over two-thirds of plants attacked each year by at least one insect or pathogen.

The Blackfoot pulverized Lomatium (*L. dissectum*) root and smudged as incense in ceremonies.

Decoctions were given as a tonic to weakened patients so that they could gain weight.

Purple-flowered Lomatium is known as Cut-leafed Angelica, Big Turnip, or Big Medicine, by the Blackfoot. It was formerly assigned the botanical designation of *Leptotaenia multifida*. The flowers are sometimes yellow.

The Blood of southern Alberta brewed the plant for chest troubles or for spitting up of blood. The plant was chewed and slapped on broken limbs to help relieve pain.

The Thompson of BC infused the dried root for colds, and fresh root as a poultice for sprains and broken bones.

The dried root powder was sprinkled on wounds, boils and other skin sores, or mixed with skunk fat and smeared on burns. They call it Bitter Head Top.

The Nez Percé referred to this powerful herb as Sacred Root. They used the shoots traditionally as a tonic, and to treat colds, flu, coughs, tuberculosis, arthritis, rheumatism, and dandruff. A root decoction was used for poor appetite, or it was combined with tobacco for sinus congestion. The root was poulticed and applied to bruises, burns, boils and various swellings. The root oil was dropped in sore eyes, and to treat horse distemper, kills ticks, fleas and revive exhausted animals.

Prairie Parsley (*L. triternatum*) is known as **OPIHTAHTSI** by the Blood, who used extracts of the roots to both induce abortions and stop nosebleeds. The neighboring Blackfoot stuffed animal pelts with the fruit during tanning to keep them from smelling too rank.

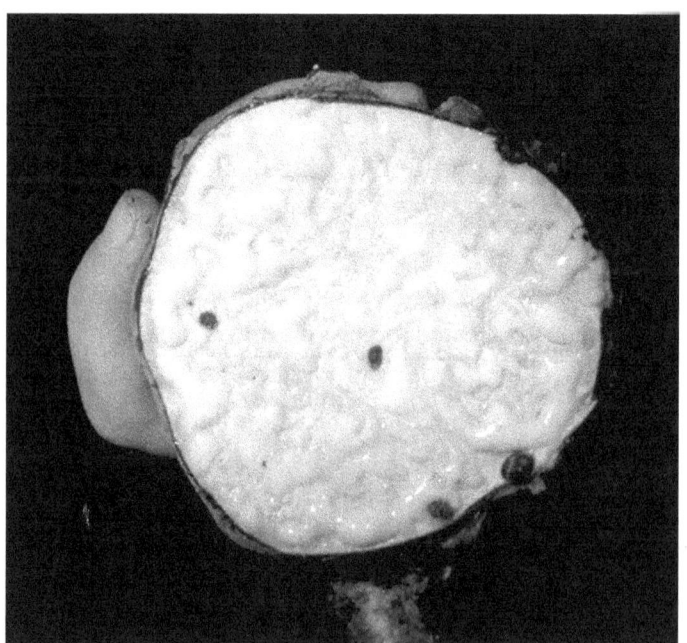

FRESH LOMATIUM ROOT OOZING SAP

The flowers were used in pemmican, and the seeds chewed by runners. A strong paste of the root was applied externally to the area of broken bones to help alleviate pain. It was considered a Big Medicine for respiratory conditions.

A porcupine foot stuffed with the fruits, and attached to a young girl's hair was a good luck charm.

The Interior Salish Natives of British Columbia used the flowers, leaves, stems and seeds of *L. triternatum*, and *L. ambiguum* for flavoring soups, teas, meat stews and tobacco. The tea was often used for sore throats and colds.

The seeds add a nice menthol taste to pipe tobacco.

Nine-leaved Desert Parsley root was decocted by the Blackfoot and used for treating coughs and sore throats. Long distance runners would chew on the seeds to prevent side aches.

The root was chewed by Blackfoot healers and spit through an eagle bone tube onto the patient's injury. The spray was thought to penetrate at that spot of the body.

Horses stricken with distemper were made to inhale the smoke of Lomatium root, by smoking roots over hot coals.

Lomatium root was mixed with the brains of the buffalo and used for tanning hides.

The highly scented stems, after drying, were cut into small pieces and worn as necklaces around the neck by various Native tribes.

The Thompson traditionally powdered the dried roots to dust wounds and sores.

Numerous tribes used root decoctions for various respiratory problems, such as flu, coughs, sinus, asthma, pneumonia and tuberculosis, as well as urinary tract and eye infections. The dried root was also combined with tobacco, and smoked for sinus and other respiratory trouble.

The fresh root was squeezed until one drop of oil fell into sore eyes.

The fresh root pulp was placed on the cut umbilical stump of newborns in the Washoe tribe.

When fresh root was unavailable, the oil was skimmed off the decoction.

Hairy Fruited Parsley is a short perennial with any stem, and small yellow flowers on very short stalks.

The Pawnee called it Flat Herb, or **PEZHE BTHASKA**, and used the seeds as a love charm.

They believed the seeds "rendered the possessor attractive to all persons, so he would have many friends, all people would serve him well, and if used in connection with certain other plants would make him winning to women, so he might win any woman he might desire", according to Gilmore. Red Cardinal Flower (*L. cardinalis*) was other part of a favourite combination, given as a love charm.

Indian Carrot or Sweet Potato (*L. macrocarpum*) is one of the tastier roots, although still strong and peppery. The Natives of British Columbia dug up the non-flowering (female) plants, saying the "male" plants with flower were too bitter.

The plant is called **QW'EQW'ILA** by several Interior tribes with many stories involving the root in Salish mythology.

According to one tradition, the meadowlark sings, "don't spoil my Qw'eqw'ila!"

The Crow and Cherokee call it Bear Root, and used it for medicine, after first burning off the outer root bark. For sore throats, a piece of the root was chewed; while for colds a tea was prepared from root shavings combined with animal fat. For swellings, a poultice of shaved and boiled root was laid on the affected area, while a salve was prepared from root shavings and tallow tea that was boiled until the water was gone.

The Blackfeet made a tea of the root that was taken for weakened conditions. As ceremonial incense, the root was sprinkled on fire coals.

White Flowered Parsley is similar in appearance to *L. macrocarpum*, but with white or pink flowers. It is confined to southern Manitoba on the Canadian prairies, but is also known as North Idaho Biscuitroot.

The Cheyenne call it Bear's Food, and used root and leaf infusions for intestinal pain and diarrhea in both children and adults.

Biscuitroot (*L. cous*) is a yellow flowered member of the genus found on dry hillsides and coulees. The roots are the best tasting of the genus. They were dug up by Native people in April and May, during or just after flowering; and eaten raw, boiled or pit-steamed. The roots were split and dried on mats in the sun, and then formed into flour for cakes, or stored for later use. It was a principal food of the Nez Perce tribe, who made cakes of the root flour.

To make the cakes, flour was moistened, and formed into bricks suspended and partially baked over a fire. The cakes were pierced with holes, through which they could string a thong to hang from saddles. Larger cakes lasted about one year; while smaller finger cakes, when properly dried, lasted up to two years.

Bare Stem Desert Parsley (*L. nudicaule*) is a yellow flowered species with a blue white bloom on leaves. The leaves were eaten fresh, or cooked in stews, while the seeds were used to flavour beverages, tobacco, and chewed to relieve colds.

The Sanich (WSÁNEC) of Vancouver Island call it **KEXMIN**. They would burn the seeds on a fire when smoking salmon. Other British Columbia indigenous people used the seeds as incense at funerals, or singers chewed the seeds to soothe their throat.

The seed smoke relieved headaches, and seed infusions were taken internally for colds and coughs. The term **KEXMIN** may derive from **SKEX**, meaning "to put a curse on someone", but was usually used to protect someone from a curse or evil thoughts.

Ryan Drum, noted west coast herbalist, believes this species is as good as others. The young roots are sweet and tender, and only contain medicinal value when more mature.

*Lomatium dissectum* seed germination up to 99.2% can be achieved with RIBAV˜, a microbial seed pretreatment for 20 minutes. Lechamo et al, *Hort Sci* 1998 33.

## MEDICINAL

**CONSTITUENTS-** *L. dissectum* root- 20% gum resins, coumarin glycosides, including nodaketin, luvangetin, columbianin, columbianin-6"-apioside, 2-(7Z-pentadecenyl) and 2-(7Z-heptadecenyl)-3-hydroxy-penta-2,4-dien-4-olide (0.2%) psoralen, cynaroside, pyrano-coumarin, volatile oils, valeric acid, and methylamine, and exceptionally high (22.8%) ascorbic acid content. Several tetronic acids (color-less oils) and a glycoside of luteolin have been shown to be the principal anti-fungal and anti-bacterial metabolites; but may also contribute to skin irritation. *L. dissectum var. multifidum* contains about 20% longifolene in essential oils, while *L. dissectum var dissectum* contains just 3%.
*L. dissectum var. dissectum* root contains 2-methylbutyrates, pellandrene, limonene, beta-caryophyllene, palmitic acid, E-beta-ocimene, linolenic acid, octanol, octyl acetate, myrcene, 4-methylpentyl 2-methylbutyrate, alpha-bisabolol, cuparene, Z-S-hexanol, decyl acetate, longifolene, palmitoleic acid, Z-ligustilide and E-2-methyl-3-octen-5-yne.
Apiose, a sugar uncommon in the coumarins is also present.
*L. macrocarpum*- root- osthole; 7-O-methylpeucenin from roots and tops; macrocarpin and sibiricin from the tops.

Lomatium was widely used by Native peoples during the great flu epidemic of 1917. This led several doctors, including E.T. Krebs, Sr. (of B15 and B17 fame) to suggest lomatium "is destined to become one of the most important antibiotic herbs known to man". At the time, it was marketed under the trade name **BALSAMEA**. He wrote a report in the *Bulletin of the Nevada State Board of Health* in 1920.

"A preparation was…employed in a great many cases among the whites, from the mildest to the most virulent type of influenza, and it proved itself to be a reliable agent in preventing pulmonary complications…The cases in which it has been used run into the hundreds. There is probably no therapeutic agent so valuable in the treatment of influenzal pneumonia…It is a bronchial, intestinal and urinary antiseptic, and is excreted by these organs."

Studies by Carlson showed varying degrees of inhibition of all 62 strains of bacteria and fungi tested. *Journal of Bacteriology* 1948 55(5): 615-21.

Lomatium contains immune-stimulating polysaccharides that decrease inflammatory response in the body.

It can be used in viral infections like Epstein-Barr, herpes, SARS, encephalitis and meningitis; and it used extensively by HIV positive patients. Lee et al, *Bioorganic and Medicinal Chemistry* 1994 10 indicated suksdorfin found in *Lomatium suksdorfii* inhibits HIV-I replication.

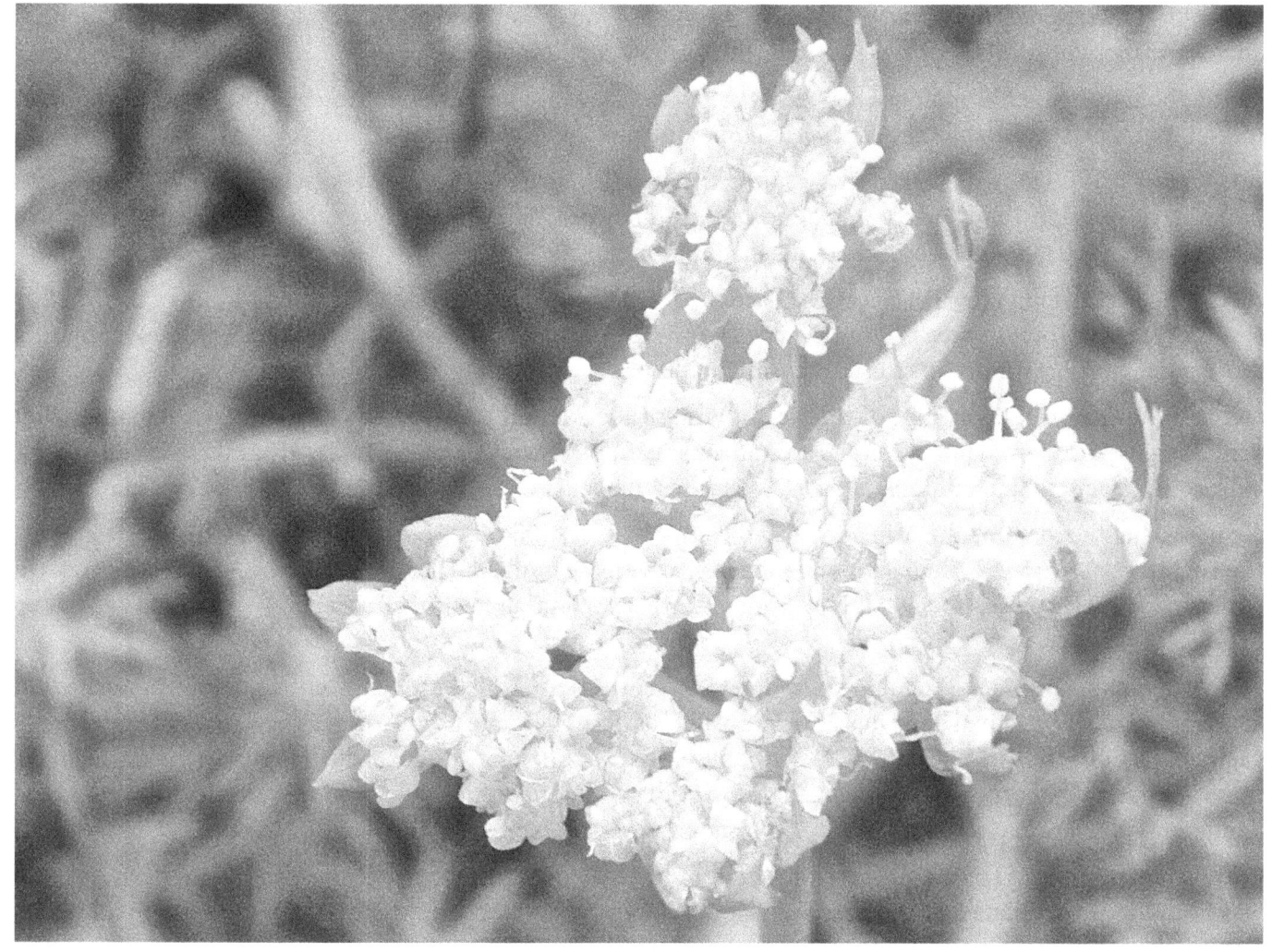

*LOMATIUM NUDICAULE* FLOWER

Psoralens are known to be able to pass through the viral envelope that normally protects a virus from damage. Columbanin has been shown to be anti-spasmodic; its potency is 140% of papaverine HCL in studies reducing uterine spasms.

Psoralen, for example, inactivates viruses, rendering them non-infectious. Schneider K et al, *Viruses* 2015 7(11): 5875-88.

It has been found to lower viral load in Hepatitis C, and help in chronic fatigue syndromes. Longifolene is as active as the drug nifurtimox against *Trypanosoma cruzi*, which causes Chagas' disease. The compound is also present in the roots of Purple Sagebrush (*Artemisia tridentata*).

It combines well with licorice root, red root and/or pleurisy root if the picture pattern fits.

Studies indicate it is active in stimulating white blood cell production. Several of the aromatic compounds have shown ability to limit viral replication, or shorten their life.

In 1995, McCutcheon et al, at the University of British Columbia, conducted research into *Lomatium dissectum* root and found it completely inhibited the cytopathic effects of bovine rotavirus. This causes gastroenteritis in humans. *J Ethnopharm* 1995 49 101-110.

Other viral infections where lomatium will help are mononucleosis, herpes virus, influenza, viral pneumonia and cervical or vulva condyloma associated with human papilloma.

And although thought of mainly as an anti-viral, it was shown, in another McCutcheon study, to completely inhibit the growth of *Mycobacterium tuberculosis,* and allied *M. avium.*

It is partially effective against *Neiserria gonorrhea,* and effective in *Shigella,* Lyme disease, various urinary and pulmonary infections, and against *Streptococcus* and *Staphylococcus bacteria.* It is effective against gram-positive bacteria at a 1:100,000 dilution; and gram negative at 1:10,000 ratio.

McCutcheon et al, found roots of *L. dissectum* active against 9 of 11 bacteria tested, including MRSA, or methicillin-resistant *Staphylococcus aureus. J Ethnopharm* 1992 37 213-223. Studies have found the root pyranocoumarins more potent against influenza viruses than amantadine.

Stephen Buhner writes. "In spite of the lack of viral studies, I, and many others, have found the plant highly active against most viral and bacterial respiratory infections, including pneumonia, avian flu, swine flu, West Nile, or incapacitating pneumonia. In some instances the people were bedridden, very weak and debilitated."

He notes that the pyranocoumarin and related compounds inhibit the M2 ion channel protein. At the present time only a few pathways including this one and neuraminidase inhibitors are clinically proven. Highly aggressive strains such as H1N1, H5N1 and H7N9 are major threats to human health. Wu X et al, *Theranostics* 2017 7(4): 826-45.

The plant is anti-fungal and useful in finger and toenail infection, Athlete's foot as well as internally for *Candida albicans* and other intestinal infections. Cold infusions or decoctions are useful for treating *Gardnerella* and other vaginal yeast infections. Follow up with acidophilus or yogurt douche to re-establish pH. In some individuals, there is a skin rash that could be prevented by including with lomatium a liver or kidney drainage herb such as dandelion root, couch grass, goldenrod, or pipsissewa.

Osthole, found in root of *L. macrocarpon* is present in other members of parsley family. In one study, osthole was found to up-regulate 214 genes and down-regulate 97. Eleven of these are related to the mitochondrial respiratory chain. By inhibiting ATP production, it inhibits growth of fungi and other microbes. Wang Z et al, *Curr Microbiol* 2017 74(3): 389-95.

One study found a combination of osthole and baicalin (Scullcap species) protected mice from methicillin resistant *Staphylococcus aureus* (MRSA) pneumonia. Liu S et al, World *J Microbiol Biotechnol* 2017 33(1): 11.

Luvangetin inhibits nitric oxide and $PGE_2$ production in LPS-stimulated BV2 cells, suggesting neuro-inflammatory activity. Tuan Anh HL et al, *Pharm Biol* 2017 55(1): 1195-1201.

Cynaroside (luteoloside) exhibits activity against enterovirus 71, and blocks 3C protease enzymatic activity. Cao Z et al, *PLoS One* 2016 11(2).

In fact, the latter combines well, one part lomatium to four parts pipsissewa for urinary tract infections. Use 90 drops four times daily.

It combines well with boneset in equal amounts for flu and colds.

Paul Bergner mentions that corticosteroid creams have no effect on the rash, indicating it is not an allergy. Michael Moore says that the rashes "seem to be short term nitrogenous waste product overload from immunologic stimulation, cytokine excess, or the waste products of viral die-off. If you use other herbs to stimulate waste product metabolism and excretion, you get no rashes." I have noted this rash to be worse in an individual with an alkaline system. It can be eased somewhat by soaking in a bathtub of warm water to which 500 grams of baking soda has been dissolved.

Also, by taking two tablespoons of apple cider vinegar in water three times daily for several days prior to using the herb, rashes will not occur.

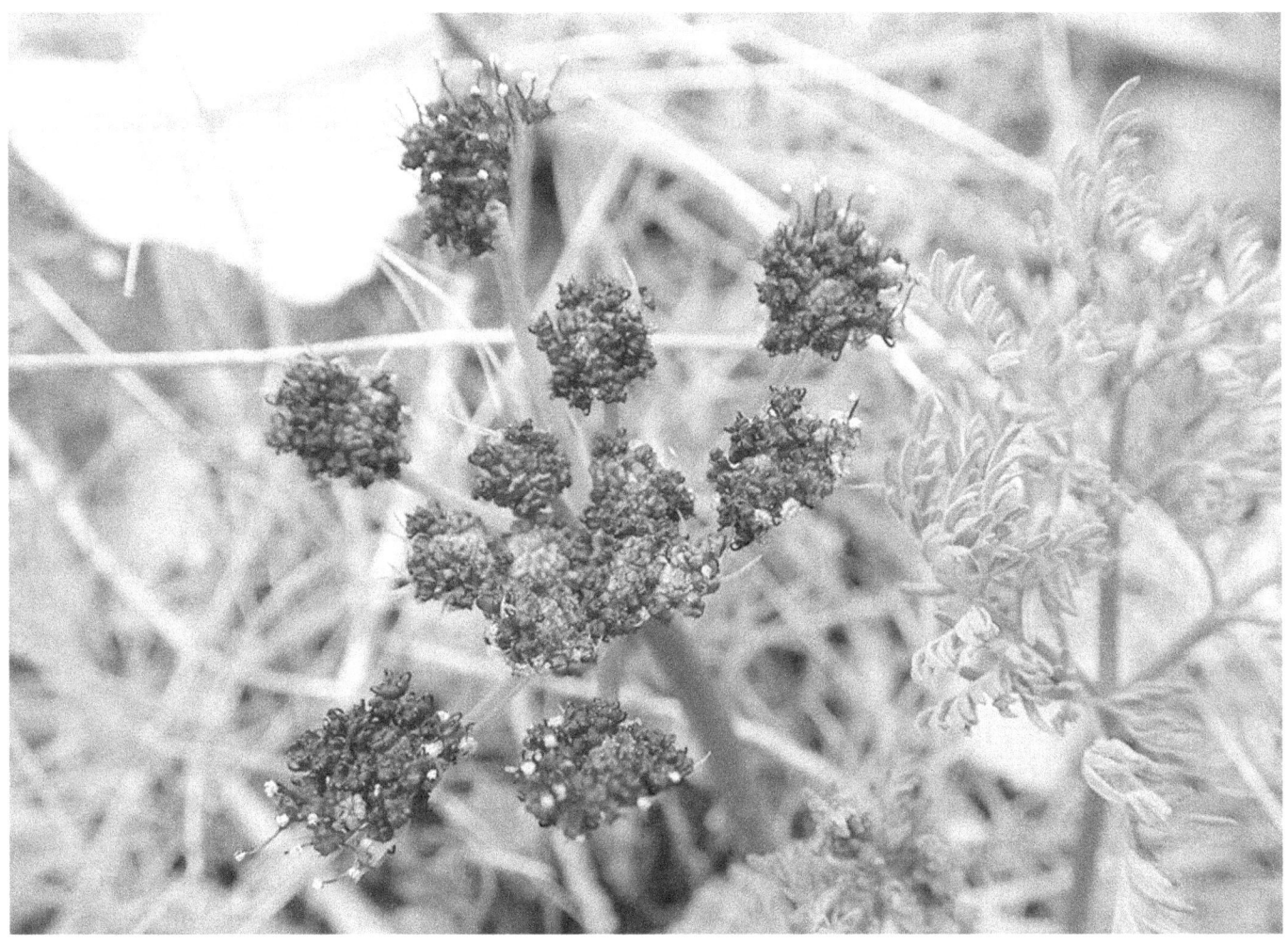

*LOMATIUM DISSECTUM* FLOWER AND LEAF (Courtesy of Tyler Ehlers)

## SEED OIL

The seeds of *L. dissectum* var. *multifidum* contain oils composed mainly of unsaturated fats, especially C16, richer than macadamia nut. These include 12% palmitic acid, 9% palmitoleic acid, and 7.6% decylacetate.

## ROOT OIL

The root contains rich, red oleoresins of various terpenes and sesquiterpenes, and the rich carrot/celery odour could probably be captured by steam distillation in a similar manner to lovage root. You can produce a root oil by using a 1:5 ratio with dry root and good quality monosaturated oil in a low temperature crock pot for 4-6 hours. In this case, keep the lid on, to avoid loss of volatiles.

## ESSENTIAL OILS

A yellow volatile oil (1%) with a mixture of sesquiterpenes, sucrose and an isomer of furanocoumarin nodakenetin, has been distilled from *L. dissectum var. mutifidum*.

Roots have been steam distilled, producing a light-yellow oil (0.6-0.9%) and colour-less oil fraction. Both have shown to be anti-bacterial (gram positive and negative) but ineffective against Candida species.

The oil is composed mainly of sesquiterpenoids that possess anti-viral activity. Valeric acid comprises 20-30%, as well as longifolene 20.4% and mycrene 23%.

The steam distilled root oil contains 4% (E)-Z-methyl limonene 3-octen-5-yne.

Complete record is found in Bairamian et al, *J Ess Oil Res* 2004 16:5.

The leaf and stem of *L. macrocarpum* contain peucenin, methyl ether, beta caryophyllene, (Z)-3 hexenol, palmitic acid and linoleic acid.

The fruit essential oil contains alpha and beta pinene.

*L. torreyi* (*L. californicum*) stems, leaves and fruits have been analyzed and found to contain limonene, mycrene, beta phellandrene, (Z)-beta-ocimene, (F)-beta ocimene, and ligustilide as major components. Ligustilide content is 5.23%, whereas typical Celery seed oil is 2.41%. The roots essential oil was 88% R-(-)-falcarinol.

Ligustilide has potential for its celery like flavour in soups and other commercial food products. Ligustilide is, according to Arctander, "very powerful, warm, spicy-herbaceous and sweet odour of excellent tenacity. In concentrations below five ppm the flavour is warm spicy, herbaceous, often described as soup-like.

## FLOWER ESSENCE

Lomatium flower essence (*L. dissectum*) is made from the large purple-brown blossoms in late spring. It is useful to individuals with the need for more magic in their lives. Everything has sameness, associated with the expression, "the trouble with normal, is it always gets worse". There is a greater need for lateral points of view and problem solving. The essence helps one seek answers with the blinders off.          **PRAIRIE DEVA**

## SPIRITUAL PROPERTIES

This plant found a place very early in Blackfoot mythology, as we are told in one legend of the beaver bundle.

When the chief of the Beavers came ashore to present the Beaver Bundle and all the details for the celebration of the Beaver Ceremonial to the Blackfoot chief who had set up his doge on the banks of the Kis-is-ska-tche-wam (Saskatchewan) or Swift Flowing River, he entered the tipi and handed the red-painted willow tongs and a sack of incense to the chief. The incense was dried lomatium leaf.

With sacred willow tongs, the Blackfoot chief would lift a coal from the fire to the altar. Then, laying on it a piece of the incense, he would purify himself in the smoke so that he might listen to the sacred things that the Beaver chief had to tell him.          **A. BROWN**

A maiden who lived in the Shuswap country refused all offers of marriage telling her numerous suitors none were good enough. Later she became anxious to marry and no one would have her. She married the root of Lomatium and soon after delivered a son. The boy did not know his father, and one day when older was taunted by other boys that he was the son of Lomatium.

He asked his mother who told him this was true, at which he became very ashamed and ran off into the mountains. He began to study and learn magical powers, at which he became quite proficient.

He left the mountain and began to meet other people of power and strength. No one could defeat him. Wherever he travelled the Lomatium root grew.          **TEIT**

## RECIPES

**COLD INFUSION-** Take one tbsp of dried root to one pint of water. Let steep overnight, and gently warm in morning. The aromatic constituents are very volatile. The dried root will last about eighteen months. Note- When collecting the root, especially in spring, dry for a few days in a paper bag, and then slice like oriental stir fry vegetables, and dry on cardboard. If sliced immediately the profuse white sticky sap would be absorbed on the cardboard; so letting them wilt a little makes the sap harden.

**HARVEST AND PROPAGATION-** Save the plant crowns, and replant in your garden. At one time, I thought it could easily be a cultivated commercial crop, but now I realize how slowly these plants grow. Ten year-old plants have a root the size of a pencil with a few leaves. Those fist-sized and flowering could be well over one hundred years old.

Natives of British Columbia used the seeds of *L. nudicaule* for sore throat and colds. Our prairie species could be tested for seed constituents, as taking the seeds only makes perennial roots grow larger and produce more seed the following year.

**TINCTURE- FRESH ROOT-** 10-30 drops up to five times daily. The fresh root tincture is 1:2 at 80% alcohol; the dry root at 1:5 and 60%. Michael Moore preferred spring roots for fresh tincture and fall roots for dry extractions.

Seed tinctures are just as good. Use ratio of 1:3 and 50% alcohol. Crush seeds first.

**CAUTION-** Safety during pregnancy is unknown, so best avoided. It can case skin rashes, or sensitivity in about 1% of individuals. Nothing helps alleviate it except a week or so. A resin free isolate is available for the sensitive. The dried root tincture does not appear to cause rash.

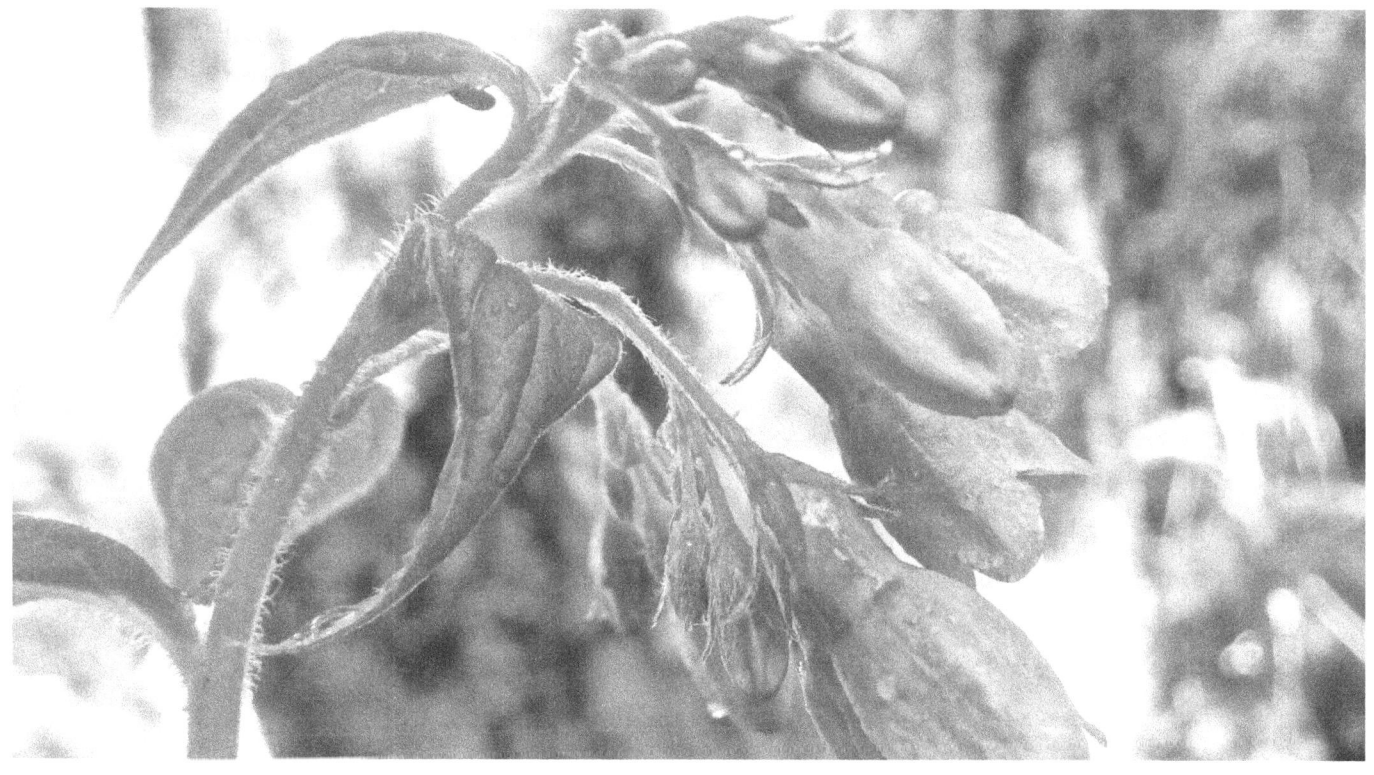

TALL LUNGWORT

**TALL LUNGWORT**
(*Mertensia paniculata* [Aiton] G. Don)
**LONG FLOWERED LUNGWORT**
(*M. longiflora* Greene)
**LANCE LEAVED LUNGWORT**
**NARROW LEAF BLUEBELL**
(*M. lanceolata* [Pursh] DC.)
**OYSTER LEAF**
**SEA LUNGWORT**
(*M. maritima* [L.] Gray)
**PARTS USED**–leaves and flowers

The king's plant is found in the boreal. The Cree named it a long time ago…It is the bluebell of the Boreal and if ever the Cree nation had an item to barter with the rest of the world, this is it.

**BERESFORD-KROEGER**

Mertensia honored the German botanist Franz Mertens, a professor at Bremen, via his son, Karl. Paniculata refers to the panicle arrangement of the flowers on the stem, where the new and younger flowers are in the middle.

The plant is affiliated with the planet Jupiter. Lungwort is from the old English *LUNGENWYRT* and pertains to another plant.

Lungwort is a beautiful blue-flowered member of the borage family. It is often called bluebell, but should not be confused with the lichen Lungwort.

Mertensia split from Asperugo in the late Oligocene to mid-Miocene (26-12 million years ago), and spread to North America when Bergenia was connected.

The lovely, drooping bells begin as tightly bunched pink buds that turn blue as they unfold. Anthocyanins which give the flowers their color, stay red when the cell sap is acidic. As the buds open and the trapped carbon dioxide escapes, the sap becomes more alkaline and the flowers turn blue. This is possibly an adaptive process in that many insects cannot see the red spectrum and will pollinate the open blue flowers, while ignoring the others. The fresh blossoms make an attractive fish lure.

They possess a mild perfume that is sweet and fleeting. Native bees love the nectar.

By the third year, from seed, the new plants will begin to flower.

The Cheyenne tribe used related *Mertensia ciliata* leaf infusions for smallpox and measles; and to increase breast milk supply. For the latter it was combined with red baneberry root and pleurisy root.

The Cherokee used bluebells for whooping cough and tuberculosis. The Iroquois decocted the roots in a battle against venereal disease.

The Northern Cree called it Bluebells, or **KASASIYOYAKANSIYOHK**.

Some Cree call it **OGU-MALASK**, or "king's plant".

The large leaves, of non-flowering plants were gathered, sun dried and used with tobacco as a smoke. The dried root is also powdered and mixed in smoking mixtures.

Lungwort makes an acceptable oyster-flavoured potherb, but it is a little hairy for salads. The steamed aerial parts, before flowering, are wonderful with a small amount of butter and balsamic vinegar.

The dried leaves can be saved for addition to herbal tea mixtures, especially when treating the lungs.

The roots make a very good edible bush food, steamed, boiled or roasted like parsnips.

Both long and lanced-leafed Lungworts are somewhat rare, and confined to the alpine slopes of southwestern Alberta.

Oyster Leaf is found in the northern hemisphere, including Canada, mainly on coastal regions, from British Columbia to Alaska, and on the east coast from Nova Scotia to Baffin Island to Greenland and northern Europe.

## MEDICINAL

**CONSTITUENTS–mucins,** silicic acid, tannin, saponin, allantoin, quercitin, kaempferol.
*M. maritima-* allantoin, rabdosiin, rosmarinic acid.

This herb is sedating to the respiratory system, much like its close relative Borage. Congestion and deep-seated emotional issues can be resolved with the use of both the herb and the flower essence.

The astringent qualities of this herb make it effective in relieving diarrhea and hemorrhoids.

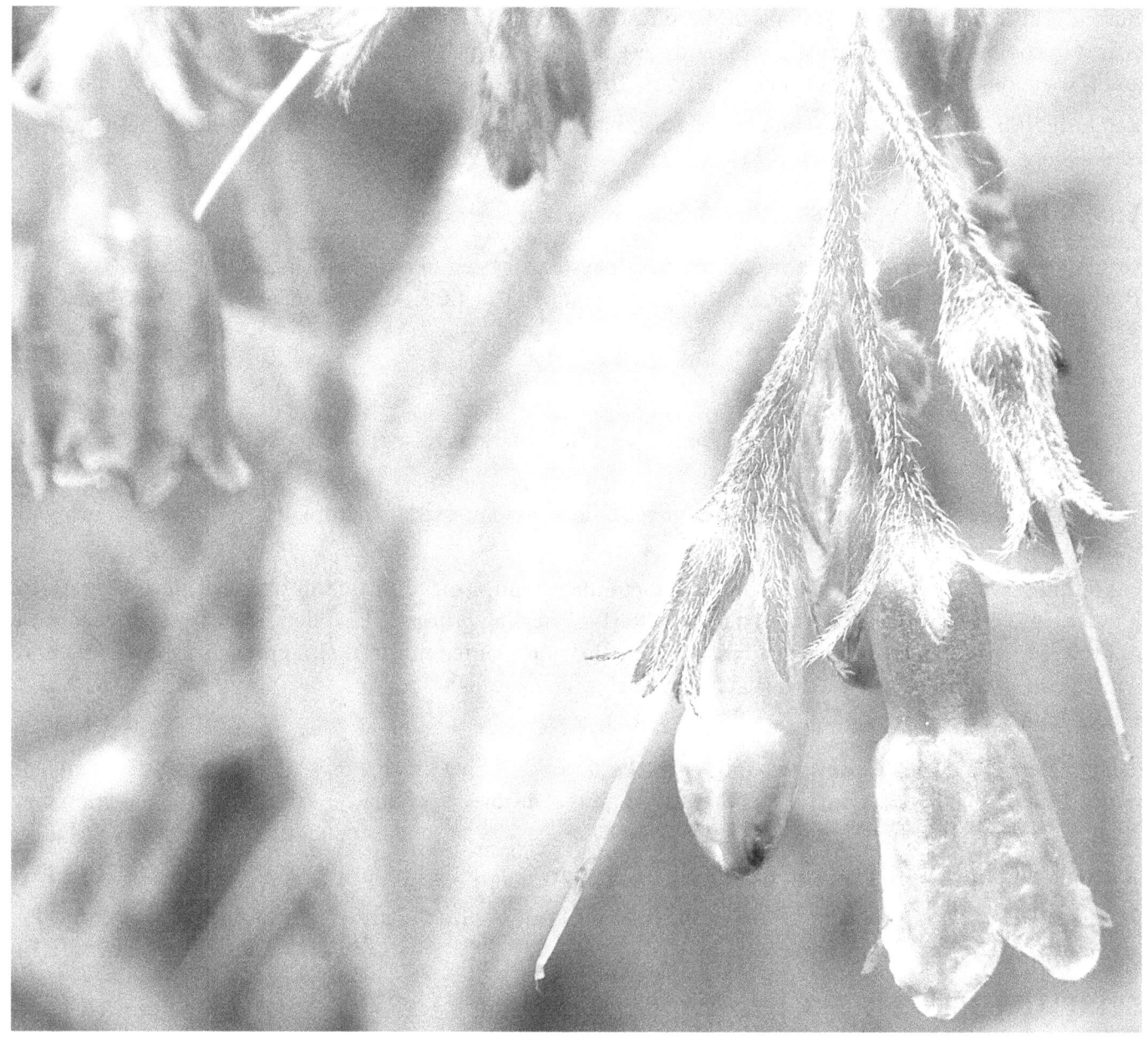

LUNGWORT FLOWERS

The leaves make useful poultices for external cuts and wounds; as well as over the lung region for respiratory problems.

The cool, moist nature of the leaves helps alleviate hot, dry inflamed conditions of the lungs, as well as skin.

Allantoin is present in comfrey, and is a cell proliferator, assisting skin healing.

The compound has peripheral antinociceptive activity that involves the opioid receptor and ATP-sensitive K(+) channels. Florentino IF et al, *J Ethnopharm* 2016 186: 298-304.

Allantoin reduces inflammation, and stimulates fibroblastic proliferation and extracellular matrix synthesis, and thus improves skin wound healing.

Rosmarinic acid is a powerful anti-oxidant. Taken internally, it is known to improve hepatic insulin sensitivity in type 2 diabetes. It also inhibits insulin resistance in skeletal muscle cells by enhancing mitochondrial biogenesis. Jayanthy G et al, *J Cell Biochem* 2017 January 6.

Russell Willier, noted Cree healer, calls the herb **KASASIYOYAKANSIYOHK**, meaning "King's Plant." The root is used in combinations for breaking spells and as a good luck charm. The root serves as a protector for the healer and is used in combinations for heart conditions. The dried root is mixed with tobacco for pipe ceremonies.

Rabdosiin inhibits hyaluronidase and beta-hexasomanidase, suggestive of benefit in anti-allergic activity. Ito H et al, *Bioorg Med Chem* 1998 6(7): 1051-6.

## ESSENTIAL OILS

Oyster leaf (*M. maritima*), also known as vegetarian oyster has been steam-distilled. The essential oils contains 109 compounds, but mainly (Z)-3-nonenal, (Z)-1,5-octadien-3-ol, (Z, Z)-3,6-nonadienal and (Z)-1,5-octadien-3-one.

## FLOWER ESSENCES

Lungwort has the special gift of spiritual song. It's gentle vibrations raise the human experience by putting us in touch with the mother earth.

This flower essence teaches our heart the language of love, as expressed by nature. It helps us be in touch with love in all our relationships.

It is for those who feel they have lost touch with their inner feelings; especially in transitions of life. Like fireweed, it moves into recently burned areas of nature to start the healing process. The difference between the magenta of fireweed and the blue of lungwort best explains the subtly difference in their approach. Fireweed is more dynamic in terms of energy pattern shifts; lungwort more maternal. **ALASKA**

Lungwort flower essence is for those dealing with physical pain. **ROCKY MOUNTAIN**

Tall Lungwort Bluebell (*M. paniculata*) flower essence is for centering into the present that one may contemplate in peace; and open to the source of forgiveness. To retune, restore, re-evaluate, so that harmonious action may result in one's relationships. **CANADIAN**

Narrow Leaf Bluebell essence is for handling peer pressure in any age group. **ROCKY MTN**

Lungwort (*M. ciliata*) is for depression registered in the body as physical gravity; listless, languid or drained— often localized in the respiratory system. **FLOWER ESSENCE SOCIETY**

## SPIRITUAL PROPERTIES

Lungwort is about the air element. The funnel shape of the flower allows one to almost see the plant breathing. All who work with meditation and the use of prana would benefit from the use of this plant.

Spiritually, this is important, due to the difficulties today in fully using prana. When using this herb as a tea, take it anytime up to one hour after exercise, and it will help in the transfer of energy. Prana is a circuit that moves through people and out into the world and is then re absorbed again.

From the lungs, this energy focuses into the brain; and becomes transferred as light into the mind. This is the reverse of the usual, where light moves into thought and then into the brain.

The mind is stimulated, with a similar movement of energy into the body. The movement of flowers from pink to blue is similar to the change in energy patterns in the body.

Those who have difficulty visualizing blues will find they can at least absorb the reddish hues that affect the lower chakras.

There is release of blockages created by anger. Those with high blood pressure should not move energy from breath to the third eye.

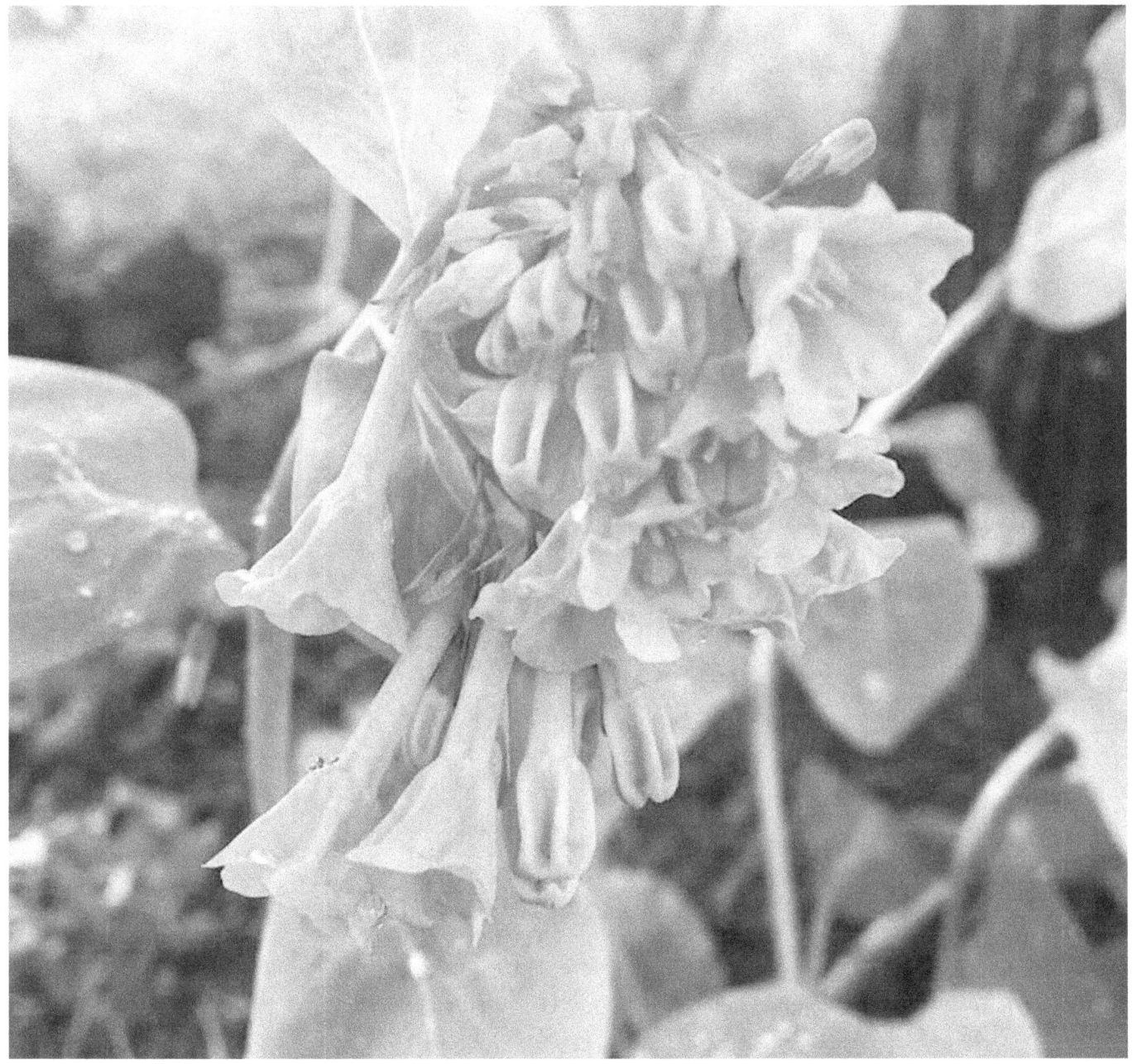

VIRGINIA LUNGWORT

The karmic lesson of lungwort is to remain intertwined with humanity and grow with it. The tuberculosis miasm is eased.

Individuals who experience lung difficulties when Mars is negatively aspected, (such as Saturn, or when it moves through the first house), will find lungwort helps the transition. **GURUDAS**

## RECIPES

**INFUSION**- Pour one cup of boiling water onto on or two tablespoons of dried herb. Drink two to three times daily.

**TINCTURE**- Take one to four mls three times daily. The tincture is made from fresh leaf and flowers at 1:4 and 80% alcohol.

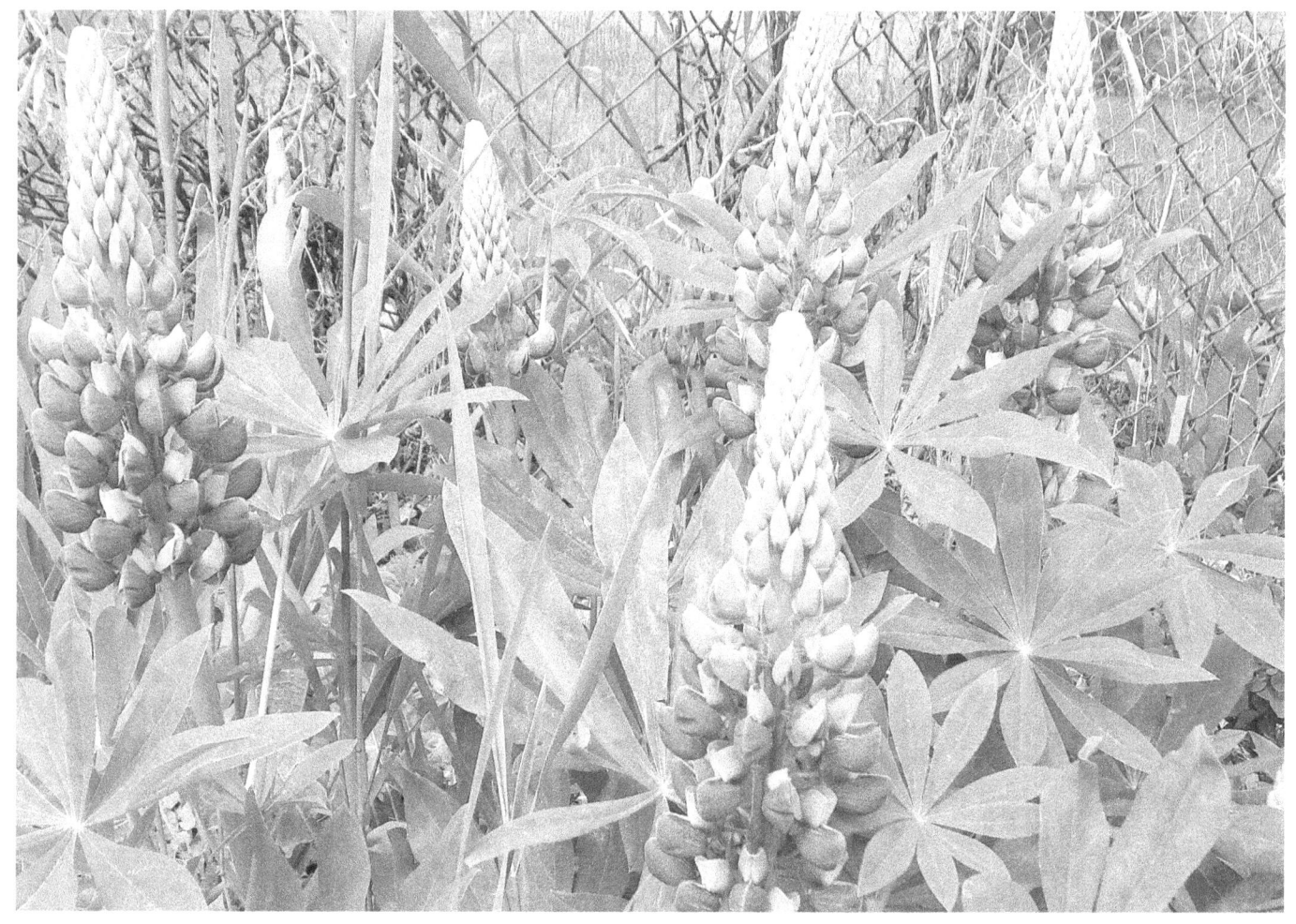

LUPINES

**WIIITE LUPINE**
**WOLF'S BEAN**
(***Lupinus albus*** L.)
(***L. albus ssp. termis*** [Forsk.] Ponert) not accepted
**EUROPEAN YELLOW LUPINE**
(***L. luteus*** L.)
**SMALL LUPINE**
**ANNUAL LUPINE**
(***L. pusillus*** Pursh.)
**LARGE LEAVED LUPINE**
**BLUE POD LUPINE**
**MARSH LUPINE**
(***L. polyphyllus*** Lindl.)

**PERENNIAL LUPINE**
**SILVERY LUPINE**
**SILVER STEM LUPINE**
(***L. argenteus*** Pursh)
**SILKY LUPINE**
**FLEXILE LUPINE**
(***L. sericeus*** Pursh)
**NOOTKA LUPINE**
(***L. nootkatensis*** Donn ex Sims)
**BLUE LUPINE**
**SWEET LUPINE**
**NARROW LEAF LUPINE**
(***L. angustifolius*** L.)
**PARTS USED**- seeds, flowers, roots

Sometimes in June, when I see unearned dividends of dew hung on every lupine, I have doubts about the real poverty of the sands. **ALDO LEOPOLD**

Lupine unsteep'd, to harshness doth incline, and like old Cato, is of temper rough. But drench the pulse in water, Him in wine, They'll lose their sourness, and grow mild enough. **ABRAHAM COWLEY**

Lupine is from the Greek **LUPE** meaning grief. This may be in reference to the facial expression of anyone who has eaten the bitter seeds. Or, it may be from the Greek **LOPOS**, a husk; or **LEPO**, a hull or peel, in reference to the pods.

Later, a false assumption was made between lupine and the Latin **LUPUS**, for wolf. It was, ironically, believed to devour the fertility of the soil with "wolfish voracity".

In Holland, Germany and Sweden, the common names translate as "wolf's bean". Several native tribes of North America included wolf as part of the name for their local species.

Sericeus is from the Latin, meaning silky; argenteus means silvery.

Those seeking to communicate with the dead at the Oracle of Epiros ate a diet of lupine seeds, which induced intoxication and perhaps, made communication much closer. On the banks of the river Acheron sat the Oracle of the Dead, a secret shrine that attracted pilgrims from all of Greece.

The symbolic meaning of lupine is voraciousness. In Ikebana-Japanese flower arranging- the lupine symbolizes avarice.

The reference to wolf-devouring of good soil, is of course, incorrect, as Lupines are nitrogen fixing legumes that help enrich the soil. The ancient Romans grew the lupine as a green manure in the manner of buckwheat to be plowed under, as fodder for animals and seed oil.

It has been used for human and animal feed for over four millennium.

The lupine was said cursed by the Virgin Mary, for when she fled the assassins of Herod, the plants made a noise that attracted the soldiers.

Darwin, in his Movements of Plants, says that the leaves of lupine are remarkable for "sleeping" in three different ways; from being in the form of horizontal star by day, the leaflets either fall and form a hollow cone with their bases upwards, or rise, and the cone is inverted, or the shorter leaflets fall and the longer rise; the object in every case to protect their surfaces from radiation and wetting with dew.

During the day, they are in constant motion, rotating 90 degrees to follow the sun. The name Sundial came from this interesting movement.

The Arctic Lupine (*Lupinus arcticus*) seeds are the oldest discovered seeds in the world to be successfully germinated.

Lupine seeds over 10,000 years old were found in Yukon soil in 1966. Their viability is thought due to the oxygen-depleted soil in which they were found frozen. When planted, they germinated within 48 hours.

The blue lupine was imported to Iceland for erosion control. When I visited this beautiful country in 2014, a blue carpet was found everywhere along the major highways.

An interesting study on the plant and its relationship with hares was conducted by Sharam and Turkington, *Can J Bot* 2005 83:10. They found the Arctic Lupine increased its sparteine content to maximum levels at night, and reduced to minimal in mid-afternoon. As the hares feed at night, this makes perfect sense as a survival mechanism. Coyotes and wolves love to eat rabbits.

Lupines dislike both wet feet and acidic soil. They are well suited to the dry, alkaline prairie soils. The perennials lose their vigor after 3-4 years. The weaker ones can be pulled, and others allowed to self-sow.

The Blood call Silvery Lupine, **AISATTSIKOHTAKO** or "Wolf Turnip". The dried leaves were burned as incense in the Ghost Dance. Those who were sponsoring the dance chewed the leaves of lupine, before undertaking any face painting, to reinforce their powers.

The hairy leaves were decocted for coughs and gas pains, helping relieve flatulence by expelling the pressure. It was also given to those suffering painful or chronic hiccups. They are given a mouthful of tea to swallow while stretching their neck and plugging their ears.

Leaf decoctions were sprayed on the tender sores of horses to protect from them from flying, and biting insects.

The roots were heated and used as a poultice to reduce the swelling of mumps. The Cree call Lupine, **WAPIKWANEYA**.

Small Lupine (*L. pusillus*) was used by the Navaho-Kayenta for both headaches and nosebleeds. They burned the plant as a fumigant for insects.

An unspecified part of lupine was made into a tea taken by Navaho women for fertility. It was believed that the birth of a baby girl was more favored if taken for several days before conception.

Silvery Lupine leaves were made into an external lotion, by the Navaho to treat poison ivy blisters. They also used the plant in the Male Shooting Way and Evil Way ceremonies.

The English herbalist Parkinson said that burning lupine seeds drive away gnats and fleas.

Culpepper said that lupine seeds ease the pains of the spleen, and kill worms. Externally, the seeds cleansed putrid skin ulcers, and gangrenes, as well as scabs, itch and inflammation.

The seeds were used, as pieces of money, by Roman actors in their plays leading to the saying "nummus lupinus", which means "a spurious bit of money".

Roman ladies used the powdered seeds; as did women of the 18th century for face creams. Lupine ointments and facemasks are good for all kinds of skin problems, invigorating tired skin and removing freckles.

The Roman herbalist, Pliny writes, "eating lupines was thought to brighten the mind, and quicken the imagination."

Protogenus, the famous 3rd century painter of Rhodes, is said to have subsisted on a diet of only lupine and water for seven years while working on the famous hunting piece of Ialysus.

Roasted, the seeds make a suitable coffee substitute.

Natives and northern Inuit cooked the roots of Nootka Lupine (*L. nookatensis*); and ate them raw after scraping off the exterior part. Consumed raw, the alkaloids sometimes produced a state resembling drunkenness. See below.

The Haida and Nuxalk of British Columbia dug the spring rhizomes and roasted them on embers.

The Gitksan ate the root in spring before leaves. Heated stones were put in a hole in the ground and covered with grass. Water was added to steam the root placed on top of the grass, and then covered with red cedar mats and dirt for the night.

When the Chinese arrived to work the railway, they taught them how to boil the beans for food, according to Smith.

Traditionally, the seed infusions are used for washing various skin ailments.

The Navaho used the lupine as a remedy for sterility. They also believed, ironically, that taking lupines before conception encouraged the birth of female children.

Other tribes used cold leaf infusions to treat nausea and internal hemorrhage.

Historically, both natives and early pioneers fed small amounts of lupine pods to horses to make them spirited.

It was said that if a horse was too spirited you rubbed lupine seeds in your palm before grabbing the reins.

Nootka Lupine root is a favourite of Grizzly bears, and you can find large feeding excavations in lupine patches, similar in size and appearance to those of bear root (*Hedysarum alpinum*).

In North Africa, the square, yellow seeds of *L. albus* are soaked in brine and eaten as an appetizer called TERMIS.

In Corsica, the seeds are placed in a canvas bag and placed in a stream for a week to remove the poisonous nature. The lupine is grown as fodder for cattle.

The seeds of Tawri (*L. mutabilis*) are soaked in water and eaten in Peru but the water is used as an insecticide and fish poison. The seeds can produce nervous disorders, as well as inflame the stomach and intestine. Several native tribes used lupine seeds for expelling worms and to bring on menstruation.

In the 1930s, George Russell, at age 60, began crossing our native Large leaved lupine (*L. polyphyllus*) with the European *Lupinus bicolour*, and others, to produce the famous Russell hybrids common today. He simply planted every variety for which he could find seed, and let bees do the work. After 15 years, he created a whole new category of plant.

He refused numerous requests to donate his flowers to funerals, saying they were for the living, not the dead.

The original Large-leaved Lupines were noted by the botanist/explorer David Douglas, who sent seeds back to England in 1825.

In 1917, a Lupine banquet was given in Hamburg, Germany, at a special botanical gathering by Dr. Thoms.

On a tablecloth made from lupine fibre, a lupine soup was served, After the soup a Lupine beefsteak, roasted in Lupine oil and seasoned with Lupine extract; then Lupine bread containing 20% lupine, lupine margarine and cheese of lupine albumin; and finally Lupine liqueur and Lupine coffee. Lupine soap served for washing the hands, while Lupine paper and envelopes with Lupine adhesive were available for writing.

Alkaloid free, or sweet strains of *L. albus* are grown largely in South Africa as a grazing crop, or for harvesting and as a stubble crop. The seed is fed to livestock as a protein concentrate.

In Australia, lupine meal is used as a protein supplement in pet foods. Caution is advised in using lupine stubble for livestock feed.

A particular fungus, *Phomopsis leptostromiformis*, produces phomopsins, linear hexapeptides, that are toxic and destructive to microtubules and interfere with absorption of iron, copper and zinc; and metabolism of vitamin E and selenium. Vaccination against lupinosis is showing some success in sheep.

Lupines, at up to 42% protein, could be fed to aquaculture fish, according to Gordon Frank, with AAFRD.

Sweet blue lupines contain hydrolyzed protein peptides that can be used by the cosmetic industry. The variety *Arabella* shows promise as a new crop for Alberta.

Two gram-negative bacteria have been found capable of using lupanine, the predominant quinolizidine alkaloid in wild *L. albus*. Work by Santana et al, in Portugal found two strains growing in the soil around the plants, and suggest they have the ability to remove toxins from QA rich lupine seeds using various biotechnologies.

Work by Gorecka et al, *Nahrung* 2000 44:4 showed that 10% hull or flour of lupine (*L. albus* or *L. luteus*) be added to foodstuffs without sacrificing sensory quality.

Modern breeding of lupines for grain and forage dates back to Sengbusch in 1937, when they obtained the first sweet, or alkaloid free seeds. In South America, the *L. mutabilis* predominates, and Chile has led the breeding of the first stable low alkaloid lines of this species.

In Peru, lupine flour is added to biscuits, breads, noodles, soups and sauces. In Chile, a bland yellow flour from the seeds of *L. luteus* and *L. albus* is nearly 60% protein and added as protein supplement to a gruel, **ULPO**.

Yellow Lupine is an annual that has been used traditionally for treating ulcers externally as a poultice. Internally, it was used for urinary tract infections and ridding the body of parasites.

Why Lupines are not grown more widely is baffling? They can grow in a wide variety of climatic conditions, and require minimal fertilizer.

The seeds contain high concentrations of protein, which is nutritious, functional and cheaper than conventional animal proteins. And the new, sweet varieties are extremely safe, with very low levels of anti-nutritional factors compared to other legumes.

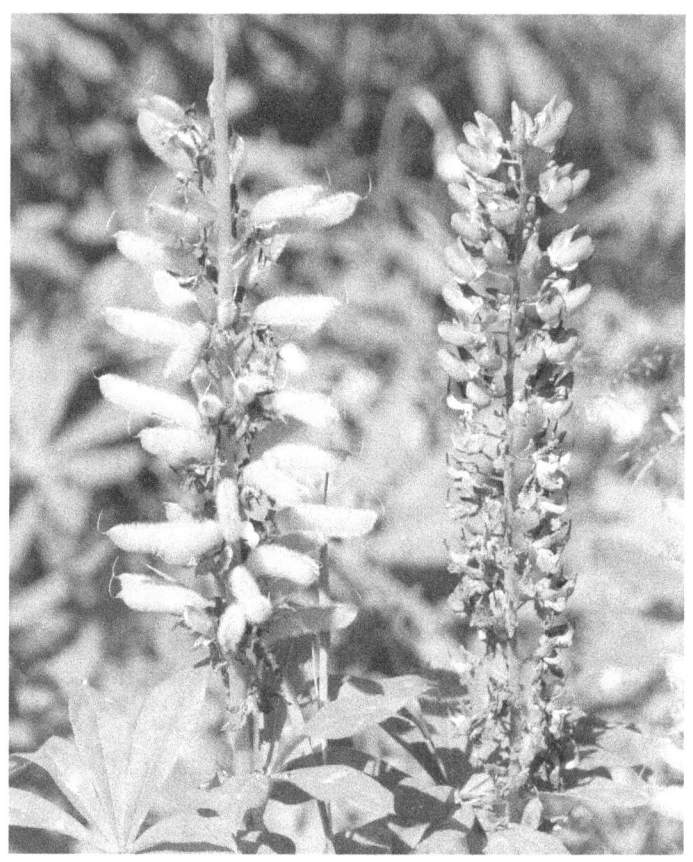

LUPINE SEED PODS

The root nodules of Lupines, especially in spring, contain symbiosomes that possess anti-oxidant and skin cell vitality properties prized for cosmetics.

Leghemoglobin, which mimics human hemoglobin is another natural anti-oxidant, as well as containing peroxidases, SOD, and homoglutathione that help retard the aging process of skin.

Lupines are nitrogen-fixing legumes that can utilize a bacterial inoculant such as *Bradyrhizobium* for maximal yields.

Lupine production is increasing in some countries. Australia, for example, increased cultivated area from 55000 hectares in 1980, to nearly a million hectares in just seven years. The seeds do not require heat treatment before use as animal feed. Milk from lupine feed animals contains more unsaturated fatty acids, than those fed soybean meal.

More recently, they have made a comeback in England. In a *Times of London* newspaper article of May 2000, "England's 'green and pleasant land' is to be transformed into a sea of blue, white and yellow in the fight against genetically modified food.

Lupines will provide the protein for GMO-free animal feed, with 150 farmers signed up to trials of lupine as the feed of the future. New varieties are being used, more suited to the English climate.

Some work has been done in Ontario, where the crop requires 120 days to maturity. Research in Prince Edward Island, indicates lupine silage showed no differences between feed intake and total weight gain of beef steers compared to traditional grass silage.

Blue Lupines are an annual that are more winter hardy than yellow but less than white lupine. It is used in many areas as a green manure. In India, for example, when planted as a green manure between successive crops of potatoes, it increased yields by nearly 4 MT/hectare.

Annual Lupines are an excellent green manure before planting strawberries, as their roots have phosphorus-gathering mycorrhizal fungi. Sow in early summer, and plow under before flowering.

Seeded at a rate of 65-90 kg/ha, blue lupine is cultivated and harvested like white lupine.

A perimeter of Lupines will deter rabbits from your herb, flower or vegetable garden.

Lupines are tolerant of aluminum, and may lead to some use as bio-accumulators of the toxic metal, and excess pesticides. They were planted around Chernobyl, Ukraine, to absorb the radiation created by the nuclear disaster. Recent work by Esteban et al at the U of Madrid has found lupines hyper-accumulate arsenic in roots.

Lupine leaves follow the sun, increasing their exposure to sunlight by up to 40%.

The seeds of *L. albus, L. luteus, L. varius, L. mutabilis,* and *L. terminis* are roasted to remove toxins, and used as a flour or coffee substitute.

White lupine seeds may be useful substitute for soy in broiler chickens. Laudadio V & V. Tufarelli, *J Sci Food Agric* 2011 91(11): 2081-7. And, egg-laying hens. Lee MR et al, *Vet Anim Sci* 2016 1-2: 29-35.

Burning lupine seeds is supposed to drive gnats and other insects away. Aphids usually avoid high alkaloid plants, but the aphid, *Macrosiphon albifrons* lives on lupines with high concentrations. It does this to gain protection from a beetle, *Carabus problematicus* that preys on it. Occasionally, the beetles make a mistake and consume an aphid with high alkaloid levels, and are literally put on their backs by the toxins and do not recover for at least forty-eight hours.

## MEDICINAL

**CONSTITUENTS-** *L. albus* seeds- lupanine (1.47%), lupinin, sparteine, oils, protein (36-52%) lecithin, beta sitosterol, fat (5-20%) and iso-sitesaphosphoric acid. Lysine is rich at 5.2%; but the seeds are typically deficient in sulfur amino acids like methionine.
*L. albus*- (-)-delta5-dehydroalbine, albine, luteone (-0-11,12-seco-12, 13-dide-hydromultiflorine, and (-)13 alpha-hydroxymultiflorine. Also contains raffinose family of oligosaccharides.
Various quinolizidine alkaloids are present that are cause for concern. As with many plant toxins, they are metabolized in animals by undergoing biotransformation in the liver, usually mediated by the cytochrome P-450 system.
*L. argenteus*- alpha isosparteine, alpha-isolupanine, thermopsine, sparteine, delta-5-dehydrolupanine; lupanine, anagyrine.
*L. luteus* foliage- (0.6-1.6%) sparteine, 13-hyroxylupanine, lupinines, lupinidin, rechts-lupinine, d-lupiane, genistein 8-C-glucoside and p-cumaroyllupinine, stachyose
Seeds- (0.4-3.3%) lupinine, lupulidin, sparteine, beta galactan; D-pinitol (0.13 mg/gram) and in some cultivated strains gramine.
*L. polyphyllus*- total alkloids (5.3%), ammondendrine, lupanine, angustifoline (3.28%).

Low alkaloid, or sweet lupine varieties are useful for animal consumption, but have the disadvantage that they can only be cultivated if predators are kept away with fences and pesticides. Protein efficiency ratio of 2.48 has been achieved in *L. albus* with the supplementation 0.3% methionine, the limited amino acid.

Medicinally, the seed are used as an alterative, anthelmintic, carminative, de-obstruent, discutient, diuretic, emmenagogue, pectoral and tonic.

The bruised seeds are soaked in water and applied to sores.

In old England, lupine meal was mixed with goat gall and lemon juice to form an ointment.

Seed decoctions of *L. albus* have been shown in laboratory studies to lower blood sugar levels. It contains high protein, low fiber and monosaturated fatty acids.

This may be due to a low content of monosaccharides and di-saccharides and no starch; leading to a number of functional food product possibilities surrounding diabetes.

Extracts of whole seeds of *L. albus and L. termis* possess hypoglycemic activity. Knecht et al, *J Heb Pharmacother* 2006 6:3-4.

Both white and sweet lupine seeds, when germinated, increase their genistein and cinnamic acid derivatives. Andor B et al, *Evid Based Complement Altern Mcd* 2016: 7638542.

Sweet Lupine (*L. angustifolius*) beta-conglutin protein may be useful in the prevention and treatment of diabetes, as well as ameliorate inflammatory disease. Lima-Cabello E et al, *Mol Nutr Food Res* 2016 Dec 24.

Conglutin-gamma may regulate muscle energy metabolism, protein synthesis and muscle specific MHC gene transcription, through modulation of the insulin-resistant conditions. Terruzzi I et al, *Nutr Metab Cardiovasc Dis* 2011 21(3): 197-205.

Lupin protein was tested on 72 high cholesterol subjects in a randomized, double-blind, controlled three-phase crossover study. Three diets included 25 grams per day of lupin protein, milk protein, or milk protein plus 1.6 grams of arginine for twenty-eight days.

The lupin group had lower total and LDL cholesterol, triglycerides, homocysteine and uric acid, and was strongest in those with severe hypercholesterolemia. Bahr m et al, *Clin Nutrition* 2015 34(1): 7-14.

Lupine protein does not influence weight loss, but does provide benefit in terms of insulin sensitivity and blood pressure. Belski R et al, *Int J Obesity* (London) 2011 35(6): 810-9.

An extract of *L. termis* has been used successfully in treating chronic eczema. Antoun et al, *J Nat Prod* 1981 44:2. Alcohol extracts of the seeds may help prevent diabetes mellitus associated DNA damage from oxidative stress. Farghaly AA & ZM Hassan, *Eur Rev Med Pharmacol Sci* 2012 16 (suppl 3): 126-32.

Seed tinctures of 1:10 ratio and 1:1 fluid extracts are available from European herbal firms.

Multiflorine, isolated from *L. albus* has been found to possess hypoglycemic effect in diabetic induced mice, and is a CNS depressant. Sheweita et al, *Toxicology* 2002 174:2.

Seeds of *L. albus and L. caudatus* lower blood sugar levels in work by Knecht et al, *Journal Herb Pharm* 2007 6:3-4.

The compound 13-hydroxylupanine is both hypotensive and anti-arrhythmic.

More recent work by Kubo et al, in *Bio and Pharm Bulletin* 2000 23:9 found compounds possessing the quinolizidin-2-one ring, may lead to new basic structure for diabetic drugs. Luteone has been found to possess anti-fungal activity, and lupanine shows activity against malaria.

Alpha galactosides, also known as raffinose family oligosaccharides, are prebiotics. These sugars encourage the growth of friendly intestinal bacteria, and are of interest in producing functional foods, such as soft drinks, cookies, cereals and candies.

Work by Martinez-Villaluenga et al, *J Ag Food Chem*, 2004 52 prepared RFOs with 99.4% purity from *L. albus* seeds.

Work by Andersen et al, *J Ag Food Chem* 2005 53 identified the raffinose, stachyose, verbascose and ajugose content of four Lupine species.

The sprouts were previously used to detect cancer, and to determine either an increase or decrease in malignant cells while under treatment.

Research by Kapusta et al, from the Institute of *Bioorganic Chemistry of the Polish Academy of Sciences*, in Poznan, Poland, utilized Yellow Lupine (*L. luteus*) as an edible vaccine against the hepatitis B virus. They introduced a DNA fragment encoding hepatitis B virus surface antigen into *Agrobacterium tumerifacience* LBA4404, to obtain transgenic lupine tissue.

Mice were then fed the transgenic lupine tissue and developed significant levels of hepatitis B virus-specific antibodies.

In the same experiment, human volunteers were fed with transgenic lettuce plants expressing hepatitis B virus surface antigen, and they developed specific serum-IgG response to plant produced protein. This is very exciting work that should be followed more closely.

In a double blind study comparing a 10% ointment from lupine seeds, with a 0.02% flumethasone pivalate ointment and a placebo, it was shown that the lupine seed extract was effective in the treatment of chronic eczema. The result was statistically comparable to those obtained with corticoid therapy. *Journal of Natural Products* 1981 44.

Luteone shows activity against sensitive and resistant strains of *Staphylococcus aureus*. Akter K et al, *J Ethnopharmacology* 2016 185: 171-81.

Yellow lupine (*L. luteus*) flowers, leaves and root all inhibit mycobacterium. Genistein 8-C-glucoside, found in the flowers, possesses anti-atherosclerotic activity.

The whole plant is used in Traditional Chinese Medicine, as a diuretic, insecticidal, febrifuge and for respiratory complaints. It is known as **YU SHAN DOU.**

The Andean lupine contains high levels of magnesium and potassium, as well as copper, zinc and iron. It also contains high levels of alpha linolenic acid, a precursor to omega 3 fatty acid. Grela ER et al, *Biol Trace Elem Res* 2017 March 29.

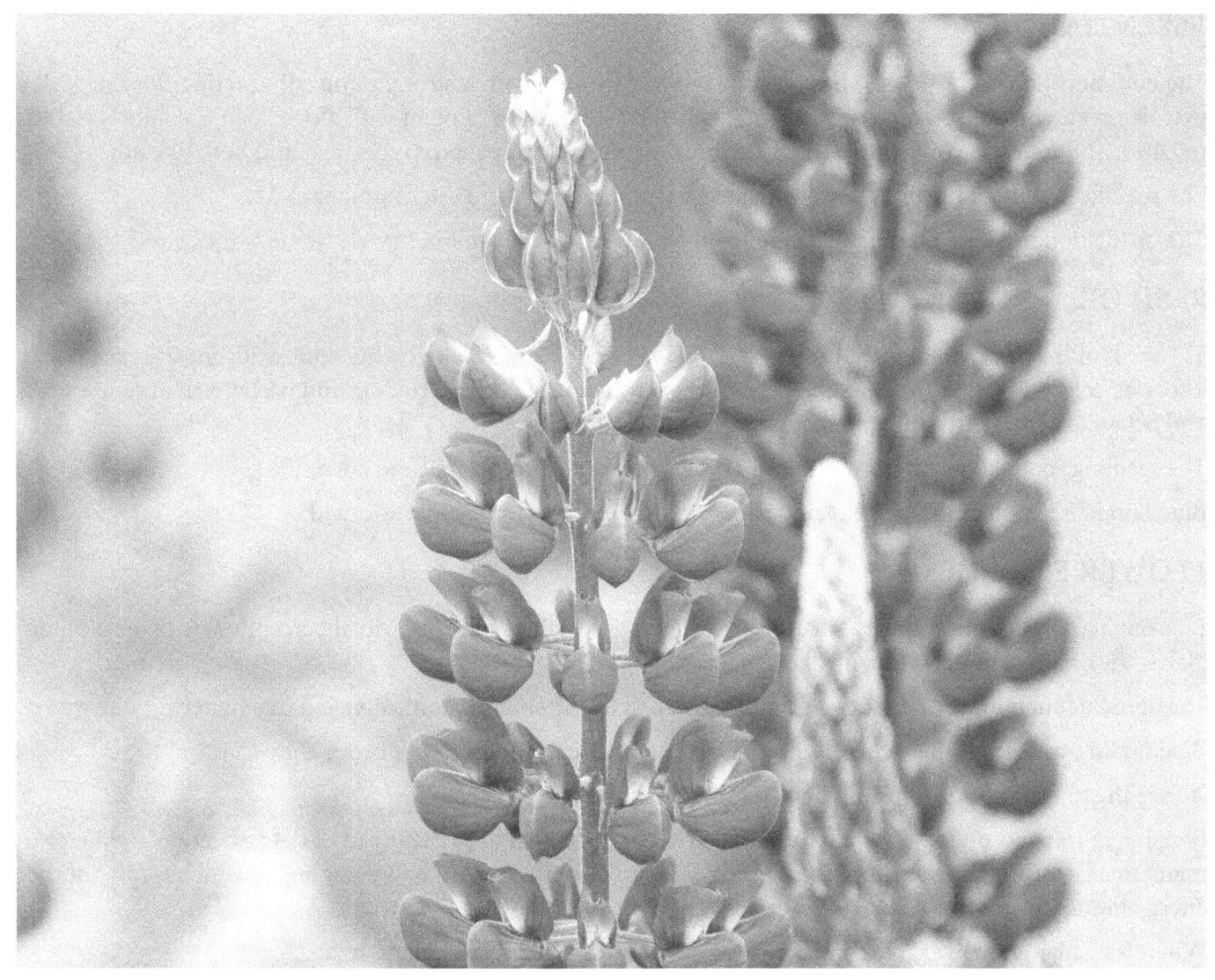

LUPINE FLOWER- CLOSE UP

The germinating seeds of Blue Lupine are rich in asparagine, used in culture media for the commercial production of tuberculin, for laboratory research.

Silver Lupine (*L. argenteus*) contains isoflavones that potentiate the anti-bacterial activity of berberine, found in Gold Thread, Oregon Grape Root and Goldenseal. The isoflavones increased the uptake of berberine into *Staphylococcus aureus* cells, suggesting inhibition of a multidrug resistance pump. Morel et al, *J Agric Food Chem* 2003 51:19.

Our native *L. polyphyllus* has been studied for anti-bacterial activity. Work by Bishop and MacDonald, *Can J Botany* 1956 29 found both alcohol and acetone extracts inhibit *Staphylococcus aureus*.

Lupeol, a lupine triterpene, markedly inhibited tumor progression canine melanoma-bearing mice. Ogihara K et al, *Springerplus* 2014 3:632. This compound is also found in birch bark. Betulinic acid, as well, is a lupine-type pentacyclic triterpenoid saponin.

Sparteine possesses anticonvulsant activity against seizures and epilepsy. Villalpando-Vargas F et al, *Seizure* 2016 39: 49-55. The compound is toxic, depressing the central nervous system and producing anti-muscarinic effects.

## ESSENTIAL OIL

The common Lupine (*L. luteus*) has beautiful yellow flowers with a strong odour. Extracting flowers with a petroleum ether results in obtaining a concrete (0.0205%). After treatment with alcohol, an absolute is yielded (60.4%). The concrete contains 0.95% of a steam volatile oil with penetrating, sweet and herb like notes.

The specific gravity of the oil is 0.900 with an acid number of 38 and ester number of 31.

The distillation of the seeds obtained among other constituents, vanillin.

## SEED OIL

The seeds of *L. luteus* contain 10% saturated, 61% oleic acid, 20% linoleic, 2% linolenic acid, and 7% erucic acid. The triacylglycerols are similar to sunflower oil. Also contains high sterol content and is very rich in campesterol and beta-sitosterol. Also contains over 90% gamma tocopherol.

The seedlings contain allantoin, a skin cell proliferator found in comfrey and corn silk.

Blue Lupine seeds contain 45.7% oleic acid, 33.7% linoleic acid, and 7% eruric acid.

## FLOWER ESSENCES

Blue Lupin (*L. rivularis*) flower essence links the pineal gland, the organ of spiritual perception, with the pituitary gland, the organ of metabolic control and balance.

The optimal functioning of these two glands is essential for eliminating confusion and remembering who we are.

Blue Lupin can help to alleviate feelings of depression which arise from not being able

"to see the forest for the trees", and helps us focus our attention.

Blue Lupin impacts on the Liver channel, which is often referred to as the organ of detoxification and helps to maintain clarity and purity within the physical system. The emotion of the liver is anger, which is just another energy in motion.

When we hang onto anger it becomes frustration, depression and even, despair.

Blue Lupin flower essence works to purify the emotional body of anger residue so that we can fully access our mental potential.                                    **PEGASUS**

White Lupine (*L. nootkatensis*) stimulates the release of familial or tribal karmic patterns; and supports the emergence of a new archetype of male spiritual energy.

It also promotes a willingness to release old patterns of behavior without reactivity or attachment to our treasured wounds and grievances.                                    **ALASKA**

Silvery Lupine flower essence may be useful for those who are unable to access spiritual vision, intuitive perception, clairvoyance, or higher wisdom; or those unable to or struggle to internally see memories, dreams, ideas, or insights; lack a higher life purpose, or have abnormal sleep patterns, sensitivity to light, frontal sinus infections, or inability to maintain body temperature.                                    **LIVING FLOWER**

Blue Pod Lupine (*L. polyphyllus*) deals with higher thought forms of the innate perfections of all things.
                                    **HIGH SIERRA**

Blue Pod Lupine (*L. polyphyllus*) essence helps to re-clear thoughts with mental overload and strain, and when concentrated thinking is not possible.                                    **MIRIANA**

Lupine (*L. latifolius*) is for selfishness, greed; intense identification with petty concerns or narrow interests that stymie community welfare.                                    **FLOWER ESSENCE SOCIETY**

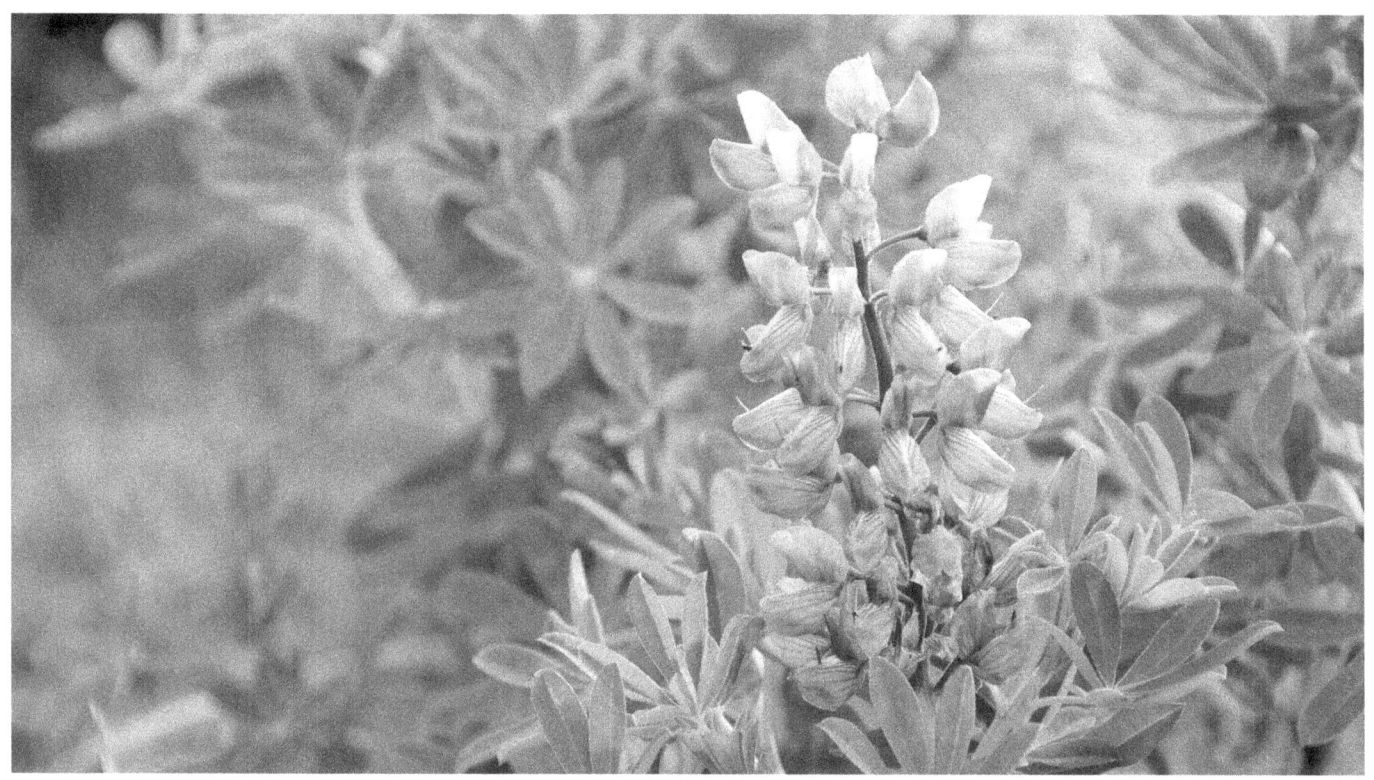

WILD BLUE LUPINE

## SPIRITUAL PROPERTIES

The Lupine helps us understand that we will pass through as many stages to the supreme as it is necessary to take, but we will arrive. **THE MOTHER**

Nature is a perfect example of harmonious balance. The spirit of the Lupin flower presents us with its simple message: to seek a more balanced approach to living.

Take note of the exquisite balance in the make-up of this flower and let it be a perfect reminder of our own potential for balance and calm. **ECLARE**

## DOCTRINE OF SIGNATURES

A distinct signature of the lupine is the open palm shaped leaflets that face the sun throughout the day. When our hands are open and not clenched, we are able to feel the power of light enter and energize our bodies. Open hands also depict giving as well as receiving, balance, openness, and willingness to surrender.

The leaflet's trough-like centre holds water and nurtures the plant.

The broad folded flower petals offer an impression of openness with protection. The lavender colour of the lupine represents the sixth chakra, and along with the plant journey and plant experience, the flower carries a deep sense of inner vision and of following one's path to higher evolvement.

Sitting in a field surrounded by lupines, my friends and I all felt an incredible opening in our sixth and seventh chakras. We were filled with visionary aspirations.

The nodules of the roots obtain nitrogen from the air, which enables them to enrich the soil. I believe this signature symbolizes our ability to attain our visions and aspirations and bring those visions into practical application, thus enriching ourselves, others, and the way we live. **PALLASDOWNEY**

## PERSONALITY TRAITS

When the woman and her husband eat too much of the lupine roots they become really drunk. Their eyes are heavy, and they cannot keep them open, and their bodies are like dead, and they are really sleepy. Then they go and lie down and sleep; and when they wake up they feel well again, because they are no longer drunk.

**BOAS**

Prairie Lupine was one of the first plants to establish itself following the devastating volcanic eruption of Mount St. Helens in 1980.

A short-lived perennial herb, it managed to establish itself quickly on the pumice plain left by the volcano.

Its pioneering spirit allowed it to flourish and influence the subsequent 15 years of plant succession.

While growing vigorously, Prairie Lupine keeps out competitors because it grows so densely. But when it dies, it leaves behind a rich substrate in which other species will thrive.

There is a tendency to resent others who arrive on the scene before we do, seemingly getting the best of the markets, most of the profits, or credit for a discovery. That's the wrong way to look at it.

Pioneers usually leave behind a legacy after they have done their work- a legacy that benefits those who follow and provide a rich medium for fresh ideas, new developments, and sometimes even greater contributions.

**G. MOHAMMED**

Few plants are so restless as the lupine, which provided a perfect subject for Darwin and other scientists in their study of the movement of plants. The leaves especially are continually on the move, the many long fingers opening and closing, or moving horizontally with every passing change of light and going quite obviously to sleep at the approach of nightfall.

**ANNORA BROWN**

## RECIPES

**CAUTION**- allergies to lupine foods are reported in the literature. The estimated prevalence is 0.27-0.81%, and may be related to cross sensitivity with peanuts.

# ABOUT THE AUTHOR

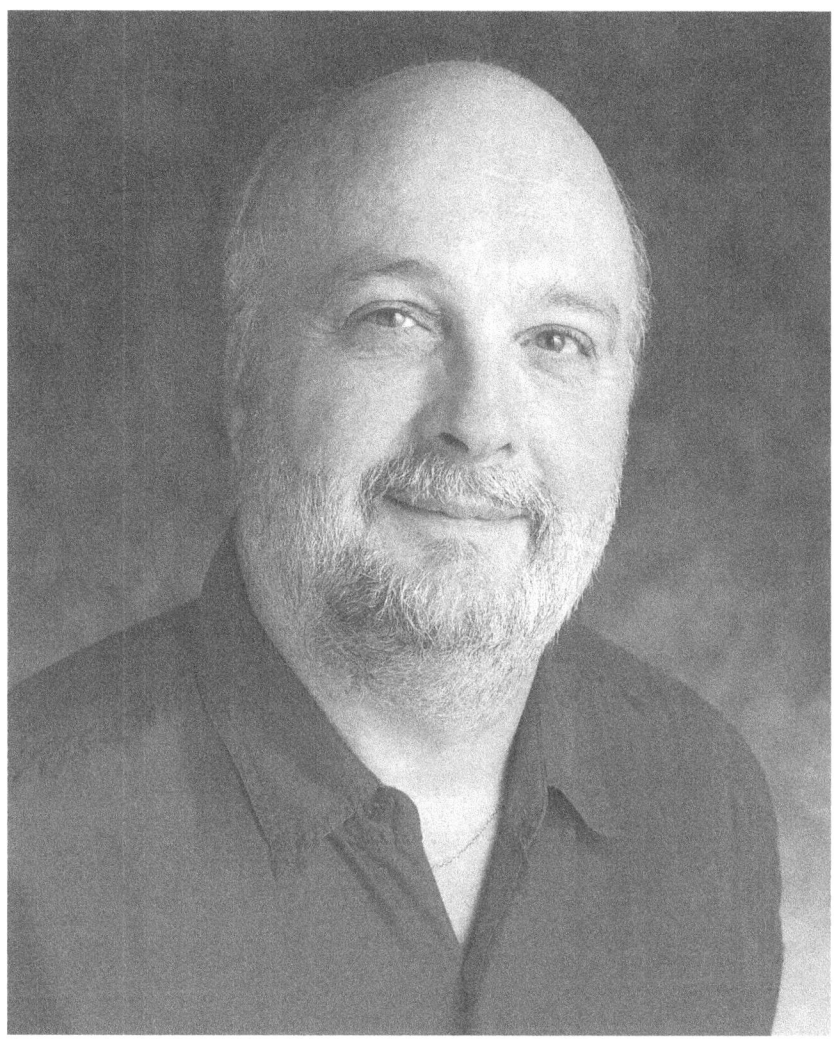

Robert Dale Rogers has been an herbalist for over forty-five years. He has a Bachelor of Science from the University of Alberta, where he is an assistant clinical professor in Family Medicine. He teaches plant medicine, including herbology and flower essences in the Earth Spirit Medicine Program at the Northern Star College of Mystical Studies in Edmonton, Alberta, Canada.

Robert is past chair of the Alberta Natural Health Agricultural Network and Community Health Council of Capital Health. He is a Fellow of the International College of Nutrition, past chair of the medicinal mushroom committee of the North American Mycological Association and on the editorial board of the International Journal of Medicinal Mushrooms. He writes occasional article for Fungi magazine.

Robert co-hosts The Alberta Herb Gathering held every second year (www.albertaherbgathering.com)

He lives on Millcreek Ravine in Edmonton with his beautiful and talented wife, Laurie Szott–Rogers and out of control cat Ceres.

You can email him at scents@telusplanet.net
or visit
www.selfhealdistributing.com

# BIBLIOGRAPHY

Abbe, Elfriede, *The Fern Herbal,* Cornell University Press, Ithaca, 1981

Acorn, J. Bugs of Alberta, Lone Pine Publishing, Edmonton, AB, 2000.

Adams, J. *Les Plantes Medicinales.* Bulletin 23, Agriculture Canada. 1916

Adams, Jean. *Insect Potpourri, Adventures in Entomology.* Sandhill Crane Press, FL. 1992

Aggarwal, Bharat. Healing Spices. Sterling Pub. New York 2011.

Albert-Puleo, Michael. *Economic Botany, 32, Jan-Mar, 1978.*

Allaby, Michael. *Temperate Forests.* Facts on File. New York. 1999.

Allen, D & Hatfield, G. *Medicinal Plants in Folk Tradition.* Timber Press, Portland. 2004

Allen,E, Morrison,D, &Wallis,G. *Common Tree Diseases of B.C. Canada Forest Service,* '96

Allende, Isabel. *Aphrodite- A Memoir of the Senses.* Harper Flamingo. New York. 1998.

Alstat, Ed. *Electic Dispensatory of Botanical Therapeutics.* Ecl Med. Oregon. 1989.

Anderson, Anne, *Some Native Herbal Remedies,* Pub 8A, Devonian Botanical Gardens 1980

_____*Plants in Cree.* Duval House Pub. Edmonton AB 2000.

Anderson, C.&Tischer,T. *Poinsettias, the December Flower,* Waters Edge Press, CA, 1997

Andoh, Anthony. *The Science & Romance of Selected Herbs used in Medicine and Religious Ceremony.* North Scale Institute. San Francisco. 1986.

Andre, Alestine & Fehr, Alan. *Gwich'in Ethnobotany.* Gwich'in Social and Cultural Institute, Box 46, Tsiigehtchie, NWT, X0E 0B0, fax 1867-953-3820.

Andrews, Tamra. Nectar and Ambrosia. ABC-CLIO Box 1911 Santa Barbara CA. 2000.

Andrews, Ted. *Animal Speak- The Spiritual and Magical Powers,* Llewellyn. Minn. 1996.

_____*Animal Wise,* DragonHawk, Jackson, TN, 1999.

Antol, Marie. *The Incredible Secrets of Mustard.* Avery Pub. New York. 1999.

Aronson J K Ed. Meyler's Side Effects of Herbal Medicines. Elsevier Amsterdam. 2009.

Arrowsmith, Nancy. Essential Herbal Wisdom. Llewellyn Pub. Woodbury, Minn. 2009.

Arsdall, Anne Van. *Medieval Herbal Remedies.* Routledge, New York. 2002.

Arvigo & Balick, *Rainforest Remedies,* Lotus Press, Twin Lakes, WI. 1993

Arvigo & Epstein. *Rainforest Home Remedies,* Harper SanFrancisco, 2001.

Assiniwi, Bernard. *La Medecine des Indiens d' Amerique,* Guerin Literature, 1988

Atal C.K. & Kapur B. *Cultivation and Utilization of Medicinal Plants,* Jammu-Tawi, 1982

Attenborough, David. *The Private Life of Plants.* Princeton U Press. Princeton NJ 1995.

Ausubel, K. *Seeds of Change The Living Treasure.* HarperSanFrancisco, 1994.

Aversano, Laura. *The Divine Nature of Plants.* Swan•Raven & Co. Columbus, NC, 2002.

Ayensu, Edward,S. *Medicinal Plants of the West Indies,* Reference Publications, 1981

Baïracli Levy, Juliette *Herbal Handbook for Farm and Stable,* Faber&Faber, London, 1952

Baker, Phil. The Dedalus Book of Absinthe. Dedalus 2001.

Barl, Branka et al, *Saskatchewan Herb Database,* U. of Sask. Saskatoon, 1996.

Barlow, Max. *From the Shepherd's Purse.* 1990

Barnes J, Anderson L, &Phillipson J. *Herbal Medicines, A guide for healthcare professionals.* Pharmaceutical Press, London, 2002.

Barnett, Robert A. *Tonics,* Harper Collins, New York, N.Y. 1997

Bartram, Thomas. *Bartram's Encyl. of Herbal Medicine,* Robinson Pub. London, 1998.

Bascom, Angella. *Incorporating Herbal Medicine into Clinical Practice.* F. Davis Co. 2002

Beals, Katherine, M. *Flower Lore and Legend,* Henry Holt, 1917

Beers, Susan-Jane. *Jamu The ancient Indonesian Art of Herbal Healing,* Periplus, 2001.

Belcourt, Christi. Medicines to Help Us. Gabriel Dumont Instit. Saskatoon, SK 2007.

Béliveau, R & Gingras,D. *Foods That Fight Cancer.* McClelland & Stewart Toronto. 2006.

Belsinger S & Dille C. *Cooking with Herbs.* CBI- Van Nostrand Reinhold, N.Y. 1984.

Benjamin, D.R. *Mushrooms: Poisons and Panaceas.* WH Freeman, San Francisco, 1995.

Bennet, Doug & Tiner, Tim. *Up North.* Reed Books Canada. Markham, Ont. 1993.

_____*Up North Again.* McClelland and Stewart. Toronto, 1997.

Bennet, J & Rowley S. *Uqalurait An Oral History of Nunavut.* McGill Queens, Mont. 2004

Benyus, Janine. *Biomimicry Innovation Inspired by Nature.* William Morrow. 1997.

Berenbaum,May R. *Buzzwords, A Scientists Muses on Sex, Bugs and Rock N Roll,* Joseph Henry Press, Washington, D.C. 2000.

_____*Bugs in the System.* Helix Books, Addison-Wesley Pub. 1995.

Beresford-Kroeger, Diana. The Global Forest. Viking Penguin. 2010.

_____Arboretum Borealis. U Michigan Press. 2010.

Berliocchi,Luigi. *The Orchid in Lore and Legend.* Timber Press, Portland Oregon, 2000.

Berlund B & Bolsby C. *The Edible Wild* Pagurian Press, Toronto, Ont. 1971.

Berkowsky, Bruce. *Mount Julius Flower Remedies. Mt. Vernon Washington, 1986*

Bermejo, J & Leon,J. *Neglected Crops-1492 ...* FAO Series 26, United Nations, Rome, 1994.

Bernhardt, P. *The Rose's Kiss, A Natural History of Flowers* . Island Press, Covelo CA 1999

Bianchi, Ivo. *Geriatrics and Homotoxicology.* Aurelia-Verlag GmbH, Baden Baden, 1994.

Bianchini, F. *The Complete Book of Health Plants.* Crescent Books, New York, 1975.

Biship, Carol. *The Book of Home Remedies &Herbal Cures,* Jonathan-James, Toronto, 1979.

Bisset, Norman G. *Herbal Drugs and Phytopharmaceuticals.* 2nd Ed. CRC Press, 2001.

Blackburn, Thomas. *December's Child: A Book of Chumash Oral Narratives* , U of California Press, Berkeley, 1975.

Blanchan, Neltje. *Nature's Garden.* Doubleday, Page&Co. New York, 1900.

Bland, John. *Forests of Liliput.* Prentice Hall, Englewood Cliffs, New Jersey, 1971.

Bliss, Anne. *Rocky Mountain Dye Plants.* Juniper House, Boulder, Colorado, 1976

Blouin, Glen. *Weeds of the Woods.* Goose Lane, Fredericton, New Brunswick 1992.

_____*An Eclectic Guide to Trees, east of the Rockies.* Boston Mills, 2001.

Boas, F. *Ethnology of the Kwakiutl.* Bureau of Am. Ethnology, 35th annual report, 1921.

Boericke, Wm. *Materia Medica with Repetory.* B. Jain Publishers. 1976

Boik, John. *Natural Compunds in Cancer Therapy.* Oregon Med Press, Princeton,Minn 2001

Boland, Bridget. *Gardener's Magic &Other Old Wives' Lore.* The Bodley Head, London, 77.

Bolton, Brett L. *The Secret Powers of Plants.* Berkley Pub Co. New York. 1974.

Bolton, J.L. *Alfalfa, Botany, Cultivation &Utilization.* Interscience Pub, New York, 1962.

Bone, Kerry. *A Clinical Guide to Blending Liquid Herbs.* Churchill Livingstone. 2003

Borrel, Marie. *Healing Plants.* Cassell & Co. Wellington House, London. 2001.

Bouchardon, Patrice. *The Healing Energies of Trees.* Journey Editions, Boston, 1999.

Bossenmaier, Eugene. *Mushrooms of the Boreal Forest.* U. of Saskatchewan Press, 1997

Boulos, Loutfy. *Medicinal Plants of North Africa,* Reference Pub. Algonac, Mich. 1983

Bowles, E. Joy. *The Chemistry of Aromatherapeutic Oils.* Allen & Unwin, Crow's Nest, Australia, 2003.

Bowman, Daria. *Hydrangeas.* Friedman/Fairfax Pub. New York. 1999.

Bradley, Peter. British Herbal Compendium Vol 2 Brit Herb Med Assoc. Bournemouth 2006.

Brahmachari, Goutam Ed. Natural Products, Alpha Sci Int Ltd. Oxford UK 2009.

Brandeis, Gayle. *Fruitflesh.* Harper Collins, San Francisco. 2002.

Brennan, M. *Complete Holistic Care & Healing for Horses*. Trafalgar Sq. Pub. VT. 2001.

Bringhurst, Robert. *A Story as Sharp as a Knife*. Douglas&Mc Intyre Vancouver, 1999.

Brinker, Francis N.D. *Herb Contraindications and Drug Interactions* .Third Edition Eclectic Medical Publications, Sandy, Oregon, 2001

_____*The Toxicology of Botanical Medicines,* revised 2nd. Eclectic Med, Oregon, 1996.

_____*Eclectic Dispensatory of Botanical Therapeutics,* Vol 2, Ecl. Med . Oregon, 1995.

Brodo, Irwin & Sharnoff. *Lichens of North America*. Yale University Press, 2001.

Brown, Deni. *Encyclopedia of Herbs and Their Uses*. Reader's Digest Press, Que. 1995.

Bruneton, J *Pharmacognosy, Phtyochemistry, Medicinal Plants,* Lavoisier Pub. Paris, 1995

_____*Toxic Plants Dangerous to Humans and Animals*. Editions TEC&Doc, Paris, '99.

Brunschwig, Hieronymus. *Book of Distillation*. Johnson Reprint Co No. 79. New York, 1971.

Brynaherb Essences  29, Kells Meend Berry Hill, Gloucestershire GL16 7AD

Bubar, Carol et al. *Weeds of the Prairies*. Alberta Agriculture Pub. Edmonton, 2000.

Buchanan, Carol. *Brothers Crow, Sister Corn*. Ten Speed Press, Berkeley, 1997.

Buckle, Jane. *Clinical Aromatherapy. 2nd ed*. Churchill Livingstone, Toronto, 2003.

Buhner, Stephen H. *Sacred and Herbal Healing Beers,* Siris Books, Boulder, Co, 1998

_____*Sacred Plant Medicine*. Robert Rinehart, Boulder, Co. 1996.

_____Herbal Antibiotics. Storey Books, Vermont, 1999.

_____*The Lost Language of Plants*. Chelsea Green Pub. White River, Vt. 2002

_____Secret Teachings of Plants. Bear & Co. Rochester, Vt. 2004.

_____The Natural Testosterone Plan. Healing Arts Press, Rochester VT. 2007

Burbridge, Joan. *Wildflowers of the Southern Interior of B.C.* U. of B.C. Press, 1989.

Burger, W. Flowers- *How they changed the world. Prometheus Books*. Amherst NY 2006.

Burgess, Isla. *Weeds Heal*. Viriditas Pub Group. Cambridge NZ 1998.

Burlando, Bruno et al, Herbal Principles in Cosmetics. CRC Press Boca Raton 2010.

Caius, Rev. Fr. Jean F., *The Medicinal and Poisonous Plants of India,* Scientific Pub, 1986.

Cameron, Elizabeth. *A Floral ABC*. John Wiley and Sons. Toronto. 1980.

Carpenter D. Snr Pub. *Nursing Herbal Medicine Handbook,* Springhouse Corp. 2001.

Carpinella, Maria et al. Novel Therapeutic Agents from Plants. Sci Pub. Enfield NJ 2009.

Carr, Emily. *Wild Flowers*. Royal BC Museum, Victoria, B.C, 2006

Carroll, Roisin. *The Crane Bag Celtic Tree Ogam Oils* , Feasibility Pub. Dublin

Carter, Bernard F. *The Floral Birthday Book*. Bloomsbury Books, London. 1990.

Casselman, Bill. *Canadian Garden Words*. Little, Brown & Co. Toronto, 1997.

Castleman, Michael. *The Healing Herbs*. Bantam Books. 1995.

Castro, Miranda. *The Complete Homeopathy Handbook*. MacMillan, 1990

Catty, Suzanne. *Hydrosols the next Aromatherapy,* Healing Arts Press, Vermont, 2001.

Cavers, Paul ed, *The* Biology *of Canadian Weeds* 62-83,Ag Institute of Canada, Ottawa, 1995

_____84-102 Ag Inst. of Canada, Ottawa, 2000.

_____103-129 Ag Inst. of Canada, Ottawa 2005

Ceres. *Herbal Teas for Health and Healing*. Healing Arts Press, Rochester, Vermont, 1984.

Chan, K, and Cheung L. *Interactions between Chincese Herbal Medicinal Products and Orthodox Drugs.* Harwood Academic Publishers, Canada, 2000.

Chandler, F. *Herbs-Everyday Reference for Health Professionals,* Can. Pharm Assoc. 2000

Chang & But. *Pharmacology &Applications of Chinese Materia Medica,* World Scientific, 86

Chang Chao-liang et al, *Vegetables as Medicine,* Pelanduk Pub, Malaysia, 1999.

Chappell, P. Emotional Healing with Homeopathy. North Atlantic Books. Berkeley, 2003.

Charissa's Cauldron. www.charissacauldron.com

Chase, Pamela & Pawlik, J. *Newcastle Trees for Healing*, Newcastle Pub. Van Nuys,1991

Chatroux, Sylvia. *Botanica Poetica*. Poetica Press 2004 1-877-POETICA.

_____*Materica Poetica*. Poetica Press 1998.

Chen, John K & Chen, Tina T. Chinese Medical Herbology & Pharmacology. Art of Medicine Press, City of Industry, CA 2004.

Chevalllier, Andrew. *The Encyclopedia of Medicinal Plants*. Reader's Digest, 1996.

Chishti, Hakim. *The Traditional Healer*, Healing Arts Press, Vermont,1988.

Christchurch Flower Essences. www.christchurchfloweressences.com

Clark, Ella E. *Indian Legends of Canada*. McClelland & Stewart. Toronto, 1960.

Coats, Peter. *Flowers in History*. Weidenfeld and Nicolson, London. 1970.

Coffey, Timothy.*The History and Folklore of North American Wildflowers,* Houghton-Mifflin, 1993.

Cohen, Kenneth. *Honoring the Medicine*. Random House, Toronto. 2003.

Conrad, Chris, *Hemp for Health,* Healing Arts Press, Rochester, Vermont, 1997.

Cook, Wm.H. *The Physio-Medical Dispensatory*. 1869. Reprinted by Eclectic Medical Publications, Portland, Oregon, 1985.

_____A compendium of the new Materia medica together with additional descriptions of some old remedies. Wm. Cook Publisher, Chicago, 1896.

Cooper, J.C. *Dictionary of Symbolic & Mythological Animals,* Thorsons, London, 1992.

Cormack, R.G.H. *Wild Flowers of Alberta*. Hurtig Publishers, 1977

Coupland, Francois. *The Encyclopedia of Edible Plants of N. America*. Keats Pub. 1998.

Cousin, Pierre J. *Eat Well, Be Well*. Thorsons, London. 2001.

Cowan, Eliot. *Plant Spirit Medicine*. Swan Raven & Co. Box 726 Newberg, Oregon, 1995.

Cowan, Thomas. The Fourfold Path to Healing. New Trends Pub. Washington DC 2007.

Crane, Eva. *Honey- A Comprhensive Survey* , Heinemann Pub. London 1975.

Craydon D. & Bellows W. Floral Acupuncture. The Crossing Press Berkeley CA 2005.

Creekmore, H. *Daffodils are Dangerous*. Walker and Co. New York. 1966.

Crow, Tis Mal. *Native Plants, Native Healing*. Native Voices Book Pub. Box 99 Summertown, Tennessee, 2001 1-888-260-8458.

Crowell, Robert L. *The Lore & Legends of Flowers*. Thomas Crowell, New York, 1982.

Crowfoot & Baldensperger. *From Cedar to Hyssop*. Sheldon Press, London, 1932.

Cruden, Loren. Medicine Grove. Destiny Books. Inner Traditions Vermont. 1997.

Cummings, S. and Ullman, Dana. *Everyone's Guide to Homeopathic Medicines,* St. Martins

Cupp, Melanie. *Toxicology and Clinical Pharmacology of Herbal Products*. Humana P. 1999

Curtin, LSM. *Healing Herbs of the Upper Rio Grande*. SouthWest Museum, Los Angeles 1965

Cutler & Cutler Eds. Biologically Active Natural Products: Agrochemicals, CRC Press 1999.

Dai Yin-fang&Liu Cheng-jun. *Fruit As Medicine*. Rams Skull Press, Kuranda, Aust. 1987

Dalton, David. Stars of the Meadow. Lindisfarne Books. Great Barrington, Mass. 2006.

D'Amelio Sr. Frank. *Botanicals A Phytocosmetic Desk Reference* CRC Press, Boca Raton, 99

Darby,Wm et al. *Food: The Gift of Osiris,* Vol 1. Academic Press, San Francisco, 1977

Darwin, Tess. The Scots Herbal, the Plant Lore of Scotland. Birlinn Ltd, Edinburgh 2008

Davidow, Joie. *Infusions of Healing, A Treasury of Mexican-American Herbal Remedies,* Fireside Books, New York, 1999.

Davis,W. *El Gringo, New Mexico and Her People*. Harpers, New York, 1857.

Demargaux, N. *Phytotherapy*. Herbal Health Publishers Ltd. 1989

De Bairacli Levy, Juliette. *Herbal Handbook for Farm and Stable,* Faber and Faber 1952

Deer Lame, J & Erdoes, R. *Lame Deer Seeker of Visions.* Washington Sq Press, 1976.

Deer, Thea Summer. Wisdom of the Plant Devas. Bear&Company Vermont 2011.

Delta Gardens Flower Essences. www.deltagardens.com

De Smet et al. *Adverse Effects of Herbal Drugs.* Springer-Verlag, Berlin. 1997.

Der Marderosian, Ara & Liberti L. *Natural Product Medicine,* George Stickley Co, Philadel.

DeRios, Marlene D. *Hallucinogens: Cross Cultural Perspectives.* U. New Mexico Press, 1984

DeSmet, P. et al. *Adverse Effects of Herbal Drugs. vol 2* Springer-Verlag

Devi, Lila. The Essential Flower Essence Handbook. Crystal Clarity Pub. Nevada City 2007.

Dewey, Laurel. *Plant Power- revised.* Safe Goods/New Century Pub, Markham Ont, 2001.

Dewick, Paul M. *Medicinal Natural Products.*3rd Ed John Wiley and Sons, West Sussex, 2009.

Diederichsen, Axel. *Coriander.* Int. Plant Genetic Resources Institute. Rome, Italy. 1996.

Dixon, Bernard.*Power Unseen, How Microbes Rule the World.* W.H. Freeman, Oxford, 1994

Dow, Elaine. *Simples and Worts.* Historical Presentations, Topsfield, MA. 1982.

Duke, James. *Handbook of Medicinal Herbs.* CRC Press, Boca Raton, Florida, 1985

_____*Handbook of Edible Weeds.* CRC Press. 1992

_____*The Green Pharmacy,* Rodale Press, Emmaus, Pennsylvania, 1997.

_____*The Green Pharmacy Herbal Handbook,* Rodale Press, 2000.

_____*Anti-aging Prescriptions.* Rodale Press. 2001.

Dumas, Anne. Book of Plants and Symbols. English Ed. Octopus Pub. London 2004.

Dymock,Wm. *Pharmacographia Indica, Vol 2*, Kegan Paul, Trench, Trubner and Co. 1891

Earle, Liz. *Vital Oils*, Ebury Press, London, 1991.

Eason, Cassandra. Fabulous Creatures, Mythical Monsters... Greenwood Press, CT. 2008.

Eastman, John. *The Book of Swamp and Bog...* Stackpole Books, Mechanicsburg, Penn, 1995

Ebadi, M. *Pharmacodynamic Basis of Herbal Medicine,* CRC Press, Boca Raton. 2002.

Eckey, E.W. *Vegetable Fats and Oils,* Rheingold Publishing Co, New York, 1954.

Eclare, Melanie. *Flower Spirit Cards.* Quadrille Publishing, London, England, 2004.

Edwards, Lawrence. *The Vortex of Life.* Floris Books. Edinburgh 2nd Ed. 2006.

Eisner T et al. *Secret Weapons.* Belknap Press, Harvard U Press. Cambridge & London 2005.

Ellingwood F. *American Materia Medica,* Eclectic Med. Pub. Portand, Oregon, reprint, 1983

Elliot, Douglas B. *Roots .* Chatham Press, Old Greenwich Conneticut.

Ellis, Hattie. *Sweetness & Light.* Hodder and Stoughton, London, 2004.

Erdoes & Ortiz. *American Indian Myths and Legends,* Pantethon Books, New York, 1984.

Erichsen-Brown,Charlotte. *Use of Plants for the Past 500 Years,* Breezy Creeks Press, 1979

_____*Medicinal and Other Uses of North American Plants,* General Pub, 1979.

Erickson, David, Wai Kit Nip *Food uses of whole oil and protein seeds,* Amer. Oil Chemists Society, 1989.

Eskin, N. A. Michael, Tamir, S. *Dictionary of Nutraceuticals and Functional Foods.* CRC Press, 2006.

Etkin, Nina. Edible Medicines, An Ethnopharmacology of Food. U Arizona Press. 2006.

Evans, W.C. *Trease and Evans' Pharmacognosy.* WB Saunders Co. Toronto, 2000.

Fang Jing Pei, Dr. *Natural Remedies from the Chinese Cupboard.* Weatherhill, 1998.

Farmer-Knowles,Helen. *The Healing Garden.* Sterling Publishing, New York, 1998.

Fielder, Mildred. *Plant Medicne and Folklore,* Winchester Press, New York, 1975.

Felter, Harvery and Lloyd, John. *King's American Dispensatory .* 1898. Reprinted by Eclectic Medical
        Publications, Portland Oregon, 1983.

Ferguson, Gary. *Spirits of the Wild.* Clarkson Potter/Random New York, 1996.

Fernie, W.T. Dr. *Old Fashioned Herbal Remedies.* Coles Pub. Toronto, 1980. Reprint.

Fingerman M. et al editors. *Bioremediation of Aquatic and Terresrial Ecosytems.* Sci Pub. Enfield NH 2005.

Fischer-Rizzi, S. *Complete Aromatherapy Handbook,* Sterling Pub. New York. 1990.

_____*The Complete Incense Book,* Sterling Pub. New York. 1998.

_____*Medicine of the Earth,* Rudra Press, Portland, Oregon, 1996

Florey, H.W. et al. Antibiotics vol 1. Oxford University Press. London 1949.

Ford, Gillian. *Plant Names Explained*. Friends of the Devonian Botanic Garden, #16, 1984

Foster, Steven. *Herbal Renaissance,* Gibbs Smith Pub. Salt Lake City

_____& Yue Chongxi. *Herbal Emissaries,* Healing Arts Press, Vermont, 1992

_____& Johnson R. *Desk Reference to Nature's Medicine.* Nat Geographic. Washington, D.C.

Fox, H. M. Gardening with Herbs. Macmillan Pub. New York 1933.

Freeman, D. & Mongeau D. Nettles and More…Vol One. Self published 2nd printing 2009.

Freeman, Lyn. *Mosby's Complementary & Alternative Medicine.*3rd Ed. Mosby Elsevier 2009

Friedman, Sara Ann, *Celebrating the Wild Mushroom,* Dodd, Mead & Co. New York, 1986

Friend, Tim. The Third Domain: the Untold Story of Archaea. Joseph Henry Press. 2007.

Fugh-Berman, Adriane. *The 5-minute Herb &Dietary Supplement Consult.* Lippincott Williams &Wilkins, Philadelphia 2003.

Gaertner, Erika. *Reap without Sowing.* General Store Publishing, Burnstown, Ont. 1995

Galun, Margalith. *Handbook of Lichenology,* CRC Press, 1988

Garran, Thomas. *Western herbs according to Traditional Chinese Medicine.* Healing Arts Press. 2008.

Garrett, J.T. *The Cherokee Herbal.* Bear&Company, Rochester, Vermont. 2003.

Genders, Roy. *Floral Scents of the World* . St. Martin's Press, London, 1977

Geuter, *Herbs in Nutrition.* Bio-Dynamic Agricultural Assoc. London. 1978.

Gildemeister, E. *The Volatile Oils.* John Wiley and Sons, New York. 1916

Gifford, Jane. The Wisdom of Trees. Sterling Pub. New York 2000.

Gill S. & Sullivan I. *Dictionary of Native American Mythology.* Oxford U Press 1992.

Gilmore, M.R. Uses of Plants by Indians of the Missouri river region. 33rd Annual Report Bureau American Ethnology, 1911-12, Washington D.C. 1919.

Gladstar R & Hirsch P. *Planting the Future.* Healing Arts Press, Rochester, Vt. 2000.

Gladstar, Rosemary. *Family Herbal.* Storey Books, North Adams, Mass. 2001

Glasby, J.S. *Dictionary of Plants Containing Secondary Metabolites,* Taylor & Francis, London 1991.

Godfrey, A & Saunders P. Principles and Practices of Naturopathic Botanical Medicine, Vol 1, CCNM Press Toronto ON 2010.

Goodrick-Clarke, Clare. Alchemical Medicine for the 21st Century. Healing Arts Press. 2010.

Gordon, David G. *The Compleat Cockroach.* Ten Speed Press, Berkeley, CA. 1996.

Gordon, Lesley. The Mystery and Magic of Trees & Flowers. Grange Books. London 1993.

Gottesfeld, Leslie M. Johnson. *Plants, Land and People, A Study of Wet'suwet'en Ethnobotany.*U of A, 1993.

Grae, Ida. *Nature's Colors, Dyes From Plants.* Macmillan Pub. New York, 1974.

Graham, Frances K. *Plant lore of an Alaskan Island.* Alaska Northwest Pub. 1985

Grandparents of the Forest flower essences. www.grandparentsoftheforest.com

Grange, Michael etal, *Handbook of Plants with Pest Control Properties,* J. Wiley& Son 1988

Gray, Bev. The Boreal Herbal. Wild Food & Medicine Plants of the North. Aroma Borealis Press 2011

Green, James. *The Male Herbal* . Crossing Press, Freedom, California, 1991.

_____*The Herbal Medicine-Maker's Handbook.* Crossing Press, Freedom CA 2000

Green, Jonathan. *Consuming Passions.* Sphere Books, London, 1985.

Grey Wolf. *Earth Signs,* Raincoast Books, Vancouver, B.C. 1998.

Grieve, M. *A Modern Herbal.* Jonathan Cape. 1931

Griffiths, Deirdre. *Elk Island National Park.* U. of Alberta Press, 1979.

Grigson, Geoffrey. *A Herbal of All Sorts.* Phoenix House, London

Grimaud, Baptiste,Paul. *TAROT DES FLEURS*, France Cartes, France 1989

Grimshaw, John. *The Gardener's Atlas.* Firefly Books, Willowdale, Ont. 2002.

Grohmann,Gerbert. *The Plant Vol 2,* Bio-Dynamic Farming & Gardening Assoc. 1989.

Gruenwald et al, Ed. PDR for Herbal Medicines. 4th Ed. Thomson Pub. 2007.

Guillet, Alma. *Make Friends of Trees and Shrubs.* Doubleday & Co. New York, 1962.

Gumbel, Dietrich. *Principles of Holistic Skin Therapy with Herb Essences.* Haug Pub. Heidelberg 1986.

Gurudas. *The Spiritual Properties of Herbs* , Cassandra Press, 1988

_____*Flower Essences and Vibrational Healing,* Cassandra Press, 1983

Hageneder, Fred. The Spirit of Trees. Continuum. NY and London. 2005.

Hale, Mason. *The Biology of Lichens.* Edward Arnold Pub. London, 1967.

Hall, Dorothy. *Creating Your Herbal Profile* , Keats, 1988

Hallworth, B & Chinnappa CC. *Plants of the Kananaskis Country* U of A Press 1997.

Hanchuk, Rena. *The Word and Wax.* Can Inst of Ukrainian Studies Press, Edmonton, 1999.

Hanson, J, & Morrison D. *Of Kinkajous, Capybaras, Horned Beetles...*Harper Collins, NY '91

Harbourne & Baxter. *The Handbook of Natural Flavonoids Vol 1&2.* John Wiley & Sons, 1999

_____*Phytochemical Dictionary.* Taylor & Francis 1993.

Harrington, Geri. *Growing Your Own Chinese Vegetables,* MacMillan, N.Y. 1978.

Harrington, H.D. *Edible Native Plants of the Rocky Mtns.* U. of New Mexico Press, 1967.

Harris, Ben C. *Eat the Weeds,* Keats Pub. New Cannan, Conneticut 1973.

_____*Make Use of Your Garden Plants.* General Pub. New York. 1978.

Harris, Marjorie. *Botanica North America.* Harper Collins, New York, 2003.

Harrison, Nora. *Flower Remedy Rhymes* , self published, England, 1990.

Hart, Jeff. *Montana Native Plants and Early Peoples,* Montana Historical Society Press. '92

_____The Ethnobotany of the Northern Cheyenne Indians of Montana. Journal of Ethnopharmacology 1981 4.

Hartung, Tammi. *Growing 101 Herbs That Heal.* Storey Books, Pownal, Vt. 2000.

Hartwell, Jonathan, *Plants Used Against Cancer.* Quarterman Pub. 1982

Hartzell, Jr. H. *The Yew Tree A Thousand Whispers.* Hulogosi, Box 1188, Eugene, OR 1991.

Harvey, C & Cochrane A. *The Healing Spirit of Plants.* Godsfield Press, Sterling Pr N.Y. 1999

Harvey Clare. The New Encyclopedia of Flower Remedies. Watkins Pub. London 2007.

Hatfield, Gabrielle. *Encyclopedia of Folk Medicine.* ABC CLIO Santa Barbara. 2004.

Haughton, Claire. *Green Immigrants.* Harcourt Brace Jovanovich. New York and London.

Hawksworth, Frank & Wiens, D. Dwarf Mistletoes, Ag Handbook 709, USDA, Wash, DC, '96

Health Canada, Native Foods and Nutrition. Medical Services Branch, 1995.

Heatherington, M. and Steck,W. *Natural Chemicals from Northern Prairie Plants,* Ag West Biotech Publishers, Saskatoon, Canada. 1997.

Heilmeyer, Marina. The Language of Flowers-Symbols & Myths. Prestel Pub. Munich 2001.

Heinerman, John. *Encyclopedia of Nuts, Berries and Seeds,* Parker Publishing, 1995.

_____*Encyclopedia of Healing Herbs & Spices.* Parker Pub. N.Y. 1996.

Heinrich, Bernd. *Winter World The Ingenuity of animal survival.* HarperCollins. NY 2003.

Heinrich, Clark. *Magic Mushrooms in Religion and Alchemy.* Park St. Press, VT. 2002.

Heiser, Charles B. Jr. *Of Plants and People.* U. of Oklahoma Press, 1985.

Hellson, John C, *Ethnobotany of the Blackfoot Indians* No. 19, National Museums of Canada, Ottawa 1974.

Henderson, Robert K. *The Neighborhood Forager.* Key Porter Books, Toronto, 2000.

Hendrickson, Robert. *Encycl of Word and Phrase Origins.* Facts on File Inc. NewYork, 1997.

Hendry, G. *Natural Food Colorants* , Blackie and Son, Glasgow Scotland, 1992.

Henry, J. David. *Canada's Boreal Forest.* Smithsonian Institute. 2002.

Hilarion. *Wildflowers, Their Occult Gifts.* Marcus Books, Queensville, Ont. 1982.

Hobbs, Christopher. *Usnea : The Herbal Antibiotic.* Botanica Press. 1986.

_____*Medicinal Mushrooms*, Botanica Press, Santa Cruz, 1995.

Hoffman, David. *The Holistic Herbal.* Findhorn Press, 1983.

_____*Welsh Herbal Medicine.* Abercastle Publications, Dyfed, 1978.

_____*Medical Herbalism.* Healing Arts Press, Rochester, VT, 2003.

Hole, Lois. *Favorite Trees and Shrubs.* Lone Pine Pub. Edmonton Alta. 1997.

_____*Perennial Favorites.* Lone Pine Pub. 1995.

Holm, LeRoy G. *World Weeds,* John Wiley and Sons, 1997.

Holmes, Peter. *The Energetics of Western Herbs, Vol 1 and 2,* Artemis Press, 1989.

_____*Jade Remedies, Vol 1 and 2,* Snow Lotus Press, Boulder 1996.

Hopman, Ellen. *A Druid's Herbal,* Destiny Books, Rochester, Vermont. 1995.

Howarth, D& Kahlee Keane. *Wild Medicines of the Prairies* Self Published, 1995.

_____*Native Medecines* Self Published , 1995

Hozeski, Bruce. *Hildegard's Healing Plants.* Beacon Press. Boston, Mass. 2001.

Hsu, Hong-Yen. *Oriental Materia Medica,* Keats Publishing,Connecticut, 1986.

Huang, Kee Chang. *The Pharmacolocy of Chinese Herbs.* 2ⁿᵈ Edition, CRC Press, 1999.

Hu-Nan. *A Barefoot Doctor's Manual.* Running Press, Philadelphia, 1977.

Hudson, James B. *Antiviral Compounds from Plants*, CRC Press, Florida, 1990

Hudson, Rick. *A Field Guide to Gold, Gemstone and Mineral Sites.* Orca Pub, Victoria, 1999

Hurley, Judith. *The Good Herb* Wm. Morrow and Co. New York, 1995.

Hutchens, Alma. *Indian Herbology of North America.* Merco. 1969

Ingram, Cass. *Supermarket Remedies.* Knowledge House, Buffalo Grove, Ill. 1998.

Injoynow essences.

Inkpen W & Van Eyk, R. *Guide to the Common Native Trees and Shrubs of Alberta,* Government of Alberta, Environmental Protection, 1995.

James & Keeler, *Poisonous Plants- 3ʳᵈ Int. Symposium,* Iowa State U. Press, 1992.

Jason, Dan & Nancy. *Some Useful Wild Plants,* Talon Books, Vancouver, 1972.

Jiao Shu-De. *Ten Lectures on the Use of Medicinals.* Paradigm Pub. Brookline, Mass. 2003.

Johnson, Kershaw, MacKinnon & Pojar *Plants of the Western Boreal Forest and Aspen Parkland,* Lone Pine Press, Edmonton, Alberta 1995.

Johnson, L. *Tending the Earth A Gardener's Manifesto.* Penguin Books, Toronto, 2002.

Johnson, Leslie. Journal of Ethnobotany and Ethnomedicine. 2006 2:29.

_____*Health, Wholeness & the Land: Gitksan Traditional Plant Use and Healing.* U of Alberta 1997.

Jones, Alison. *Larousse Dictionary of World Folklore.* Larousse, New York, 1995.

Jones, Pamela. *Just Weed, History, Myths and Uses.* Prentice Hall Press, Toronto, 1991.

Kamm, Minnie W. *Old Time Herbs for Northern Gardens* Little Brown & Co. 1938.

Kane, Charles W. Herbal Medicine of the American Southwest. Lincoln Town Press. 2007.

_____Herbal Medicine: trends and traditions. Lincoln Town Press 2009.

Kapoor, L.D. *CRC Handbook of Ayurvedic Medicinal Plants,* CRC Press, Boca Raton, 1990.

Kari, Priscilla. *Tanaina Plantlore.* National Park Service, Alaska Region 1987.

Kaur, Sat Dharam. *The Complete Natural Medicine Guide to Breast Cancer.* Robert Rose Inc Toronto, 2003.

Kavash E, Barrie & Barr K, *American Indian Healing Arts.* Bantam Books, Toronto 1999.

_____*The Medicine Wheel Garden.* Bantam Books, N.Y. 2002.

Kay, Margarita Artschwager. *Healing with Plants in the American and Mexican West,* The University of
   Arizona Press, Tucson. 1996

Kays, S & Nottingham S. Biology and Chemistry of Jerusalem Artichoke. CRC Press 2008.

Keane, Kahlee & Howarth,D. *The Standing People.* Saskatoon, Saskatchewan. 2003.

Kee Chang Huang, *The Pharmacology of Chinese Herbs,* 2nd Edition, CRC Press, 1999.

Kemp, Cynthia. *Cactus and Company.* Desert Alchemy, Tucson, Arizona, 1993.

Kenner D &Requena Y. *Botanical Medicine:* .Paradigm Pub. Brookline, Mass, 1996.

Kerik, Joan. *Living with the Land:Use of Plants by the Native People of Alberta,* Alberta Culture, Circulating
   Exhibits Program, National Museums of Canada Fund, 1981.

Kershaw, Linda. Edible & Medicinal Plants of the Rockies, Lone Pine, Edmonton 2000.

_____*Alberta Wayside Wildflowers.* Lone Pine, Edmonton, 2003.

_____*Saskatchewan Wayside Wildflowers.* Lone Pine, Edmonton, 2003.

_____*Manitoba Wayside Wildflowers.* Lone Pine, Edmonton, 2003.

Kershaw, L. et al. *Rare Vascular Plants of Alberta.* U. of Alberta Press, Edmonton, 2001.

Kershaw, MacKinnon & Pojar. *Plants of the Rocky Mountains.* Lone Pine, Edmonton 1998.

Keys, John. D. *Chinese Herbs,* Charles E. Tuttle Co. 1976.

Kimmerer,Robin. *Gathering Moss.* Oregon State University Press, Corvallis, 2003.

Kindscher, Kelly. *Medicnal Wild Plants of the Prairies.* Univ. Press of Kansas. 1987.

King, Francis X. *Rudolf Steiner and Holistic Medicine.* Rider & Co. England, 1986.

Klein, Carol. Plant Personalities. Timber Press, Portland, Oregon. 2005.

Klein, Richard. *The Green World.* 2nd edition. Harper Collins, 1987.

Kloss, Jethro. *Back to Eden.* Woodbridge Press Pub.Co. Santa Barbara, Ca. 1975.

Knab, Sophie H. *Polish Herbs, Flowers and Folk Medicine.* Hippocrene Books, N.Y. 1999.

Knowles, Hugh. *Woody Ornamentals for the Prairies.* U. of Alberta , 1995.

Knudtson,P & Suzuki D. Wisdom of the Elders. Greystone Books. Vancouver BC 2006.

Kraft, K & Hobbs C. *Pocket Guide to Herbal Medicine.* Thieme, N.Y. 2004.

Kranich, Ernst M. Planetary Influences Upon Plants. Bio-Dynamic Lit. Wyoming RI 1984.

Krymow, V. Healing Plants of the Bible. Wild Goose Pub. Glasgow, UK 2002.

Kuhnlein, Harriet and Turner, Nancy. *Traditional Plant Foods of Canadian Indigenous Peoples.* Gordon and
   Breach Science Publishers. 1991.

Kuijt, Job. *The Biology of Parasitic Flowering Plants,* U. of California Press, 1969

Kunkele, U. & Lohmeyer, T. *Herbs for Healthy Living.* Parragon Pub. Bath UK 2007.

Lacey, Laurie. *Micmac Medicines Remedies and Recollections.* Nimbus Pub. Halifax, 1993.

Lahring, Heinjo. *Water and Wetland Plants of the Prairie Provinces,* Can Plains Research Center, U. of Regina,
   2003

Lambert, Grant. *Falling Leaf Essences.* Healing Arts Press, Rochester Vermont, 2002.

Lamont, SM. *The Fisherman Lake Slave and their environment: a story of floral and faunal resources.* Master's
   thesis. U. of Saskatchewan, Saskatoon, 1977.

Langenheim, Jean. *Medicinal Plant Resins.* Timber Press Portland Oregon 2003.

Larsen,Henning. *An Old Icelandic Medical Miscellany,* Norske Akademi, Oslo, Norway '31

Lavabre, Marcel. *Aromatherapy Workbook.* Healing Arts Press, Vermont. 1990.

Lawless, Julia, *The Encyclopedia of Essential Oils* , Element Books, 1992.

LeClaire,N &Cardinal,G. *Alberta Elders' Cree Dictionary,* U of Alberta Press, 1998.

Leduc, M.A. *The Explorers Guide to Boreal Forest Plants,* Hwy Book Shop, Cobalt, Ont. 1997

Leighton, Anna L. *Wild Plant Use by the Woods Cree ( NIHITHAWAK) of East-Central Saskatchewan .* Paper
   no. 101, National Museums of Canada, Ottawa, 1985

Lepore, Donald. *The Ultimate Healing System.* Woodland Books, Provo, Utah, 1988.

Le Strange, Richard, *A History of Herbal Plants.* Arco Pub. New York. 1977.

Leung, Albert. *Chinese Herbal Remedies.* Universe Books, New York, 1984.

Leung & Foster, *Encyclopedia of Common Natural Ingredients,* J. Wiley&Sons, N.Y. 1996.

Levey,M. *The Medical Formulary or Aqrabadhin of Al-Kindi* U of Wisconsin Press, 1966

Leyel, C.F. *Elixirs of Life,* Faber and Faber, London.1948

Li, Thomas. *Medicinal Plants, Culture, Utilization & Phytopharmacology.* Technomic Publishing, Lancaster, Pennsylvania, 2000.

Li, Thomas. *Chinese and related North American Herbs.* CRC Press, Boca Raton, 2002.

Libster, Martha. *Delmar's Integrative Herb Guide for Nurses.* Delmar, 2002.

Lininger et al. *The Natural Pharmacy.* Healthnotes, Prima Pub. Rocklin Ca, 1999.

L'Orange Darlena, *Herbal Healing Secrets of the Orient.* Prentice Hall, New Jersey, 1998.

Lock, Carolyn. *Country Colours.* Nova Scotia Museum. 1981

Lovejoy, Sharon. *Sunflower Houses.* Workman Pub Co. New York 2001.

Lu, Henry. *Using Foods to Stay Young,* Sterling Press, New York, 1996.

_____*Chinese Natural Cures.* Black Dog & Leventhal Pub. New York, 1994

Luetjohann, Sylvia. *The Healing Power of Black Cumin.* Lotus Light, Twin Lakes, WI, 1998

Lyle, Katie Letcher. *The Wild Berry Book,* NorthWord Press, Minocqua, WI, 1994.

Mabey, Richard. *Plantcraft.* Universe Books. 1978.

MacKinnon, Pojar, Coupe. *Plants of Northern British Columbia.* Lone Pine Press, 1992.

Mailhebiau, Philippe. *Portraits in Oils.* C.W. Daniel Company, Essex, England, 1995.

Malmud, René. *The Amazon Problem,* trans by M. Stein, Spring Pub. Dallas TX, 1980.

Maloof, Joan. *Teaching the Trees, Lessons from the Forest.* U Georgia Pr, Athena GA. 2005.

Manandhar, N.P. *Plants and People of Nepal.* Timber Press, Portland, Oregon, 2002.

Maple, Eric. *The Secret Lore of Plants and Flowers.* Robert Hale Ltd. London 1980.

March, Kathryn & Andrew. *The Wild Plant Companion.* Meridian Hill Pub. 1986.

Marles, Robin. *The Ethnobotany of the Chipewyan of Northern Saskatchewan,* 1984. Thesis.

_____et al. *Aboriginal Plant Use in Canada's Northwest Boreal Forest.* UBC Press, Vancouver, and Natural Resources Canada, 2000

McBride, L.R. *Practical Folk Medicine of Hawaii.* Petroglyph Press, Hilo,Hawaii, 1975.

McCune B. & Geiser L. *Macrolichens of the Pacific Northwest.* Oregon State U. Press, 1997

McFarland, Phoenix. *The Complete Book of Magical Names.* Llewellyn Pub. St Paul 1996

McGrath, Judy. *Dyes from Lichens and Plants.* Van Nostrand Rheinhold, 1977.

McGuffin, Nancy. *Spectrum: dye plants of Ontario.* Burr House Spinner, Richmond Hill '86

Mc Intyre, Anne. *The Complete Woman's Herbal,* Henry Holt, New York, 1995.

Mears, R & Hillman,G. Wild Food. Hodder and Stoughton

MELODY. *Love is in the Earth, A Kaleidoscope of Crystals.* Earth Love Pub. Col. 1995.

Mercatante, A. S. The Facts on File Encyclopedia of World Mythology. New York 1988

Merriam, C. Hart. *Dawn of the World, Weird Tales of Mewan Indians.* Arthur H. Clark, Cleveland, 1910

Meyer, George et al. *Folk Medicine and Herbal Healing,* Charles Thomas, Springfield, 1981

Meyerowitz,Steve. *Sprout It!* The Sprout House, Box 1100,Great Barrington, MA, 1993.

Meyers, Edward C. *Basic Bush Survival,* Hancock House, Surrey, B.C. 1997.

Miller, L &Murray,W. *Herbal Medicinals A Clinician's Guide.* Hawthorn Press, N.Y. 1998.

Miller, Sandra. Editor Echinacea- Medicinal and Aromatic Plants. CRC Press, 2004.

Mills S. & Bone,K. *Principles and Practice of Phytotherapy.* Churchill Livingstone, 2000.

_____*The Essential Guide to Herbal Safety.* Churchill Livingstone, 2005.

Mills, Simon. *Out of the Earth.* Viking Penquin Books, Toronto. 1991.

Millsbaugh, Charles. *American Medicinal Plants,* Dover Pub. New York, 1974

Milne, Courtney. *Visions of the Goddess,* Penguin Studio, Toronto, 1998

Minnis & Elisens. *Biodiversity and Native America.* U. Oklahoma Press, 2000.

Mitchel, Jr. Wm. *Plant Medicine in Practice.* Churchill Livingstone, St. Louis, 2003.

Moerman, Daniel, *Medicinal Plants of Native America.* U of Michigan No. 19, 1986

Mohammed, G. *Catnip & Kerosene Grass* Candlenut Books, Sault Ste. Marie, Ont, 2002.

Montgomery, Pam. *Plant Spirit Healing.* Bear and Company, Rochester, VT 2008.

Moore, Michael. *Los Remedios.* Red Crane Books, 1990

_____*Medicinal Plants of the Desert and Canyon West.* Museum of New Mexico Press 1989

_____*Medicinal Plants of the Mountain West,* Museum of New Mexico Press '79

_____Med Plants of the Mountain West. Revised, expanded. 2003

_____*Medicinal Plants of the Pacific West,* Red Crane Books, 1993

More, Daphne. *The Bee Book,* Universe Books, New York, 1976.

Morelli, I. et al. *Selected Medicinal Plants.* University of Pisa. FAO 53/1

Morton, Julia. *Major Medicinal Plants* . Charles Thomas, Springfield, Illinois 1977

_____*Atlas of Medicinal Plants of Middle America, Bahamas to Yucatan.* 1981

Moss, E.H. *Flora of Alberta.* University of Toronto Press. 1983

Mother, The. *Flowers and their Messages.* Sri Aurobindo Ashram Trust, India 1979.

Mourning Dove. Coyote Stories. Caxton Press Caldwell Idaho. 1933.

Mowrey, Daniel. *The Scientific Validation of Herbal Medicine.* Cormorant Books, 1986.

Mucz, Michael. *Baba's Kitchen Medicines.* U of Alberta Press, Edmonton, 2012.

Mulders, Evelyn. *Western Herbs for Eastern Meridian & 5 Element Theory. Self publ. 2006.*

Mulligan, G editor *The biology of Canadian Weeds,* 1-32 Pub. 1693 Ag Canada 1979

_____33-61 Pub. 1765 Ag Canada 1984

Murphy, Cristine Editor, *Practical Home Care Medicine,* Lantern Books, New York, 2001

Murray, Michael. *The Pill Book Guide to Natural Medicines.* Bantam Books, April, 2002.

_____& Pizzorno, J. The condensed Encycl of Healing Foods. Pocket Books NY 2005.

Naegele, Thomas A. *Edible and Medicinal Plants of the Great Lakes Region,* Wilderness Adventure Books, Davisburg, Michigan. 1996.

Naiman, Ingrid. *Cancer Salves, A Botanical Approach to Treatment.* N. Atlantic Books, 99.

Nesse R & Williams G. *Why We Get Sick.* Vintage Books/Random House, New York, 1996.

Neuwinger H.D. *African Traditional Medicine.* Medpharm Sci. Pub. Stuttgart 2000.

_____African Ethnobotany, Poisons and Drugs. Chapman & Hall, London 1996.

Newcombe C.F. unpub notes on Haida plants. Dept of Anthro. Am Mus Nat Hist. NY 1897

_____unpublished papers. Prov Archives B.C. Victoria. 1898-1913.

Nicander. *The Poems and Poetical Fragments.* Cambridge U. Press, New York, 1953.

Norman,Howard. *Northern Tales.* Pantheon Books, New York, 1990.

Northcote, Rosalind. *The Book of Herbs.* John Lane: The Bodley Head, London, 1912.

Null, Gary. *The Clinician's Handbook of Natural Healing.* Kensington Books, N.Y. 1997.

Olive, Barbara. *The Flower Healer.* Cico Books, London and New York. 2007.

Ollsin, Don. *Herbal Healing Journey-Playful Workbook.* Aquiline Comm, Victoria,BC 1998.

Ootoova I. et al. *Interviewing Inuit Elders, Perspectives on Traditional Health.* Vol 5, Nunavut Arctic College, Box 600, Iqaluit, Nunavut X0Z 0H0.

Page, George. *Inside the Animal Mind.* Doubleday, New York, 1999.

Pallasdowney, Rhonda. *The Complete Book of Flower Essences.* New World Library, 2002.

Pappalardo, Joe. Sunflowers (the secret history). The Overlook Press. Woodstock NY 2008.

Parish, Coupé & Lloyd. *Plants of S. Interior British Columbia*. Lone Pine Edmonton 1996

Park, Willard Z. *Ethnographic Notes on the Norhern Paiute of Western Nevada, 1933-40* compiled by Catherine Fowler, U. of Utah, Salt Lake City, 1989.

Parvati, J. *Hygieia, A Woman's Herbal*. Freestone Collective. 1978

Paturi, Felix *Nature, Mother of Invention*. Harper and Row Pub. New York. 1976.

Peirce, Andrea. *Practical Guide to Natural Medicines*. Stonesong Press. 1999.

Pelikan, W. Healing Plants. Mercury Press, Spring Valley NY 1997.

Pellowski, Anne. *Hidden Stories in Plants*. MacMillan Pub. New York. 1990.

Penoel, Daniel & Franchomme, P. *L'Aromatherapie Exactement* , Roger Jollois, France, 1990

Peneol, Daniel. *Medecine Aromatique, Medecine Planetaire*. Roger Jollois France 1991.

_____& Peneol, Rose-Marie. *Natural Home Health Care Using Essential Oils*. Osmobiose Pub. 1998.

People of 'Ksan, The. *Gathering What the Great Nature Provided*. Douglas & Mc Intyre. Vancouver, B.C. 1980.

Peters, Josephine & Ortiz B. After the First Full Moon in April. Left Coast Press. Walnut Creek CA, 2010.

Pettitt, Sabina. Energy Medicine, Healing from the Kingdoms of Nature, Pacific Essences, Box 8317, Victoria, B.C. V8W 3R9 Canada, 1999

Phaneuf, Holly. Herbs Demystified. Marlowe and Company, New York. 2005

Pielou, E.C. *The Naturalist's Guide to the Arctic*. U. of Chicago Press. 1994.

Pieroni, A & Price L. Eating and Healing, Trad Food as Medicine. Haworth Press. N.Y. 2006.

Pfeiffer E. *The Earth's Face and Human Destiny,* Rodale Press, Emmaus, Pa. 1947.

Plotkin, Mark. *Medicine Quest*. Viking Penguin Books, New York, 2000.

Pojar, J & MacKinnon, A. *Plants of Coastal British Columbia* Lone Pine Edmonton 1994.

Pollock, L. With Faith and Physic: the life of a tudor gentlewoman. Collins & Brown,1993.

Polya, Gideon. *Biochemical Targets of Plant Bioactive Comp.* CRC Press, Boca Raton 2003

Pond, Barbara, *A Sampler of Wayside Herbs,* Chatham Press, Riverside, Conn.

Pressor, Arthur, *Pharmacist's Guide to Medicinal Herbs,* Smart Pub. Petaluma, CA,2000

Price, Len & Shirley. *Understanding Hydrolats*. Churchill Livingstone, Toronto, 2004.

_____Aromatherapy for Health Professionals, Churchill Livingstone 1995.

Purvis, William. *Lichens*. Smithsonian Institution Press. Washington D.C. 2000

Quin, Frederick F. *The Flora Homoeopathica*. B. Jain Pub. New Delhi, India. 1997.

Radin, Paul. *The Winnebago Tribe,* Bur of Am Ethnology, Smithsonian Inst. 37th. 1923.

Rätsch, C. *Plants of Love, The History of Aphrodisiacs.* Ten Speed Press, Berkeley,1997.

_____The Dictionary of Sacred & Magical Plants. ABC-CLIO St Barbara 1992.

_____The Encyclopedia of Psychoactive Plants. Park St Press. 2005.

Raven Essences. www.ravenessences.com

Ravenworks flower essences. www.ravenworksministries.weebly.com

Reaume, Tom. 620 Wild Plants of North America. Nature Manitoba. Canadian Plains Research Center, U of Regina, U of Toronto Press. 2009.

Reckeweg, Hans-Heinrich, *Materia Medica, Vol 1. Aurelia-Verlag GmbH, Baden Baden* 1996.

Reich, Lee. *Uncommon Fruits Worthy of Attention,* Addison-Wesley Pub. 1991.

Reid, Daniel, *A handbook of Chinese Healing Herbs,* Shambala, Boston, 1995

Rhode, David. Native Plants of Southern Nevada. U of Utah Press. 2002.

Richards B & Kanecko A. *Japanese Plants- Know Them &Use Them.* Shufunotomo, Tokyo 1995

Richardson, David. *The Vanishing Lichens*. David and Charles, Vancouver, BC, 1975

Riddle, John M. *Eve's Herbs*. Harvard U Press. Cambridge Mass. 1997.

_____Goddesses, Elixirs and Witches. Palgrave MacMillan. England 2010.

Rister, Robert. *Healing Without Medication.* Basic Health Pub. N. Bergen, N.J. 2003.

Roberts, Jonathan. *The Origins of Fruit and Vegetables.* Universe Pub. New York. 2001.

Robicsek, F. *The Smoking God: Tobacco....*Norman: U. of Oklahoma Press, 1978.

Robinson, Peggy. *Profiles of Northwest Plants.* Far West Book Service. Portland, OR 1979

Rogers, Dilwyn. *Edible, Medicinal, Useful & Poisonous Wild Plants of the Northern Great Plains —South Dakota Region.* Buechel Memorial Lakota Museum, St. Francis,SD, 1980.

Rogers, Pattiann. *Firekeeper:New & Selected Poems.* Milkweed Editions, 1994.

Rogers, Robert Dale. *Sundew Moonwort Vols-1-7, self-published.* Edmonton 1995-present.

_____Rogers' Herbal Manual. Karamat Wilderness Ways, Edmonton, 2000.

_____& Capital Health, Herbal Drug Interactions. Mediscript Comm. 2003.

_____The Fungal Pharmacy, The Complete Guide to Medicinal Mushrooms and Lichens of North America, North Atlantic Books 2011.

Rombi, Max. *Phytotherapy.* Herbal Health Publishers. U.K. 1990.

Rosengarten,Jr. F. *The Book of Edible Nuts.* Walker and Co. New York. 1984.

Ross, Gary. *Nature's Guide to Healing.* Freedom Press, Topanga, Ca. 2000.

Ross, Ivan. *Medicinal Plants of the World.* Vol 1 Humana Press, Totowa, New Jersey. 1999.

_____ Vol 2 Humana Press, Totowa, N. J. 2002.

Rotella, Rev. Alexis. *The Essence of Flowers,* Jade Mountain Press, N.J. 1991.

Royer F. & Dickinson R. *Plants of Alberta.* Lone Pine Pub. Edmonton, AB. 2007.

Rudginsky, Marlene *The Flower Speaks.* U.S. Games Systems, Stamford, Conn. 1999.

Rupp, Rebecca. *Red Oaks and Black Birches* , Storey Comm. Garden Way Publishing. 1990

Russell, Sharman Apt. *Anatomy of a Rose.* Perseus Pub. Cambridge, Mass. 2001.

_____An Obsession with Butterflies. Perseus Publishing 2003.

Ryan, J et al, *Traditional Dene Medicine.* Lac La Martre NWT, 1993.

Ryden, Hope. *Wildflowers around the year.* Clarion Books, New York. 2001.

Ryrie, Charlie. Garden Folklore That Works. Reader's Digest. Pleasantville, NY 2001.

Sagadic O. & Ozcan M. *Food Control* 2003 14.

Salmon, Wm. *Botanologia: The English Herbal.* London: I. Dawkes, 1710.

Sandberg & Corrigan. *Natural Remedies, their origins and uses.* Taylor & Francis 2001.

Sanders, Jack. *The Secrets of Wildflowers.* The Lyons Press, Guilford, CT, 2003.

Sapolsky, Robert. *The Trouble with Testosterone.* Scribner, New York. 1997.

Sauer, Johann Christopher, Compendious Herbal-see Weaver below.

Savage, Candace. Bees, Nature's Little Wonders. Greystone Books. Vancouver 2008.

Schalkwijk-Barendsen, Helene. *Mushrooms of Western Canada* . Lone Pine Pub. 1991.

Schar, Douglas. *The Backyard Medicine Chest.* Elliott&Clark Pub. Washington, DC. 1995.

Scheffer, Mechthild, *Bach Flower Therapy, Theory and Practice,* Healing Arts Press, 1988

Schenk, George. *Moss Gardening.* Timber Press, Portland Oregon. 1997.

Schnaubelt, Kurt. *Medical Aromatherapy.* Frog Ltd. Berkeley CA. 1999.

Schneider, Anny. *Wild Medicinal Plants.* Key Porter Books, Toronto. 2002.

Schnell, Donald. *Carnivorous Plants.* 2nd Ed. Timber Press, Portland, Oregon, 2002.

Schofield, Janice. *Discovering Wild Plants.* Alaska Northwest Books. 1989.

_____*Nettles.* Keats Publishing, New Canaan, Conneticut, 1998.

Schulman, Robert. *Solve It With Supplements.* Rodale Press. New York. 2007.

Shapiro, R & Rapkins J. Awakening to the Plant Kingdom, Cassandra Press 1991.

Shauenberg, Paul and Paris. *Guide to Medicinal Plants.* Keats Publishing, 1977.

Shook, Edward Dr. *Advanced Treatise on Herbology* . Reprint Health Research.

Shosteck,Robert. *Flowers and Plants*. Quadrangle/The New York Times Book Co. 1974.

Siegfried, EV. Masters Thesis, Ethnobotany of the Northern Cree of Wabasca/Desmarais. U of Calgary, Alberta. 1994.

Silverman, Maida. *A City Herbal*. David R. Godine , 1990.

Silvertown, Jonathan. An Orchard Invisible. U of Chicago Press. 2009.

Simonot, Danielle. *Bio-Manufacturing in Saskatchewan-* Assessment of the Manufacturing Potential of Select Saskatchewan Plants, Sask. Nutraceutical Network, Saskatoon, 2000

Simpson, Brenan, M. *Flowers At My Feet,* Hancock House, Surrey, B.C. 1996.

Sionneau, P. *An Introduction to the Use of Processed Chinese Medicinals*. Blue Poppy Press, Second Printing 2003, Translated by Bob Flaws.

Smagghe, Guy Ed. Ecdysone: Structures and Functions. Springer Sci 2009.

Small, E & Catling, P. *Canadian Medicinal Crops,* NRC Research Press, Ottawa 1999.

Small, Ernest. *Culinary Herbs, Second Ed.* NRC Research Press, Ottawa, 2006.

_____*Medicinal Herbs,* NRC Research Press, Ottawa, 2000.

_____Top 100 Food Plants. NRC Press, Ottawa. 2009.

Smith, Andrew. *Strangers in the Garden, the Secret Lives of Our Favorite Flowers.*McClelland & Stewart 2004.

Smith, Annie Lorrain. *Lichens,* Cambridge at the University Press, 1921.

Smith, Harlan, *Ethnobotany of the Gitksan Indians of B.C.* Edited by B. Compton, B. Rigsby, and M.L. Tarpent, Mercury Series, Can Ethno Service, Paper 132, Can Mus of Civil. 1997.

Smith, Huron H. Manataka American Indian Council. www.manataka.org.

Snell, Alma Hogan. A Taste of Heritage. Crow Indian Recipes and Herbal Medicines. University of Nebraska Press 2006.

Soule, Deb. *The Roots of Healing, A Woman's Book of Herbs.* Citadel Press, 1995.

Spencer, Kate. *The Magic of Green Buckwheat ,*Richard Clay, England, 1987.

Spinella, Marcello. *The Psychopharmacology of Herbal Medicine.* MIT Press, 2001.

Steedman, E.V. *The Ethnobotany of the Thompson Indians of British Columbia.* 1930.

Stein, Sara. *My Weeds, A Gardener's Botany.* Harper and Row, 1988.

Stern, Gai. *Australian Weeds.* Harper and Row, Australia 1986

Stern Wm. *Stern's Dictionary of Plant Names for Gardeners.* Cassell Pub, London, 1972

Stewart, Hilary. *CEDAR.* Douglas & Mc Intyre. Vancouver/Toronto, 1984.

Storl, Wolf D. Healing Lyme Disease Naturally. NorthAtlantic Books, Berkeley, CA 2010.

Strehlow,W & Hertzka,G. *Hildegard of Bingen's Medicine* Bear & Co. Santa Fe 1988

Stuart, David. *Dangerous Garden.* Harvard University Press, Cambridge, Mass. 2004

Sturdivant L.&Blakley,T. *Medicinal Herbs in the Garden, Field and Marketplace* Bootstrap Guide, San Juan Naturals, Friday Harbor,WA, 1999.

Sumner, Judith. *The Natural History of Medicinal Plants.* Timber Press, Oregon, 2000.

Sun Bear & Wabun, *The Medicine Wheel* Prentice Hall, NJ 1980.

Swanton, J.R. *Haida Texts and Myths.* Bureau Am Ethnol, Bull #29. Smithsonian Inst. Washington, D.C. 1905.

_____*Bureau of Am Ethno 26th Ann Report.* Smithsonian Inst. Washington, 1908.

Szczeklik, Andrzej. Kore: On Sickness, the Sick and the Search for the Soul of Medicine. Counterpoint Berkeley 2012.

Tainter, D& Grenis A, *Spices and Seasonings ,* VCH Pubishers, New York, 1993.

Talalaj,S.& Czechowicz,A S. *Herbal Remedies,* Hill of Content Press, Melbourne, 1989

Taylor, Wm &Farnsworth,N. The Vinca Alkaloids, Marcel Dekker, New York, 1973.

Teeguarden, Ron. *The Ancient Wisdom of the Chinese Tonic Herbs.* Warner Bros. 1998.

Telesco, Patricia. *The Victorian Flower Oracle,* Llewellyn Pub. St. Paul 1994

Temple, Robert. *The Genius of China.* Simon and Schuster. New York. 1986.

Thompson, Gerry, *Astral Sex to Zen Teabags.* Findhorn Press, 1994.

Thoreau, Henry David. *Wild Fruits.* W. W. Norton & Co. New York, 2000.

Throop, Priscilla. *Hildegard von Bingen's Physica.* Healing Arts Press, Vt. 1998.

Tick, Edward. *The Practice of Dream Healing.* Quest Books Wheaton, Illinois, 2001.

Tierra, Michael. *The Way of Herbs- revised Pocket Rooks,* New York, 1998.

Tigner, Daniel. *Canadian Forest Tree Essences,* self published,1998. ISBN 0968365809

Tilford, Gregory. *Edible and Medicinal Plants of the West.* Mountain Press, Missoula 1997.

Timbrook, Jan. Chumash Ethnobotany. St. Barbara Mus, Heyday Books, Berkeley Ca 2007.

Traill, E.C. *Studies of Plant Life in Canada.* A. S. Woodburn, Ottawa, 1885.

Traill, C. P. *The Backwoods of Canada.* McClelland and Stewart. Toronto. 1846.

Tobyn, G., Denham, A., Whitelegg, M. The Western Herbal Tradition. 2000 years of medicinal herbal knowledge. Churchill Livingstone Toronto 2011.

Toop, Edgar W & Williams, Sara. *Perennials for the Prairies.* U of A&Saskatchewan. 1991.

Treben, Maria. *Health Through God's Pharmacy.* Wilhelm Ennsthaler. 1982.

Tresidder, Jack. Symbols and Their Meaning. Friedman/Fairfax Pub. 2007.

Tucker A. & DeBaggio,T. *The Big Book of Herbs.* Interweave Press. Loveland CO. 2000.

_____The Encylcopedia of Herbs. Timber Press, Portland. 2009.

Turkington, Carol. *The Home Health Guide to Poisons and Antidotes,* Facts on File 1994

Turner, Nancy J. *Food Plants of Interior First Peoples.* UBC Press, Vancouver, 1997.

_____*Food Plants of Coastal First Peoples.* UBC Press, Vancouver, 1995.

_____*Plant Technology of First Peoples in B.C.* UBC Press, Vancouver, 1998.

_____et al. *Thompson Ethnobotany.* Memoir #3, Royal B.C. Museum, 1996.

_____*Plants of Haida Gwaii.* Sononis Press, Winlaw, B.C. 2004.

_____The Earth's Blanket. Douglas & Mc Intyre. Vancouver. 2005.

Turner, N & von Aderkas, P. Common Poisonous Plants and Mushrooms. Timber Press 2009

Turner, W.B. *Fungal Metabolites,* Academic Press, London and New York, 1971.

Twitchell, Paul. *Herbs The Magic Healers.* Eckankar, Box 3100 Menlo Park, CA, 1986.

Vermeulen, Nico. *Encyclopedia of Herbs.* Whitecap Books, Vancouver B.C. 1998.

Viereck, Eleanor, G. *Alaska's Wilderness Medicines.* Alaska Northwest Pub. 1987

Vitt, Marsh and Bovey, *Mosses, Lichens, and Ferns,* Lone Pine Press, 1988.

Vogel, A. *Swiss Nature Doctor.* A. Vogel, Switzerland. 1952

_____*Nature-Your Guide to Healthy Living.* Verlag A. Vogel, Teufen, Switzerland 1986.

Vogel, Virgil. *American Indian Medicine,* U. of Oklahoma Press, Norman, 1970

Vortex Essences (Mt. Shasta Essences) www.vortexessences.com

Walker, Barbara. *The Woman's Dictionary of Symbols&Sacred Objects.* Csstle Books, 1988.

Walker, Marilyn. Wild Plants of Eastern Canada. Nimbus Pub. Halifax NS. 2008.

Ward, Bobby J. The Plant Hunter's Garden. Timber Press, Portland. 2004.

Ward-Harris, Joan.*More Than Meets the Eye, The Life and Lore of Western Wildflowers* Oxford University Press, Toronto, 1983

Watanabe & Shibuya. *Pharmacological Research on Traditional Herbal Medicines.* Harwood Academic Publishers, 1999.

Watt, John, and Breyer-Brandwijk, Maria *The Medicinal and Poisonous Plants of Southern and Eastern Africa* . E and S. Livingstone. Edinburgh and London. 1962.

Watts, Donald. Elsevier's Dictionary of Plant Lore. Elsevier. 2007.

Waugh, F.W. *Iroquois Foods and Food Preparation* #12 Anthropological Series, Ottawa. 1916. Reprinted by Iroqrafts, RR #2, Ohsweken, Ontario N0A 1M0, 1991.

Weaver, Wm. *100 Vegetables & Where They Came From.* Workman Pub. New York, 2000.

_____*Sauer's Herbal Cures America's First Book of Botanic Healing 1762-1778,* Routledge, New York, 2001.

Weed, Susan. *Menopausal Years, The Wise Woman Way.* Ash Tree Pub. Woodstock NY, 1992

Weigle, Marta. *Spiders and Spinsters.* U. of New Mexico Press, Albuquerque, 1982.

Weiner, M. *The People's Herbal, A family guide.* Putnam Publishing, New York, 1984.

Weiss, Rudolf. *Herbal Medicine.* Beaconsfield Publishers, 1988.

_____*Herbal Medicine* 2nd Edition. Thieme, Stuttgart, New York, 2000.

Wells, Diana.*100 Flowers and How They Got Their Names,* Algonquin Books, Chapel Hill,97

Westcott, Frank. *The Beaver Nature's Master Builder.* Hounslow Press, Willowdale, ON '89.

Westrich, LoLo, *California Herbal Remedies,* Gulf Pub Co. Houston, TX, 1989.

Wetzel, Suzanne et al. Bioproducts from Canada's Forests. Springer Netherlands 2006.

WHO monographs on selected medicinal plants, vol 1, 1999; vol 2, 2002.

White, Ian. *Australian Bush Flower Essences.* Bantam Books, 1991

White, Florence. *Flowers as Food* . Jonathan Cape. 1934

Whitmont, Edward. *Psyche and Substance.* North Atlantic Books. 1980

Wilkinson, Kathleen. *Trees and Shrubs of Alberta.* Lone Pine Books, Edmonton 1990.

_____*Wildflowers of Alberta.* U of A/Lone Pine Books, Edmonton 1999.

Williams, Jude. *Nature's Gentle Cures.* Sterling Publishing. New York. 1997.

Williamson, Darcy. 130 Medicinal Plant Monographs of the NW. self pub. E-book. 2011.

Williamson, E. *Major Herbs of Ayurveda.* Churchill Livingstone, Elsevier Science, 2002.

# FLOWER ESSENCE RESOURCES

Aditi Himalaya Flower Essences, 15,Jaybharat Society, 3rd Road, Khar (W), Bombay 400 052, India.

Alaskan Flower Essence Project, P.O. Box. 1369, Homer, Alaska USA 99603-1369. www.alaskanessences.com.

Australian Bush Flower Essences. Australia. www.ausflowers.com.au.

Bach- Healing Herbs English Flower Essences- in Canada by Self Heal Distributing, Box 95008, Whyte Postal Outlet, Edmonton, AB T6E 0E5, 1800-593-5956 or www.selfhealdistributing.com Also www.healingherbs.co.uk or www.fesflowers.com

Bailey Flower Essences, 8 Neslon Road, Ilkley, West Yorkshire England, LS298HN. www.flowervr.com

Bloesem Remedies. Netherlands. www.bloesem-remedies.com

BrynaHerb Essences. www.brynaherbessences.uk

Canadian Forest Essences, PO Box 29128,1996 W. Broadway, Vancouver, BC V6J 1Z0

Canadian Forest Tree Essences. Ottawa. www.essences.ca. 613-725-9764.

Choming Flower Essences. www.mkprojects.com

Clear Path Essences. www.clearpathessences.com

Dancing Light Orchid Essences. Fairbanks, Alaska. www.orchidessences.com

Desert Alchemy, PO Box 44189, Tucson, Arizona, USA 85733. www.desert-alchemy.com.

Deva Flower Essences BP3 38880, Autrans, France. www.lab-deva.com

Eastern Flower Herbal Essences. julied@hfx.eastlink.ca.

Falling Leaf Essences. Box 78, Kallista, Victoria 3791, Australia. www.advancedalchemy.com.au.

Findhorn Flower Essences, Morayshire, Scotland IV36 0TY. www.findhornessences.com

Florais des Minas, Rua Albita, 194-Sala 408, Cruziero, CEP 30310-160,BH, MG, BRAZIL

FlorAlive', Brent Davis. Contact info@floralive.com

FES Flower Essence Society, PO Box 1769, Nevada City, California, USA, 95959. www.fesflowers.com Canadian Distributor- Self Heal Distributing, Box 95008, Whyte Postal Outlet, Edmonton, AB T6E 0E5 – www.selfhealdistributing.com

Green Hope Farm Flower Essences, PO Box 125, Meriden, New Hampshire USA 03770

Green Man Tree Essences. www.greenmantrees.demon.co.uk.

Habundia Flower Essences. c/o Peter Aziz. PO Box 90, Totnes, Devon, England TQ11 0YG.

Harebell Remedies. Scotland. ellie@harebellremedies.co.uk.

Hawaiian Gaia Flower Essences. www.gaiaessences.com

High Sierra Flower Essences. PO. Box 4275 Truclee, CA 96160. holly.hsb@highoctavehealing.com

Horus Flower Essences- horus@floweressences.de.

Hummingbird Remedies, PO Box 50161, Eugene, Oregon, USA 97405

Icelandic Flower Essences. www.kristbjorb.is.

Jade Mountain Flower Essences, Box 125, Mountain Lakes, New Jersey USA 07046-0125

Korte Phi. www.PHIessences.com

Light Heart Essences. England. www.lightheartessences.co.uk.

Light Mountain Flower Essences, Michael A. Vertolli, 1-800-667-HERB.

Living Essences of Australia, Box 355, Scarborough, 6019, Perth, Australia. www.livingessences.com.au

Living Flower Essences, www.livingfloweressences.com . Rhonda Pallasdowney.

Master's Flower Essences, 14618 Tyler Foote Rd Nevada City, California, USA, 95959. www.masteressences.com

Miriana fortem Flower Essences. www.mirianaflowers.com and info@miraflowers.com.

NaturaSacredplay, PO Box 32, Buckhorn, New Mexico, 88025, (505-535-2255).

New Millenium Flower Essences of New Zealand. info@nmessences.com.

New Zealand New Perception Flower Essences, PO Box 60-127,Titirangi, Auckland 7, NZ

Pacific Essences, Box 8317, Victoria, B.C. V8W 3R9. www.pacificessences.com.

Pegasus Products, PO Box 228, Boulder, Colorado, USA 80306-0228. 1-800- 527-6104.

Perelandra, Box 3603, Warrenton, VA. 22186. www.perelandra-ltd.com

Petite Fleur Essence, 8524 Whispering Creek Trail, Fort Worth, Texas, USA 76134. www.aromahealthtexas.com

Prairie Deva Flower Essences, Box 95008, Whyte Postal Outlet, Edmonton, AB T6E 0E5  1-(780) 433-7882. www.selfhealdistributing.com

Ravenworks- joni@ravenworksministries.org

Running Fox Farm PO Box 381,Worthington, Maryland USA 01098

Star Peruvian Flower Essences. Santa Barbara. www.starfloweressences.com

Stars of the Meadow, David Dalton, Lindisfarne Books, Mass. 2006.

Sun Essences. Norfolk, England. www.sunessence.co.uk

Sweetwater Sanctuary Essences. www.plantspirithealing.com

Tree Frog Farm Flower Essences. www.treefrogfarm.com

Whole Energy Essences, PO Box 285, Concord, Mass. 01742

Wild Rose Essences. www.wildrose.com

Woodland Essence, PO Box 206, Cold Brook, New York, USA 13324.